Medical Anthropology
and the World System

Medical Anthropology and the World System

Critical Perspectives, Third Edition

HANS A. BAER, MERRILL SINGER, AND IDA SUSSER

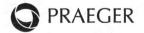 PRAEGER

AN IMPRINT OF ABC-CLIO, LLC
Santa Barbara, California • Denver, Colorado • Oxford, England

Library of Congress Cataloging-in-Publication Data

Baer, Hans A., 1944–
  Medical anthropology and the world system : critical perspectives / Hans A. Baer, Merrill Singer, and Ida Susser. — Third edition.
       pages.   cm
  Includes bibliographical references and index.
  ISBN 978-1-4408-0255-3 (hardcover : alk. paper) — ISBN 978-1-4408-2915-4 (paperback : acid free paper) — ISBN 978-1-4408-0256-0 (ebook)
  1. Medical anthropology.   I. Singer, Merrill.   II. Susser, Ida.   III. Title.
  GN296.B34 2013
  306.4′61—dc23   2012049606

ISBN: 978-1-4408-0255-3 (case)
       978-1-4408-2915-4 (pbk)
EISBN: 978-1-4408-0256-0

17 16 15 14 13   1 2 3 4 5

This book is also available on the World Wide Web as an eBook.
Visit www.abc-clio.com for details.

Praeger
An Imprint of ABC-CLIO, LLC

ABC-CLIO, LLC
130 Cremona Drive, P.O. Box 1911
Santa Barbara, California 93116-1911

This book is printed on acid-free paper ∞
Manufactured in the United States of America

Contents

Preface   vii

I.   **What Is Medical Anthropology About?**   1

1   Medical Anthropology: Central Concepts and Development   3

2   Theoretical Perspectives in Medical Anthropology   35

II. **The Social Origins of Disease and Suffering**   67

3   Health and the Environment: From Foraging Societies
     to the Capitalist World System   69

4   The Impact of Climate Change, Environmental Crises,
     and Disasters on Health   103

5   Poverty, Injustice, and Health in the World System   137

6   Reproduction, Biotechnologies, and Inequality   167

III. **Social Diseases and Social Suffering**   199

7   Violence and War   201

8   Legal and Illegal Drugs: Experience, Behavior, and Society   225

9   AIDS and Infectious Diseases   267

10   Syndemics and the Biosocial Nature of Health   301

IV. Medical Systems in a Social Context   **331**

11 Medical Systems in Indigenous and Precapitalist and
    Early Capitalist State Societies   333

12 Biomedical Hegemony in the Context of Medical Pluralism   359

V. Toward an Equitable and Healthy Global System   **395**

13 Health Praxis and the Struggle for a Healthy, Socially Just,
    and Environmentally Sustainable World System   397

Bibliography   435

About the Authors   499

Index   501

Preface

Medical anthropology is one of the youngest and, some would even boldly claim, most dynamic of the various subdisciplines of anthropology. It concerns itself with a wide variety of health-related issues, including the etiology of disease, the preventive measures that humans as members of sociocultural systems have constructed or devised to prevent the onset of disease, and the curative measures that they have created in their efforts to eradicate disease or at least to mitigate its consequences. In some ways, the term "medical anthropology" is a misnomer that reflects the curative rather than preventive nature of health care in modern societies. After all, anthropologists who study religious beliefs and practices generally refer to their subdiscipline as the "anthropology of religion" rather than "religious anthropology." Taking their cue from sociologists who speak of the "sociology of health and illness" rather than "medical sociology," some anthropologists interested in health-related issues have suggested substituting the label "anthropology of health and illness" rather than "medical anthropology." Indeed, one of the interest groups (of which Baer and Singer were among the cofounders) of the Society for Medical Anthropology after one year of existence changed its name from the Political Economy of Health Caucus to the Critical Anthropology of Health Caucus. Undoubtedly the preference for the label "medical anthropology" over "anthropology of health and illness" constitutes yet one more example of the powerful influence of M.D. medicine (generally referred to by medical anthropologists as biomedicine) in the modern world. Although we adopt the more common usage of the term "medical anthropology" in this textbook, the perspective that informs our work is far from conventional.

In a long overview of medical anthropology, David Landy (1983: 185) observes "that the human group that calls itself by the name medical anthropology is a lively, heterogeneous community, busily engaged in myriad activities, studying, and writing about behaviors of human collectivities and individuals in understanding and coping with disease and injury." In the United States, medical anthropology has grown in recent decades to the extent that the Society for Medical Anthropology constitutes the second largest unit of the American Anthropological Association. Although experiencing its most rapid pattern of development in this country, medical anthropology has embarked on a process of growth in Canada, Britain, Germany, Denmark, Italy, Japan, and South Africa, as well as other countries around the globe. Four journals, *Medical Anthropology, Social Science and Medicine, Culture, Medicine and Psychiatry,* and the *Medical Anthropology Quarterly,* serve as the major forums for anthropologists interested in health-related issues. In addition, many medical anthropologists publish in other anthropological journals as well as sociological behavioral science, medical, nursing, public health, and health policy journals. As should be the case, medical anthropologists have borrowed the frameworks that guide their teaching, research, and applications from a larger corpus of anthropological theory as well as a number of other perspectives that cut across disciplinary boundaries.

Our own perspective has been in large measure, but not exclusively, informed by critical anthropology as well as by other critical perspectives in the social sciences. Relying primarily but not exclusively on the perspective of "critical medical anthropology" (CMA), *Medical Anthropology and the World System* examines health-related issues in precapitalist indigenous and state societies, capitalist societies, and postrevolutionary or socialist-oriented societies. Although it draws heavily on neo-Marxian, critical, and world systems theoretical perspectives, critical medical anthropology attempts to incorporate the theoretical contributions of other theoretical perspectives in medical anthropology, including biocultural or medical ecology, ethnomedical approaches, cultural constructivism, poststructuralism, and postmodernism.

This textbook can be used in introductory medical anthropology courses both at the undergraduate and graduate levels. In that in its second and third editions it has grown in length, Merrill Singer and Hans Baer were approached several years ago to write a shorter medical anthropology designed primarily for undergraduate students (Singer and Baer 2007, 2012). In addition to anthropology students, this book can be used by health science and public health students and practitioners.

Part I ("What Is Medical Anthropology About?) consists of two chapters that discuss central concepts in and the development and scope of medical anthropology, as well as the critical perspective that we use. Chapter 1 discusses the concepts of health, disease, the sufferer experience, the medical system, medical pluralism, biomedicine, medicalization, and medical hegemony. It also expands on the earlier discussion in the second edition of the concept of syndemics to that one that includes a discussion of the concepts of eco-syndemics, pluralea, and environmental crises and their health impacts. Finally, Chapter 1 examines the history of medical anthropology in the United States and elsewhere. Chapter 2 examines the various theoretical perspectives in medical anthropology, including the medical ecological or biocultural and cultural interpretive perspectives. It highlights critical medical anthropology and examines its concepts, historic debates, and dialogues with the other theoretical perspectives in medical anthropology. Chapter 2 also discusses the limitations of the "social determinants of health" and "global health" perspectives that have become fashionable in public health.

Part II, "The Social Origins of Disease and Suffering," consists of eight chapters and in a sense forms the heart of this textbook. Chapter 3 ("Health and the Environment: From Foraging Societies to the Capitalist World System") discusses health and the environment in preindustrial societies and in the context of the capitalist world system. It also examines the environmental devastation in postrevolutionary societies—not only the former Soviet Union but also China—under a rapid program of modernization and industrialization. This chapter includes a "Closer Look" titled "Motor Vehicles Are Dangerous to Your Health" that touches on the rapid increase of motor vehicles in China and India and serves as a portal for the next chapter in that motor vehicles are a major source of greenhouse gas emissions and contributor to climate change. Chapter 4 ("The Impact of Climate Change, Environmental Crises, and Disasters on Health") draws on the book *Global Warming and the Political Ecology of Health* as well as various environmental health essays written by the first two authors of this textbook. It constitutes the first such chapter found in a medical anthropology textbook.

Chapter 5 ("Poverty, Injustice, and Health in the World System") discusses not only homelessness, as an extreme manifestation of poverty, but also the worldwide processes of growing inequality of housing, which have resulted from the centrality of real estate investment to the global economic arena. It discusses the ways in which the dismantling of the welfare state and the growing inequalities in both the global North and the South have contributed to an increasing gap in health outcomes between rich and poor. The chapter then draws on recent ethnographies of homelessness and poverty in the United States and elsewhere to show

how recent policies have contributed to or undermined the health of men, women, and children. Chapter 6 ("Reproduction, Biotechnologies, and Inequality") discusses the different aspects of reproduction that have been studied by anthropologists in the global North and South. It contrasts issues of the biotechnologies of birth that have been significant for middle-class women in the North with the problems of maternal morbidity and mortality more significant in the global South. Chapter 7 ("Violence and War") draws on Rudolf Virchow's observation over 150 years ago that "war, plague and famine condition each other" and is concerned with the issues of war and violence as understood through the window of health. Especially since the War in Vietnam, anthropologists have studied local violence, including domestic, intimate partner, and community violence as well as war at the local and global levels within broader frameworks produced by the political-economic forces of state, power, and finance.

Chapter 8 ("Legal and Illegal Drug Use: Experience, Behavior, and Society") examines human interaction with psychotropic drugs, which stretches deep into human history and is found across all societies. It examines human use of mind- and mood-altering drugs of all kinds and their impact on health across societies in light of the evolution of social inequality, globalization, and the transformation of drugs from a cultural vehicle for spiritual experience into commodities produced and distributed by legal and underground corporations for profit. Chapter 9 ("AIDS and Infectious Diseases") discusses the explosion beginning in the early 1980s of HIV/AIDS on the world scene, causing extensive suffering and exposing underlying social inequalities in health and health care access, thus reshaping medical and public health conceptions of the continued importance of infectious disease in human health. It examines the AIDS pandemic as an intertwined health and social issue and the response of medical anthropologists over time (and evolving medical treatments) and place to this notable and complex global health threat.

Chapter 10 ("Syndemics and the Biosocial Nature of Health") explores the concept of syndemics (synergistic interaction among diseases within oppressive social contexts that increase the health burden of populations) that was developed and introduced to public health and the health social sciences and clinical sciences by medical anthropology. It examines the nature and historic and contemporary health impacts of several notable syndemics (e.g., interacting viral and bacterial infection as the cause of the deadly influenza pandemic of 1918–1919, the multiple and impactful syndemics of HIV [e.g., HIV/TB, HIV/malaria, HIV/malnutrition, SAVA], the smoking/drinking syndemic, chronic noncommunicative/infectious disease syndemics). In addition to exploring how diseases interact and the various biological and social pathways and mechanisms of unidirectional and multidirectional interaction, the chapter reveals how such interaction can significantly magnify the deleterious impact of diseases and the critical role of social inequality in advancing disease clustering and entwinement in vulnerable populations.

Part IV, "Medical Systems in a Social Context," consists of two chapters. Chapter 11 ("Medical Systems in Indigenous and Precapitalist State Societies") discusses ethnomedicine as a response to disease in indigenous societies. It particularly gives attention to the shaman as the prototypical healer in indigenous societies. It examines the rise of medical pluralism in precapitalist state societies and early modern Europe during eras in which a divide emerged between medicine for the elites and medicine for the masses. Chapter 12 ("Biomedical Hegemony in the Context of Medical Pluralism") examines the emergence of biomedicine as a global medical system. It views dominative medical systems as reflections of social relations in the larger society. This chapter also examines the encounters that shamans and other indigenous healers have with the world system and the hospital as the primary locus of biomedicine.

Part V, "Toward an Equitable and Healthy Global System," consists of only one chapter, which seeks to contextualize the agenda of critical medical anthropology within the struggle for a healthier world. Chapter 13 ("Health Praxis and the Struggle for a Healthy, Socially Just, and Environmentally Sustainable World System") examines the concept of global democratic ecosocialism, particularly in the light of anthropogenic or human-created climate change. It examines historical reasons for the discrepancies between the ideals and realities of socialism and the emergence of new social movements around the world. This chapter also discusses the concepts of socialist health and health praxis and the need for a critical bioethics in medical anthropology.

This book is the third edition of *Medical Anthropology and the World System*, which first appeared in 1997. Although numerous textbooks are now available for introductory undergraduate courses, this one and *Introducing Medical Anthropology* (Singer and Baer 2007, 2012) are the only ones that draw primarily on critical medical anthropology—a perspective that has achieved considerable prominence in the subfield over the course of the past thirty years or so. In some ways, this textbook is an expansion of a more theoretical book titled *Critical Medical Anthropology*, which draws heavily on Singer and Baer's earlier efforts, in collaboration with numerous colleagues (including Susser), to develop a "critical medical anthropology" (Singer and Baer 1995). In that critical medical anthropology (CMA) has now "come of age" and has evolved into one of the major perspectives and a popular one, particularly among younger faculty members and students, we felt that the time was more than ripe for a textbook from this perspective.

Philosophically, this volume seeks to contribute to the further development of what we call "critical anthropological realism." In modern analytic philosophy, realism is the perspective that claims that objects, events, and beings in the world exist externally to us and to our experience of them; there is, in other words, an acceptance of a reality independent of our conception of it. As anthropologists, who, by design, seek to have close encounters with the peoples of the world and their ways of being and knowing, it has long been evident in the diversity of worldly conceptions that exist that humans do not ever know the external world directly but only through theory-laden participation and observation. And culture is the source of all theories of the world and hence of all experiences of it. Indeed, even systematic observation, or what we call science (which includes our own systematic observation as anthropologists), is recognized as cultural in origin and function. Additionally, as anthropologists, we have come to appreciate a form of philosophical relativism known as "cultural relativism," which is the notion that beliefs and behaviors must be studied and understood in their natural social context. Ripped from their cultural contexts, behaviors as humane as life-saving surgery or the ritual veneration of one's ancestors can be ridiculed as practices of inferior beings or fools. Cultural relativism teaches us respect for other ways of being and knowing, as well as humility about our own approaches to worldly knowledge. Nonetheless, as scientists, our work does not stop with the observation and description of peoples and their endless array of beliefs and behaviors but moves from there to the analysis and explanation of human ways of being, that is to say, to the analysis and explanation of culture (including our own culture, and including science as culture). However, given that, in the words of Cornel West (1999: xv–xvii), our goal as critical scientists is to confront "the pervasive evil of unjustified suffering and unnecessary social misery in our world," we avoid allowing our cultural relativism to "give in to sophomoric relativism ('Anything goes' or 'All views are equally valid')" or "to succumb to wholesale skepticism ('There is no truth')." Rather, we use our anthropological respect and appreciation (indeed, our celebration) of peoples of the world to analytically critique (and, as activist scholars, to publicly oppose) beliefs, behaviors, and social structures that promote structural violence and social suffering.

PART I

What Is Medical Anthropology About?

CHAPTER 1

Medical Anthropology: Central Concepts and Development

Medical anthropology concerns itself with the many factors that contribute to disease or illness and with the ways that human populations respond to disease or illness. Although the human body is the complex product of at least five million years of a dialectical relationship among human biological, the environment, and sociocultural evolution, it is a system subject to a multiplicity of assaults as well as to the deterioration that inevitably accompanies aging. Body processes are not only shaped by physiological variables but also mediated by culture and by emotional states. Hence, our bodies and our health are greatly influenced by our experiences and social contexts. In short, our bodies are biopsychosocial in nature. More-over, most of the cells in a human body are not human, they are bacteria, fungi, viruses, and other micro-organisms. In this sense, each of us is a natural community of organisms, or a superorganism. The composition of these other cells also significantly affects our health.

In this chapter, we introduce some key concepts developed in medical anthropology that we use repeatedly in this book. These concepts should enable students to comprehend more clearly the relationship between health-related issues and the sociocultural processes and arrangements of the modern world. We also present a brief history of medical anthropology as a subdiscipline of anthropology—one that has the potential to serve as a bridge between biological anthropology and sociocultural anthropology.

As we show, medical anthropology has drawn from a variety of theoretical perspectives within anthropological theory and social scientific theory as well as from biology. While these perspectives offer important insights into health-related issues, the authors of this volume work within a theoretical framework generally referred to as *critical medical anthropology*. The authors, with many other medical anthropologists, use this critical approach in the belief that social inequality and power are primary global determinants of health and health care. Although critical medical anthropology as a theoretical perspective is discussed in greater detail in Chapter 2, along with various other theoretical perspectives active within medical anthropology, suffice to say at this point that this perspective views health issues within the context of encompassing political and economic forces that pattern human relationships; shape social behaviors; condition collective experiences; reorder local ecologies; and situate cultural meanings, including forces of institutional, national, and global scale. The emergence of critical medical anthropology reflects both the historic turn toward political-economic approaches in anthropology in general, as well as an effort to engage and extend the political economy of health approach within and beyond the discipline (Baer, Singer, and Johnsen 1986; Morgan 1987; Morsy 1990; Baer and Singer 2009; Singer and Baer 2012).

CENTRAL CONCEPTS AND CONCERNS

The concepts described in this section, which we discuss frequently in this textbook, play a central role in the way we think about health issues in medical anthropology.

Health

The World Health Organization (WHO) defines health as "not merely the absence of disease and infirmity but complete physical, mental and social wellbeing" (WHO 1978). The notion of "wellness" has also become a key concept within the field especially among those involved in the holistic health movement. The human concern with wellness, however, is not a recent one. As chiropractor-anthropologist Norman Klein (1979: 1) so aptly observes, "Well-being is a human concern in all societies—in part because humans, like other life forms, are susceptible to illness." Health, more than merely a physiological or emotional state, is a concept that humans in many societies have developed to describe their sense of well-being and threats to desired states of wellness. Many medical anthropologists regard health to be a cultural construction, the meaning of which varies considerably from society to society or from one historical period to another.

Taking a neo-Marxian perspective, Sander Kelman (1975) views health within the context of a system of production. He makes an important distinction between "functional health" and "experiential health." The former he defines as a state of optimum capacity to perform roles within society, particularly within the context of capitalism (the dominant political economy of the contemporary world), to carry out productive work that contributes to profit-making. "Experiential health" entails freedom from illness and alienation and the capacity for human development, including self-discovery, self-actualization, and transcendence from alienating social circumstances. Whereas "functional health" is an inevitable component of social life under capitalism, "experiential health" tended to occur in many simple preindustrial societies and could theoretically occur again under modern societies based on egalitarian social relations.

Before casting their attention to state or complex societies, cultural anthropologists historically focused their research efforts primarily on indigenous societies around the world. Indeed, anthropologists as well as other visitors to these indigenous societies, including explorers, traders, and missionaries, remarked on the health and vigor of the people whom they encountered. While such accounts may have exhibited a certain element of romanticism, epidemiological and ethnographic studies support the conclusion that people in indigenous societies who reach adulthood generally exhibit a general state of good health and vigor. John H. Bodley succinctly captures some of the reasons why health conditions tend to be favorable in indigenous societies:

[M]ost importantly, the generally low population densities and relative social equality of small-scale societies would help ensure equal access to basic subsistence resources so that everyone could enjoy good nutrition. Furthermore, low population densities and frequent mobility would significantly reduce the occurrence of epidemic diseases, and natural selection—in the absence of the antibiotics, immunizations, surgery, and other forms of medical intervention   would develop high levels of disease resistance. Healthy people are those who survive. Tribal societies, in effect, maintain public health by emphasizing prevention of morbidity rather than treatment. The healthiest conditions would likely exist under mobile foragers and pastoralism, whereas there might be some health costs associated with the increasing densities and reduced mobility of settled farming villages. (Bodley 1994: 124)

From the perspective of CMA, health can be defined as *access to and control over the basic material and nonmaterial resources that sustain and promote life at a high level of individual and group satisfaction.* This definition pays attention both to local cultural factors (e.g., the definition of what is considered a satisfying condition of health) as well as to material factors, such as access to health-related resources). Health is not some absolute state of being but an elastic concept that must be evaluated in a larger sociocultural and political economic context. For example, the Gnau, a Sepik Valley group on the island of New Guinea, regard health as an "accumulated resistance to potential dangers" (Lewis 1986: 128). Among the Gnau, these dangers are seen as being primarily malevolent spirits. In capitalist societies, achieving health entails struggle against class-dominated powers that do not exist in indigenous societies. Although the ultimate character of health care systems is determined outside the health sector by dominant social groups, like heads of insurance companies and other large corporations, significant forms of struggle take place within this sector and help to shape its institutions. Consequently, an examination of contending forces in and out of the health arena that impinge on health and healing becomes an essential task in building a critical approach to health issues.

Disease

Even under the best of circumstances, human beings inevitably find themselves confronted with disease or illness. A central question for medical anthropology, as it is for biomedicine, is: What is disease? It is evident why this query is important to biomedicine. The nature of its importance to medical anthropology is more complex, and thus medical anthropologists have tended to avoid the question altogether by defining disease as clinical manifestations of ill health and illness as the sufferer's experience of ill health. Many medical anthropologists (especially in the past) treat the form as the domain of biomedicine and the latter as the appropriate arena of anthropological investigation. From the perspective of CMA, however, the bracketing of disease as outside the concern or expertise of anthropologists is a retreat from ground that is as much social as it is biological in nature. Humans in all societies perceive disease as a disruptive event that in one way or another threatens the flow of daily life and, potentially, the identity of the sufferer. Disease raises moral questions such as, "Why am I sick?" or "Why am I being punished?" and may serve as a mechanism for expressing dissent from existing sociocultural arrangements.

People around the world struggle with such existential questions, including uncertainties about the etiology of disease. For example, although the Azande of the Sudan acknowledge that misfortunes, including disease and death, may have a variety of causes, they attribute almost all of them to witchcraft, sorcery, or failure to follow a moral rule (Evans-Pritchard 1937). The Azande make a distinction between witchcraft (*mangu*) and magic (*ngua*), the latter term covering not only magical procedures but also herbal and other medicines. Whereas witchcraft may be caused by the unconscious hatred, envy, or greed that an individual may feel, magic functions as a means of counteracting witchcraft through the conscious manipulation of medicines. As this example shows, illness among the Azande has the potential to become an arena for ventilating social dissatisfaction and personal distress.

Health and disease are conditions that people in a society encounter, depending on their access to basic as well as prestige resources. Disease varies from society to society, in some part because of climatic or geographic conditions but also because of the ways productive activities and reproduction are organized and carried out. Following in the analytic tradition begun by Friedrich Engels and Rudolf Virchow, it is evident that discussion of specific health problems apart from their social contexts only serves to downplay social relationships underlying environmental, occupational, nutritional, residential, and experiential conditions. Disease is not just the straightforward result of a pathogen or physiologic disturbance. Instead, a variety of social problems such as malnutrition, economic insecurity, occupational risks, industrial and motor vehicle pollution, bad housing, stressful social environments, and political powerlessness contribute to susceptibility to disease.

In short, disease must be understood as being as much social as it is biological. In this light, the tendency, be it in medicine or in medical anthropology, to treat disease as a given, as part of an immutable physical reality, contributes to the tendency to neglect its social origins. By contrast, CMA strives, in McNeil's (1976) terms, to understand the nature of the relationship between microparasitism (the tiny organisms, malfunction, and individual behaviors that are the proximate causes of much sickness) and macroparasitism (the social relations of exploitation that are the ultimate causes of much disease). For example, an insulin reaction in a diabetic postal worker might be ascribed (in a reductionist mode) to an excessive dose of insulin causing an outpouring of adrenaline, a failure of the pancreas to respond with appropriate glucagon secretion, and so on. Alternatively, the cause might be sought in the postal worker having skipped breakfast because he was late for work; unaccustomed physical exertion demanded by a foreman; inability to break for a snack; or, at a deeper level, the constellation of class forces in U.S. society that ensures capitalist domination of production, enormous gaps between company directors and the majority of workers, and the moment-to-moment working lives of most people (Woolhandler and Himmelstein 1989: 1208).

Sufferer Experience

Medical social scientists have become increasingly concerned about sufferer experience—that is, the manner in which an ill person manifests his or her disease or distress. Margaret Lock and Nancy Scheper-Hughes (1990), who refer to themselves as critically interpretive medical anthropologists, reject the long-standing Cartesian duality of body and mind that pervades biomedical theory (Lock and Scheper-Hughes 1990). They have made a significant contribution to an understanding of sufferer experience by developing the concept of the "mindful body" (Scheper-Hughes and Lock 1987). Lock and Scheper-Hughes delineate three bodies: the individual body, the social body, and the body politic. People's images of their bodies, either in a state of health or well-being or in a state of disease or distress, are mediated by sociocultural meanings of being human. The body also serves as a cognitive map of natural, supernatural, sociocultural, and spatial relations. Furthermore, individual and social bodies express power relations in both a specific society and the world system.

Sufferer experience constitutes a social product, one that is constructed and reconstructed in the action arena between socially constituted categories of meaning and the political-economic forces that shape daily life. Although individuals often react passively to these forces, they may also respond to economic exploitation and political oppression in active ways. In her highly acclaimed and controversial book *Death without Weeping: The Violence of Everyday Life in Brazil*, Scheper-Hughes (1992) presents a vivid and moving portrayal of human suffering in Bom Jesus, an abjectly impoverished *favela*, or shantytown, in northeastern Brazil. She contends that the desperate and constant struggle for basic necessities in the community induces in many mothers an indifference to the weakest of their offspring. Although at times Scheper-Hughes appears to engage in a form of blaming the victim, she recognizes ultimately that the suffering of the mothers, their children, and others in Bom Jesus is intricately related to the collapse of the sugar plantation, which has left numerous people in the region without even a subsistence income. Most of the residents of Bom Jesus have not benefited from the development of agribusiness and industrialization sponsored by both transnational corporations and the Brazilian state. Under such conditions of poverty, the death of small children is not a rare event, and one that mothers are forced to stoically accept as a routine part of life. As this example suggests, the experience of sufferers and the members of their support network is critical to understanding illness-related behavior.

Health Care Systems

In responding to disease and illness, all human societies create health care systems of one sort or another. The term "health care system" refers to the social relationships that revolve around a healer and his or her patient. The healer may be assisted by various assistants and, in the case of complex societies, may work in an elaborate bureaucratic structure, such as a clinic, health maintenance organization, or hospital. The patient likely will be supported by what Janzen (1978) refers to as a "therapy managing group"—a set of kinfolk, friends, acquaintances, and community members who confer with the healer and representatives of his or her support structure in the healing process.

All health care systems consist of beliefs and practices that are consciously directed at promoting health and alleviating disease. Health care in simple preindustrial societies is not clearly differentiated from other social institutions such as religion and politics. The reality of this is seen in the shaman, a part-time magicoreligious practitioner who attempts to contact the supernatural realm when dealing with the problems of his or her group. In addition to searching for game or lost objects or related activities, the shaman devotes much of his or her attention to healing or curing. When curing a victim of witchcraft, the shaman among the Jivaro, a horticultural village society in the Ecuadorian Amazon, sucks magical darts from the patient's body in a dark area of the house at night, because this is believed to be the only time when he can interpret drug-induced visions that reveal supernatural reality (Harner 1968). The curing shaman vomits out the intrusive object, displays it to the patient and his or her family, puts it into a little container, and later throws it into the air, at which time it is believed to fly back to the bewitching shaman who originally sent it into the patient.

Even though physicians in industrial societies purport to practice a form of science-based health care that is distinct from magic, religion, and politics, in reality their endeavors are intricately intertwined with these spheres of social life. In his classic analysis of body ritual among the Nacirema, which has been reproduced in many introductory anthropological books, Horace Miner (1979) challenges North American ethnocentrism by showing that our own customs, seen with new eyes, are no less exotic than those of less complex preindustrial societies. Nacirema is merely American spelled backward and refers in Miner's somewhat tongue-in-cheek essay to a "magic-ridden" people whose "medicine men" (i.e., biomedical physicians) perform "elaborate ceremonies" (surgery) in imposing temples, called *latipos* (i.e., hospitals). The medicine men are assisted by a "permanent group of vestal maidens [female nurses] who move sedately about the temple chambers in distinctive costume and headdress" (Miner 1979: 12). Miner's point is that by the words we use, it is easy to exoticize the health care systems of other people while making our own cultural patterns seem natural and normal.

In a somewhat more serious vein, Rudolf Virchow, the well-known nineteenth-century pathologist and an early proponent of social medicine, declared that politics is "nothing but medicine on a grand scale" (quoted in Landy 1977: 14). By this, he simply meant that, like government, medicine is filled with power struggles and efforts to control individuals or social groups. Although medical anthropologists and other medical social scientists routinely use the term "medicine" as a heuristic or analytical device, it is important to remember that the notion of medicine as a bounded system is a cultural construct. In reality, health care is intertwined with other cultural arrangements, including kinship, the polity, the economy, and religion.

As noted in Foster and Anderson's medical anthropology text (1978: 36–38), every health care system embraces a disease theory system and a health care system. The *disease theory system* includes conceptions of what health is and the causes of disease or illness. Foster and Anderson make a distinction between (1) personalistic systems and (2) naturalistic systems. The former view disease as resulting from the action of "*Sensate* agent who may be a supernatural being (a deity or a god), a nonhuman being (such as a ghost, ancestor, or evil spirit), or a human being (a witch or sorcerer)" (Foster and Anderson 1978: 53). Naturalistic systems view disease as emanating from the imbalance of certain inanimate elements in the body, such as the male and female principles of yin and yang in Chinese medicine. Personalistic and naturalistic explanations are not mutually exclusive and may be found together in the same society.

Medical Pluralism

Regardless of their degree of complexity, all health care systems are based on the *dyadic core*, consisting of a healer and a patient. The healer role may be occupied by a generalist, such as the shaman in preindustrial societies or the family physician in modern societies. It may also be occupied by various specialists, such as an herbalist, a bonesetter, or a medium in preindustrial societies or a cardiologist, an oncologist, or a psychiatrist in modern societies. In contrast to simple preindustrial societies, which tend to exhibit a more-or-less coherent health care system, state societies manifest the coexistence of an array of health care systems, or a pattern of what is called *medical pluralism*. From this perspective, *the* health care system of a society consists of the totality of medical subsystems that coexist in a cooperative or competitive relationship with one another. In modern industrial societies, one finds, in addition to biomedicine, the dominant medical system, other systems such as chiropractic, naturopathy, Christian Science, evangelical faith healing, and various ethnomedical systems, which are the healing systems developed by particular ethnic or cultural subgroups. In the U.S. context, examples of ethnomedical systems include herbalism among rural whites in Southern Appalachia, rootwork among African Americans in the rural South, *curanderismo* among Chicanos of the Southwest, *Santeria* among Cuban Americans in southern Florida and New York City, and a variety of Native American healing traditions.

Various medical anthropologists have created typologies that recognize the phenomenon of medical pluralism in complex societies. On the basis of their geographic and cultural settings, Dunn (1976) delineated three types of health care or medical systems: (1) local medical systems, (2) regional medical systems, and (3) the cosmopolitan medical system. *Local* medical systems are folk or indigenous medical systems of small-scale foraging, horticultural or pastoral societies, or peasant communities in state societies. *Regional* medical systems are systems distributed over a relatively large area. Examples of regional medical systems include Ayurvedic medicine and Unani medicine in South Asia and traditional Chinese medicine. *Cosmopolitan* medicine refers to the global medical system or what commonly has been called scientific medicine, modern medicine, or Western medicine. Complex societies generally contain all three of these medical systems. India, for example, has numerous local medical systems associated with its many ethnic groups. In addition to biomedicine, modern Japan has a variety of East Asian medical systems (Lock 1980). The most popular of these is *kanpo*, a form of herbal medicine that was brought to Japan from China in the sixth century. In addition to prescribing herbs, *kanpo* doctors administer acupuncture, body manipulation, and moxibustion therapy. They tend to treat psychosomatic ailments in which the patients' chief complaints are tiredness, headaches, occasional dizziness, or numbness—typical symptoms emanating from the somatization of distress.

Chrisman and Kleinman (1983) developed a widely used model that recognizes three overlapping sectors in health care systems. The popular sector consists of health care conducted by sick persons themselves, their families, social networks, and communities. It includes a wide variety of therapies, such as special diets, herbs, exercise, rest, baths, and massage and, in the case of industrial societies, articles such as humidifiers, hot blankets, patent medicines, or over-the-counter drugs. Kleinman, who has conducted research in Taiwan, estimates that 70 to 90 percent of the treatment episodes on that island occur in the popular sector. The folk sector encompasses healers of various sorts who function informally and often on a quasi-legal or sometimes, given local laws, an illegal basis. Examples include herbalists, bonesetters, midwives, mediums, and magicians. In the U.S. context, examples of folk healers include lay hypnotists, lay homeopaths, faith healers, African American rootworkers, *curanderas, espiritistas,* and Navajo singers. The *professional* sector encompasses the practitioners and bureaucracies of both biomedicine and professionalized heterodox medical systems, such as Ayurvedic and Unani medicine in South Asia and herbal medicine and acupuncture in the People's Republic of China. Whereas medical sociologists have tended to focus their attention on the professional sector of health, anthropologists have also given much attention to the folk and popular sectors.

Patterns of medical pluralism tend to reflect hierarchical relations in the larger society. Patterns of hierarchy may be based on class, caste, racial, ethnic, regional, religious, and gender distinctions. Medical pluralism flourishes in all class-divided societies and tends to mirror the wider sphere of class and social relationships. It is perhaps more accurate to say that national medical systems in the modern or postmodern world tend to be plural, rather than pluralistic, in that biomedicine enjoys a dominant status over heterodox and ethnomedical practices. In reality, plural medical systems may be described as dominative in that one medical system generally enjoys a preeminent status vis-à-vis other medical systems (Baer 2004, 2009g). Within the context of a dominative medical system, one system attempts to exert, with the support of social elites, dominance over other medical systems; nevertheless, people are quite capable of the dual use of distinct medical systems. Based on her research among the Manus in the Admiralty Islands of Melanesia, Lola Romanucci-Ross (1977) identified a "hierarchy of resort" in which many people utilize self-administered folk remedies or consult folk healers before visiting a biomedical clinic or hospital for their ailments. Although this sequence is the most prevalent one, more acculturated Manus, in contrast, often rely on biomedicine initially or first after home remedies; if these two fail, they may finally resort to folk healers.

Biomedicine

In attempting to distinguish the Western health care system that became globally dominant during the twentieth century from alternative systems, social scientists have employed a variety of descriptive labels, including regular medicine, allopathic medicine, scientific medicine, modern medicine, and cosmopolitan medicine. Following Comaroff (1982), Hahn (1983), and Lock and Nguyen (2010), most medical anthropologists have come to refer to this form of medicine as "biomedicine." Michel Foucault (1975) argues in *The Birth of the Clinic* that biomedicine emerged around 1800 in Europe as it systematically began to classify diseases into families and species and focused more on the body and its parts and subparts (externally and internally), thus the term "clinical gaze," than on the sick person as a whole, complex emotional, psychological, physical, and social being. In later writings, Foucault portrayed biomedicine as one of a series of social control mechanisms of modern societies, along with the state, asylums, and prisons.

Furthermore, Hahn (1983) argues that in diagnosing and treating sickness, biomedicine focuses primarily on human physiology and even more specifically on human pathophysiology. Perhaps the most glaring example of this tendency to reduce disease to biology is the common practice among hospital physicians of referring to patients by the name of their malfunctioning organ (e.g., "the liver in Room 213" or "the kidney in Room 563"). A fourth-year chief resident interviewed by Lazarus (1988: 39) commented, "We are socialized to—disease is the thing. Yeah, I slip. We all do and see the patient as a disease." As these examples illustrate, commonly the central concern of biomedicine is not general well-being nor individual persons per se but rather simply diseased bodies. Biomedicine is highly specialized, which means that patients may visit numerous specialists for a single disease. According to Seefeld and Landman (2008: 17),

This makes it difficult to ensure that any single provider has access to a patient's complete medical record, including clinical notes, lab results for such things as blood work, or imaging results such as X-rays. A universal electronic medical record would help, but that's years, if not decades, away from becoming a reality.

In essence, biomedicine subscribes to a type of physical reductionism that radically separates the body from the nonbody. Hahn notes that biomedicine emphasizes curing over prevention and spends much more money on hospitals, clinics, ambulance services, drugs, and "miracle cures" than it does on public health facilities, preventive education, cleaning the environment, addressing malnutrition, and eliminating the stress associated with modern life. Biomedicine too is an ethnomedicine. It constitutes the predominant ethnomedical system of European and North American societies although it has become widely disseminated and dominant throughout the world.

Within the U.S. context, biomedicine incorporates certain core values, metaphors, beliefs, and attitudes that it communicates to patients, such as self-reliance, rugged individualism, independence, pragmatism, empiricism, atomism, militarism, profit-making, emotional minimalism, and a mechanistic concept of the body and its repair (H. Stein 1990). For example, U.S. biomedicine often speaks of the war on cancer. This war is portrayed as a prolonged attack against a deadly and evil internal growth, led by a highly competent general (the oncologist) who gives orders to a courageous, stoical, and obedient soldier (the patient) in a battle that must be conducted with valor despite the odds and, if necessary, until the bitter end. Erwin (1987) aptly refers to this approach as the "medical militarization" of cancer treatment. Conversely, according to Hanteng Dai, a Chinese physician who had worked with cancer patients in Arkansas, told Hans Baer sometime in the late 1990s that both health personnel and members of the therapy management group in the People's Republic of China tell cancer patients a white lie by referring to their condition as being something less serious to spare them from purported mental anguish. Given that cancer constitutes a breakdown of the immune system, it is interesting to draw attention to Emily Martin's (1987: 410) observation that the main imagery employed in popular and scientific descriptions of this system portrays the "body as nation state at war over its external borders, containing internal surveillance systems to monitor foreign invaders."

It is important to stress that biomedicine is not a monolithic entity. Rather, its form is shaped by its national settings, as is illustrated by Payer's (1988) fascinating comparative account of medicine in France, Germany, Britain, and the United States. He argues that French biomedicine, with its strong orientation toward abstract thought, results in doctor visits that are much longer than in German biomedicine. French biomedicine also places a great deal of emphasis on the liver as the locus of disease, including complications such as migraine headaches, general fatigue, and painful menstruation. Conversely, German biomedicine regards *Herzin-suffizienz,* or poor circulation, as the root of a broad spectrum of ailments, including hypotension, tired legs, and varicose veins. Both German and French biomedicine rely more heavily than U.S. biomedicine on the capacity of the immunological system to resist disease and therefore deemphasize the use of antibiotics. In contrast to U.S. biomedicine, they also exhibit a much greater acceptance of soft medicine or alternative medical systems such as naturopathy, homeopathy, hydropathy (a system that relies on a wide variety of water treatments), and extended stays at spas in peaceful, parklike surroundings. German patients tend on the average to visit the doctor's office more than twice as often as their counterparts in France, England, and the United States. U.S. biomedicine relies much more—than biomedicine in France, Germany, and England—on invasive forms of therapy, such as cesarean sections, hysterectomies, breast cancer screenings, and high dosages of psychotropic drugs. As we saw in the case of cancer treatment, U.S. biomedicine manifests a pattern of aggression that seems in keeping with the strong emphasis in American society on violence as a means of solving problems—a pattern undoubtedly rooted in the frontier mentality that continues to live on in what has for the most part become a highly urbanized, postindustrial society. In this sense, the war on cancer and the war on drugs are symbolic cultural continuations of the war against Native Americans that cleared the frontier for white settlement.

It should also be noted that biomedicine varies by region within a nation. In the United States, for example, Pilote and coworkers (1995) found substantial regional variation in how doctors manage heart problems. New England physicians were found to be atypical of doctors in other regions of the country in their relatively limited use of various cardiac medications and surgical procedures. This same pattern of regional difference in medical practice has been found for many other health problems.

Biomedicine achieved its dominant position in the West and beyond with the emergence of industrial capitalism and with abundant assistance from the capitalist class whose interests it commonly serves. Historian E. Richard Brown argues that the Rockefeller and Carnegie foundations played an instrumental role in shaping "scientific medicine" by providing funding only to those medical schools and research institutes that placed heavy emphasis on the germ theory of disease. According to E. R. Brown (1979), "The medical profession discovered an ideology that was compatible with the world view of, and politically and economically useful to, the capitalist class and the emerging managerial and professional stratum." Biomedicine focused attention on discrete, external agents rather than on social structural or environmental factors. In addition to its legitimizing functions, the Rockefeller medicine men believed that biomedicine would create a healthier workforce, both here and abroad, which would contribute to economic productivity and profit. Biomedicine portrayed the body as a machine that requires periodic repair so that it may perform assigned productive tasks essential to economic imperatives. Even in the case of reproduction, as Martin (1987: 146) so aptly observes, "birth is seen as the control of laborers (women) and their machines (their uteruses) by managers (doctors), often using other machines to help."

Indeed, although the Soviet Union emerged as the first nationwide movement against the capitalist world system, the ideological influence of biomedicine was so strong that Navarro (1977) applied the label "bourgeois medicine" to the "mechanistic" and "curative" orientation of the Soviet medical paradigm. Although certain other professionalized medical systems, such as homeopathy, Ayurveda, Unani, and traditional Chinese medicine, function in many parts of the world, biomedicine became the preeminent medical system in the world not simply because of its curative efficacy but as a result of the expansion of the global market economy.

Medicalization and Medical Hegemony

Biomedicine has fostered a process that many social scientists refer to as *medicalization*. This process entails the absorption of ever-widening social arenas and behaviors into the jurisdiction of biomedical treatment through a constant extension of pathological terminology to cover new conditions and behaviors. Health clinics, health maintenance organizations, and other medical providers now offer classes on managing stress; controlling obesity; overcoming sexual impotence, alcoholism, or drug addiction; and smoking cessation. The birth experience, not just in the United States but also in many countries that pride themselves on undergoing modernization, has been distorted into a pathological event rather than a natural physiological one for childbearing women. Aspects of the medicalization of birthing include (1) the withholding of information on the disadvantages of obstetrical medication, (2) the expectation that women give birth in a hospital, (3) the elective induction of labor, (4) the separation of the mother from familial support during labor and birth, (5) the confinement of the laboring woman to bed, (6) professional dependence on technology and pharmacological methods of pain relief, (7) routine electronic fetal monitoring, (8) the chemical stimulation of labor, (9) the delay of birth until the physician's arrival, (10) the requirement that the mother assume a prone position rather than a squatting one, (11) the routine use of regional or general anesthesia for delivery, and (12) routine episiotomy (Haire 1978: 188–94). Fortunately, the women's liberation movement has prompted women to challenge many of these practices and has contributed to a heavier reliance on home births conducted by lay midwives.

One factor driving medicalization is the profit to be made from discovering new diseases in need of treatment. Medicalization also contributes to increasing social control on the part of physicians and health institutions over behavior. It serves to demystify and depoliticize the social origins of personal distress. Medicalization transforms a "problem at the level of social structure—stressful work demands, unsafe working conditions, and poverty— . . . into an individual problem under medical control" (Waitzkin 1983: 41).

Underlying the medicalization of contemporary life is the broader phenomenon of medical hegemony, the process through which capitalist assumptions, concepts, and values come to permeate medical diagnosis and treatment. The concept of *hegemony* has been applied to various spheres of social life, including the state, institutionalized religion, education, and the mass media. In the development of this concept, Antonio Gramsci, an Italian political activist who fought against fascism under Mussolini, elaborated on Marx and Engels's observation that the "ideas of the ruling class are, in every age, the ruling ideas." Whereas the ruling class exerts direct domination through the coercive organs of the state apparatus (e.g., the parliament, the courts, the military, the police, the prisons, etc.), hegemony, as Femia (1975: 30) observes, is "objectified in and exercised through the institutions of civil society, the ensemble of educational, religious, and associational institutions."

Hegemony refers to the process through which one class exerts control of the cognitive and intellectual life of society by structural means as opposed to coercive ones. Hegemony is achieved through the diffusion and reinforcement of certain values, attitudes, beliefs, social norms, and legal precepts that, to a greater or lesser degree, come to permeate civil society. Doctor–patient interactions frequently reinforce hierarchical structures in the larger society by stressing the need for the patient to comply with a social superior's or expert's judgment. Although a patient may be experiencing job-related stress that may manifest in various diffuse symptoms, the physician may prescribe a sedative to calm the patient or help him or her cope with an onerous work environment rather than challenging the power of an employer or supervisor over employees.

Despite the hegemony of biomedicine, medical pluralism persists and exhibits hybridization under which biomedical and indigenous medical systems, both professionalized and popular or folk, interact and borrow from each other. Within this process, some nonbiomedical systems, such as Chinese medicine, Ayurvedic medicine, and Tibetan medicine, have also become "cosmopolitan" medical systems, a term that Charles Leslie in the 1970s applied to biomedicine. At the same time, biomedicine seeks to contain competing medical systems by integrating them only when their knowledge and practices become standardized according to biomedical regulations and practices.

Syndemics

One effect of the kind of reductionist thinking in health that tends to dominate biomedical understanding and practice is the tendency to isolate, study, and treat diseases as if they were distinct entities that existed separate from other diseases and from the social contexts in which they are found. CMA, however, seeks to understand health and illness from a holistic biocultural, biosocial, and political economic perspective (sometimes called *critical bioculturalism*) that runs counter to the dominant reductionist orientation. This approach attempts to identify and understand the determinant interconnections between one or more health conditions, sufferer and community understandings of the illness(es) in question, and the social, political, and economic conditions that may have contributed to the development of ill health. To help frame this kind of big-picture dialectical thinking in health, critical medical anthropologists introduced the concept of *syndemic* (Singer 2009a) as a new term in epidemiological and public health thinking. At its simplest level, the term syndemic refers to two or more epidemics (i.e., notable increases in the rate of specific diseases in a population) interacting synergistically with each other inside human bodies and contributing, as a result of their interaction, to an excess burden of disease in a population. In other words, the adverse consequences of syndemic interaction among diseases in a population is greater than the mere addition of the effects of the two or more diseases involved.

As Millstein (2001: 2), organizer of the Syndemics Prevention Network at the Centers for Disease Control, notes, "Syndemics occur when health-related problems cluster by person, place or time." Importantly, however, the term refers not only to the temporal or locational co-occurrence of two or more diseases or health problems but also to the negative health consequences of the biological or other interactions among the health conditions present. Although the co-presence of two or more diseases in a population does not automatically result in their interaction and all disease interactions do not necessary worsen the health of sufferers, when adverse or syndemic interaction does occur, it can take a significant toll on human life and well-being. One example of this is the 1918–1919 influenza pandemic that may have resulted in as many as 100 million deaths globally. This deadly pandemic has been shown to be the result of the interaction of an influenza virus with pathogenic bacteria that cause pneumonia, especially *Streptococcus pneumonia* and *S. pyogenes*. As summarized by Morens and Fauci (2007: 1020), individuals suffering from viral infection during the 1918 pandemic were at risk for the development of "aggressive bronchopneumonia . . . from which pathogenic bacteria could usually be cultured at autopsy. . . . In a few autopsies, severe bronchopneumonia was seen without evidence of bacteria, but studies generally showed a close correlation between the distributions of pulmonary lesions and cultured bacteria."

Of equal importance in syndemics as the diseases involved and the pathways or mechanisms and outcomes of their interaction are the social conditions (including socially medicated environmental conditions) that promote the clustering of diseases. Thus, syndemics are defined as the concentration and deleterious interaction of two or more diseases or other health conditions in a population, especially as a consequence of social inequity and the unjust exercise of power. Inequality, discrimination, poverty, and other insults to human dignity, as well as the suffering that results from such conditions, have been shown to damage human health in ways that leave people vulnerable to disease and the likelihood of multiple disease clustering.

Awareness of the significance of syndemics in past, contemporary, and future health is being recognized across disciplines. Chapter 10 further explores syndemics and their role in shaping global health and also examines a number of related concepts that recognize the importance of interactions (among both diseases and environmental conditions).

Pluralea and Health

The term *pluralea,* which in Latin means "many threats," is a concept within environmental health that refers to the interaction and resulting enhancement of two or more health-impacting ecocrises. In other words, pluralea involve cases in which several expressions of environmental degradation (e.g., deforestation), contamination (e.g., air or water pollution), and/or restructuring (e.g., global warming) combine and as a result multiply the damage done to human health. An example of the health impact of pluralea is seen in the interaction now occurring between allergens and infectious agents that have contributed to global increases in the distribution, frequency, and severity of asthma. Although traditionally associated with developed nations, the WHO (2012) now estimates that 235 million people globally suffer with asthma, and approximately a quarter of a million people, mostly in low- and lower-middle-income countries, annually die of the disease. Increases in asthma rates in developing countries are especially evident among urban populations and reflect the intertwined impact of (1) global warming, which contributes to increasing levels of allergens by facilitating the spread, early budding, and enhanced pollen production of heat-loving plants (e.g., ragweed) and airborne particulate matter from wildfires, and (2) vehicular and other industrial air pollutants such as nitrogen dioxide.

Of considerable importance in the study of pluralea are their proximate and ultimate causes, and especially the precise role of human social and economic systems in generating health damaging environmental stresses. Also critical to the pluralea conceptualization, as discussed more thoroughly in Chapter 10, is the development of an understanding of the pathways and mechanisms through which two or more ecocrises interact to produce increasingly injurious environmental and health impacts. Introduced by medical anthropology, the concept of pluralea underlines the importance of environmental factors in the quality of human health.

A BRIEF HISTORY OF MEDICAL ANTHROPOLOGY IN THE UNITED STATES AND ELSEWHERE

Medical anthropology as a distinct subdiscipline of anthropology did not begin to emerge until the 1950s. Nevertheless, Otto von Mering (1970: 272) contends that the formal relationship between anthropology and medicine began when Rudolf Virchow, a renowned pathologist interested in social medicine, helped to establish the first anthropological society in Berlin. Indeed, Virchow influenced Franz Boas while he was affiliated with the Berlin Ethnological Museum during 1883–1886 (Trostle 1986: 45). Nevertheless, the political economic perspective that Virchow fostered became a part of medical anthropology only beginning in the 1970s. In the course of conducting ethnographic research on indigenous societies, various anthropologists have collected data on medical beliefs and practices along with the usual data on kinship, subsistence activities, religion, and forms of enculturation. W. H. R. Rivers, a physician-anthropologist who conducted fieldwork in the southwest Pacific and one of the first anthropologists to discuss health-related issues cross-culturally, argued in *Medicine, Magic, and Religion* (1924: 51) that "medical practices are not a medley of disconnected and meaningless customs" but rather an integral part of the larger sociocultural systems within which they are embedded. This observation may appear obvious today, but followers of a school of anthropology known as historical particularism tended to view culture as a thing of threads and patches or a byproduct of a complex process of contacts among many social groups.

Forrest Clements (1932) served as another precursor to medical anthropology by attempting to classify conceptions of sickness causation on a worldwide basis. During the 1940s, Erwin Ackerknecht (1971) and others wrote papers and articles on topics that would today be considered medical anthropology (e.g., folk nosology and healing). He sought to develop a systematic cultural relativist and functionalist interpretation of what he termed *primitive medicine*. Indeed, Rivers, Clements, and Ackerknecht unwittingly contributed to biomedical hegemony by bracketing biomedicine off from ethnomedicine. They accepted biomedicine as science at face value, not as a subject for social science, as do medical anthropologists and medical sociologists today. As Kleinman (1978: 408) aptly observes, biomedical science and care "in fully modern societies were, for a long while, excluded from cross-cultural comparisons, and unfortunately still are even in some fairly recent studies."

After World War II, an increasing number of anthropologists turned their attention to health-related issues, especially applied ones. Indeed, the first overview of what today constitutes medical anthropology, authored by William Caudill (1953), was titled "Applied Anthropology in Medicine." Although Norman Scotch (1963) is often credited with popularizing the term *medical anthropology*, it reportedly was first used by a Third World scholar in an Indian medical journal (Hunter 1985: 298). Much of conventional medical anthropology received its initial impetus from two main sources: (1) the involvement of various anthropologists in international health work and (2) the involvement of anthropologists in the clinical setting as teachers, researchers, administrators, and clinicians. Many of these efforts, beginning after World War II and continuing to the present day, have sought to humanize the physician–patient relationship.

Anthropological involvement in the international health field began within the context of British colonialism during the 1930s and 1940s—a period when the delivery of Western health services was seen as part of a larger effort to administer and control indigenous populations. Cora DuBois became the first anthropologist to hold a formal position with an international health organization when she received employment from the WHO in 1950 (Coreil 1990: 5). Later during the 1950s, several anthropologists received appointments to international health posts. They included Edward Wellin at the Rockefeller Foundation, Benjamin Paul at the Harvard School of Public Health, and George Foster and others at the Institute for Inter-American Affairs (the forerunner of the U.S. Agency for International Development). Benjamin Paul (1969: 29) saw anthropologists as being "especially qualified by temperament and training . . . [for] the study of popular reactions to programs of public health carried out in foreign cultural settings." In retrospect, the writings of Paul and many of his contemporaries strike many medical anthropologists, particularly those of a critical bent, as unduly naive about the nature and function of United States–sponsored international health programs. Their work, which was conducted at the peak of the Cold War, exhibited a profoundly Eurocentric ideological cast that included an implicit biomedical bias.

Some anthropologists became involved in efforts to facilitate the delivery of biomedical care to populations in the United States. For example, Alexander and Dorothea Leighton, anthropologists who conducted extensive research on the Navajo, became involved in the Navajo-Cornell Field Health Project, which was established in 1955 (Foster 1982: 190). This project resulted in the creation of the role of "health visitor," a Navajo paramedic and health educator who served as a "cultural broker" or liaison between the Anglo-dominated health care system and his people. As part of the larger effort to deliver biomedical health services and to ensure the compliance of patients, many medical anthropologists turned to ethnomedical approaches that sought to elicit the health beliefs of their subjects.

Clinical anthropology, as a distinct branch of medical anthropology, began to develop in the early 1970s as part of a larger effort to humanize the increasingly bureaucratic and impersonal aspects of biomedical care. Nevertheless, medical anthropologists such as Otto von Mering had been working in clinical settings since the early 1950s (T. M. Johnson 1987).

Arthur Kleinman (1977), a psychiatrist with a master's in anthropology, urged medical anthropologists to assume a "clinical mandate" under which they would help to facilitate the doctor–patient relationship, particularly by eliciting patient "explanatory models," or the patient's perceptions of disease and illness, that would help the physician deliver better medical care. In addition to seeking to reform biomedicine, although certainly not significantly to change it, clinical anthropology has focused attention on searching for alternative health careers for anthropologists during the 1980s and 1990s. The tight academic job market prompted many anthropology students to seek careers in medical anthropology because it held out the hope of providing employment in nonacademic settings, including clinical ones.

A long symbiotic relationship has existed between medical anthropology and medical sociology (Conrad 1997; M-J. D. Good and Good 2000). Various people, such as Peter Kong-Ming New, Ronald Frankenberg, Ray H. Elling, and Meredith McGuire, have served as disciplinary brokers between medical sociology and medical anthropology. Medical anthropologists have often relied on medical sociological research, particularly in their research on aspects of biomedicine and national health care systems. For instance, in the first medical anthropology textbook ever to be published, G. M. Foster and Anderson (1978) drew heavily on medical sociological research in their chapters "Illness Behavior," "Hospitals:

Behavioral Science Views," "Professionalism in Medicine: Doctor," and "Professionalism in Medicine: Nursing."

A steering committee formed to explore the possibility of establishing a formal organization for medical anthropologists began publishing the *Medical Anthropology Newsletter* in 1968. The committee represented a growing coterie of anthropologists interested in "carving out and defining a topical field within anthropology, that was analogous to such other topics as religion, economics, social organization, psychological anthropology, and the like" (Landy 1977: 2–3). Indeed, David Landy began at the University of Pittsburgh in 1960 to teach in the anthropology department a course titled "Primitive and Folk Medicine" and simultaneously, in the School of Public Health, a course titled "Social and Cultural Factors in Health and Disease." The Group for Medical Anthropology (GMA) debated whether it should affiliate with either the American Anthropological Association or the Society for Applied Anthropology between 1968 and 1972 (Weidman 1986). GMA evolved into the Society for Medical Anthropology (SMA), which finally became a constituent unit of the American Anthropological Association in 1975. The first doctoral programs in medical anthropology were established at the University of California at Berkeley/San Francisco, Michigan State University, and the University of Connecticut during the 1970s. Since that time, many anthropology departments have established master's and doctoral programs in medical anthropology, and some have even established postdoctoral programs in medical anthropology or on specific health issues such as social gerontology, reproductive health, or infectious diseases. Beyond the academy, many medical anthropologists work in community settings. Merrill Singer, for example, worked for twenty-five years at the community-based organization known as the Hispanic Health Council, where he directed applied studies of health and health intervention among health disparity populations in the inner city of Hartford before moving to the oldest academic program in medical anthropology at the University of Connecticut.

About three decades ago, Landy (1983: 193) asserted that medical anthropology "has begun to come of age, or at least to have left its childhood and entered its adolescence." Today, the SMA is the second largest unit of the American Anthropological Association. Furthermore, health-related issues have become a major area of study among anthropologists in the United Kingdom, continental Europe, Latin America, South Africa, Japan, and elsewhere.

Although medical anthropology as a field is most developed in the United States, it has diffused to many parts of the world. Francine Saillant and Serge Genest (2007) edited an anthology that includes chapters on medical anthropology in eleven countries—not only the United States, but also Canada, Brazil, Mexico, France, Spain, Italy, Germany, the Netherlands, the United Kingdom, and Switzerland. As Salliant and Genest (2007: xviii) observe, medical anthropology is "fragmented by its myriad national traditions," not to speak of "many disciplinary subfields that have emerged and developed within it." Although in Australia, health sociology, which is represented by a thematic group within the Australian Sociological Association and a journal titled *Health Sociology Review,* is a more identifiable endeavor than medical anthropology, there is a growing interest in medical anthropology as well, particularly at the Centre of Health and Society at the University of Melbourne. A group of Australian medical anthropologists have been pioneers in "hospital ethnography," including Anna Harris (2009), who conducted her PhD research on how "overseas doctors" have adjusted to working within the corridors of two Melbourne suburban hospitals. Since first coming to Australia in 2004 and then returning permanently in 2006, Hans Baer has worked on complementary medicine in Australia (Baer 2009b) as well on health and the *critical anthropology of global warming* (Baer and Singer 2009). Judith Littleton and Julie Park (2009) at the University of Auckland have been pacesetters in New Zealand medical anthropology including the study of syndemics. Unfortunately, however, the "contemporary influence of managerialism in the neoliberal New Zealand health care environment is . . . a local pressure which works against the increasing uptake of anthropological approaches in health research because of the very long frame in which such research takes place" (Fitzgerald and Park 2003: 18).

Outside the United States, medical anthropology has seen its greatest growth in Great Britain. A session convened by Meyer Fortes at the 1972 annual conference of the Association of Social Anthropologists (ASA) at the University of Kent played a key role in launching the subdiscipline in the United Kingdom. The papers presented at this session were eventually published in a volume titled *Social Anthropology and Medicine* (Loudon 1976). The narrow focus of medical anthropology in Britain initially is illustrated by Rosemary Firth's (1978: 244) recommendation that anthropologists interested in health-related issues confine their activity primarily to the translation of symbolic systems and avoid collaboration with other social scientists and also "social engineers and social reformers." Her advice against starting an applied medical anthropology reflects an earlier era during which many sociocultural anthropologists believed that their discipline should focus its research on simple preindustrial societies in a purportedly pristine or socially isolated form. At any rate, the 1972 ASA conference prompted the founding of the British Medical Anthropology Society in 1976. In contrast to their North American counterparts, however, medical anthropologists in the United Kingdom followed Firth and tended to eschew applied research (L. Kaufert and Kaufert 1978). In time, medical anthropology in Britain began to emerge from its "tight confinement to ethnomedicine" (Hunter 1985: 1298). The work of Ronald Frankenberg (1974) and that of socially oriented physicians such as Joyce Leeson (1974) at Manchester University served as a precursor to the later emergence of critical medical anthropology in the United States and the United Kingdom.

Also important in the development of a critical perspective in British medical anthropology was the work of the medical sociologist Mervyn Susser, a South African physician who collaborated with anthropologist William Watson during the early 1960s on the sociology of medicine.

While a professor in the Department of Community Medicine at Manchester University in England, Susser participated in discussions of health, medicine, and society with Frankenberg and Leeson. In South Africa, Mervyn Susser and Zena Stein Susser were inspired by Sydney Kark, who founded the community health center movement, later replicated in the United States. Until they were forced to leave South Africa for political reasons, they worked on issues of social medicine, including developing community health programs at Alexandra Township Clinic, exposing forms of contamination in oil cans that local people reused for water, and helping to write the health aspects of the Freedom Charter. In 1956, when Mervyn Susser was hired as a senior lecturer in the Department of Social and Preventive Medicine at Manchester University in England, the Sussers were welcomed by fellow South African Max Gluckman, then chair of anthropology, and their friendship built strong links between the two departments. Mervyn Susser worked with William Watson, a student of Gluckman's who taught in the anthropology department and wrote *Tribal Cohesion in a Money Economy* (Manchester University Press 1958). Susser and Watson wrote the first medical textbook, *Social Medicine: Sociology in Medicine* (1962, 1971, 1985), which became a key text in medical schools and schools of public health in the United States and elsewhere. The third edition was published in the 1980s, with the anthropologist Kim Hopper. Over the next fifty years, Susser and Stein's research crossed the borders of social science and public health, from a classic study of the health and development of babies whose mothers were pregnant during the Dutch Famine of 1944 to the effects of social inequality on the health of populations (Z. Stein et al. [1975] on the Dutch famine; Susser and Stein [2009] on human rights). Over the decade the Sussers were at Manchester, they participated in discussions of health, medicine, and society with Joyce Leeson, a good friend and a lecturer in social medicine.

Through the ongoing collaborations between the two departments, Joyce Leeson, who later published a book on women in medicine, met Ronald Frankenberg, and they published in medical anthropology. Frankenberg and Leeson went to Zambia together and published a joint article on medical anthropology. In later years, Ronald Frankenberg became a key figure in contributing to and shaping critical medical anthropology in the United States.

In the late 1960s, contemporary medical anthropology made its debut in the Federal Republic of Germany when Joachim Sterly established the Arbeitsgemeinschaft Ethnomedizin (Working Society on Ethnomedicine; Pfeiderer and Bichman 1986). At the same time, he founded a unit for ethnomedicine, because the term medical anthropology already designated earlier medical concerns in the Deutsche Gesellschaft für Voelkerkunde (German Society of Ethnography). German cultural anthropology, both in the Federal Republic of Germany and the former German Democratic Republic, has been divided into *Volkskunde* (the study of German populations) and *Voelkerkunde* (ethnology of peoples around the world). The term *Anthropologie* tends to be avoided because it refers to physical anthropology—a field the Nazis used to support their racial program. After World War II, physical anthropology eventually became rehabilitated in East Germany and, somewhat later, in West Germany.

For a period of time, the Institute of Tropical Hygiene and Public Health at the University of Heidelberg published the journal *Ethnomedizin*. The Arbeitsgemeinschaft Ethnomedizin (the Working Society on Ethnomedicine) publishes the journal *Curae*. Both Heidelberg University and Hamburg University offer course work in medical anthropology, with the latter offering a doctoral degree in medical anthropology.

Medical anthropology has become an area of growing interest in various other European countries, including Belgium (Devisch 1986), Italy (Pandolfi and Gordon 1986; Seppilli 2012), the Netherlands (Streefland 1986; Geest 2012), Austria (Kutalek, Muenzenmeir, and Prinz 2012: 42–43), Switzerland (Kutalek, Muezenmeir, and Prinz 2012: 43–45), and Scandinavia (Heggenhougen 1986), as well as in other parts of the world.

Medical Anthropology and Epidemiology

Medical anthropology obviously shares many common concerns with epidemiology, particularly social epidemiology, which seeks to identify social structural factors, such as social inequality, occupational hazards, employment, and workplace stress, that contribute to disease incidence and prevalence. Conversely, whereas epidemiology tends to be highly statistical and quantitative in its methodology, anthropology tends to be more qualitative and even historical. James A. Trostle (2005: 4) has been promoting an "integrated and interdisciplinary dialogue" between medical anthropology and epidemiology. He maintains "that epidemiologists should devote the same attention to culture that they have given to 'social' factors over the past few decades" and calls for a *cultural epidemiology* that draws attention to "health-related effects of behavior and belief" (Trostle 2005: 5). In reality, however, social and cultural factors are so intertwined that we might speak of sociocultural factors.

Toward the close of the twentieth century, the health arena was rocked by the sudden appearance of a host of seemingly new infectious diseases, all of them direly frightening in their sudden appearance, horrific symptoms, and often lethal power (Garrett 1994). Some of these new diseases, like AIDS or Lyme disease, have become widespread and well known to the general public. Others only garner popular attention when an outbreak suddenly occurs. For example, in 1967, the Marburg virus first appeared in the Behring Works company in Germany. Workers came down with fevers, nausea, vomiting, diarrhea, severely bloodshot eyes, rashes, and bleeding mucus membranes. Twenty-five percent of those afflicted died. Two years later, a group of American nurses in Nigeria were struck by a new disease called Lassa, which produced symptoms similar to Marburg but was found to be caused by a different pathogen. The disease now accounts for at least 5,000 deaths per year in West Africa. The first American case occurred in Chicago in 1989. Seventy percent of those struck by Lassa succumb to the disease.

In 1976, the world first became frighteningly aware of Ebola following a deadly rampage of infection that began at the Yambuku Mission Hospital in western Sudan. Named after the Ebola River, spread of the disease produced widespread fear and anxiety and helped spark contemporary global concern about emergent diseases. Families of Ebola victims watched helplessly as their loved ones developed taxing respiratory problems, total loss of appetite, intense headache, chills, abdominal pain, diarrhea, vomiting, and massive internal bleeding. As the disease progressed, the blood of victims failed to clot, and they bled from injection sites as well as into their gastrointestinal tracts, skin, and internal organs. As body systems collapsed, the victims fell into shock, and 90 percent died. As described by Preston (1994: 68) in *The Hot Zone*, his best-selling chronicle of this "emergent disease," infection hit the hospital like a bomb. It savaged patients and snaked like chain lightning out from the hospital through patients' families. The toll mounted as the virus spread to fifty-five villages surrounding the hospital. Especially hard hit were women relatives who prepared bodies for burial. Over three hundred people died in the initial outbreak, including hospital nurses, patients, and the family members of patients. Subsequent outbreaks have occurred in Sudan in 1979, western Zaire in 1995, Gabon in 1996 and late 2001–early 2002, and Uganda in 2000. Unlike other highly contagious hemorrhagic fever viruses, which tend to have an animal or insect vector that spreads the disease, Ebola (for which a vector has not yet been identified) is spread by contact with the blood or other bodily fluids and tissues of an infected person. The Ebola virus has been identified as a member of the virus family called Filoviridae, a group characterized by a threadlike appearance. However deadly they may be, these viruses are usually only 800 to 1000 nanometers (nm) long (1 nm is equal to one-billionth of a meter). There remains no known cure or vaccine for Ebola.

In their book *Ebola, Culture and Politics: The Anthropology of an Emerging Disease,* Barry and Bonnie Hewlett (2008) report on their involvement in Ebola outbreak response teams affiliated with WHO. They begin by noting that the work they eventually did with WHO, which they term *outbreak ethnography* was not originally part of the mind-set at WHO about who to involve in responding to a deadly contagious disease outbreak. It was not until twenty-five years after the first outbreak of Ebola that anthropologists began to be invited onto outbreak response teams, in no small part because WHO realized it was facing important problems during outbreaks that it did not know the answers to, such as the following:

- Why did people run away from ambulances sent to pick up Ebola cases?
- Why did people stop taking sick family members to the hospital?
- How was local culture contributing to infection?

The Hewletts argue for discovering the emic perspective on Ebola and the identification of local behaviors that might promote or prevent the spread of the disease. As part of this work, they visited several outbreaks and conducted interviews, focus groups, and observation (while wondering how badly they were putting themselves at risk).

Ebola and the other conditions mentioned here are examples of what epidemiologists today call *emerging diseases*—those that have only come to be recognized in recent years, with seemingly increasing frequency. In addition to the diseases mentioned here, other emerging diseases, most of which are caused by previously unknown viruses, include infantile diarrhea caused by Rotavirus, Legionnaires' disease, Hantavirus disease, hemorrhagic colitis caused by *Escherichia coli,* Lyme disease, gastric ulcers caused by *Helicobacter pylori,* Nipah virus disease, SARS [severe acute respiratory syndrome] A/H1N1 influenza), all of which hold potential for new pandemics and some of which have triggered acute high-mortality epidemics. Also, WHO has placed a number of reemergent infections on its international watch list, including diphtheria, cholera, dengue fever, yellow fever, and bubonic plague; these involve diseases that were previously considered controlled but have once again become significant threats to human health. Finally, the constant process of mutation (such as the species jumps in zoonotic diseases) and natural selection and the misuse of pharmacologic resources have resulted in the development of drug-resistant pathogenic species—a growing problem, for example, with tuberculosis.

Each of the cases of the disease outbreaks described in this section has been of special concern to the public health field of epidemiology. This applied discipline is concerned with understanding the "distribution and determinants of disease" (Trostle and Sommerfeld 1996: 253) and using this information to make social, physical, or other changes needed to prevent further illness. Unlike, biomedicine, which primarily focuses on the treatment of ailments in specific individuals, epidemiology addresses the larger level of the population with the intention of preventing new illness. In other words, the goal of epidemiology is assessing the distribution of disease with the intention of identifying "the risk factors that enable intervention and, ultimately, control" (Agar 1996: 391). At the first reports of a disease outbreak, epidemiologists, like those who work for the Centers for Disease Control and Prevention in Atlanta, Georgia, rush to the scene (often anywhere in the world). Their objectives include determining the cause(s) of illness, the incidence rate (numbers of new cases over time), the prevalence (total number of cases relative to the size of the population at risk), the pathways of disease spread, and possible methods for lowering disease morbidity and mortality. Specifically, as Hahn (1999: 34) relates,

In the epidemiological investigation of an outbreak of an infectious disease, the first step is to locate individuals who may be ill and obtain symptom histories. This "case finding" activity allows the epidemiologist to characterize the outbreak and construct hypotheses about the source of the infection.

In the case of the 1976 Ebola outbreak, it was found that the nuns who ran the Yambuku Mission Hospital began their work each day by putting out five syringes for use with the hundreds of patients who would need injections. Occasionally, the syringes were cleaned with warm water to clear blood clots and drying blood that interfered with needle efficiency, but often a syringe was pulled from the arm of one patient, refilled with medicine, and reinjected into another patient without cleansing. In this way, an effective (if completely unintended) method for viral transmission was created, much like the one that has allowed HIV to move rapidly among illicit injection drug users who are forced to reuse syringes used by others because of a lack of access to sterile syringes. Other routes of Ebola transmission also were identified, including mortuary practices that exposed individuals to the infected body fluids of Ebola victims. Identification of these routes of transmission led to a rapid end to the 1976 Ebola outbreak.

With its focus on observable behaviors and actual social and physical contexts of health and illness, as well as its concern with the population level rather than the individual case of disease, it is recognized that epidemiology shares features with medical anthropology. Indeed, a number of anthropologists and some epidemiologists have pointed out the benefits of close collaboration between the two disciplines. To this union, advocates of collaboration argue, epidemiology brings a rigorous scientific approach, an emphasis on quantitative data collection, and a specifically applied orientation. Anthropology's contribution includes an emphasis on intensive qualitative investigation of behaviors and social relations in context and a keen awareness of the importance of culture (and meaning) in shaping people's behavior as well as their willingness to change behaviors to accommodate public health dictates.

Over the past several decades, collaborations of this sort have become increasingly common, although they do not yet constitute standard practice. Singer, for example, has worked closely with a number of epidemiologists in assessing social context factors that contribute to the extent of HIV risk among injection drug users in three New England cities. Combining anthropological emphasis on direct observation of actual risk settings, social networks, and behaviors with an epidemiological focus on rigorous measurement (e.g., using standardized surveys and the careful structuring of participant sampling), the multidisciplinary team conducting this study has been able to identify key local context factors at both the neighborhood and city levels that contribute to differences in HIV risk and infection in different social environments. Findings such as this are important in moving the field of AIDS prevention from efforts built on a one-size-fits-all approach to the tailoring of prevention to fit the specific characteristics of local social environments.

Despite the recognized benefits of interdisciplinary collaboration, a number of anthropologists have been critical of epidemiology. Concerns about the types of data that are valued and devalued (e.g., inattention to people's behaviorally motivating beliefs and understandings of disease) and an unquestioned embrace of scientific method without sensitivity to the cultural shaping of scientific understandings have been voiced by a number of anthropologists about epidemiology (True 1996). Furthermore, Di Giacomo (1999: 451) has questioned whether genuine collaboration is occurring, noting the tendency of epidemiology to raid the storehouse of anthropological cultural knowledge in search of "bits of information about 'culture' which can then be plugged into a statistical model that generates correlations amenable to being represented as causal." From the critical perspective developed in this volume, the primary concern emerges from the intensely political nature of public health as a social practice. As Moss astutely observes:

As most practitioners know, the comfortable truism about epidemiology that public health schools teach their graduate students—that epidemiology is the basic science of public health—is not actually true. It may be closer to reality to say that politics is the basic science of public health. (Moss 2000: 1385)

All too often, public health or population health is viewed as a branch of biomedicine as certainly is the case at the University of Melbourne where the School of Population Health is embedded in the Faculty of Medicine and Dentistry. In reality, however, as Navarro (2011: 118) boldly asserts, "medicine is a branch of public health." He further argues:

There is overwhelming scientific evidence that the public's health depends primarily on political, economic, social, and cultural factors. Medical care, as its name suggests, takes care of people when they are ill or injured, but it does not do much curing. (Navarro 2011: 118)

Politics, not epidemiological findings, tends to dominate social thinking and policy making around disease, especially with regard to infectious diseases, and politics and not misguided cultural behaviors tend to be the determinant force in shaping the conditions for the spread of disease. For example, returning to the 1976 Ebola outbreak, as Farmer (1999: 46) notes, social elites and Europeans did not fall victim because "likelihood of coming into contact with . . . unsterile syringes was inversely proportion to one's social status." High-quality medical care was available to the wealthy, lesser-quality care was accessible by subordinate social classes. Similarly, on a global scale, Ebola, an African disease, garnered intense media attention in the West (propelling the very word to *Ebola* into a symbol of looming darkness and impending danger) despite the relatively small number of individuals who have been infected. Farmer's point is that epidemiological models of disease need to avoid "facile claims of causality, particularly those that scant the pathogenic roles of social inequalities. Critical perspectives on emerging infections [for example] must ask how large-scale social forces come to have their effects on unequally positioned individuals in increasingly interconnected populations; a critical epistemology needs to ask what features of disease emergence are obscured by dominant analytic frameworks" (Farmer 1999: 5).

One of the questions for medical anthropology ushered in by Ebola is how do people who are at high risk for infection perceive, explain, and, using local knowledge sets, respond to deadly epidemics. On the basis of their research on Ebola, Barry and Bonnie Hewlett (2008: 81) conclude that, although some cultural practices may amplify the spread of disease, "local people have beliefs and practices already in place that can be useful for controlling rapid-killing epidemics such as Ebola."

A blind spot among major health institutions (e.g., WHO) to the ways in which local behaviors are structured by local and global social inequality has limited the development of broader understandings of disease in epidemiology (Doyal with Pennell 1979). However, this is no less the case for medical anthropology for much of its history. This parallel limitation suggests the potential benefits of the further development of critical epidemiology and critical medical anthropology and of their collaboration in assessing and responding to disease. In this collaboration, strong focus using methodologies that collect both qualitative and quantitative data and integrate them for purposes of analysis would be applied to addressing the big questions, such as what are "the precise mechanisms by which such forces as racism, gender inequality, poverty, war, migration, colonial heritage, and even structural adjustment programs [such as those imposed by entities like the World Bank and International Monetary fund before monies will be loaned to developing countries] become embodied as [culturally shaped] increased risk" (Farmer 1997: 524). Critical medical sociologist Phil Brown (1992: 269) introduced the notion of *popular epidemiology*, which constitutes "the process by which laypersons gather scientific data and other information, and also direct and marshal the knowledge and resources of experts in order to understand the epidemiology of disease." In essence, popular epidemiology functions as an important methodological component of critical epidemiology.

Today, medical anthropology constitutes an extremely broad endeavor that no single textbook can possibly summarize. Students who are interested in further acquainting themselves with the scope and breadth of medical anthropology as a subdiscipline are advised to consult the following anthologies: (1) *Medical Anthropology: Contemporary Theory and Method*, edited by Carolyn F. Sargent and Thomas M. Johnson (1996), (2) *Training Manual in Applied Medical Anthropology*, edited by Carole E. Hill (1991), (3) *Anthropology and Public Health*, edited by Robert A. Hahn and Marcia Inhorn (2009), (4) *A Companion to Medical Anthropology*, edited by Merrill Singer and Pamela I. Erickson (2011), and (5) *Medical Anthropology at the Intersections*, edited by Marcia Inhorn and Emily A. Wentzell (2012). These volumes provide students with an overview of the continuity and changes in medical anthropological concerns over the course of the past several decades. At the theoretical level, medical anthropologists are interested in topics such as the evolution and ecology of disease, paleopathology, and social epidemiology; the political economy of health and disease; ethnomedicine and ethnopharmacology; medical pluralism; cultural psychiatry; the social organization of the health professions, clinics, hospitals, national health care systems, and international health bureaucracies; human reproduction; and nutrition. At the applied level, medical anthropologists work in areas such as community medicine; public health; international health; medical and nursing education; transcultural nursing; health care delivery; mental health services; health program evaluation; health policy; health care reform; health activism and advocacy; biomedical ethics; research methods in applied medical anthropology; and efforts to control and eradicate a wide array of health-related problems, including malaria, cancer, alcoholism, drug addiction, AIDS, malnutrition, and environmental pollution. In many ways, the work of medical anthropologists overlaps with that of medical sociologists, medical geographers, medical psychologists, medical social workers, epidemiologists, and public health people. In the past, medical anthropologists tended to focus on health problems at the local level and, less often, at the national level, but this is no longer the case; global health is a growing concern within medical anthropology, as discussed in the concluding section of this chapter.

Physician-anthropologist Cecil Helman (1994: 338) maintained that future research in medical anthropology "will involve adopting a much more global perspective—a holistic view of the complex interactions between cultures, economic systems, political organizations and ecology of the planet itself." He identifies overpopulation, urbanization, AIDS, primary health care, pollution and global warming, deforestation, and species extinction as some of the areas with which medical anthropologists will need to concern themselves. For critical medical anthropologists, the future has already arrived, in that they have for some time been urging making micro–macro connections—ones that link patients' suffering to the global political economy the focus of research in medical anthropology.

Global Health

Global health is a concept that developed over the course of the past several decades and has become a staple of conceptualization in public health, population health, and in international health circles. It echoes a broader public health discourse that a growing number of medical anthropologists have entered. According to Janes and Corbett,

Global health has emerged as a major field of research and practice, producing a growing number of academic programs, departments, conferences, and professional organizations. Yet despite its current popularity, global health is rarely defined, or if it is defined, it is not often done with the consistency and conceptual clarity that would differentiate it from its historical forebears, international public and tropical medicine. (Janes and Corbett 2011: 135)

Indeed, Jacobsen (2008: 1–2) acknowledges that the term *global health* is sometimes used interchangeably with *international health* but goes on to observe that global health also refers to "health concerns that cross national borders" and also "concerns about the continued and growing disparities in health between nations and within nations." Her textbook on global health includes chapters on health inequalities, the socioeconomic context of disease, maternal and child health, the spread of infectious diseases, HIV/AIDS, malaria, TB, globalization and emerging infectious diseases, environmental health, the health effects of environmental health, global health payers and players, and global health priorities. Ultimately, the term global health is replacing international health as a way of emphasizing the interactions that exist in health across national borders, from spreading epidemics (e.g., the H1N1 influenza pandemic) to health crises that require cooperation of multiple nations (e.g., the 2010 Haitian earthquake).

The Nossal Institute for Global Health (established in 2006) at the University of Melbourne states on its website that it is "committed to improving global health through research, education, inclusive development practice, and training of future leaders" and that it works in partnership with "other organisations who share its vision of improving health where health is at its poorest." It is committed to "translating medical research into health for all" by utilizing a multi-disciplinary perspective." The Nossal Institute consists of the following units: (1) Disease Prevention and Health Promotion, (2) Health Systems Strengthening, (3) Education and Learning, (4) Tropical Health and Infectious Diseases, and (5) Inclusive Development Practice. It focuses its research efforts on the Asia Pacific region and southern Africa, working principally in India, Indonesia, Cambodia, Vietnam, Laos, Papua New Guinea, and Mozambique. Ironically, many academic staff and researchers in the School of Population Health at the University of Melbourne also work on what might be termed global health issues, although others tend to focus on public health issues in Australia, including among Indigenous Australians. Organizationally, the Nossal Institute and the School of Population Health, despite the fact that they are situated a block from each other, function as separate entities within the same university. Academic and research staff at the former, however, tend to be biomedical physicians whereas those at the latter tend to be nonphysicians with training in public health, epidemiology, women's health, the medical social sciences, medical ethics, and Aboriginal health.

Mark Nichter (2008), an anthropologist who trained in international health at John Hopkins University in 1980, has authored a book titled *Global Health* in which calls for three new approaches to epidemiology: (1) ecosocial epidemiology, (2) the life-span perspective, and (3) popular epidemiology. In terms of the first concern, which draws from the work of Nancy Krieger, he notes that "[e]cosocial epidemiology studies the unnatural distribution of disease, like syndemic analysis, it looks beyond proximal risk factors to more distal social and political economic factors that predispose sections of a population to ill health" (Nichter 2008: 160). With regards to the life-span perspective, Nichter (2008: 161) draws on Margaret Lock's notion of *local biology*, which refers to the "manner in which one's bodily experience is mutually by biology and culture" over the course of an individual's life. For example, malnutrition and infectious diseases experienced during an individual's formative years many predispose him or her as a member of a larger population to chronic diseases in later years of the life cycle. Finally, popular epidemiology refers to a methodology developed by critical medical sociologist Phil Brown in which ordinary people share their understandings of particular diseases based on their lived experiences with professional epidemiologists to identify the political, economic, and social structural roots of those diseases. Along similar lines, the *Global Health Watch Reports 1 and 2* have been written as a collaborative effort on the part of various social movements and nongovernmental organizations that seek to provide an "alternative health report" that seeks to challenge major bodies that influence health policies, such as the WHO, UNICEF, and the World Bank (People's Health Movement et al. 2005–2006).

CHAPTER 2

Theoretical Perspectives in Medical Anthropology

Since its emergence as a distinct field of research, medical anthropology has been guided by several theoretical perspectives, although their boundaries have not always been neatly delineated. There have been disagreements about what theoretical approaches are the leading ones at any point in time. In his book *Sickness and Healing: An Anthropological Perspective*, Robert Hahn (1995), for example, notes three dominant theoretical perspectives. Byron J. Good (1994), in *Medicine, Rationality, and Experience: An Anthropological Perspective*, identifies four theoretical perspectives in medical anthropology: the empiricist paradigm, the cognitive paradigm, the "meaning centered" paradigm, and the critical paradigm. Finally, in *Medical Anthropology in Ecological Perspective*, Ann McElroy and Patricia Townsend (2003) also discuss four approaches (medical ecological theories, interpretive theories, political economy or critical theories, and political ecological theories) but, as we can see, these are not quite the same as those cited by Good. Joralemon (2010: 10) delineates four medical anthropological approaches: (1) the cultural constructivist or interpretive approach; (2) the ecological or ecological/evolutionary approach; (3) critical medical anthropology (CMA); and (4) applied medical anthropology, which he asserts "pursues more effective health interventions." In reality, however, the first three approaches do engage with applied medical anthropology. In their medical anthropology textbook titled *Culture and Healing*, Andrew Strathern and Pamela J. Stewart (2010) seek to blend the cultural interpretive and critical medical anthropological perspectives.

Despite these varying ways of grouping medical anthropology's various frames of understanding, it is clear that most medical anthropologists do tend to agree that some reasonably identifiable clusters of theory are guiding work done within the field. This book was written to help students gain a clearer understanding of the issues addressed within medical anthropology from the perspective of one of these clusters: the one labeled *critical* or *political economic medical anthropology*. In this chapter, we first present short introductions to the other two approaches, including discussion of their respective strengths and weaknesses from the critical perspective. This is followed by a more detailed discussion of the critical perspective, which in large part guides this textbook.

It bears noting that critical medical anthropologists sometimes have been accused of being "especially blunt, outspoken critics of other theories in medical anthropology" (McElroy and Townsend 1996: 65) and, further, of believing that the critical approach is "superior to other models" (McElroy 1996: 519). We plead guilty to both charges, as should anyone who embraces a theoretical frame of reference. Theory building in any discipline progresses, in part, through open discussion and debate, including pointing out shortcomings of alternative approaches. Criticism of this sort is a needed and healthy process within a field of study. Indeed, it is the absence of debate that should be cause for concern. Certainly, CMA has benefited from critiques framed from other perspectives. Similarly, as a result of the medical ecological framework, McElroy and Townsend (1996: 68) have moved toward a more thoroughgoing political ecological orientation. Moreover, it is likely that the proponents of all perspectives find their own to be superior. After all, why would one embrace a perspective he or she thought to be inferior or even equal to its alternatives? It is the sense that it can better frame important research questions and guide the explanation of research findings that leads to the promotion of a particular perspective. Because the asking of questions and the interpretation of findings is always guided by assumptions and prior understandings, having a theoretical perspective is unavoidable. In this light, prior to elaborating upon the perspective of CMA, we present two alternatives to it: medical ecological theory and cultural interpretive theory.

MEDICAL ECOLOGICAL THEORY

This approach rests on the acceptance of the concept of adaptation, defined as behavioral or biological changes at either the individual or group level that support survival in a given environment, as the core concept in the field. Indeed, from this perspective, health is seen as a measure of environmental adaptation. In other words, a central premise of the medical ecological orientation is that a social group's level of health reflects the nature and quality of the relationships "within the group, with neighboring groups, and with the plants and animals [as well as nonbiotic features] of the habitat" (McElroy and Townsend 1996: 12). McElroy and Townsend (2009: 20) conceptualize the environment as consisting of three parts: the physical, or abiotic environment; the biotic environment; and the cultural environment" which are "interdependent and continually in interaction." The biotic environment consists of predators, vectors, pathogens; the abiotic environment of climate, energy, and materials; and the cultural environment of technology, social organization and ideology (McElroy and Townsend 2009: 29).

Alexander Alland (1970), the formulator of the medical ecological perspective, pointed out that although the Mano people of Liberia lack a cultural conception or folk disease category for malaria, this disease nonetheless significantly affects Mano well-being and their ability to function and reproduce in their local environment. The presence of malaria, he argues, "is known to change gene frequencies, affect the immunological pattern, produce susceptibility to other pathologies, and lower the efficiency of affected individuals" (Alland 1970: 10). The Mano, to survive, have had to adapt both biologically and behaviorally to the challenge of malaria. Biologically, an adaptation to malaria that is commonly cited by ecologically oriented medical anthropologists is a mutation in the gene that controls the production of hemoglobin. As a result of this mutation (which involves a reversal in the order of two amino acids, valine and glutamic acid, at the sixth position in the genetic instructions for the production of the oxygen-binding blood molecule hemoglobin), red blood cells are distorted into clumps of needlelike crystals that form a crescent shape. This change inhibits the production of the malaria parasite, a protozoan of the genus *Plasmodium*, within human blood and confers protection from the worst symptoms of malaria infection. For individuals who receive the sickling mutation from both parents, however, the consequence is a life-threatening disease called sickle cell anemia, a condition that afflicts about two of every thousand African American children in the United States.

Medical ecologists also point to the importance of behavioral adaptations to health threats. McElroy and Townsend (1996, 2009), for example, note the indigenous development of snow goggles that protect the eyes of arctic dwellers from the harsh and damaging glare of sunlight reflected off ice and snow. Also from the medical ecological perspective, behavioral complexes such as medical systems, including everything from shamanistic healing of soul loss to biomedical thromboendarterictomy (the reaming out of the inner layer of a sclerotic or hardened artery) can be viewed as "sociocultural adaptive strategies" (Foster and Anderson 1978: 33). This way of understanding human biology and behavior, as an interactive set of adaptations to ecological and social challenges, makes a lot of sense to many medical anthropologists. Yet others have raised questions about this approach. B. Good (1994: 45), an interpretive medical anthropologist, argues that in ecological studies "[d]isease is often taken to be a natural object, more or less accurately represented in folk and scientific thought. Disease is thus an object separate from human consciousness." In turn, medical systems are seen as utilitarian social responses to intrusive natural conditions. B. Good (1994:46) questions both parts of this medical ecological equation, asserting that in such formulations "culture is . . . absorbed into nature, and cultural analysis consists of demonstrating its adaptive efficacy." Lost in such understanding is a full appreciation of the human cultural/symbolic construction of the world they inhabit. In other words, human communities do not respond, even in the ways they get sick and certainly in the ways that they think about and respond to sickness, to an external material reality that is independent of cultural valuation and signification. AIDS, for example, is a disease chock-full of cultural conceptions, values, and strong emotions. It is quite impossible for humans somehow to strip these away and confront AIDS in some kind of raw, culture-free natural state. Humans can experience the external material world only through their cultural frames; thus diseases, as they are known consciously and somatically by sufferers and healers alike, are packed with cultural content (e.g., believing that AIDS is a punishment from God or, as some people with AIDS have experienced it, an opportunity to turn their lives to more positive ends). Even science is not a route to a culture-free account of the physical world, because it too is a cultural construction.

In the fifth edition of their widely adopted textbook, McElroy and Townsend (2009: 15) admit that the concept of adaptation has been challenged by the new construct of resilience, "denoting the flexibility of humans to respond to problems through a hierarchy of response potentials, some genetic and physiological, others behavioral and cultural." Although recognizing that there are multiple sources of resilience that depend on ethnicity and class, they maintain that "in general resilience comes from individual and community resources for solving problems" (McElroy and Townsend 2009: 306). In the case of political refugees, *cultural brokers* who collaborate with social workers can serve as sources of resilience in adapting to the new society in a developed society such as the United States or Australia.

Critical medical anthropologists agree with much in the interpretive critique of the ecological model. The emphasis in its own critique, however, emerges from CMA's focus on understanding the specific structure of social relationships that give rise to and empower particular cultural constructions, including medical anthropological theories. CMA asks, "Whose social realities and interests (e.g., which social class, gender, or ethnic group) do particular cultural conceptions express, and under what set of historic conditions do they arise?" Furthermore, CMA has faulted medical ecological approaches for failing fully to come to grips with the fact that "it is not merely the idea of nature—the way [external reality] is conceived and related to by humans—but also the very physical shape of nature, including of course human biology, that has been deeply influenced by an evolutionary history of hierarchical social structures—that is to say, by the changing political economy of human society" (Singer 1996b: 497).

The problem inherent in conceptualizing the health aspects of the human–environmental relationship, in terms of adaptation, can be illustrated with the case of the indigenous people of Tasmania, an island that lies just off the southeastern tip of Australia. Tasmania was successfully inhabited by aboriginal people for more than ten thousand years before the arrival of Europeans at the end of the eighteenth century. Yet, building on the work of Robert Edgerton, McElroy and Townsend cite the Tasmanians as a case of maladaptation that led to the dying out of these people by 1876. They note:

In about 12,000 years of isolation from the mainland, the Tasmanians *devolved* losing the ability to make many tools, to make fire, and to construct rafts or catamarans that would have allowed them to fish and travel. The division of labor between men and women was inefficient, endangering women. Their political ecology emphasized raiding, capture of women, and competitiveness between tribal bands. During the cold season they went hungry, and their clothing and housing were inadequate. . . . [In sum] their way of life was far from ideal, and the society quickly collapsed after Europeans arrived. (McElroy and Townsend 1996: 112; emphasis in original)

The impression given by this account is that the arrival of European settlers on Tasmania in the late eighteenth century played but a small part in the disappearance of a society that was poorly adapted to its environment and paid the ultimate evolutionary price for its maladaptation. A closer examination of the historic political economic events surrounding the nature and impact of European arrival suggests rather different conclusions. Within thirty years of the arrival of the British in Tasmania, the indigenous population, which had been stable at around four thousand to five thousand before contact, dropped to a mere eleven. This shocking level of depopulation, which was occurring not just in Tasmania but throughout Britain's Third World colonies, led the British House of Commons to constitute a fifteen-member Select Committee on Aborigines, which published its findings in 1837. The committee concluded that the lands of indigenous people "had been usurped; their property seized; their character debased; European vices and diseases have been introduced" (quoted in Bodley 1975: 25). Douglas Oliver, an anthropologist with extensive experience in

Oceania, reports the exact nature of these "European vices," noting that the aboriginal peoples of Australia and Tasmania were the victims of playfulness: the sport-loving British pioneers occasionally relieved the boredom of isolation by hunting "abos" in lieu of other game. More frequently, however, these hunts were serious undertakings: now and then aborigines would be brash enough to kill or steal livestock pastured on their horde territories, and that called for systematic drives for extermination by the white owners. Aboriginal men, women, and children would be rounded up and shot; to slay a pregnant woman was accomplished by leaving poisoned food. The tragedy was played to its finish in Tasmania, where all [indigenous people] were wiped out . . . by 1876. One efficient colonial administrator even declared an open season against the Tasmanians, culminating in the infamous "Black Drive" [an open season on the hunting of Tasmanians] of 1830 (Oliver 1961: 161). Quite simply, the disappearance of the Tasmanians was not a consequence of maladaptation to their environment. They were victims of the genocidal extermination that characterized the colonial era.

Medical ecologists respond to such critiques—naively, in the view of CMA—by asking: "Should medical ecology be political?" (McElroy 1996). However, if social science is to matter, that is to say, if it is to have any impact on the world other than providing researchers with jobs, then it is inherently political (whether we as social scientists like it or not). For those who believe that AIDS is a punishment from God, for example, the scientifically supported statement that syringe exchange programs are effective in protecting drug injectors from the spread of disease is a very political position. Despite the extensive toll of AIDS and multiple studies demonstrating the effectiveness of syringe exchange, a government ban continues to block the use of federal dollars to support this public health measure. Science, including medical anthropology, cannot escape being political if it is to be part of the conflicted world of social policies and actions. It can, however, escape its untenable assertions that its reach for objectivity takes it beyond the influence of social values or that only critical theory has a political agenda (e.g., Hahn 1995: 74).

CULTURAL INTERPRETIVE THEORY

As Byron Good (1994) observes, the emergence of the cultural interpretive or meaning-centered approach in medical anthropology was a direct reaction to the dominance of the ecological perspective on health issues. Whereas ecological medical anthropologists have treated disease as part of nature and hence as external to culture, the fundamental claim of the cultural interpretive model, introduced by Arthur Kleinman, is that disease is not an entity but an explanatory model. "Disease belongs to culture, in particular to the specialized culture of medicine. And culture is not only a means of representing disease, but is essential to its very constitution as a human reality" (B. Good 1994: 53).

In other words, from the cultural perspective disease is knowable, by both sufferers and healers alike, only through a set of interpretive activities. These activities involve an interaction of biology, social practices, and culturally constituted frames of meaning (e.g., the Western cultural association between obesity and lack of self-control) and result in the construction of clinical realities (e.g., a diagnosis of AIDS or the flu). That different subspecialties of biomedicine sometimes reach quite different conclusions about the same clinical episode affirms to interpretive medical anthropologists the fundamental role of cultural construction in the making of a disease. The training of medical students, for example, as B. Good (1994) points out, does not simply involve teaching students about biology and pathology; more important, it involves enculturating a way of seeing physical reality. In anatomy classes, for example, students are taught to "see structure where none was obvious. Only with experience [do] gross muscle masses become apparent and recognizable. Veins, arteries, nerves, lymphatic vessels, and connective tissue [are] largely indistinguishable from one another until weeks into gross anatomy" (74).

The primary shortcoming, historically, of the interpretive approach from the critical perspective has been its inattention to the role of asymmetrical power relations in the construction of the clinical reality and the social utility of such construction for maintaining social dominance. For example, although B. Good (1994: 62) indicates at the beginning of his book that his intention is to articulate an interpretive approach that is "conversant with critical theory," the fulfillment of this intention seems modest at best in the remainder of the volume. The role of political economy (e.g., class relations) in shaping the formative activities through which illness is constituted, made the object of knowledge, and embedded in experience, for example, is largely ignored in Good's account.

As a result of the clash and exchange between medical ecological theory, cultural interpretive theory, and critical theory, there have been developments in all three of the primary theoretical models within medical anthropology. Medical ecologists have begun to adopt a more political ecological orientation; interpretive medical anthropologists acknowledge and are attempting—and in some cases, succeeding—in producing work that is highly sensitive to political economic issues; and critical medical anthropologists have developed a significant level of interest in political ecology (Baer 1996) and the role of political economy in the production of meaning. Nonetheless, there is much work to be done in this regard, and theoretical debate within medical anthropology—which we see as a healthy sign of the vibrancy of the discipline—is likely to continue.

CRITICAL MEDICAL ANTHROPOLOGY: AN ENGAGED BRANCH OF MEDICAL ANTHROPOLOGY

It may seem presumptuous to label our approach critical. After all, most medical anthropologists view their subdiscipline as a critical endeavor that challenges the assumptions of the disease model in biomedicine. We contend, however, that this critical perspective is primarily limited to lower levels of analysis and ignores the political economy. Much of this research concerns indigenous societies, peasant communities, and slums, where practitioners of Western biomedicine come into contact with members of a subproletariat or ethnic minority. Although we do not oppose research on social relationships and small communities (indeed, we see it as an essential component of CMA), we maintain that it must be conducted with the recognition that disease and its treatment occur within the context of the capitalist world system (Wallerstein 1979, 2004). The critical perspective we want to nourish and extend has its taproot in Marx, Engels, the critical theorists of the Frankfurt School, and C. Wright Mills (1959). We are concerned with the ways power differences shape social processes, including research in medical anthropology. Like Navarro (1976), Krause (1977), Doyal with Pennell (1979), Waitzkin (1983, 2011), and Foucault (1975), we feel that the dominant ideological and social patterns in medical care are intimately related to hegemonic ideologies and patterns outside of biomedicine. Baer and Singer were the first to coin the label *critical medical anthropology*, in a paper presented at the 1982 American Anthropological Association meeting, but others preceded them in the effort to incorporate a critical or political-economic approach into medical anthropology (Frankenberg 1974; Young 1978).

The Precursors of Critical Medical Anthropology

The initial effort to forge a critical redirection for medical anthropology can be traced to the symposium "Topias and Utopias in Health" at the 1973 Ninth International Congress for Anthropological and Ethnological Sciences, which ultimately developed into a volume with the same title (Ingman and Thomas 1975). An explicit turn toward the political economy of health tradition within medical anthropology awaited Soheir Morsy's (1979) review essay titled "The Missing Link in Medical Anthropology: The Political Economy of Health." Morsy's article—as well as an exposure to the political economy of health research, particularly the work of Vincente Navarro, a progressive physician with extensive training in the social sciences—and articles in the *International Journal of Health Services,* prompted Baer (1982) to write a short review of this corpus of literature and its relevance for medical anthropologists. Beginning in 1983, we along with others became involved in the organization of sessions at anthropological meetings and the editing of special issues of several journals on CMA.

Although a perspective on capitalism is an important starting point for a CMA, it is insufficient for a fully developed approach. CMA attempts to address the nature of health-related issues in indigenous societies as well as in precapitalist and socialist-oriented state societies. It understands health issues within the context of encompassing political and economic forces—including forces of institutional, national, and global scale—that pattern human relationships, shape social behaviors, condition collective experiences, reorder local ecologies, and situate cultural meanings. The emergence of CMA reflects both the turn toward political-economic approaches in anthropology in general and an effort to engage and extend the political economy of health approach (Baer, Singer, and Johnsen 1986; Morsy 1990; Singer, Baer, and Lazarus 1990).

In the first and second editions of this textbook, we referred to CMA as the "brash left-wing of medical anthropology." In reality, the vast majority of medical anthropologists are somewhere to the left of the political centre, which has tended to shift to right, in the various countries where they are based. Although CMA continues to be the most politically radical and engaged theoretical perspective within medical anthropology, perhaps most critical anthropologists are not as brash as they were twenty to thirty years ago when CMA was in its early stages. Although still a minority theoretical perspective within medical anthropology, CMA has become somewhat respectable, at least within the corridors of medical anthropology. Indeed, since its advent, CMA has sought to engage in a debate and dialogue with other medical anthropological perspectives, something that Joralemon acknowledges in the following quote:

Paradoxically, it was the assault launched by critical medical anthropologists on all four [we would say three] perspectives . . . that initiated conversations about the possibility of an integrative approach to medical anthropology. A central object of this text is to move close to this integration—to develop an approach to the study of health and disease which (1) pays attention to ecological, biological, *and* cultural factors; (2) considers the political and economic forces that influence disease patterns and affect access to health care resources; and (3) offers an opportunity for health-promoting interventions. (Joralemon 2010: 10–11)

Despite such acceptance of CMA, particularly in the case of its political economy/world system genre, some of its thunder has been subtly co-opted in the form of a discourse that emerged around the mid-1990s generally known as the *social determinants of health* and has entered in the public health arena (Marmot and Wilkinson 2000). In 2004, the WHO Commission on Macroeconomics and Health created the Commission on Social Determinants of Health. Unfortunately, this approach tends to ignore the political economy of health from which CMA draws heavily that preceded the former by more than twenty years. The social determinants of health that are often identified in this literature include poverty, employment and unemployment, stress, inequalities in housing, education, social inclusion, nutrition, as well as various lifestyle factors, such as ethnicity and sexual behavior. Some proponents of the social determinants of health perspective employ the notion of *social capital,* which may be defined in terms of macro-dimensions, such as countries or regions, or in terms micro-dimensions, such as individual social networks or social trust (Kawachi 1997). Although such variables certainly may have an impact on health outcomes, the social determinants of health approach tends not to look further upstream and certainly does not posit them as ultimately being rooted in the capitalist world system. As Raphael (2006: 654) observes,

[O]ne shortcoming in the work on social determinants of health is the failure to consider "a master conceptual scheme" that illuminates the political, economic, and social processes by which the quality of social determinants of health is shaped. Hence, much of the work lacks what is usually termed a "critical social science" perspective.

In an analysis of twenty-three developed and developing countries, Lindstroem and Lindstroem (2006) conclude that income inequality and absolute income levels have a much stronger impact on overall health statistics than does the social capital variable of trust. They argue that social capital theory "puts the responsibility of having low social capital on individuals with low social capital themselves—that is, blaming the victim—while ignoring the health effects of macrolevel social and economic policies and power relations between social classes" (Lindstroem and Lindstroem 2006: 680).

Biomedicine as a Starting Point for CMA

The concept of biomedicine serves an appropriate starting point for examining the perspective of critical medical anthropology. CMA seeks to understand who ultimately controls biomedicine and what the implications are of such control. An analysis of the power relations affecting biomedicine addresses questions such as the following: (1) Who has power over the agencies of biomedicine? (2) How and in what forms is this power delegated? (3) How is this power expressed in the social relations of the various groups and actors that comprise the health care system? and (5) What are the principal contradictions of biomedicine and associated arenas of struggle and resistance that affect the character and functioning of the medical system and people's experience of it?

Figure 2.1
Levels of Health Care Systems

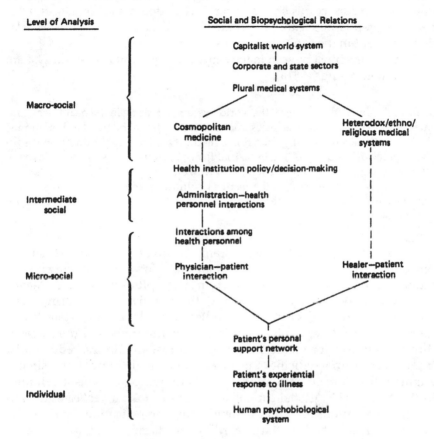

Any discussion of the impact of power relations in the delivery of health services needs to recognize the existence of several levels in the health care systems of developed capitalist, underdeveloped capitalist, and socialist-oriented societies. Figure 2.1 presents a schematic diagram of these levels and the social relations associated with them.

The Macrosocial Level

Critical medical anthropology recognizes that the development and expansion of a global economic system represents the most significant, transcending social process in the contemporary historic epoch. Capitalism has progressively shaped and reshaped social life. As a discipline, anthropology has lagged in its attention to the nature and transforming influence of capitalism. As part of the larger effort of critical anthropology in general to correct this shortcoming, CMA attempts to root its study of health-related issues within the context of the class and imperialist relations inherent in the capitalist world system.

Biomedicine must be seen in the context of the capitalist world system. According to Elling (1981a),

Some of the particular agents of the world-system operating in the health sector include international health agencies, foundations, national bilateral aid programs, all multinationals (especially drug firms, medical technology producers and suppliers, polluting and exploiting industrial firms, agribusinesses, commercial baby food suppliers, purveyors of chemical fertilizers and pesticides, and sellers of population control devices), and a medical cultural hegemony supportive of the activities of these agents on the world scene and in particular nations and locales. (pp. 24–24)

At all levels, the health care systems of advanced capitalist nations reproduce the structures of class relations. The profit-making orientation caused biomedicine to evolve into a capital-intensive endeavor heavily oriented to high technology, the massive use of drugs, and the concentration of services in medical complexes. The state legitimizes the corporate involvement in the health arena and reinforces it through support for medical training and research in the reductionist framework of biomedicine. Corporate-controlled foundations simply augment the state, at both international and national levels. Beginning in the early 1980s, global capitalism began to take a *neoliberal* turn in which corporations and international financial institutions, such as the World Bank and the International Monetary Fund, began to push governments around the world to minimize their regulation of businesses and to privatize a wide variety of enterprises and social and health services, ranging from energy utilities to hospitals and health clinics. David Harvey (2005) argues that neoliberalism essentially functioned as a project to restore power to the global capitalist class. Various think tanks, such as the Heritage Foundation and the American Enterprise Institute, promoted the neoliberal agenda in the United States and the Institute of Public Affairs played a similar role in Australia. Economists and other policy advisors from such think tanks found their way as experts not only in the corridors of governments but also the mass media, including the Public Broadcasting System in the United States and the government-owned Australian Broadcasting Corporation. Under the rubric of *globalization,* as critical physician-sociologist Howard Waitzkin observes,

The transnational capitalist class promoted trade policies and agreements concerning the environment, workplace safety, intellectual property, food, water, and professional licensing. In such efforts, the members of this class acted to reduce the capacity of governments to carry out their traditional functions in protecting public health and in providing health services. (Waitzkin 2011: 68)

To a large degree the nation-state evolved into a transnational state in which corporate and political elites met together in settings such as the Trilateral Commission, the European Union, the United States, the World Bank, the International Monetary Fund, the G7 and later the G8, the G20, and the World Trade Organization. Various sectors of civil society, however, such as nongovernmental organizations (NGOs) and social movements (particularly the anticorporate globalization or global justice and environmental movements) sought with varying success to challenge the neoliberal agenda.

The World Bank has become a key player in establishing health policies and making financial loans to health care endeavors. It loaned annually approximately $1.5 billion between 1991 and 1993, which placed it slightly ahead of WHO and UNICEF (cited in Walt 1994: 128). The World Bank has a strong influence on health policy as a result of its practice of cofinancing resources from international and bilateral agencies and matching funds from recipient governments. It also conducts country-specific health sector analyses and makes proposals for health care reform that are compatible with market-driven economies. As a result of this emphasis on capitalist solutions to health problems, Walt (1994: 157) argues, national policy makers sense "that Bank staff [appear to be] more driven by pressure to lend than a desire for successful implementation." In the case of Mexico, the World Bank promoted reforms that allowed "private patients to opt out of coverage by the social security system and into coverage by managed care organizations" (Waitzkin 2011: 118). WHO and the Pan American Health Organization also came to promote private-state partnerships (Waitzkin 2011: 136). Despite the fact that almost all Third World nations are supposed to be politically independent, their colonial inheritance and their neocolonial situation impose health care modeled after that found in advanced capitalist nations. James Paul (1978: 272) argues "medicine has from the beginning functioned in the service of imperialism, supporting logically the voracious search for ever wider markets and profitable deals." The ruling elites that control Third World countries collaborate with international agencies, foundations, and bilateral aid programs to determine health policies (Justice 1986). These elites and the agents they deal with often advocate nationalized and preventive medicine, but their actions favor curative rather than preventive approaches to health care for themselves and even for lower social strata.

Big Pharma or the pharmaceutical industry has become a major player in the "medical-industrial complex" both in the developed and developing world. According to Mehrabadi,

Pharmaceutical/biotechnology companies cannot be pinpointed to one location as they function as a transnational cooperation would: globally. As with any corporation that is transnational in scope, operations are carried out depending on where labor is cheapest, raw materials are the least expensive, where taxes can be most easily evaded, as well as where market regulations are the least strict. (Mehrabadi 2005: 1)

The emergence of chronic diseases among the poor and working-class people in developing societies is providing a new market for the pharmaceutical industry, a biomedical approach that continues to ignore the impact of ongoing deprivation and hunger. Thus, just as biomedicine had functioned as a tool of colonial empires, it is now serving as a tool of neoliberalism. The popularity of pharmaceuticals around the world has contributed to emergence of an informal sector for the distribution of commercial drugs, such as "injection doctors" who give single shots of antibiotics in community markets.

Medical anthropologists and other medical social scientists have become increasingly interested in biotechnology, often engaging in an interdisciplinary endeavor termed *science and technology studies*. Lock and Vinh-Kim Nguyen (2010: 22) describe biomedicine as technology in the sense that much of biomedicine consists of numerous relatively complicated technological devices, such as mechanical ventilators, X-ray machines, and magnetic resonance imagers, prosthetic limbs, to simple devices such as over-the-counter drugs, adhesive bandages, and cotton balls. Bodily organs, whether from dead people or living ones, have resulted in an international market that capitalizes on the poor in both legal and illegal ways. Biomedicine has promoted ARTs (assisted reproduction therapies) to such an extent that the Euro-American conflation of biological and social parenthood has broken down.

Large corporations are involved in the health sector of the Third World not only in pharmaceuticals/biotechnology but also in "hospital construction, development and outfitting, the supply of medical, surgical and diagnostic equipment, and numerous ancillary goods and services" (Doyal with Pennell 1979: 270). They, of course, ally themselves with Third World elites and, through jobs, favors, and outright bribery, influence health policies.

Despite the global hegemony of biomedicine, our scheme recognizes that complex societies exhibit a pattern of medical pluralism. Ultimately, these systems are dominative in that biomedicine enjoys a dominant status over heterodox and ethnomedical systems. This dominant status is legitimized by laws that give biomedicine a monopoly over certain medical practices and limit or prohibit the practice of other types of healing. Various heterodox medical systems such as Ayurveda and Unani in India; natural medicine in Germany; and chiropractic and naturopathy in the United States, Canada, and Britain may have their own professional associations, schools, hospitals, and clinics and thus replicate the organizational structure of biomedicine. Biomedicine systematically attempts to shore up its dominance by progressively subordinating an array of assumed competitors. Nevertheless, alternative practitioners proliferate and even flourish in certain areas, such as the San Francisco Bay Area. In much folk and popular culture, medicine is practiced and learned outside of bureaucratic settings. Especially important to recognize is the role played by class and related social struggle as a breeding ground for medical pluralism. Oppressed populations may attempt to cling to or resurrect traditional ethnomedical practices as an expression of resistance to domination or as a marker of group solidarity/identity, and countercultures may initiate new medical systems for similar reasons. Similarly, the inability of biomedicine to cure the somatized distress and sickness associated with the postmodern world creates a potent source for pluralism. Under such circumstances, it is common for popular health movements, folk healing systems, and heterodox medical traditions to rise up to fill the void. Despite elements of resistance in these alternative medical systems, it is important not to overlook the capacity of biomedicine and its patrons in the capitalist class and the state sector to co-opt them. Nevertheless, it is important to point out that the growth of NGOs has come more and more to serve as a counter-hegemonic force challenging corporate and state health policymakers. As Walt (1994: 204) observes, NGOs constitute a "sign of increased civic challenge, which may be translated into new social movements and public protest but may also create debate within existing formal institutions."

The Intermediate Level

At the intermediate level of health care systems, the hospital, which varies in size from a gigantic medical center to a rural hospital, has become the primary arena of social relations. Navarro (1976) has demonstrated the pervasive control that members of the corporate class and the upper middle class have over both "reproductive institutions" (health foundations and private and state medical teaching institutions) and "delivery institutions" (voluntary and proprietary or profit-making hospitals). The power that hospital administrators and physicians enjoy at this level is in reality a delegated power. As Freidson (1970: 5) observes, the professional dominance of biomedicine is secured by the political and economic influence of the elite that sponsors it—an influence that drives competing occupations out of the same area of work, discourages others by virtue of the competitive advantages conferred on the chosen occupation, and requires still others to be subordinated to the profession. Although physicians exert a great deal of control over their work, because of their monopoly of medical skills and the congruence between their version of disease theory and capitalist ideology, they find themselves subject to bureaucratic constraints in hospitals. Some social scientists have even argued that physicians are undergoing a process of deprofessionalization or proletarianization in their status as employees of health care corporations and health maintenance organizations (HMOs) that seek to increase their profits under the guise of managed care. In addition to a growing number of physicians employed in public agencies, hospitals, medical schools, insurance companies, and HMOs, "even those primarily in office-based practice are dependent on their hospital affiliations to pursue their work, and increasingly face restrictions under the rules of the hospital as a social and legal entity" (Mechanic 1976: 49).

The wide array of other health workers means that the medical hierarchy replicates the class, racial/ethnic, and gender hierarchy. The nurse as a relatively high-status subordinate traditionally was supposed to exhibit docility toward physicians and the top administration, although the impact of the feminist movement had, at least until recently, altered these patterns in certain places to some extent. According to Leonard Stein (1967), early in her training, the nurse learned to play the "doctor-nurse game," in which "she must communicate her recommendation statement" to the physician. Despite their stereotypic nurturing role, many registered nurses now serve as lower-level managers who must carry out policies made at higher levels. The ironic twist of this development is that the health workers with the lowest status and least power are those persons who come into the most continuous and intimate contact with patients in hospital settings. The medical hierarchies of advanced capitalist countries are replicated in Third World nations, although various accommodations are made to local customs and traditions.

Class struggle has become an explicit aspect of the intermediate social level. Although the trend toward unionization in U.S. hospitals first occurred among its underpaid unskilled and semiskilled workers, it has spread to technicians, nurses, and even physicians. Factors serving to mitigate demands by unionized hospital workers, however, include the shift of costs from higher wages to consumers and the emergence of a "new professional managerial class of hospital administrators" who are sometimes willing to arbitrate with unions in return for disciplined workers (Krause 1977: 68–77). Furthermore, professionalization continues to be seen by many health workers as a more viable approach for socioeconomic advancement, thus preventing them from forming an alliance with lower-status workers. In recent years, many hospitals have turned to downsizing their full-time nursing staffs by using either temporary registered nurses or licensed practical nurses and nurses' aides as cheaper forms of health care providers.

The Microlevel

The microlevel primarily refers to the physician-patient relationship and what Janzen (1978) calls the "therapy management group." The major initial diagnostic task of the physician is heavily mediated by social factors outside the examining room. Similarly, medical treatment, the other major task of the physician, is not determined solely by the needs of the patient. It also serves the special needs of physicians and other powerful sectors within and outside the health care system. The physician role, in fact, performs two key functions for the encompassing social system and its existing distribution of power: (1) controlling access to the special prerogatives of the sick role and (2) medicalizing social distress. In the first, the physician may limit access to the sick role by judging whether an individual may or may not be excused temporarily from work. It must be noted, however, that his or her power in this area is far from absolute, in that most people adopt the sick role without consulting physicians. They frequently consult with lay members of the therapy management group in arriving at this decision. In the second function, according to the reductionist model of disease in which physicians assign the source of disease to pathogenic or related factors, personal stress emanating from social structural factors such as poverty, unemployment, racism, and sexism is secluded from the potentially disruptive political arena and secured within the safer medical world of individualized treatment. As Zola (1978) argues, the ultimate function of both the gatekeeping and the medicalizing activities is social control. Research and analyses at the microlevel must begin to locate the physician-patient relationship "in the broader political and economic framework" (McKinlay 1976: 155).

The individual level entails consideration of the patient's response to sickness or sufferer experience. Critical medical anthropology is sensitive to what Scheper-Hughes and Lock (1987) term the *mindful body*. In their view, an individual's body physically feels the distress that its bearer is experiencing. The critical approach to the individual level begins with the recognition that sufferer experience is constructed and reconstructed in the action arena between socially constituted categories of meaning and the political-economic forces that shape the context of daily life. Recognizing the powerful influence of such forces, however, does not imply that individuals are passive or impersonal objects but rather that they respond to the material conditions they face in light of the possibilities created by the existing configuration of social relations. Medical anthropology needs to generate awareness of the ways in which sufferer experience produces challenges to medical hegemony at both the individual and collective level. For these reasons, the study of sufferer experience and action is an important corrective to the tendency to assume that, because power is concentrated in macrolevel structures, the microlevel is mechanically determined from above. Missing from this understanding of the construction of daily life is an appreciation of the capacity of the microlevel to influence the macrolevel.

Influenced by the argument of Sheper-Hughes and Lock (1987) that human experience is embodied, since the 1980s, the body has become a central topic in the medical anthropology study. Central to this work is the realization that we not only know the world through our bodies but, in addition, we know ourselves and others not as freestanding minds or personalities, but as personalities within specific bodies. In that illness and disease occur within bodies and are experienced by sufferers as bodily sensations, and, further, in that treatment of illness and disease is focused, at least to some degree, on the healing system and on changing the body, how we conceptualize the human body is a critical issue for medical anthropology. Yet our bodies are not self-evident; they are not merely biology straightforwardly perceived through an objective, culture-free lens. Rather, they are a focal site for the coming together and entwinement of biology, lived experience, culture, and social relationship.

In other words, the body, as we know and experience it, is culturally and socially constructed. This statement is not intended to deny the material existence and physical properties of the body as a biological system that has a reality separate from human consciousness, but rather to say that (1) we do not have awareness of our bodies independent of our cultural frames of understanding and valuing, (2) human societies physically shape the human body to conform to cultural expectations, and (3) social relationships are inscribed directly on the body in both intentional and unintentional ways. Each of these aspects of embodiment are now discussed in turn.

All cultures develop an understanding of the human body. Adams (1998: 84), for example, provides the following description of bodily understanding from Tibet within the context of a patient diagnosed as suffering from *rlung* ("heart wind"). "In Tibetan medicine, *rlung* is the most important of the body's humors. Just as with winds outside of the body, winds inside of the body are responsible for any and all movement. . . . As such, winds take a variety of forms. . . . Winds are the responsible force that moves the body and substances through and out of the body."

A different conception of the body is found in the Caribbean island of Haiti. According to Brodwin, many Haitians believe that

Certain strong emotions, especially anger and shock, can cause a person's blood to heat, thicken, or rise in the body. Blood can accumulate in the head, causing headaches, stroke, or madness; it can lodge in the throat, causing suffocation; or it can pass into the breast of a nursing mother, spoiling her milk and causing illness to her baby. Blood can change color or become too "sweet" or "sour" as a result of unsettling emotional experience as well as exposure to certain "hot" and "cold" foods and environmental agents. (Brodwin 1996: 86)

As these two accounts suggest, traditional Tibetan and Haitian conceptions of the body differ in marked ways from the body as known in contemporary scientific anatomy or in Western society generally. It should not be assumed, however, that other people's cultural conceptions about the body are misinformed folk notions and our own ideas are rooted in empirical knowledge free of cultural influence. For example, Martin (1996) has analyzed conceptions of the body's immune system in the United States. With reference to the image of the immune system portrayed in the mass media, she found that the body is depicted frequently as a highly defended nation-state with a clear and rigid boundary between the self and the external world, with the latter being described as foreign, hostile, and a constant threat. Always at the ready to fend off a horde of foreign invaders that seek to take over the body, the immune system is visualized in militaristic terms as a hierarchical and well-coordinated army that is always in a state of war. In light of the frequency of U.S. involvement in wars around the globe during the recent evolution of human immunology it is not difficult to identify the source of the body at war imagery that dominates media portrayals. Similarly, hierarchical corporate structures, ruled by decision-making upper-class CEOs and boards of directors at the top and populated by working-class functionaries carrying out menial tasks at the bottom, would seem to be the model adopted in both professional and popular understandings of the organization of the immune system. In this depiction, smart T cells (lymphocytes) control the immune system, giving biochemical orders to obedient B cells to carry out specific activities, and with dumb macrophage cells at the bottom doing the dirty work of cleaning up the vanquished bodies of foreign invaders and other debris.

Importantly, Martin found the war motif present in the immune system understandings of many immunologists (and immunology textbooks) and among the lay public, although often tempered by other conceptions as well. For many of the physicians, researchers, and representatives of the general public that she interviewed, the military model of the immune system was "not just a metaphor, but 'how it is'" (Martin 1996: 96)—that is, not just a useful analogy for describing the immune system but a factual representation of its actual nature. Some immunologists, however, pointed out the problems with this socially dominant conception: (1) many "foreign" (i.e., nonhuman) organisms live in the human body without being targeted for elimination by the immune system, including organisms capable of causing disease; (2) newly emergent pathogens, like HIV, could not successfully link up biochemically, effectively unlock, enter, and reorganize human cells if they were truly foreign; and (3) top-down, corporate-like, notions of hierarchy within the immune system do not fit well with the recognized interdependency of the various types of cells that play a role in human immune response. In short, Western understandings of the body, even those held by scientists, are as culturally influenced as any other folk system of bodily knowledge (see Critical Medical Anthropology and Science later in the chapter).

In addition to images and ideas, cultural influence on our experience of the human body includes the impact of values, that is, beliefs about good and bad, right and wrong. As Freund and McGuire (1991: 4) observe:

Every society has many levels of sharing ideas about bodies: What is defined as healthy, in one society might be considered unhealthily fat and ugly in another; what is seen as thin and lean in one group might be defined as sickly in another. Aging may also be defined as something to be either conquered, feared, accepted, or revered.

As this statement suggests, attitudes about body size and fatness vary considerably across societies. In North America, fatness is seen as both unattractive and unhealthy and is interpreted as a sign of moral laxness if not self-hatred. Studies show that American women who diet have strong concerns about their self-control and associate weight gain with greed (Counihan 1990). By contrast, among the traditionally nomadic Moors of Mauritania, fatness, especially in women, is considered quite attractive. The ability of a man to produce a fat daughter or to sustain a fat wife demonstrates his wealth and secures him highly valued social prestige. Consequently, daughters are force-fed large quantities of fatty camel milk to help them gain weight. Girls generally accept this practice because they know it will enhance their ability to attract a wealthy husband. This sentiment is captured in a Moorish folk saying: "To be a woman of quality, it is necessary to be a woman of quantity" (Cassidy 1991: 197). Hearing about such beliefs and practices, North Americans are quick to raise questions about the health risks of being overweight. As contrasted with Moorish folk sayings, an American quip is that "No woman can be too rich or too thin." However, blanket statements about slimness and health confuse cultural desires with clinical realities in several ways.

First, research shows that from a health standpoint, the ideal weight for a specific height increases with age (the best weight for someone at age 25, for example, is too thin for the same person at age 65). Second, although morbidity increases with high weights, it does so for low weights as well. Third, there is a broad range for ideal weight for height ratios, with relatively little change in health risk in increases within a thirty- to fifty-pound range. Finally, the key relationship between body fat and morbidity is not degree but distribution (i.e., where body fat is stored), with accumulation of adipose in the abdominal area being notably riskier (for cardiovascular disease, hypertension, and cancer) than on the hips and thighs (Rittenbaugh 1991).

The differing ways people conceive and value the human body are evident not only in variations across societies but also within societies. Bourdieu (1984), for example, has analyzed critical differences in ideas about body image across class and gender lines in Western society. Illustratively, he notes that the percentage of women who consider themselves to be below average in beauty or think that they look older than they really are is directly related to social class, with upper-class women feeling "superior both in the intrinsic, natural beauty of their bodies and in the art of self-embellishment" with working-class women, who have fewer resources and time to invest in cultivating their bodies, being more likely to express alienation from their body image (Bourdieu 1984: 206). In that weight is linked culturally in the United States with self-control and with personal value, the tendency of upper-class individuals to be slimmer than members of the working class (a reversal of nineteenth-century weight distribution patterns) serves not only as a visual marker of one's class standing but as an embodied affirmation and constant reminder of the innate superiority of dominant social classes.

The work of culture on bodies is not merely conceptual, it is also physical. Tattooing and body piercing are contemporary illustrations of the ways people actively engage in recreating their physical bodies to conform to desired appearances. Although participants often explain these practices as a form of self-expression, their relatively sudden and widespread appearance, especially in certain age and social groups, suggests that cultural forces and not merely individual tastes and values are at work. In fact, throughout history, humans have reconfigured their bodies to conform to cultural standards. Historically, among the Kwakiutl Indians of the northwest coast of North America, babies spent many hours fastened to cradle boards to create a culturally valued flattened head shape. Foot binding of girls—to create a tiny and nonfunctional foot—as practiced among wealthy families in China traditionally, is another example of culturally dictated body shaping. Other examples, such as orthodontia and plastic surgery, indicate that bodies are not only shaped by cultural values but that cultural values about the body can be ensnared by and shaped by for-profit commercial processes. Consequently, body reconfiguring has become big business, generating billions in new wealth for a variety of industries from workout gyms and tanning salons to cosmetics and hair product manufacturers to weight loss programs and dietary supplement distributors. Rather than merely meeting a cultural demand for beauty-enhancing products and procedures, critics argue that corporate commodification of body imagery generates feelings of inadequacy and worthlessness, resulting in diseases such as anorexia and bulimia among vulnerable populations. As critical medical anthropologists Mark and Mimi Nichter observe, promoting

[d]issatisfaction and envy constitute important ingredients in the business of selling transformation. Progress is an ideal basic to the American dream, an ideal exploited by those engaged in marketing by transforming the work ethic from work site to body and from the pursuit of virtue to the pursuit of beauty as commodity fetishism. Being "self made" has given way to being "made over." (Nichter and Nichter 1991: 249–250)

Further, as Martin (1990) asserts, medicalization of the body (including the tendency of biomedicine to focus narrowly on individual organs), commercialization of body parts (including the buying and selling of organs for transplant), and commodification by the beauty industry have left people experiencing their bodies not as an inherent component of their immutable selves but as fragmented collections of reworkable organs and improvable appearances imprinted with a public exchange value. We have reached, Martin maintains, the end of the body as we once knew it. In its place, from the standpoint of the capitalist market, is the profitable body, one that can and should constantly be improved through the purchasing of body products, procedures, and activities.

The shaping of bodies is driven not only by cultural notions of ideal appearance but also by class, gender, and other hierarchical social relationships. Social inequalities find direct expression in the shape and appearance of the human body in various ways. One pattern, found in many societies, is that people from upper classes tend to be taller than those from the lower classes in their society, often several inches taller on average. These differences, which are linked to diet, access to health care, and other factors, are first evident before birth and are well established by age six years (Cassidy 1991).

Worksite exposure to toxic substances produces another type of bodily difference between the classes. Reviewing the literature on this issue, Millen and Holz (2000) note, for example, that half of the workers in factories that produce industrial chromates have been found in both

Mexico and South Africa to have perforated nasal septa. Indeed, exposure to toxins in manufacturing, mining, and farming is quite common among workers in developing nations, producing a wide range of disease impacts on lives and bodies. Environmental exposure to toxic substance also differentiates the bodies of upper and lower classes. Dumping of toxins is much more common in the poorer areas of poor countries than in wealthier locations, even if the substances are produced in wealthy countries and shipped for disposal to poorer ones. A wide range of industrial toxins, such as mercury and lead, are dumped into the environment of poor countries each year resulting in a host of damaging effects on the bodies of poor and working-class individuals. Similarly, poor neighborhoods are much more likely than wealthy ones to be sited for garbage dumps or other waste disposal locations.

Oths (1999) calls attention to another expression of the embodiment of social relations in her analysis of the folk disease called *debilidad* among highland peasants in Peru. The most common symptom experienced by those who suffer from this culture-specific illness is pain in the brainstem area, with pain in the cranium being the second most common complaint. Other symptoms include numbness, dizziness, and fatigue. These discomforts tend to be endured stoically by sufferers without much public complaint. Looking at *debilidad* in its social context, Oths concludes that it is an "expression of the embodiment of life's accumulated hardships. In the highlands of northern Peru, reproductive and productive stresses generated primarily by the pressures of maintaining a living under hard social and economic conditions lead to a culture-specific complaint of *debilidad*, or exhaustion. . . . Those with debilidad can be shown to have suffered more physically and psychologically over their lifetimes" (Oths 1999: 309).

The study of the mindful body in interconnected experiential, cultural, social, and political economic contexts, with particular concern for the ways social inequality is inscribed in bodies and bodies, in turn, are transformed into consumers of self-improvement commodities (or themselves become commodities for sale for the improvement of others) are key topics for critical medical anthropology. Implied in this wide range of concerns is the belief that a critical perspective provides the conceptual framework needed to analyze macro-micro connections (e.g., between individual experience, decision making, and action and powerful social forces like global commodity and labor markets, social stratification, and transnational geopolitical domination).

We view CMA as providing a perspective and set of concepts for analyzing macro-micro connections. At the theoretical level, some maintain that critical medical anthropology has developed two contending camps, the so-called political economy/world system theorists and the Foucaultian poststructuralists (Morgan 1987). Scheper-Hughes and Lock

(1986: 137), principal proponents of the latter camp, although granting that the political economy of health perspective served as a useful corrective to conventional medical anthropological studies, asserted—perhaps prematurely—that it has "tended to depersonalize the subject matter and the content of medical anthropology by focusing on the analysis of social systems and *things*, and by neglecting the particular, the existential, the subjective content of illness, suffering, and healing as *lived* events and experiences" (emphasis in original). The orientation of this volume, written from the political economic/world system perspective embraced by its authors, we believe, throws into question the alleged neglect of the individual level of analysis. The study of lived experience, embodiment, social suffering, and individual agency are all-important to the CMA approach. What is distinctive with regard to CMA's approach to the individual level is its recognition of the degree to which issues of power, inequality, oppression, exploitation, and the like create the social environments within which the individual level is actualized and intimately contributes to the social shaping of individual experience, the social construction of human bodies, and the social production of potential pathways of personal action.

Scheper-Hughes argues for the creation of what she terms a "third path between the individualizing, meaning-centered discourse of the symbolic, hermeneutic, phenomenologic medical anthropologists, on the one hand, and the collectivized, depersonalized, mechanistic abstraction of the medical Marxists, on the other. To date, much of what is called *critical* medical anthropology refers to . . . the applications of marxist political economy to the social relations of sickness and health care delivery" (Scheper-Hughes 1990: 189; emphasis in original).

Despite some theoretical differences between the two genres of CMA, they share a commitment to the development of appropriate practical expression. CMA rejects a simple dichotomy between the "anthropology of medicine" and the "anthropology in medicine" that separates theoretical from applied objectives (Foster and Anderson 1978). Rather, critical medical anthropologists seek to place their expertise at the disposal of labor unions, peace organizations, environmental groups, ethnic community agencies, women's health collectives, health consumer associations, self-help and self-care movements, alternative health efforts, national liberation struggles, and other bodies or initiatives that aim to liberate people from oppressive health and social conditions. In sum, through their theoretical and applied work, critical medical anthropologists strive to contribute to the larger effort to create a new health system that will serve the people. This system will not promote the narrow interests of a small, privileged sector of society. Its creation requires a radical transformation of existing economic relationships.

Ironically, there are still some hints that some conventional medical anthropologists, while recognizing the existence of critical medical anthropology, continue to sideline it, particularly a CMA that emphasizes political economy of health and world systems theory as we seek to do in this textbook. For example, in their *A Reader in Medical Anthropology*, Byron Good et al. assert:

By the early 1980s, diverse critical theories, including both Marxist-inspired writing and post-structuralism, had become increasingly influential within anthropology and post-structuralism, had become increasingly influential within anthropology and ethnographic writing. . . . We have chosen not to include here the polemical debates about what constitutes a "critical medical anthropology," in which some argued that interpretive medical anthropologists failed to attend adequately to macrosocial forces and the play of power, or some of the earliest writings influenced by Michel Foucault. Instead, we include essays that represent more recent efforts to draw on decades of writing about biopolitics, biosociality, governmentality, citizenship and subjectivity, all a part of the post-structuralist vocabulary, in order to think through topics such as contemporary prison psychiatry, nuclear disaster, HIV treatment, communal violence, and migrant health. (Good et al. 2010: 4)

Yet many of the topics listed in this quote are ones that we touch on in this textbook, which emphasizes the political economy/world systems genre of CMA.

Critical Medical Anthropology and Science

As inscribed in its 1902 Articles of Incorporation, the mission of the American Anthropological Association is to "advance anthropology as the science that studies mankind in all its aspects." Yet in recent years, the issue of science in anthropology has become highly contentious. To some degree, this reflects an older debate as to whether anthropology is a science or belongs to the humanities. However, the character of this debate has become more intense, and science is now portrayed by some in increasingly negative terms. Consequently, the question sometimes becomes, "Is CMA science or antiscience?" Those who raise this question are interested to know whether medical anthropologists who embrace a critical perspective believe that their work is conducted within the framework and canons of science or within an alternative, nonscientific mode of understanding reality, such as radical social constructionism, which might be viewed by some as antiscientific in its perspective. Perhaps the starting point for answering this question is to raise another: "What is science?"

It is generally agreed that science views itself as an approach to the discovery of knowledge that adheres to certain rules commonly called the scientific method. Two key rules of the scientific method are *empiricism* (scientific questions are answered through systematic research) and *objectivity* (research must be replicable by others and controlled for bias). The believability of scientific claims to knowledge about the world rests on acceptance that the knowledge it produces is gained through a fair and scrupulous adherence to these rules.

One approach to critiquing science involves showing the high level of bias found in work presented under the banner of scientific objectivity. An example relevant to the concerns of CMA is the book *The Bell Curve: Intelligence and Class Structure in American Life* by Richard Herrnstein and Charles Murray. This work, one in a long line of books that have attempted to show scientifically that African Americans inherently have lower IQs than whites, created an enormous stir when it was published in 1994. The book was celebrated and embraced by those with a conservative political orientation as strong proof that social programs to redress social inequality are a waste of time and money: Biology is destiny—and the ultimate cause of social disparities.

Unfortunately for the authors of *The Bell Curve*, as many have pointed out, the book is a case of bad science. For example, Leon Kamin (1995), a professor at Northeastern University, has shown how the book relies on concocted data, research findings contrary to those reported by Herrnstein and Murray, non-IQ data reported as IQ findings, and similar distortions that are made to serve a predetermined set of conclusions about African American inferiority. Based on his analysis, Kamin (1995: 103) concludes, "The book has nothing to do with science." The problem here is not science per se but the rotten apple in an otherwise healthy barrel.

Radical social constructionism takes a different approach in its critique of science. As Haraway (1991: 186) explains, the goal of this perspective is to find "a way to go beyond showing bias in science (that proved too easy anyway), and beyond separating the good scientific sheep from the bad goats of bias and misuse." Instead, social constructionists seek to deconstruct "the truth claims of . . . science by showing the radical historical specificity, and so contestability, of every layer of the onion of scientific . . . constructions." In other words, social reconstructionism is concerned with showing that scientific knowledge (including that which falls into the realm of good science) is produced under a particular and influencing set of cultural and historic conditions and that the insights of science are not discovered but socially crafted. As Latour and Woolgar (1986: 243) argue, based on a careful ethnographic study of daily life in a scientific laboratory, "Scientific activity is not 'about nature,' it is a fierce fight to construct reality." The underlying objective of science is to create order out of the disorder of experience. But, Latour and Woolgar emphasize, the order of science is constructed by scientists and is not inherent in nature. In this view, the scientific method is a set of rules for constructing an order that is so endowed with an aura of facticity and authority that it is embraced and treated by other scientists as fundamentally true.

In this light, it is the view of CMA that it is just as problematic not to see the cultural (and political economic) in science as it is to see only the cultural (and political economic) in science. A failure to see science as an activity that emerged and operates within a given set of cultural circumstances is influenced by the worldview and values peculiar to those circumstances, and serves particular social needs and groups found therein is to treat science as a special case, different from other forms of human activity. There is no justification for this kind of privileging of one form of human endeavor over all others. Conversely, if science is to be treated as nothing but culture, then surely it cannot be brought to bear in discerning the accuracy or validity of any claim to truth. The Nazi claim, for example, that Jews constitute a subhuman group cannot be refuted scientifically if science is deconstructed as culture only. Franz Boas, a leader of modern anthropology during its development in the United States, undertook precisely this kind of work. His books were burned by the Nazis in Germany because he mobilized scientific research to show that Nazi slanders against the Jews and other people whom the Nazis viewed as inferior to Aryans were as full of holes as are the latter-day claims made by Herrnstein and Murray about African Americans.

In sum, CMA views its approach as scientific (and built on the scientific method), while recognizing that its perspective on reality is no less conditioned by social circumstance and no less open to critical examination and debate than any other perspective. The scientific method is built on, indeed demands, open and constant critique, and self-examination. This book presents some of the critique developed within CMA of scientific medicine and medical anthropology, the sources of health problems in contemporary society, and a range of other issues pertinent to the field of medical anthropology. To this examination, CMA brings a special concern with the political economic context in which all ideas and behaviors emerge and have an impact on the world.

The Social Origin of Disease

CMA seeks to understand the social origin of disease, all disease. It shares this concern with other critical medical social scientists and public health researchers. Like the latter, critical medical anthropologists endeavor to identify the political, economic, social structural, and environmental conditions in all societies that contribute to the etiology of disease.

CMA views disease as a social as well as a biological product. Friedrich Engels and Rudolf Virchow were nineteenth-century theorists who recognized this reality. In *The Condition of the Working Class in England* ([1845] 1969), Engels, Karl Marx's confidante and frequent collaborator, observed firsthand the conditions of the working class in his position as a middle-level manager in his father's textile mill in Manchester. He maintained that disease in the textile workers was rooted in the organization of capitalist production and the social environment in which they had to live as a result of their meager wages. In contrast to most orthopedists and chiropractors, who generally neglect the social origins of the musculoskeletal problems that their patients experience, Engels recognized that they often derive from the nature of factory work:

The operatives . . . must stand the whole time. And one who sits down, say upon a window-ledge or basket, is fined, and this perpetual upright position, this constant mechanical pressure of the upper portions of the body upon spinal column, hips, and legs, inevitably produces the results mentioned. (Engels [1845] 1969: 190–193)

Rudolf Virchow, a renowned German pathologist and an elected member of the German Reichstag or parliament, also was a pioneer in social medicine—a concern that most biomedical physicians completely ignore. He argued that the material conditions of people's daily life at work, at home, and in the larger society constituted significant factors contributing to their diseases and ailments. On the basis of his studies of a typhus epidemic in Upper Silesia, a cholera epidemic in Berlin, and an outbreak of tuberculosis in Berlin during 1948 and 1949, Virchow concluded that these health problems were in large measure shaped by adverse social environmental conditions. He concluded that "[t]he improvement of medicine would eventually prolong life, but improvement of social conditions could achieve this result even more rapidly and successfully" (Virchow 1879: 121–122). In recognition of this insightful medical scientist, the Critical Anthropology of Health Caucus of the Society for Medical Anthropology annually presents the Rudolf Virchow Award for the best article in CMS submitted to a panel of three judges.

The study of the social origins of disease is referred to under a number of rubrics, including historical materialist epidemiology, the political economy of illness, and the political ecology of disease. Regardless of its designation, attention to the social origins of disease is an integral part of critical medical anthropology. In keeping with this interest, CMA strives, in McNeil's (1976) terms, to understand the nature of the relationship between microparasitism (the tiny organisms, malfunctions, and individual behaviors that are the proximate causes of much disease) and macroparasitism (the social relations of exploitation that are the ultimate causes of much disease).

Dangerous Liaisons

We close this chapter with a visit to an issue of controversy—namely, the role of cooptation of the anthropological vision. If, as some have maintained throughout its history, anthropology is inherently a troublesome, even dangerous, discipline, that sees and at times exposes that the emperor is naked (or, adversely, armed to the teeth with deadly and oppressive weapons), then it might be fair to ask, is anthropology at risk from forces of social power, the very sources so prominent in the making of illness and disease? Certainly attacks on anthropology have occurred over the years. Most recently, this attitude was expressed in the words of a Florida governor who publically claimed in 2011 that his state does not need anthropologists and that it was his intention to shift funding to science, technology, and math departments, and away from departments like psychology and anthropology. For much of its history, the focus of anthropology has been on people "without history" or often without much visibility in the halls of global or national power. But the field has changed, and increasingly anthropology is addressing pressing public issues including global warming, other environmental degradation, human rights, the social origins of disease, mistreatment of women, unhealthy health policy, killer commodities, war, and similarly controversial topics that require an assessment of power and inequality and their role in human suffering. If the goal of anthropology should always be to speak truth to power, how will power speak back? One way, as we detail in this section with reference two of the most prominent critical voices in medical anthropology, is through cooptation.

Paul Farmer and Jim Kim, both born in 1959, earned their MDs and their PhDs in medical anthropology at Harvard University and have collaborated on various projects as well as conducted ones of their own. Along with Ophelia Dahl, Thomas J. White, and Todd McCormack, in 1987 they cofounded Partners in Health (PIH), a Boston-based NGO whose motto is "providing a preferential option for the poor," that from its initial program, Zanmi Lasante in Haiti, has expanded to a sizeable organization that employs some 14,000 people worldwide and has, in addition to Haiti, projects in Chiapas (Mexico), Guatemala, Boston, Russia, Burundi, Lesotho, Rwanda, Malawi, Kazakhstan, and Dominican Republic. Both Kim and Farmer have worked closely with the Institute for Health and Social Justice based in Cambridge, Massachusetts, which serves as PIH's advocacy and policy arm.

At least until recently, Farmer, has been more visible both within medical anthropological circles and in the public arena, than Kim, largely due not only to his globetrotting activities as an engaged physician/anthropologist, which have earned him the reverential title of "Saint Paul" among some of his admirers, but also his numerous published books and a book-length biography about him titled *Mountains beyond Mountains* (Kidder 2003). Within medical anthropology, Farmer's most significant books are *AIDS and Accusation* (Farmer 1992), *Infections and Inequalities* (1999), and *Pathologies of Power* (2003). The devastating earthquake that rocked Haiti on January 12, 2010, propelled his fame and that of PIH even further because of PIH relief efforts in the aftermath of this tragic event. As Farmer (2011) discusses in his most recent book *Haiti after the Earthquake*, he worked closely with and as an envoy for Bill Clinton, who became a UN Special Envoy for Haiti and whose organization, the Clinton Health Access Initiative, provided financial and moral support to earthquake victims. PIH arranged for supplies, including medications, generators, water, and portable ultrasound machines to be transported by private jets to Haiti (Farmer 2011: 69). In reflecting on issues relating to natural disasters, social inequality, and global health, Farmer asserts:

The earthquake and our responses to it posed anew questions I'd struggle with while spanning the uneven world between Harvard and Haiti. Broadly, how could we diminish the growing inequalities in the world, which lead to, and (for those shy about claims of causality) are associated with, so much death, disability, and social instability? More specifically, just how "natural" a disaster was the one that struck this vulnerability was social, rather than natural, and caused by bad policies, foreign and homegrown? (Farmer 2011:117)

Later in the book Farmer (2011: 217) concludes the "growing inequality, both within countries and between them, is the linchpin of modern servitude." Although such arguments fit well into the spirit of critical medical anthropology, over the years in his various writings, Farmer has chosen to maintain a certain, undefined distance from this theoretical perspective. Only occasionally does he refer to capitalism or neoliberalism; he prefers to talk about structural violence emanating from racism, gender inequality, and other inequalities that of course are part and parcel of the capitalist world system.

Although Jim Kim has not been as much of a household name within medical anthropological circles as has his good friend and longtime collaborator Paul Farmer, nonetheless, he has proven to be a formidable figure in the universe of global health. Before serving as the seventeenth president of Dartmouth College, Kim served as the chairperson of the Department of Global Health and Social Medicine at Harvard Medical School and the director of the Francois-Xavier Bagnoud Center for Health and Human Rights. He also served as the director of the World Health Organization's (WHO's) Department of HIV/AIDS, which ultimately provided some three million HIV patients with antiretroviral drugs.

Kim was propelled into the international limelight in March 2012 when President Barrack Obama nominated him to head the World Bank, a position he began on July 1, 2012. Kim's nomination met with stormy opposition both from parties in the developing countries as well as from neoliberal economists. His involvement as the lead coeditor of an anthology titled *Dying for Growth* (Kim, Millen, Irwin, and Gershaman 2000) prompted some economists to assert that he is "antigrowth." In its various chapters, the book explores the linkages between neoliberalism and health problems among the poor in various countries. In his review of *Dying for Growth*, Baer (2001a) wrote a generally positive assessment but faulted the editors for failing to provide readers with a vision that will not simply ameliorate the worst effects of global capitalism on the health of poor. Consistent with the critical medical perspective, this vision would entail the creation of health for all that entails constructing an alternative global political economy oriented toward meeting social needs rather than to profit making, a vision that we discuss in the final chapter of this textbook.

Perhaps this omission provided Kim with the wiggle room he may have needed when during his nomination process for the presidency of the World Bank many questions were asked about whether, as some presumed by his role as lead editor of *Dying for Growth*, he was antigrowth or anticapitalist. In a BBC interview, he asserted that capitalist "market-based growth is a priority for every single country" in that it will create jobs and lift people out of poverty" (www.bbc.co.uk/news/business-17757480, April 18, 2012). In a *Washington Post* editorial, Farmer defended his friend by arguing that "any reasonable reading of the book indicates that *Dying for Growth* is pro-growth, raising questions about particular policies and patterns of growth that exclude the great majority of people living in poverty. Hence the double entendre in the title" (Farmer and Gershman 2012). Anthropologist Jason Hickel (2012: 1) doubts whether Kim will be able to get the World Bank to accept needed reforms such as forgiving Third World debts and eradicating structural adjustment policies "because they would run up against enormously powerful interests."

In reality, both Kim and Farmer appear to be overlooking the increasing number of scholars and activists who are challenging the growth paradigm associated with the capitalist world system, especially in light of the increasing evidence that the treadmill of production and consumption highly dependent on fossil fuels is not only contributing to increasing social inequality around the world but also the depletion of natural resources and environmental impact, of the which the most profound is climate change, topics that we raise in Chapters 3 and 4 of this textbook. At this point, it is unclear whether Kim and Farmer never fully embraced the perspective advocated by critical medical anthropologists, a perspective that sees an inherent contradiction between market economics and both social equality and environmental sustainability, or whether aspects of their view have been co-opted by their admittance to the world stage and the heartfelt desire to achieve meaningful impact by being high up in powerful systems rather than challenging them from the outside. Consequently, while recognizing the tremendous contributions to improved global health of both Kim and Farmer we, like others, know that powerful systems always seek to have the last word, and cooptation of leading critics is one way of achieving this goal. Indeed, some have pondered whether academia itself serves this function in muting the critiques of many scholars.

In the next part of this book, we examine the relationship between health and the environment in general and the social origins of several diseases and forms of suffering, including hunger, malnutrition, homelessness, alcoholism, drug addiction, and AIDS.

PART II

The Social Origins
of Disease and Suffering

CHAPTER 3

Health and the Environment: From Foraging Societies to the Capitalist World System

Since their emergence some five million years ago, humans have lived in a delicate interaction with the rest of the natural habitat. Humans, of course, are a part of nature. In contrast to other animal species, however, we engage nature not directly but through our sociocultural systems. According to Godelier (1986: 28), the natural environment is a "reality which humanity transforms to a greater or lesser extent by various ways of acting upon nature and appropriating its resources." In other words, humans are situated in an environment that entails both a natural dimension and a culturally constructed one. This social environment is an intricate system of interaction between nature and culture, which is created under specific physical limits and imposes various material constraints on human populations. Experientially, of course, we cannot separate nature and culture. As humans we can only experience nature as we culturally construct it, imbue it with meaning, and interact with it in ways that fit within our particular cultural frames of understanding and emotion.

Technological innovations have enabled humanity to adjust to habitats other than the savannah of East Africa, where it appears that the first bipedal primates or hominids emerged. In the past, most anthropologists believed that the adoption of farming or food production constituted an evolutionary advance: the overforaging or food collection that resulted in an improvement in human health and well-being. Research by Richard Lee and Irven DeVore (1976) among the San in the Kalahari Desert of Southwest Africa, however, revealed that people in this desert-dwelling foraging society worked fewer hours per day to provision themselves than most farmers but were better nourished and generally healthier than their horticultural neighbors. As a result of such findings about contemporary foragers, many prehistorians began to revise their theories about living conditions in societies relying on foraging, horticulture (farming that relies on simple implements, such as a digging stick or hoe), and agriculture (intensive farming that relies on more sophisticated implements such as an animal-drawn plow and elaborate techniques such as large-scale irrigation systems and terracing in mountainous areas).

Particularly in foraging societies that lacked contact with civilization or have had minimal contact with it, it appears their members enjoyed good health and long lives while they fulfilled their material desires without endangering the natural environment. As a result of such favorable living conditions, Marshall Sahlins (1972) referred to foragers as the "original affluent society." Conversely, the new interpretation viewed farming as a subsistence strategy necessitated by increasing population densities and declining animal and plant resources among foragers. This new theory argued, "farming permitted more mouths to be fed without necessarily increasing leisure time or lessening the demands of the food quest, while resulting in a general decline in the quality and desirability of food" (Cohen 1984: 2).

Anthropologists and other social scientists have presented a wide array of schemes for delineating the evolutionary trajectory of human societies. In his cultural anthropology textbook, John Bodley (1994) classifies the world's cultures into three broad categories: small, large, and global. Small cultures include nomadic foragers, village horticulturalists, and tribal pastoralists. These societies tend to be relatively egalitarian and to place a great deal of emphasis on reciprocity. Large-scale cultures include both chiefdoms and early states and empires. These societies exhibit a considerable amount of social ranking, or stratification, and centralization of power but lack a developed market economy or industrial production. According to Bodley,

A relatively new scale of organization, [the] global culture has emerged within only the past 200 years. . . . This global system has systematically absorbed large-and small-scale cultures and is itself so homogenous that it could be treated as a single culture. Industrialization has enriched, impoverished, and destabilized the world. The global system was created by a commercialization process that reversed the relationship between political and economic organization. Political organization is now in the service of ever more powerful economic interests. The global economy is primarily dedicated to the production of profit for the stockholders of corporations. When the costs and benefits of global-scale culture are considered, poverty must be added to inequality and instability, because the global system contains economically stratified nations, which are themselves highly stratified internally. (Bodley 1994: 16)

Following the work of Wallerstein (1979, 2004) and others, we prefer, as is apparent in this textbook, to refer to the global culture that Bodley describes as the capitalist world system. At any rate, the evolution of sociocultural systems has been accompanied, as Bodley (1996: 25) asserts, by "a remarkable increase in the human sector of the global biomass (humans and domestic plants and animals) and a corresponding reduction in the earth's natural biomass" or what environmental scientists refer to as biodiversity. The advent initially of agrarian state societies and later of capitalist industrial societies was accompanied by patterns of differential power, social stratification, urbanization, population growth, increasing production and consumption, resource depletion, and environmental degradation. Indeed, John Bennett (1974: 403) alludes to an "ecological transition" in sociocultural evolution that entails a "progressive incorporation of Nature into human frames of purpose and action" and evolution from societies that were in relative equilibrium with the natural environment to those that are in disequilibrium with it. According to Bodley (1985: 31), "Social stratification, inequality, urbanization, and state organization . . . set in motion a system that is almost inherently unstable." Agricultural practices in ancient states or civilized societies often were factors in environmental degradation. Large-scale irrigation in ancient Mesopotamia, the area between the Tigris and Euphrates Rivers in what is present-day Iraq, resulted in the gradual accumulation of salts in the soil, which in turn contributed to the collapse of Sumerian civilization after 2000 B.C. The development of mercantile and later of industrial capitalism resulted in an expanded culture of consumption that even further strained the environment. Juergen Habermas describes the destructive impact of capitalism upon the global ecosystem as follows:

The indifference of a market economy to its external costs, which it off-loads on to the social and natural environment, is sowing the path of a crisis-prone economic growth with the familiar disparities and marginalizations on the inside; with economic backwardness, if not regression, and consequently with barbaric living conditions, cultural expropriation and catastrophic famines in the Third World; not to mention the worldwide risk caused by disrupting the balance of nature. (Habermas 1991: 41)

HEALTH AND THE ENVIRONMENT
IN PREINDUSTRIAL SOCIETIES

Critical medical anthropology recognizes that since antiquity human interaction with the environment has created opportunities for the production of disease. Human health is affected by an environment that is the product of the dialectical interaction of natural and sociocultural forces. According to P. Brown and Inhorn (1990: 190), disease is "not a thing but a process triggered by an interaction between a host and an environmental insult." Various scholars have argued that people in foraging societies have generally enjoyed cleaner environments and better health than the majority of peoples in agrarian civilizations (Cohen 1989). Epidemiological studies indicate that disease became a more rampant and devastating problem for human populations with the advent of agrarian state societies or civilization.

Foraging Societies

Ancient foragers appear on the whole to have enjoyed surprisingly well-nourished and fulfilling lives. Table 3.1 presents data that compare life expectancies in ancient foraging societies to later, more complex societies.

Although early hominids carried parasitic diseases that had also existed among their pongid or ape ancestors, their low population densities and migratory patterns tended to mitigate the disease load of specific foraging bands. Nevertheless, despite a relative abundance of food and a low incidence of infectious and chronic diseases, it appears that life, in terms of life expectancy, during the Paleolithic or "Old Stone Age" (the vast period from the earliest stone tools to the period just before the advent of farming) was often precarious. A heavy reliance on a fluctuating and unpredictable supply of large game and the existence of predators posed a significant risk for human populations, who had to rely on handmade weapons and fire as forms of protection. Big-game hunting itself was a highly dangerous endeavor that undoubtedly took the lives of many hunters. The retreat of the glaciers of the last Ice Age or Fourth Glacial period (about ten thousand years ago) converted grasslands to forests, thus leading to the extinction of most of the big game animals that had subsisted on grass and on which foragers had relied heavily for their food.

These climatic and environmental changes ushered in a period that archaeologists refer to as the Mesolithic, associated with a broad-spectrum revolution that entailed a greater reliance on a wide assortment of small and medium-sized game, such as deer and rabbit (which were far less dangerous to hunt), as well as a wider diversity of plant foods. According to Hunt (1978: 56) and as we can see from Table 3.1, "the evidence from paleopathology indicates a quantum jump in the expectation of human life at birth in the Mesolithic stage of cultural evolution (about ten thousand years ago) followed by a plateau that lasted until medieval times."

Table 3.1
Life Expectancies of Various Preindustrial Human Populations

Group	Mean Life Expectancies at Specific Ages		Range in Additional Life Expectancy at 15 Years
	Birth	15 Years	
Paleolithic	19.9	20.6	15.0–26.9
Mesolithic	31.4	26.9	15.0–34.8
Copper Age	28.4	22.2	15.2–34.8
Bronze Age	32.1	23.7	20.4–27.0
Iron Age	27.3	23.4	18.0–32.4
Classical period	27.2	24.7	15.0–34.5
Ancient foragers		16.5	15.0–19.1
Proto-agricultural averages		19.8	15.0–28.7
Urban agricultural averages		25.3	16.9–34.6
Contemporary indigenous averages		26.3	19.2–34.0

Adapted from Kerley and Bass (1978: 56).

Furthermore, ancient as well as contemporary foraging societies lived or continue to live in relative harmony with their respective econiches. Nonetheless, it is important not to romanticize these societies or to believe that we may return to a life of nomadic hunting, fishing, and gathering. Additionally, these societies do leave their footprints on their environments. For example, foragers historically have used fire to clear the landscape of brush and trees to hunt game more effectively. This has led to deforestation in many settings. Bison drives on the North American plains, in which the Indians stampeded large herds over cliffs, led to mass deaths of animals. In contrast to later societies, however, the adverse ecological impact of the earliest human societies was minimal. The Mbuti pygmies of the Ituri Forest in Zaire, central Africa, for example, base their tendency to limit the consumption of animal protein on their belief that eating animals such as deer and elephants shortens their life span. They maintain that in the primeval past they were vegetarians who could have lived forever, but with the adoption of meat eating, they embarked on a path that ultimately led to death.

Epidemiologist Frederick Dunn (1977: 102–3) makes several key generalizations about the health status of foraging populations:

1. Patent malnutrition is rare.
2. Starvation occurs infrequently.
3. Chronic diseases, particularly those associated with old age, are relatively infrequent.

4. Accidental and traumatic death rates vary greatly among hunter-gatherer populations.
5. Predation, excluding snakebites, is a minor cause of death in modern foragers and may have been relatively more important in the past.
6. No generalizations about mental illness among foragers can be made due to lack of sufficient evidence.
7. Ample evidence is available that "social mortality" [homicide, suicide, cannibalism, infanticide, gerontocide, head-hunting, etc.] has been and is significant in the population equation for any foraging society.
8. Parasitic and infectious disease rates of prevalence and incidence are related to the type of econiche.

Dunn's first two generalizations appear to apply better to foragers living in tropical rain forests, savannahs, and even deserts than they do to foragers living in arctic areas. Although starvation was reportedly not a frequent cause of death among the Inuit, McElroy and Townsend (1989: 3) contend that "it is certain that mortality increased among old people and small children during serious food shortages."

Humans appear to have inherited various infectious diseases from their primate ancestors. Under certain environmental conditions, infectious diseases are caused by biological agents ranging from microscopic, intracellular viruses to large, structurally complex helminthic parasites. Foragers probably acquired diseases such as head and body lice, pinworms, and yaws from prehominid populations. Livingstone (1958) discounts the likelihood that early hominids had malaria because they lived in savannahs rather than in humid areas in close proximity to still bodies of water. Contemporary primates often carry viral, bacterial, and protozoan infections, including malaria, yellow fever, dysentery, yaws, filariasis, herpes, poliomyelitis, tuberculosis, hepatitis, and rabies (C. Wood 1979: 42). Humans also became infected by intestinal worms and protozoa carried by hunted animals.

Human susceptibility to disease depends in part upon geography—a reality illustrated in Table 3.2. Whereas groups who live in semiarid or arid conditions, such as the San and the aborigines of the Central Australian desert, encounter few or no species of helminths (intestinal worms) and protozoa (microscopic organisms), those who live in tropical rain forests, such as the Mbuti pygmies and the Semang of Malaysia, encounter numerous species of these parasites.

In the following, "A Closer Look," we explore what lessons the health profile of ancient and contemporary foraging peoples may have for us today.

Table 3.2
Parasitic Helminths and Protozoa in Four Foraging Groups

Terrain	San of Kalahari Desert savannah	Central Australian Aborigine desert	Semang of Malaysia tropical rain forest	Mbuti Pygmy of Zaire tropical rain forest
No. Species				
Helminths	2	1	10	11
Intestinal Protozoa	–	–	9	6
Blood Protozoa	1	–	3	3
Total No. Species	3	1	22	20

Adapted from Dunn (1977: 105).

"A Closer Look"

WHAT DO PREHISTORIC AND CONTEMPORARY FORAGERS TELL US ABOUT EATING AND LIVING RIGHT?

In *The Paleolithic Prescription*, physician S. Boyd Eaton, anthropologist Marjorie Shostak, and physician-anthropologist Melvin Konner propose a general plan for healthy living in the modern world by adopting certain dietary and exercise habits from prehistoric and contemporary foraging societies (Eaton, Shostak, and Konner 1988). Indeed, they argue that our biochemistry and physiology are much more in tune with an active nomadic foraging lifestyle than with one in which most people are engaged in relatively sedentary occupations (e.g., repetitive assembly-line work, office work, or attending lectures and studying) and sedentary leisure activities (e.g., spectator sports and television and movie viewing). As part of their program for healthy living, Eaton et al. suggest that modern people adopt a "stone age diet." They contend that among foragers

[d]ietary quality is generally excellent, providing a broad base of proteins and complex carbohydrates along with a rich supply of vitamins and nutrients. Dietary quantity is occasionally marginal or deficient, but this is true of most agricultural cultures as well—probably even more so. Maintenance of the forager diet is accomplished with a moderate work load, leaving ample time for the pursuit of leisure activities. (Eaton, Shostak, and Konner 1988: 28)

Table 3.3 compares the nutritional content of a late Paleolithic to that of a contemporary U.S. diet. The high level of meat consumption among

Table 3.3
Late Paleolithic and Contemporary U.S. Dietary Compositions

	Late Paleolithic Diet	Contemporary Diet
Forms of Dietary Consumption		
Protein	33	12
Carbohydrate	46	46
Fat	21	42
Polyunsaturated:Saturated Ratio	1.41	0.44
Cholesterol (mg)	520	300–500
Fiber (gm)	100–150	19.7
Sodium (mg)	690	2,300–6,900
Calcium (mg)	1,500–2,000	740
Ascorbic Acid (mg)	440	90

Adapted from Eaton, Shostak, and Konner (1988: 84).

foragers resulted or continues to result in a high cholesterol intake. According to Eaton et al. (1988: 86), the fact that contemporary foragers seem to "escape cardiovascular complications may be due to their different patterns of fat intake; they eat much less of it, and the fats they do eat—derived from wild game and vegetable foods—have a higher ratio of polyunsaturated to saturated fats." They obtain roughage, or dietary fiber, from wild plant foods. Foragers drank water as their major and generally only beverage. By and large they began to consume alcohol only after contact with civilized societies. Indeed, alcohol served as an important vehicle used by European societies for conquering not only foragers but also indigenous populations in North America and the Pacific Islands.

Paleontological evidence indicates that prehistoric foragers exhibited strength, muscularity, and leanness on par with outstanding contemporary athletes. Both hunting and gathering demand great stamina. Men track, stalk, and pursue game; and women walk long distances with heavy loads of wild plants, wood, water, and young children. Although blood pressure and blood sugar levels tend to rise with age among contemporary North Americans, they remain low throughout life among foragers, even among those who live to an advanced age. Cholesterol levels typically are much lower among foragers, as well as among horticulturalists and pastoralists, than they are among people in industrial societies. The San of Southwest Africa who are still able to live some semblance of a traditional foraging lifestyle reportedly exhibit a low incidence of hypertension, heart disease, low cholesterol, obesity, varicose veins, and stress-related diseases such as ulcers and colitis (Lee 1979). The life expectancy of San adults exceeds that of adults in many industrial societies. Conversely, they are more vulnerable to infant mortality, malaria, and respiratory infections, as well as to accidents, because of the limited availability of biomedical facilities. In the case of the Inuit, McElroy and Townsend (1989: 28) report that although their diets are high in fat, they exhibit low cholesterol levels, low blood pressure, and low rates of heart disease.

Eaton et al. propose a "discordance hypothesis" as an explanation for many modern illnesses, especially the chronic "diseases of civilization" that account for approximately 75 percent of mortality in industrial societies. They contend that modern humans function with a "40,000-year-old model body" that is "essentially out of synch with our life-styles, an inevitable discordance . . . between the world we live in today and the world our genes 'think' we live in still" (Eaton, Shostak, and Konner 1988: 43). Conversely, Eaton et al. fully recognize that foragers never lived in the Garden of Eden. They argue:

The late Paleolithic *was* a period when human existence was in accord with nature and when our life-styles and our biology were generally in harmony. . . . [It was also] a time when half of all children died before reaching adulthood, when posttraumatic disfigurement and disability were distressingly common, and when the comfort and basic security of life were orders of magnitude less than they are at present [at least for the majority of people in the middle and upper classes in industrial societies]. (Eaton, Shostak, and Konner 1988: 283)

Although some observers of foraging peoples have reported that they have seen few elderly people in their ranks, others have reported the presence of active, healthy elderly individuals. In contrast, whereas biomedicine has been able to prolong the length of life with medication, surgery, and expensive technology, it has been able to do little for the quality of life in the later years.

Given the paucity of foraging peoples in the world today, Eaton et al. argue that people in industrial societies could also draw insights from the lifestyles of pastoralists, rudimentary horticulturalists, and simple agriculturalists because these populations continue to resemble Paleolithic populations in fundamental ways. In reality, their program for healthy living in the hectic, modern world—or what many describe as the postindustrial, postmodern world with its emphasis on high-tech living and intensive consumption—is easier for affluent and professional people to follow than it is for working-class and, particularly, poor people. The latter generally are much less likely to have the financial resources, time, and educational opportunities that strict adherence to such a regimen dictates. Indeed, health itself has been transformed from a normal dimension of the human condition to yet another commodity. People with disposable incomes invest billions of dollars in diet programs, exercise machines, megavitamin tablets, and even holistic health care, or what in some cases may be termed "yuppie medicine."

The program that Eaton et al. call for places the responsibility for good health upon the individual rather than the community or the larger society. Although indeed certain foraging dietary practices, such as eating lots of fiber, may counteract the development of various forms of cancer, that program neglects the role that the heavy use of pesticides, preservatives, radioactive materials, various forms of pollution, and other social environmental factors play in the etiology of cancer. Furthermore, we must ask why so many people in modern societies, including physicians and nurses, engage in eating patterns and other forms of behavior, such as smoking, heavy drinking, and overeating, that they know unequivocally contribute to disease. It appears that many unhealthy behaviors constitute mechanisms for coping with modern problems—alienating work, unemployment or the fear of it, social isolation, lack of a sense of personal fulfillment, and the frantic pace of life in which time has become equated with money and in which full membership in a supportive community has been replaced by partial membership in diverse social groups and activities such as churches, hobbies, and self-help organizations.

Horticultural Village Societies

The semi-sedentary encampments of the Mesolithic and the more sedentary villages of the Neolithic provided new breeding places for domesticated animals that harbored infectious diseases (Armelagos and Dewey 1978). The Neolithic refers to an archeological period associated with the domestication of plants and animals. It first appeared in the hilly regions of the Fertile Crescent of the Near East about ten thousand years ago, but it developed either independently or as a result of diffusion in other parts of the Old World as well as the New World. The clearing of land for cultivation, the domestication of animals, and an increase in sedentary living provided ideal conditions for many of the helminthic and protozoal parasites.

Although domesticated animals act as scavengers that remove human waste and recycle garbage, Cohen argues that domestication of animals has probably contributed greatly to human exposure to infectious diseases:

Domestication forces human beings to deal at close range with animals throughout their life cycles and to encounter their body fluids and wastes, as well as their carcasses. Domestic dogs, as well as wild ones, can transmit rabies. In fact, they are the major source of human infection. Domestic cats may harbor toxoplasmosis. . . . Tetanus, one of the most dreaded diseases of recent history, is spread by domestic horses and to a lesser extent by cattle, dogs, and pigs. It can also spread to soil, but soil that has never been grazed or cultivated is generally free from bacteria. (Cohen 1989: 45–46)

In large part, greater susceptibility to disease in sedentary communities results from a higher population density and greater exposure to fecal contamination and household vermin. At any rate, research from Neolithic sites in both the Old and New Worlds demonstrates a recurrent pattern of decreased stature, higher infant mortality, and increased physiological stresses associated with malnutrition.

The nutritional quality of food in horticultural village societies tends to be inferior to that of foraging societies. The major foods (e.g., manioc, cassava, sweet potatoes, yams, bananas, plantains, etc.) among slash-and-burn horticulturalists are high in bulk but low in nutrients. Although these starchy tropical crops are good sources of food energy, they are poor sources of protein. As a result, horticulturalists sometimes raise domesticated animals, such as pigs in the case of highland populations in Papua New Guinea. Most horticulturalists, however, lack domesticated animals and rely instead upon hunting or fishing for their supply of animal protein. They also tend to work harder than foragers. Slash-and-burn horticulturalists need considerable time and energy to clear land and plant, tend, and harvest their crops as well as hunt or raise domestic animals.

Agrarian State Societies

The foremost characteristic of state societies—ancient or modern—is a marked pattern of social stratification in which an elite or ruling class dominates economic, political, social, and cultural endeavors. Although the ruling class in state societies has generally relied heavily on ideological or hegemonic methods of social control to maintain its domination over subordinate social categories, its monopoly over agencies of coercive force (e.g., the military, the police, legal codes, courts, and prisons) serves to ensure its domination in the event that members or segments of the lower classes resist or revolt against their subjugation.

Because of differential access to resources, including land and food, peasants in agrarian state societies subsist in large part on a limited number of cultivated crops. These crops have historically been highly vulnerable to droughts, floods, and pests. The need for arable land and lumber for building houses, furniture, wagons, tools, and ships induced the inhabitants of agrarian state societies to engage in a large-scale clearing of forests and to develop a world view in which they came to regard nature as a force to be conquered and subdued. Increasing social stratification, resulting from the emergence of a small managerial class in archaic state societies, created the conditions that resulted in a more than adequate food supply for elites and serious and often chronic food shortages for poor urbanites, peasants, and slaves.

The dawn of agrarian states resulted in a significant transformation of societal-environmental relations. The emergence of social mechanisms for harnessing large amounts of energy from the environment produced the emergence of predatory ruling classes. As Hughes (1975: 29) observes, "The rise of civilizations depended upon the increasing ability of people to use and control their natural environment, and the downfall of these same civilizations was due to their failure to maintain a harmonious relationship with nature."

Population density played an even more crucial factor in human susceptibility to disease in agrarian state societies than it did in horticultural village societies. For example, Cohen (1989: 49) contends that measles, which may have come from a virus of dogs or cows, constitutes a "disease of civilization" in that its "origins must be related to the growth of the human population and its coalescence into dense aggregates or widespread and efficient networks." The appearance of the first cities in archaic state societies made access to clean water and the removal of human wastes problematic. Agriculture in many of these early states was based on large-scale irrigation systems, which often created the conditions for vector-borne diseases such as malaria and schistosomiasis. Unequal access to food supplies contributed to the emergence of malnutrition and, as a consequence, greater susceptibility to disease among the economically exploited masses, particularly in urban areas.

In his classic *Plagues and Peoples,* historian William H. McNeill (1976) demonstrates that epidemics have played a major role in the expansion of agrarian states throughout history, especially in their incorporation of indigenous societies. He suggests that three major waves of disease in the past two thousand years can be related to three major events of population movements: the formation of trade linkages by sea and land early in the Christian era, the militaristic expansion of the Mongols in the thirteenth century, and European expansion beginning in the fifteenth century. The depopulation of North and South American societies was a by-product of European colonization that introduced alien infections from the Old World. McNeill describes such imperialistic and mercantile processes as expressions of "macroparasitism." Whereas the term microparasites refers to disease organisms, such as viruses, bacteria, protozoa, and helminths, macroparasites are large organisms, including humans, that expropriate food and labor from conquered or low-status groups. Although macroparasitism as a sociocultural phenomenon emerged during the Neolithic period, Peter Brown (1987: 160) maintains that it took on its most elaborate form in state societies where it became manifested in "terms of tribute, rent, sharecropping contracts, and other forms of 'asymmetrical economic exchange.'"

Although agriculture served to support an increased population, the rise of civilization also contributed to a net loss of dietary diversity and nutritional quality, particularly among peasants and economically marginal urbanites. As Cohen (1989: 69) notes, the "power of the elite not only affects the quality of food for the poor but may undermine their access to food, their very right to eat." At the very same time that elites came to enjoy sumptuous supplies of food imported from far-flung areas as well as seemingly unlimited luxuries, masses of people were denied fulfillment of their basic subsistence needs—a tragedy of the human condition that historically has contributed to a wide variety of diseases and premature death in the laboring classes. It is no wonder that Stanley Diamond (1974) has argued that ever since the emergence of civilization, humans have been in "search of the primitive"—that is, the ability to satisfy their basic needs for food, clothing, and shelter and a sense of community, all of which are crucial to the maintenance not only of "functional health" but also of "experiential health," a distinction made in Chapter 1.

HEALTH AND THE ENVIRONMENT IN THE CONTEXT OF THE CAPITALIST WORLD SYSTEM

Agrarian states, with their patterns of social stratification and urbanization, set in motion an inherently unstable societal-environmental dynamic and the basis for massive malnutrition, susceptibility to infectious diseases, and social mortality resulting from large-scale and systematic warfare. The emergence of capitalism as a world economy—a global network of productive and market activities aimed at profit making—around the fifteenth century planted the seeds for a global environmental crisis. The dangers of local ecological self-destruction that plagued archaic and feudal state societies became universal with the advent of capitalism.

In the nineteenth century, Karl Marx and Friedrich Engels presented in a wide array of works the most thorough and critical analysis of capitalism ever written. Although they did not give a great deal of attention to ecological issues, they were certainly cognizant of the dialectical relationship between sociocultural systems and the natural environment. Colonialism as a mechanism for capitalist expansion in the Americans, Asia, and Africa disrupted traditional farming practices that had achieved some semblance of sustainable adjustment to local environmental conditions. The advent of the capitalist Industrial Revolution in England during the late eighteenth century resulted in increased water and air pollution and, as peasants were pushed off the land and migrated to emerging factory towns seeking work in horribly unsanitary and overcrowded slums. In *The Condition of the Working Class in England*, Engels ([1845] 1969) describes the devastating impact of industrialization on the natural environment. Furthermore, as Merchant (1992: 140) observes, "Marx gave numerous examples of capitalist pollution: chemical by-products from industrial production; iron filings from machine tool industry; flax, silk, wool, and cotton wastes in the clothing industry; rags and discarded clothing from consumers; and the contamination of London's River Thames with human waste."

Capitalist development projects in the Third World in the form of dam construction, land reclamation, road construction, and resettlement of populations have contributed to the spread of infectious diseases such as trypanosomiasis, malaria, and schistosomiasis. The rapid spread of schistosomiasis, which is acquired when larval parasites are released in water from snail vectors, is in large measure a direct consequence of water development projects such as the construction of high dams, artificial lakes and reservoirs, and irrigation canals. It has infected an estimated 200 to 300 million people worldwide (Inhorn and Brown 1990: 98).

As opposed to relatively minor environmental modifications wrought by indigenous societies, the capitalist world system, with its emphasis on ever-expanding production and a culture of intensified consumption, introduced completely new environmental contaminants that interfered with natural biochemical processes. Indeed, the precursors of this transition occurred with the transition to agrarian state societies beginning some six thousand years ago. Armelagos and Harper (2010) delineate three epidemiological transitions in human sociocultural development. The first epidemiological transition, which we already discussed, began around ten thousand years ago with appearance of Neolithic diseases that accompanied the domestication of plants and animals. The second epidemiological transition began with the Industrial Revolution and entailed "a decrease in pathogen-induced infections and an increase in chronic, man-made diseases" (Armelagos and Harper 2010: 299). According to Armelagos and Harper (2010: 300), the third epidemiological transition is relatively recent and is the "direct result of social, economic, and technological change on a global level." They identify six factors contributing to the reemergence of infectious disease in recent decades: "ecological change, human demographics and behavior, international travel and commerce, technology and industry, microbial adaptation and change, and the breakdown of public health measures" (Armelagos and Harper 2010: 300). From our perspective, it is interesting that the second and third epidemiological transitions occurred at different historical junctures of the capitalist world system, during a period of emerging industrialization in the case of the second transition and in a period of ongoing expansion and globalization in the case of the third transition.

Capitalism has historically assumed that natural resources—not only minerals but also air, water, fertile soil, and trees—exist in unlimited abundance. Moreover, industrial capitalism has expanded into a world system of unequal exchange between developed and underdeveloped countries, with significant implications for global ecological destruction.

Immanuel Wallerstein (1979, 2004), a comparative sociologist who incorporates ideas from history, anthropology, and political economy, argues that the capitalist world system emerged in sixteenth-century Europe and now incorporates the entire globe. He maintains that capitalism "as a system for production for sale in a market for profit and appropriations of this profit on the basis of individual or collective ownership has only existed in, and can be said to require, a world system in which the political units are not coextensive with the boundaries of the market economy" (Wallerstein 1979: 66). Capitalism is an economic system of production and exchange that exploits technology, natural resources, and labor in the pursuit of profit making. Although the contemporary world system consists of some 192 nation-states and several thousand nations or ethnic groups, its economic division of labor consists of three units: (1) the core, (2) the semiperiphery, and (3) the periphery. The core includes strong stable states characterized by a high degree of bureaucratization and large, technologically sophisticated militaries. It serves as the base for multinational or transnational corporations owned and managed by a powerful and wealthy capitalist class or bourgeoisie that tends to dominate state policies. The core also has a large professional class, a large working class or proletariat, and a smaller semiproletariat consisting of semiskilled, menial workers and unemployed or underemployed people. The core is the site of the most technologically advanced, capital-intensive production and in recent decades has undergone a transformation from heavy industry to information technology. The periphery includes relatively weak, unstable states characterized by inefficient and oftentimes corrupt bureaucracies and unsophisticated and often repressive militaries. Its small national bourgeoisies and professional classes tend to be closely linked with an international capitalist class. Peripheral countries have small proletariats and large semiproletariats. The semiperiphery consists of relatively strong states with increasing bureaucratization and relatively technologically sophisticated militaries that are often dependent on core states for arms production. It has relatively small national bourgeoisies and a roughly even mixture of proletarian and semiproletarian labor force. In keeping with a pattern of unequal exchange, the core exploits the semiperiphery and periphery, whereas the periphery is exploited by both the core and the semiperiphery. The periphery and, to a lesser degree, the semiperiphery serve as sites of cheap raw materials and cheap labor for the core. The semiperiphery is situated in an intermediate status as being exploited by the core and exploiting the periphery.

Scholars disagree as to which countries fit into the three main divisions of the capitalist world system. Shannon (1996: 87) differentiates between major core countries (e.g., the United States, Japan, Germany, France, and Britain) and minor core countries (e.g., Canada, Australia, Italy, the Switzerland, and the Scandinavian countries). Whereas some scholars classified the Soviet Union as a core country, others viewed it as a member of the semiperiphery. Furthermore, some scholars regard Canada, Australia, and New Zealand as semiperipheral countries because of their economic subservience to various core countries, particularly the United States and Britain. Examples of semiperipheral countries include Italy, Spain, Russia, Poland, Mexico, Brazil, Argentina, Saudi Arabia, Israel, Egypt, Indonesia, the Philippines, and South Korea. Examples of peripheral countries include Bolivia, Honduras, Haiti, Zaire, Tanzania, Ethiopia, Afghanistan, and Kampuchea. Whereas some scholars regard China as a semiperipheral country, others regard it as a member of the periphery. At any rate, over time, countries may move up or down in the division of labor of the capitalist world system. Over the course of the development of the capitalist world system, the gap between the rich countries and poor countries has tended to widen. Watkins (1997), an Oxfam policy analyst, says that whereas in 1966, the richest fifth of the world's population earned an income 30 times greater than the poorest fifth, by 1997 the gap had increased to 78:1. As Cohen and Kennedy so aptly observe:

Indeed, a measure of income disparity may not even be the most salient. The significant differences between the global winners and global losers may turn on such basic issues as the provision of clean water, access to shelter and health care and the chances of surviving infanthood. (R. Cohen and Kennedy 2000: 151)

Although there has been a tremendous amount of economic development in East Asia, South Asia, and Southeast Asia in recent decades, much of it has been accompanied by widening social stratification and environmental degradation. Africa, despite being endowed with tremendous natural resources, has become the home of the poorest people in the world. The *Human Development Report* of 2005 stated: "During the 1990s, 25 countries in Sub-Saharan Africa and 10 in Latin America experienced a sustained period of economic stagnation" (quoted in Surin 2009: 98). One scholar reports that whereas the top 20 percent of the world's population receives 75 percent of all income, the bottom 20 percent of the world's population receives a mere 1.5 percent of all income (G. Taylor 2008: 71). Invariably, wealth as opposed to income is always more concentrated, with the top 1 percent of the world's population owning 40 percent and bottom percent owning 40 percent of all wealth (G. Taylor 2008: 1). Derek Wall (2010: 13) reports:

Despite losing some of their wealth because of the recession, the world's three richest individuals—Bill Gates, Warren Buffet and Carlos Slim Helu—were worth $112 billion in 2009, according to the Forbes list of the world's billionaires. *Forbes* recorded a total of 793 billionaires in 2009. (Wall 2010: 13)

Although the super-wealthy tend to be concentrated in developed countries, one also finds a growing number of the super-wealthy in developing societies. Despite its stated commitment to social parity as an allegedly *socialist market economy*, since the late 1970s, China, under its modernization program, has experienced a marked increase in social inequality. Whereas inequality in China in 1980 was comparable to that of social democratic Germany (Gini coefficient = 0.250), by 2005, it was less equal than Russia (Gini coefficient = 0.45). The wealthiest 10 percent of the Chinese population earned seven times that of the poorest 10 percent of the Chinese population in the 1980s, but by 2005, that inequality had risen to a factor of 18. The richest 10 percent of the population now accounts for 45 percent of the country's wealth, the poorest only 1.4 percent (N. Smith 2010: 256).

As Table 3.4 indicates, the capitalist world system has a strong impact on the health profiles of its various nation-states. Countries with high gross national products per capita tend to have low infant mortality rates and high life expectancies, whereas countries with low gross domestic products per capita tend to have high infant mortality rates and low life expectancies. Certain postrevolutionary countries, such as China and Cuba, situated in the periphery or semiperiphery, exhibit a relatively healthy populace because of the commitments that they have made to eradicate malnutrition, improving sanitation, and providing both preventive and curative health services. Although Cuba remains a relatively poor country and has faced enormous economic difficulties following the collapse of the Soviet Union, it has an infant mortality rate of 5.1 per 1,000 live births and a life expectancy of 79.0 years, health statistics that compare favorably with those of the United States, the leading and richest member of the core. In reality, there is a considerable amount of variation in terms of health statistics of countries in the various sectors of the capitalist world system. Whereas the United States exhibits a relatively high GDP (PPP), it has the worst health statistics of any of the core countries in the world, in part because it is the only core country without some kind of national health plan, and it has the highest degree of social inequality of any country in the core. Although Spain is in the upper echelon of the semiperiphery, it boasts better health statistics than the United States. In addition to having a national plan, Spaniards tend to include a lot of fish, vegetables, and fruit in their diets and follow a relatively relaxed lifestyle compared with many Americans who consume a substantial amount of "junk food," are overworked, and/or live hectic lives. Table 3.4 is only a rough comparative overview of health within the context of the capitalist world system. A detailed comparison of disparities in terms of health outcomes within the system would require a systemic analysis of its various nation-states, taking into consideration numerous factors, including the degree of social

Table 3.4
A Profile of Health in the Capitalist World System—Selected Countries

	GDP per capita (PPP, 2008, $US)	Infant Mortality (per 1,000 live births)	Life Expectancy at Birth (years) for 2005–2010
Core			
Norway	58,810	3.0	81.0
USA	47,094	6.81	79.6
Switzerland	39,849	3.75	82.2
Australia	38,692	4.66	81.9
Canada	38,668	5.22	81.0
Germany	35,308	3.77	80.2
Japan	34,692	2.62	83.2
Semiperiphery			
Spain	29,661	3.76	81.3
Saudi Arabia	24,726	18.5	73.3
Russian Federation	15,258	11.3	67.2
Mexico	13,974	16.7	76.7
Turkey	13,359	24.0	72.2
Brazil	10,607	23.5	72.9
China	7,258	22.0	73.5
Periphery			
Bolivia	4,357	45.6	66.3
Indonesia	3,957	28.8	71.5
India	3,337	52.9	64.4
Nigeria	2,156	96.1	48.4
Nicaragua	2,567	21.5	73.8
Kenya	1,628	64.7	55.6
Bangladesh	1,587	49.0	66.9
Ethiopia	992	72.4	56.1
Haiti	949	63.1	61.7
Cuba	—	5.12	79.0

Sources: GDP and life expectancy data: *Human Development Report 2010—20th Anniversary Edition.* United Nations Development Report. Infant mortality data: List of Countries by Infant Mortality Rate. Available at www.wikipedia.org. Accessed January 31, 2012. The World Bank employs a conversion called the purchasing power parity that takes into account differences in U.S. dollars from country to country.

inequality, the existence or absence of a national health plan, exposure to HIV/AIDS, lifestyle, and national and community cohesiveness.

Australian epidemiologist Anthony McMichael and C. Butler observe:

[T]he seeming paradox is that, while these collective disruptions to the global environment increase, the national indices of population are most improving. These health gains, reflect, in part, the continuing (often time-lagged) benefits from earlier health-related scientific and social advances; including public and domestic hygiene, vaccination, housing quality, antibiotics, primary health care, and, more recently, the benefits from antismoking campaigns, screening programs, and life-saving tertiary care. (McMichael and Butler 2011: 181–182)

Although conversely, there may a time lag between environmental degradation and human impacts. For example, the intensification of the HIV/AIDS epidemic in certain regions of the world, particularly sub-Saharan Africa, has already contributed to declining life expectancies in those regions. Furthermore, urbanization and increased geographic mobility are contributing to widespread decline of social support systems, such as extended family structures, and thus to increasing psychological depression.

Although globalization has been a feature of the capitalist world system since its inception, corporate and government policy makers throughout the globe have increasingly relied on a political-economic perspective referred to as *neoliberalism* that essentially maintains that corporate profit making will result in a trickle-down improvement of socioeconomic and health conditions, with minimal state intervention, to address the health and social needs of the poor. The World Bank's neoliberal policy of *structural adjustment,* however, has fostered privatization of social and health services that in turn has adversely affected the poor around the globe. The deleterious impact of neoliberalism on the poor is documented in *Dying for Growth* (Kim, Millen, Irwin, and Gershman, 2000), an ambitious and encyclopedic project emanating from the collaborative efforts of an interdisciplinary team, which includes several medical anthropologists, based at the Institute for Health and Social Justice in Cambridge, Massachusetts.

Private multinational corporations and state corporations in both capitalist and postrevolutionary or socialist-oriented societies have created not only a global factory but also a new global ecosystem characterized by extensive motor vehicle pollution, acid rain, toxic and radioactive waste, defoliation, and desertification. Anthropologist John Bodley (1996) contends that the environmental crises provoked by "industrial civilization" produces many social problems, including overpopulation, overconsumption, poverty, war, crime, and many personal crises, including a wide array of health problems. Indeed, some analysts, such as Andre Gorz, argue that capitalism is on the verge of self-destruction because of its emphasis on ever-expanding production:

Economic growth, which was supposed to ensure the affluence and well-being of everyone, has created needs more quickly than it could satisfy them, and has led to a series of dead ends which are not solely economic in character: capitalist growth is in crisis not only because it is capitalist but also because it is encountering physical limits. . . . It is a crisis in the character of work: a crisis in our relations with nature, with our bodies, with future generations, with history: a crisis of urban life, of habitat, of medical practice, of education, of science. (Gorz 1980; 11–12)

To a greater or lesser degree, all human societies encroach on and modify the natural environment. Foragers contributed to the creation of grasslands, pastoralists overgrazed their lands, and peasants caused deforestation. The emergence of social mechanisms for harnessing large amounts of energy from the environment contributed to what Ruyle (1977: 623) terms "predatory ruling classes." The dangers of ecological self-destruction that plagued ancient state societies became even more pronounced with the advent of industrial capitalism around 1800, growing ever greater with the passage of time. The Industrial Revolution allowed for the harnessing of nonrenewable fossil fuels—namely, coal, petroleum, and natural gas—and humans came to rely increasingly on machine power rather than the energy derived from humans, animals, and even water and wind.

In *The Accumulation of Capital*, Rosa Luxemburg (1959, orig. 1913) argued that capital accumulation would lead to environmental degradation. This has been recognized even by non-Marxian scholars. Nearly forty years ago, Meadows et al. (1972), in their seminal book *The Limits to Growth*, recognized that capital accumulation would prove to be environmentally unsustainable by 2100 if unchecked. A thirty-year update for the book essentially confirms the original findings (Meadows, Randers, and Meadows 2004). The Limits to Growth project was part of a larger study called the Project on the Predicament of Mankind sponsored by the Club of Rome, a collection of prominent business executives and mainstream economists from the United States, Western Europe, and Japan who were assembled by Fiat executive Auerlio Peccei. The Limits of Growth project advocated a no-growth economy and a redistribution of income sufficient to guarantee everyone a subsistence income while maintaining a capitalist economic system, a stance that contradicts the need for capitalism to grow or die out. According to Resistance, an Australian-based socialist group,

Under capitalism, no-growth periods are produced by the inherent tendency of capitalist production to outstrip the market. During such crises (commonly called recessions) the owners of industry show no inclination to distribute the necessities of life to workers thrown on the scrapheap by production cutbacks. (Resistance 1999: 43)

In essence, capitalism lacks a concept of sufficiency, of individuals having enough and demands continual growth. If it does not grow, it may implode into an economic crisis, as occurred during the Great Depression of the 1930s.

Table 3.5 depicts the annual energy consumption for various world regions in 2004.

Table 3.5
Annual Energy Consumption for Various World Regions, 2004

Region	Percentage Share
Asia and Oceania	31
North America	27
Europe	19
Eurasia	10
Middle East	5
Central and South America	5
Africa	3

Source: Adapted from Burman (2007: 20).

Chivers (2009: 103) reports the following approximate figures of energy use per capita (kWh) in selected countries in 2008: Canada, 96,000; United States, 89,000; Australia, 75,000; European Union, 48,000; China, 19,000; Tanzania, 4,000; and Nepal, 3,500. Bear in mind, in all of these countries, there are class differences in terms of energy utilization. Klare (2008: 33) observes that the "worldwide requirement for primary energy is expected to rise by 57 percent between 2004 and 2030," with much of the growth occurring in Asia, particularly China and India.

Table 3.6 depicts that ecological footprint of various categories of countries, regions, and selected specific countries. The term *ecological footprint* refers to a measurement in global hectares, which aggregates six types of productive areas: (1) cropland, (2) grazing land, (3) forest, (4) fishing ground, (5) built-up land, and (6) land area required to absorb CO_2 for fossil fuel use (Wackernagel and Rees 1996). The United States has the highest per capita ecological footprint of any country, considerably higher than many developed societies, particularly in Europe. Specific countries vary widely in the ecological footprints of specific individuals. Even in a developed country, a wealthy family with multiple residences and motor vehicles and frequent holidays in far-off places leaves a much greater ecological footprint than a slum dweller or homeless person does. A profound form of environmental degradation around the world is deforestation. Deforestation once was primarily a phenomenon of temperate regions, such as Europe and North America but occurs now primarily in the tropical zones of the developing countries, such as Brazil, Indonesia, and other Southeast Asian countries. The 3.6 billion hectares (a hectare is 2.41 acres) in existence in 1980 declined by 5 percent to 3.2 billion hectares by 1995 (Rosa and Dietz 2010: 23). Urban sprawl has been a major factor accounting for deforestation.

Table 3.6
Ecological Footprint of World Regions, and Selected Countries, 2007

	Population (millions)	Ecological Footprint (Global Hectacres per capita)
World	6,671.6	2.7
High-income countries	1,031.4	6.1
Middle-income countries	4,323.4	2.0
Low-income countries	1,303.3	1.2
Unclassified countries	13.5	
Africa	963.9	1.4
Congo, Democratic Republic of	62.5	0.8
Egypt	80.1	1.7
Ethiopia	78.6	1.1
Kenya	37.8	1.1
Nigeria	147.7	1.4
South Africa	49.2	2.3
Asia	4,031.2	1.8
Afghanistan	26.3	0.6
Bangladesh	157.8	0.6
China	1,336.6	2.2
India	1,164.7	0.9
Indonesia	224.7	1.2
Japan	127.4	4.7
Kuwait	2.9	6.3
Nepal	28.3	3.6
Pakistan	173.2	0.8
Qatar	1.1	10.5
Timor-Leste	1.1	0.4
United Arab Emirates	6.2	10.7
Europe	730.9	4.7
Albania	3.1	1.9
Denmark	5.4	8.3
Germany	82.3	5.1
Russian Federation	141.9	4.4
Spain	44.1	5.4
United Kingdom	61.1	4.9
Latin America/Caribbean	69.5	2.6
Bolivia	9.5	2.6
Brazil	190.1	2.9
Cuba	11.2	1.9
Haiti	9.7	0.7
Peru	28.5	1.5
Uruguay	3.3	5.1
Venezuela	27.7	2.9
North America	341.6	7.9
Canada	32.9	7.0
Mexico	107.5	3.0
USA	308.7	8.0

Table 3.6
(continued)

	Population (millions)	Ecological Footprint (Global Hectares per capita)
Oceania	34.5	5.4
Australia	20.9	6.8
New Zealand	4.2	4.9
Papua New Guinea	6.4	2.1

Source: Adapted from Ecological Footprint and Biocapacity, 2007. Global Footprint Network, www.footprintnetwork.org, extracted on October 12, 2010.

We refer to the approach we find most useful—in considering the complex interaction of political economy and environment, particularly under capitalism—as *political ecology*. Conventional biocultural medical anthropology tends to downplay political and economic factors and thus fails to fully "consider the relation of people to their environment in all its complexity" (Turshen 1977: 48). We believe that, on the contrary, critical medical anthropology needs to treat political economy and political ecology as inseparable. As Howard L. Parsons has argued,

Economy is a matter of ecology: it has to do with the production and distribution of goods and services in the context of human society and nature. . . . [It recognizes that] under the ecological practices of monopoly capitalism, the natural environment is being destroyed along with the social environment. (Parsons 1977: xii)

Like critical medical anthropology, political ecology is committed to praxis—the merger of theory and social action. In other words, political ecology recognizes that humans not only can comprehend the complexities of their social reality but also ultimately must find a way to end those practices and patterns of social relation that exploit and oppress human populations, causing disease, malnutrition, and injury and destroying the fragile ecosystem of which they are a part. As Turshen (1977: 17) maintains, political ecology "gives central importance to human agency in the transformation of the complex, interacting web that characterizes the environment." As critical medical anthropologists, we seek to contribute to a larger interdisciplinary endeavor that can be termed the *political ecology of health* (Baer 1996; Singer 1998a) and to collaborate with various biocultural anthropologists, who in their efforts to incorporate the political economy of health, seek to develop a "critical biocultural anthropology" (Goodman and Leatherman 1998; Singer 2001).

Scholars interested in the political economy/political ecology of health, among whose ranks critical medical anthropologists are increasingly represented, have considered a wide array of political/ecologically-induced health problems, including malaria, occupational accidents, and cancer. The social production of black-lung disease among coal miners in eastern Kentucky is the focus of Barbara Kopple's Academy Award–winning *Harlan County USA*, an excellent 1976 documentary film (Criterion Collection, http://www.criterion.com/films/777-harlan-county-usa). Fortunately, the miners portrayed in the film became part of a larger black-lung movement that emerged in southern Appalachia in the late 1960s. The national debate over health and safety conditions in U.S. coal mines, much worse than in countries such as Britain, Germany, and Australia where the labor movement historically has been much stronger, eventually pressured Congress to pass in December 1969 the Coal Mine Health and Safety Act, "which detailed to an unprecedented degree mandatory work practices throughout the industry and offered compensation to miners disabled by black lung and the widows of miners who died from the disease" (B. Smith 1981: 352).

In the following "Closer Looks," we examine two health problems. The first of these is malaria, a long-standing infectious disease that continues to be endemic in many Third World countries. The second is related to a relatively recent technological development, the motor vehicle—a form of transportation that continues to spread around the globe.

"A Closer Look"

MALARIA IN THE THIRD WORLD: A PERSISTING DISEASE OF POVERTY

Despite repeated campaigns to eradicate or control it, malaria continues to plague massive numbers of people in certain parts of the Third World. Of an estimated 200 million victims of this dreaded disease, some two million people die of it annually (McElroy and Townsend 1989: 84). In Africa alone, an estimated one million people, mostly children under six years of age, die from malaria each year (Mascie-Taylor 1993: 30). The most common form of malaria is transmitted by a protozoan parasite called *Plasmodium falciparum*, which lives in red blood cells and is transmitted from person to person by various species of mosquitoes. The symptoms of malaria include a fever, which sometimes recurs every second or third day, anemia, splenomegaly, headaches, and a wide array of other symptoms. The human host requires many years of repeated infections before he or she becomes more or less immune to the disease. Although malaria appears to be an ancient disease, the environmental conditions for its transmission are greatly enhanced when a human population clears the forest environment to the extent that pools of stagnant water are created.

Frank Livingstone (1958) conducted a now-classic study that demonstrated that malaria became endemic in sub-Saharan Africa about two thousand years ago when Bantu peoples entered the sub-Saharan tropic rain forest and introduced horticulture. The Bantu horticultural villages transformed the African ecology by creating sunlit, stagnant pools of water that allowed mosquitoes to breed. The introduction of horticulture and agriculture in other parts of the world, including South Asia, Southeast Asia, the Mediterranean area, and the Americas, also contributed to endemic outbreaks of malaria. Falciparum malaria was probably introduced to the Americas when slave ships transported mosquitoes that followed many of their passengers, most of whom were slated to work on plantations. Malaria is not confined to tropical and semitropical environments. Outbreaks of malaria also occurred in temperate areas, such as southern Canada and New England during the seventeenth century and the frontier of the Pacific Northwest during the nineteenth century.

Initially European colonialists often ignored the impact of malaria on indigenous populations. Conversely, as indigenous peoples and peasants in conquered state societies were recruited for agricultural work on plantations, colonial powers and corporate-funded foundations came to implement extensive public health campaigns to ensure a productive labor force. The Rockefeller Foundation played a key role in malaria and hookworm control in both the U.S. South and in China (E. R. Brown 1979). According to Cleaver (1977: 567), such campaigns to control malaria and other infectious diseases in China were part and parcel of an effort to stem peasant uprisings. Conversely, public protests often prompted corporate interests and states to undertake public health projects. Turshen (1989: 57) delineates four basic approaches that corporate interests, states, and, more recently, international health organizations such as the WHO have utilized in their efforts to eradicate or control malaria: (1) the use of drugs or chemotherapy to kill the disease in its human host, (2) the use of insecticides such as DDT to kill the parasite along with its insect vector, (3) the adoption of lifestyle changes such as the proper use of mosquito netting on beds, and (4) an environmental approach—one implemented before the invention of DDT—that "deprives the mosquito of its habitat by draining pools of stagnant water, by filling in ditches and open drains where water collects, and by draining or eliminating swamps and marshes." Although constituting a source of profits for the pharmaceutical industry, chemotherapy as a method of malaria control is of limited value because parasites quickly develop resistance to drugs. DDT, which was used in a global malaria campaign undertaken by the WHO and many Third World states beginning in the 1950s, had adverse effects on the environment, created other health problems, and also was counteracted by the development of resistant strains of mosquitoes.

Despite initial success, the international effort to eradicate malaria underwent a reversal in the 1970s, with new outbreaks of the disease occurring in places such as India, Pakistan, Afghanistan, Southeast Asia, Central America, and Haiti. The WHO identified several reasons for the resurgence of malaria, including the increasing resistance of mosquitoes and parasites to pesticides and drugs, the inadequate administration of eradication programs, insufficient medical research on malaria itself, a paucity of adequately trained public health personnel, limited supplies of pesticides and drugs, the lack of malaria-control strategies in hydraulic development projects, and poor health care facilities. Furthermore, the WHO recognized that the overall economic underdevelopment of Third World countries contributed to the eruption of a malaria epidemic.

Critical social scientists have offered a variety of explanations for the upsurge of malaria. Harry Cleaver (1977) maintains that various sectors of business and a number of national governments have allowed malaria to spread to counteract the protest efforts of workers who have challenged exploitative economic practices and political oppression. He asserts corporate interests and various governments tried to undercut wage struggles by creating international inflation through shortages, especially in energy and food. The austerity measures used to counteract inflation resulted in cutbacks in public health measures, including those for malaria eradication or control. In 1973, the government of the Philippines, under the notorious dictator Ferdinand Marcos, responded to the demands of Moslem rebels in Mindanao and the Sulu Archipelago by deciding to "stop malaria control spraying on at least one important island in order to help the sickness spread among the insurgent population" (Cleaver 1977: 576).

Chapin and Wassertrom (1981) maintain that the increase of malaria resulted from growth of agribusinesses on a global scale. They conclude that malaria tends to be resurgent or appear in epidemic proportions for the first time in areas where pesticide-intensive cash cropping has occurred. In her study of a long history of campaigns to eradicate or control malaria in the Sudan, a country with a high prevalence of malaria, anthropologist Ellen Gruenbaum (1983) argues the ongoing economic dependence of that poor country on export agriculture for foreign currency serves to trap it in a never-ceasing battle against this debilitating disease. At the global level, as Turshen (1989: 162) so aptly observes, a meaningful antimalarial campaign has to date "come into conflict with overriding political and economic considerations, namely the opposition of urban elites to rural improvements and of agribusinesses to any restraints, such as restrictions on the use of DDT, which would affect the profitable green revolution." Furthermore, pharmaceutical companies and insecticide-producing chemical companies have a heavy investment in conventional approaches to malarial control. Finally, effective malaria eradication requires the existence of adequate national health services, which Third World countries are not in a position to support as long as they are embedded as peripheral political-economic entities of the capitalist world system.

"A Closer Look"

MOTOR VEHICLES ARE DANGEROUS TO YOUR HEALTH

The motor vehicle, with its internal combustion engine, perhaps more than any other machine embodies the ecological contradictions of capitalism. However, as Sweezy (1973) notes, the "political economy of the automobile" remains a relatively unexplored topic. The reality that North Americans love their cars is captured in James J. Flink's book *The Car Culture*. He observes, "During the 1920s automobility became the backbone of a new consumer-goods-oriented society and economy that has persisted into the present" (Flink 1973: 140). By this time, as Barnet and Cavanaugh (1994: 262) so aptly note, "the car became a primary locus of recreation, a badge of affluence, a power fantasy on wheels, a gleaming sex symbol," all images that have been heavily promoted by the automobile industry through intensive advertising. Automobiles constitute the second most expensive commodity (after homes) that Americans purchase. In 1990, Americans spent 31.3 percent of their incomes on housing and 18.1 percent of their income on motor vehicles (Freund and Martin 1993: 16). In recent decades, automobile firms have been searching for new markets in the Third World and, with the collapse of the Soviet bloc, in Eastern Europe. According to Dicken (2003: 359),

in the Americas, both Canada and Mexico are tightly enmeshed with the US automobile industry . . . while Brazil remains the major automobile production centre in Latin America. The most striking new development of recent years has been the sudden emergence of South Korea as an important producer. As recently as the early 1980s, Korea was producing only 20,000 automobiles. In 2000 Korean output was 2.4 *million* (6 percent of the world total). Thailand has evolved into the "car capital" of Southeast Asia with many major foreign companies having manufacturing facilities there.

The Chinese automobile industry consists of state companies as well as a number of joint operations between these companies and foreign companies, including Volkswagen, Toyota, Nissan, Honda, Hyundai, and General Motors (Dicken 2003: 396–397). The most dramatic instance in the growth of motor vehicles in the developing world is China. Jared

Diamond (2005: 362) reports that the "number of motor vehicles (mostly trucks and buses) increased 15-fold between 1980 and 2001, cars 130-fold." According to Sachs (2008: 76), "China's annual production is now soaring, up to around 7 million per year as of 2006 as compared with just 2 million in the year 2000." Various studies project that China will have approximately 200 million cars by 2020 and nearly 400 million cars by 2030 (Montgomery 2010: 37).

Whereas in 1951 India had an estimated 300,000 cars, this number had increased to about 85 million by 2005 (Shiva 2008:52). Tata launched the mini-car Nano in 2008 as an alleged "people's car" and projected producing a million of them per annum in 2011. Even in Singapore, which has an excellent public transport system, many affluent people are being seduced by the culture of automobility. Although Singapore has a lower private motor vehicle ownership than cities of similar size in the core, this bustling and prosperous city in the semiperiphery went from about 100 cars per 1,000 people in 1970 to 130 cars per 1,000 people in 2008, excluding foreigners (M. A. Brown and Sovacool 2011: 279). Undoubtedly, if it had not been for numerous schemes such as levies on new vehicles and restricted access of cars to the CBD during peak travel hours, the increase probably would have been more dramatic as it has been in China, India, and other developing countries. Sperling and Gordon (2010: 4) project there will be more than 2 billion motor vehicles worldwide, at least half of them cars, by 2020.

Motor vehicles have had major impacts on not only patterns of consumption but also energy utilization, the environment, settlement patterns, social relations, public policy, congestion, and last, but not least, health. During the Cold War era of the 1950s and early 1960s, General Motors urged patriotic U.S. citizens to "see the USA in your Chevrolet." Such advertisements on the part of the automobile industry served to seduce North Americans away from what was once a relatively well-developed mass transportation system, which included passenger trains, numerous intercity bus lines, and extensive urban and interurban trolley lines. Indeed, a consortium, called National City Lines, consisting of General Motors, Standard Oil of New Jersey, and the Firestone Tire and Rubber Company, spent $9 million by 1950 to obtain control of street railway companies in sixteen states and convert[ed] them to less efficient GM buses.

The companies were sold to operators who signed contracts specifying that they would buy GM equipment. . . . National City Lines in 1940 began buying up and scrapping parts of Pacific Electric, the world's largest interurban electric rail system, which by 1945 served 110 million passengers in fifty-six smog-free Southern California communities. Eleven hundred miles of Pacific Electric's track were torn up, and the system went out of service in 1961, as Southern California commuters came to rely narrowly on freeways. (Flink 1973: 220)

In describing the economic situation in U.S. society during the 1970s, Sweezy (1973: 7) contended that the "private interests which cluster around and are directly or indirectly dependent upon the automobile for their prosperity are quantitatively far more numerous and wealthy than those similarly related to any other commodity or complex of commodities in the U.S. economy." Automobile advertisements frequently have promised and continue to promise their target populations that they will achieve power, prestige, freedom, sexual desirability, and prowess if they choose to become the proud owners of a highly individualized form of transportation. In conjunction with automobile driving, Freund and McGuire (1991: 60) note, "Many young males are socialized into taking lots of risks and into feeling or appearing invulnerable; media messages glorify speed and risk-taking."

Despite the messages conveyed by advertisements promoting its sale as well as by the mass media as a whole, the automobile is not merely a toy or an extension of the male genitalia but a highly lethal machine. Visitors to other countries, particularly Western Europe and Japan, have noted that "automobilization" (Sweezy 1973: 7) has become a global phenomenon. Along with industrial pollution, motor vehicles have transformed many cities around the world, particularly ones in the Third World such as Mexico City, into environmental disaster areas accompanied by a wide array of health problems. Of the estimated 4.4 million tons of human-generated pollutants emitted into the air of Mexico City in 1989, 76 percent were produced by motor vehicles (Freund and Martin 1993: 67). In contrast, of the 3.5 million tons of human-generated pollutants emitted into the air of Los Angeles—America's most polluted city—in 1985, 63 percent were created by motor vehicles. The rush-hour motor vehicle speeds have been reported to be 7 miles per hour in London, 12 miles per hour in Toyko, 17 miles per hour in Paris, and 33 miles per hour in Southern California (Freund and Martin 1993: 2). Indeed, Sweezy (1973: 4) compares auto congestion and pollution to the "outward symptoms of a disease with deep roots in the organs of the body." In other words, the automobile has become a major form of assault on the social and ecological body.

Motor vehicles also are a major contributor to climate change (Alvord 2000: 70–71). The Environmental Defense Fund (2007) released the following sobering statistics on motor vehicles and their contribution to greenhouse emissions in the United States alone:

- There are 232 million registered vehicles.
- The average U.S. car consumes 600 gallons of gasoline per year.
- The average U.S. car emits 12,000 pounds of CO_2 each year.
- U.S. cars and light trucks traveled 2.7 trillion miles in 2004.

- 30 percent of the world's automobiles are situated in the United States.
- The United States accounts for 45 percent of the world's automotive CO_2 emissions.

One of the major by-products of gasoline exhaust is benzopyrene, a carcinogenic chemical that is suspended in urban air. Motor vehicles emit carbon monoxide, sulfur oxides, and nitrous oxides, which in turn contribute to acid rain and human respiratory complications. The American Lung Association estimated that in 1985 motor vehicle pollution contributed to some 120,000 deaths in the United States (Freund and Martin 1993: 29). Sixty percent of the residents of Calcutta, India, were found to have pollution-related respiratory problems (Freund and Martin 1993: 67).

In addition to their destructive impact on the environment, motor vehicles are a major source of accidents around the world. Freund and McGuire (1991) present the following sobering statistics on auto accidents in the United States country:

While the death rate due to auto accidents in the United States is by no means the highest among the industrialized countries, some 43,000 to 53,000 Americans die each year in such accidents, producing a death rate of over 26 deaths per 100,000 population. Worldwide, some 200,000 people died in traffic accidents in 1985. There are approximately 4 to 5 million injuries related to motor vehicles in the United States. Of these, 500,000 people require hospitalization. . . . Auto accidents are a leading cause of death for young people between the ages of five and twenty-four; young males between the ages of fourteen and twenty-four are at highest risk. Per passenger mile, cars are more dangerous than trains, buses, or planes. (Freund and McGuire 1991: 59)

Forman, Watchko, and Segui-Gomez (2011) refer to deaths and injury from automobile collisions as an "overlooked epidemic" deserving of medical anthropological study. Automobile accidents reportedly result in more than 1.2 million deaths per year worldwide and an estimated 25 million to 50 million injuries (Brown and Sovacool 2011: 27). An epidemiological study revealed that in the United States in 2008, 36,710 deaths resulted from automobile fatalities and another 65,638 deaths resulted from particulate-matter pollution, much of it due to motor vehicle exhaust fumes (Sovacool 2010). The motor vehicle accident appears to be the highest in developing countries, which have more recently acquired cars and other motor vehicles compared with developed countries. According to Smeed's Law following research conducted by a R. J. Smeed, a British statistician and road-safety expert, the number of motor fatalities tend to rise as the number of motor vehicles on the road rise up to a certain point, but then the fatality rates begin to drop and even the absolute numbers of fatalities drop (Vanderbilt 2008: 231). Eventually governments pass regulations that promote safety, such as the requirement to wear seat belts and restrictions on the amount of alcohol that a driver may consume shortly before driving, and drivers become more cautious in their road behavior. According to Vanderbilt (2008: 231–232), "In China, one sees things . . . like bicycles traveling on restricted highways, scooter drivers carrying several children without helmets, and drivers stopping on the highway to urinate—but presumably, a number of years down the road, these things will largely be only memories." Hopefully so, but driver safety regulations will not eradicate the pollution and greenhouse gases emitted by motor vehicles in a country with a rapidly growing number of motor vehicles.

Motor vehicles also pose hazards for pedestrians and cyclists. The National Safety Council reported some 6,600 pedestrian deaths and 800 cyclist deaths in 1989 in the United States (Freund and Martin 1993: 102). Motor vehicle driving, particularly under congested conditions, also induces stress and heightened blood pressure, contributes to medical complications such as lumbar disk herniation, or motorist's spine, and contributes to sedentarization. Truck drivers in particular suffer a high rate of back injuries. City bus drivers around the world experience a great deal of stress, particularly during peaks hours. Reportedly, "[m]edical ailments send more than half of them into early retirement" (Vanderbilt 2008: 141).

Auto transportation discourages patterns of sociability that are vital to mental health in that most motorists, especially in First World countries, drive alone. With the decline of public transportation, especially in the United States, mothers in particular function as chauffeurs for their children as they transport them hither and yon in sprawling suburban developments. Low-income people often find themselves without adequate transportation in cities where an increasing number of jobs are located in the suburbs.

Public awareness of some aspects of motor vehicle transportation reached new heights with the publication of Ralph Nader's (1965) book *Unsafe at Any Speed*. Although there have been efforts to reduce motor vehicle accidents with the installation of seat belts and other safety devices and, at least until 1995, a lowering of speed limits, such measures tend to focus on altering individual behavior. Furthermore, the automobile industry lobby has consistently resisted the passage of regulations to require air bags in cars. In reality, as Jacoby (1975: 141) observes, the victim of an automobile accident is a "victim of an obsolete transportation system kept alive by the necessities of profit." Unfortunately, a powerful lobby consisting of the automobile industry, petroleum companies, and trucking companies, poses a power barrier to the development of effective public transportations, especially in most American urban areas. Whereas heavy trucks contribute more than 95 percent of the highway deterioration in the United States, trucking firms pay only 29 percent of the country's highway bill (Freund and Martin 1993: 2).

It follows, following Freund and McGuire (1991: 60), that an ecological approach to addressing the health consequences of the automobilization of society requires "changing the social and physical environment (e.g., building safer highways), producing safer cars, and making many alternative ways of traveling available to drivers." Unfortunately, the sanctity of the automobile as an integral component of U.S. culture has virtually gone unchallenged. In contrast, the Green movement in Western Europe has mobilized as a counterhegemonic opposition to the automobilization of society by emphasizing the need for people to rely on other forms of transportation, including cycling. Environmentalists in Germany, for example, attempt to promote cycling as a form of transportation by sponsoring demonstrations consisting of bikers riding through city streets to slow or halt traffic. However, although cycling constitutes an "environmentally friendly" mode of transportation as well a healthy means to provide the body with aerobic exercise, it will remain a highly dangerous activity as long as the streets and highways are filled with fast-moving motor vehicles (increasingly occupied by distracted drivers busily cutting business deals or socializing on car telephones and thus endangering lives even further) and exhaust fumes.

ENVIRONMENTAL DEVASTATION IN POSTREVOLUTIONARY SOCIETIES

Critics of neo-Marxian theory often argue that although capitalism may indeed have had a devastating impact on the environment, postrevolutionary or socialist-oriented societies have a dismal record of environmental destruction. Indeed, it is essential that critical medical anthropologists and other critical social scientists come to grips with the realities of environmental destruction in these societies. Some of the contributors to journals such as *Capitalism, Nature, and Socialism; Society and Nature: The International Journal of Political Ecology;* the *Journal of Political Ecology;* and *EcoSocialist Review* (sources unfortunately rarely cited in the medical anthropology literature) have attempted to grapple with these realities.

Postrevolutionary societies have had, by and large, a poor environmental record. The fast-paced drive for industrialization, in part rooted in the threat posed by the capitalist countries, contributed to serious environmental damage. The managerial objective of producing maximum output at minimum cost resulted in high levels of air, water, and soil pollution and a lack of safety precautions in industrial and nuclear power plants. Feshbach and Friendly (1992: 40) maintain that the "plan and its fulfillment became engines of destruction geared to consume, not conserve, the natural wealth and human strength of the Soviet Union." The Soviet Union exhibited the worst instances of radioactive contamination, the most spectacular being that of the Chernobyl nuclear plant, and Czechoslovakia and Poland had the highest levels of industrial pollution in Europe and perhaps in the world (Commoner 1990: 219–220).

According to Yih, such instances of environmental devastation are rooted in the conditions under which postrevolutionary societies developed:

relative underdevelopment, external aggression, and, especially for the small, dependent economies of the Third World, a disadvantaged position in the international market. The corresponding pressures to satisfy the material needs of the populations, ensure adequate military defense, and continue producing and exporting cash crops and raw materials for foreign exchange, have led to an emphasis by socialist policy-makers on the accumulation by the state, the uncritical adoption of many features of capitalist development, and a largely abysmal record vis-à-vis the environment (although there are exceptions, of course). (Yih 1990: 22)

Furthermore, the weak development of democratic institutions in postrevolutionary societies and bureaucratic suppression of information about the environmental impact of agricultural and industrial practices had until recently inhibited the emergence of an independent environmental movement (O'Connor 1989: 99). Although *glasnost* permitted the emergence of a small Green movement in the Soviet Union, the official policy of *perestroika*, with its emphasis on production, and the serious disruption of the Soviet economy in what proved to be its last days served as impediments to the implementation of environmental protection regulations. The ongoing emphasis on capitalist practices and penetration of foreign capital into the new Commonwealth of Independent States, which encompasses the territory of the former Soviet Union without the Baltic republics and Georgia, may continue to exacerbate environmental problems rather than to resolve them.

CHAPTER 4

The Impact of Climate Change, Environmental Crises, and Disasters on Health

Almost all climate scientists, as well as all professional organizations of disciplines concerned with the environment, have come to the conclusion that climate change is both real and largely the result of human (i.e., anthropogenic) activities, particularly beginning with the Industrial Revolution. Thus, scholarly organizations such as the American Meteorological Society, the American Geophysical Union, and the American Association for the Advancement of Science have all reviewed the evidence and drawn the conclusion that the case for climate change and human modification of Earth's climate is compelling. As summarized by the American Public Health Association (2011), "The evidence is unequivocal; the Earth is warming and our climate is changing." Moreover, the evidence is growing that climate change has already had a serious impact on natural systems of the planet as well as visited significant economic, political, and health consequences on humanity and will continue to do so, at ever more rapid rates, as the twenty-first century unfolds.

Human populations have never faced an environmental problem on this scale before, certainly not since the end of the last glacial period about 12,500 years ago (a time when the total human population was quite small compared with the 7 billion people on the planet today). Climate change and its repercussions have become topics of increasing public awareness, although this awareness varies considerably from society to society, as well as within societies and over time, and has been affected by denials of global warming. Awareness of abrupt climate change has found its way into popular culture, the mainstream media, and science fiction. Al Gore's

2006 documentary film, *An Inconvenient Truth*, and accompanying book (Gore 2006) and the "Stern Report," authored by Nicholas Stern (2007), a former World Bank economist, in particular helped propel climate change into public consciousness around the world. No doubt, events such as Hurricane Katrina in 2003 and Hurricane Sandy in 2012; the intense and deadly heat waves in Europe in 2003, in Russia in 2010 and the intense drought in the U.S. in 2012; as well as increases in massive flooding in various locations have also heightened popular concern. Certainly all of the well-known environmentalist and conservationist organizations, including the Sierra Club, the World Wildlife Fund, Nature Conservancy, the National Audubon Society, Environmental Defense, and Green Peace, among many more, have pushed for action to slow or stop the global climate trend. A growing number of business leaders and politicians as well have come to embrace a form of *green capitalism*, which asserts that climate change poses a serious threat to the existing global economy but that capitalism has the capacity to reform itself, adopt new forms of energy and environmentally sustainable technologies, and continue to achieve economic expansion and profit-making. Conversely, various radical environmentalists, eco-socialists, and certain critical social scientists view climate change as yet one more of the contradictions, perhaps the most profound contradiction, of global capitalism and one that green capitalism cannot fix.

Although humans have been emitting greenhouse gases for centuries, the Industrial Revolution, with its heavy reliance on fossil fuels and capitalist treadmill of production and consumption, contributed to a new type of climatic change, not one generated so much by natural events but by human-induced or anthropogenic activities. Capitalism (even in its green form) is a global economic system that in its drive for profits requires ongoing accumulation and expansion. It fosters ever-expanding production and consumption (and waste) primarily for the making of profits for a few and, in the process, because they are rated of lesser importance than profit, sacrifices meeting basic human needs and achieving environmental sustainability.

Archeologist Brian Fagan (2008: xvii) asserts that "we've entered a time of sustained warming, which dates back to at least 1860, propelled in large part by humanity—by the greenhouse gases from fossil fuels." Although climate scientists debated for a long time whether recent climate change has been primarily a natural phenomenon rather than an anthropogenic one, the vast majority now agree that it has been largely created by the emission of various greenhouse gases, particularly carbon dioxide, which has increased from 280 parts per million (ppm) at the time of the Industrial Revolution to 390 ppm in 2010. In contrast, the level of CO_2 "varied between a minimum of 180 ppm and a maximum of 280 ppm" with the lower levels having occurred during glacial advance periods and the higher levels having occurred during interglacial periods over the course of some 400,000 years before 1800 (Ward 2010: 56).

The Australian Academy of Sciences (2010: 3) reports that climate models "estimate that by 2100, the average global temperature will be between 2°C (3.6°F) and 7°C (12.6°F) higher than preindustrial temperatures, depending on future greenhouse gas emission and on the ways that models represent the sensitivity of climate to small disturbances." Although most projections of climate change tend to focus on the twenty-first century as the point at which effects will become undeniable, climate models also indicate the climate change will continue well after 2100. Given that humanity has been on the face of the planet for some five to six million years, ongoing global warming and associated climatic and environmental changes raise the question of how long humanity can thrive, at least at its present numbers and social configurations and occupying much of its present-day places of habitation, into and beyond the 2100.

Although environmental sociologist John Bellamy Foster at the University of Oregon, who also serves as the editor of *Monthly Review* (a well-read socialist magazine), acknowledges that climate change constitutes the most serious ecological threat facing both humanity and planet, he views it as a manifestation of a larger global environmental crisis with its interrelated components. He asserts:

Independently of climate change, tropical forests are being cleared as a direct result of the search for profits. Soil destruction is occurring due to current agribusiness practices. Toxic wastes are being diffused through the environment. Nitrogen run-off from the overuse of fertilizer is affecting lakes, rivers, and ocean regions, contributing to oxygen-poor dead zones. (Foster 2010: 3)

In this chapter, we examine the nature and extent of the changes that are occurring; the human role in producing these changes; the kinds, sources, and global distribution of greenhouse gas emissions; the nature of the treadmill of commodity production and the world system in creating greenhouse emissions; social attitudes about climate change; the multiple health and social consequences of climate change; and other anthropocentric ecocrises and their unhealthy interactions with climate change.

HUMAN-INDUCED CLIMATE CHANGE

In the language of climate science, *forcings* are external boundary conditions or inputs to a climate model which affect climate. They include numerous agents, ranging from greenhouse gases to air pollution to reforestation or deforestation to carbon sinks, such as the ocean. Current forcings that can affect climate include (1) changes in the sun's energy output;

(2) variations in the distance of Earth from the sun, and in the angles at which solar radiation reaches various parts of Earth; (3) changes in the atmospheric and oceanic circulation systems; (4) changes in the earthly surface's absorption or radiation of energy as influenced by extent of the cloud cover and the nature of Earth's surface; (5) possibly volcanoes; and (6) the greenhouse effect (Farley 2009:69; Officer and Page 2009: 109). All of these forcings except for the last one are natural. Atmospheric CO_2 hovered between 180 and 300 ppm over the course of the past 650,000 years before recent times (Maslin 2009: 8). CO_2 hovered around 280 ppm during the past 10,000 years until the onset of the Industrial Revolution, which was heavily reliant on fossil fuels.

The greenhouse effect can be seen in temperature trends over time. In the Northern Hemisphere, the average temperature rose about 1°F (1.8°C) from 1900, declined 0.5°F (9.0°C) between 1940 and 1970, and then began to rapidly increase again (Officer and Page 2009). The period from 1940 to 1970 appears to be a deviation from the broader pattern. Indeed, many climate scientists in the early 1960s wondered if the temporary cooling phase was the onset of a new glacial stage of the last Ice Age or the start of a new Ice Age. In time and with new data, however, it became apparent that this short period of global cooling was a result of what has been called *global dimming,* as a result of various anthropogenic activities that hindered the penetration of sunlight from reaching Earth's surface. These anthropogenic activities included the effects of urbanization and manufacturing and increased motor vehicle and aircraft exhausts. Motor vehicles and aircraft contribute particulates to the atmosphere, which contribute to global dimming but also contribute greenhouse gases to the atmosphere, which in turn contribute to global warming. Global dimming diminished in developed societies as they shifted from heavy industrial activities but then outsourced these to various developing societies, such as China, that have embarked on paths of industrialization that "account for local cooling by reflecting considerable amounts of solar radiation back into the atmosphere" (Luke 2008: 125).

According to Ruddiman (2005: 172), "Industrial-era emissions of sulphate aerosols have probably cancelled part of the warming that greenhouse-gas emissions would have otherwise have caused." Furthermore, the decline in the intensity of sunspots during the 1960s and 1970s contributed to the cooling trend (Maslin 2009: 211). Even today, global dimming may be occurring in various places, such as in China, which have embarked on paths of intense industrialization that "account for local cooling by reflecting considerable amounts of solar radiation back into the atmosphere" (Luke 2008: 125).

According to the Intergovernmental Panel on Climate Change (IPCC; 2007), a UN body that periodically summarizes assessments of the state of climate change around the world, the current rate of warming has been about ten times faster than any rate in the past 10,000 years. Unless drastic steps are taken, the atmospheric CO_2 level will continue to rise rapidly during the course of the twenty-first century. The 2007 IPCC synthesis report predicts that global temperatures could rise further between 1.1°C and 6.4°C by 2100 and sea level could rise between 28 cm and 79 cm by 2100, even more if the melting of Greenland and Antarctica accelerate, which is a real possibility. The National Aeronautical and Space Administration reports that temperatures started to climb in 1977 and have been above the norm every year since. The twentieth century was the warmest century of the past millennium. NASA reports that 2005 and 2010 were tied for the status of the warmest year on record to date. The World Meteorological Organization maintained that 2005 was the hottest year since records began to be kept in 1850. According to NASA, the hottest temperature on record in Asia occurred in Pakistan, when the temperature hit 53°C in July 2010.

In early summer 2012, many parts of the United States experienced record-breaking temperatures, which had been preceded by the warmest March, the third warmest April, and the second warmest May on record. Freedman reports: "In Colorado, June 2012 was the warmest June on record, with temperatures averaging 6.4°F above the average. Seven other Western States had a top warm June" (Freedman 2012: 2).

Temperatures also soared in more easterly states and cities. For instance, St. Louis set an all-time June monthly high temperature on June 28 at a whopping 108°F. U.S. federal scientists claimed that July 2012 was the hottest month ever recorded in the lower 48 states, breaking a record set during the Dust Bowl of the 1930s (http://bigstory.ap.org/article/ouch-july-us-was-hottest-ever-history-books). In 2012, the United States repeatedly set new records for weather extremes based on the precise calculations that include drought, heavy rainfall, unusual temperatures, and storms. The average temperature in July 2012 was 77.6°F (43.1°C), thus breaking the old record, starting with record keeping in 1895, from July 1936 by 0.2°F, according to the National Oceanic and Atmospheric Administration. Along with Superstorm Sandy that blasted the northeastern United States, the "contiguous U.S. experienced the warmest year in the 1895–2012 period of record for the nation" (NOAA National Climatic Data Center 2012: 1). Outside of the United States, in May of 2012, temperatures soared in parts of India, claiming more than one hundred lives (Hindustan Times 2012). Down Under, Australia experienced its hottest month on record with a nationwide heat wave in January 2013, with an average mean maximum temperature of 36.92°C (Australian Bureau of Meteorology 2013). During that month, Sydney hit a record high of 45.8°C on January 18 and Hobart a record high of 41.8°C. Moona in South Australia had the highest temperature (49.6°C on January 12) recorded during the heat wave. Although parts of interior Australia were experiencing ravaging bushfires, coastal Queensland and New South Wales experienced heavy rainfall and flooding.

Australian atmospheric scientist A. Barrie Pittock (2008: 19) argues that given the uncertainties in climate science, "many scientists have consciously or unconsciously downplayed the more extreme possibilities at the high end of the uncertainty range in an attempt to appear moderate and 'responsible' (that is, to avoid scaring people)."

The Copenhagen Diagnosis, a report that seeks to synthesize most policy-relevant climate science published since the 2007 IPCC report, was released in time for UN Copenhagen conference in December 2009 (Allison et al. 2009: 5). The report indicates that 2008 constituted the ninth warmest year on record, one in which La Niña caused a temporary dip in average global temperature (Allison et al. 2009). Despite the fact that the sun exhibited extremely low brightness over the course of the previous three years (Allison et al. 2009), numerous temperature records were broken during this period. Years 2007, 2008, and 2009 saw the lowest summer Arctic sea ice cover ever recorded. The Northwest Passage and Northeast Passage simultaneously were ice-free for the first time in 2008, a phenomenon that was repeated in 2009. Every single year of the twenty-first century has been among top ten warmest years since instrumental records began, with winters warming faster than summers (Allison et al. 2009). Continuing marked increases in hot extremes and decreases in cold extremes are expected in most areas across the world (Allison et al. 2009: 15). *The Copenhagen Diagnosis* reports that the mean global temperature is expected to increase 2° to 7°C [3.6.2°–12.6°F] by 2100 (Allison et al. 2009: 49).

The warming trends noted above are having the following effects:

- The cryosphere is losing ice at an unusually rapid rate, with the rapid and general retreat of glaciers, and collapse of ice shelves.
- The oceans are warming, becoming more acidic, and rising.
- Animal species (plants too) are retreating to higher altitudes and latitudes.
- The most profound warming is occurring at the poles, with the Northern Hemisphere leading the Southern Hemisphere.

Greenhouse Gas Emissions

The principal greenhouse gases include carbon dioxide, nitrous oxide, methane, water vapor, the chlorofluorocarbons, and ozone. Carbon dioxide comes mainly from the burning of fossil fuels, deforestation, and the destruction of carbon-rich soils, and production of cement from limestone.

Current atmospheric CO_2 levels are higher than they have been in the past million years. Global CO_2 emissions have been growing at about 3 percent a year since 2000. Global emissions of CO_2 from fossil fuel combustion and cement production rose from 22.6 billion tons in 1990 to 31 billion in 2008, a 37 percent increase (Flavin and Engelman 2009:). U.S. CO_2 emissions from fossil fuel combustion grew by 27 percent between 1990 and 2008 and in China an astounding 150 percent, from 2.3 billion to 5.9 billion tons. While Russia, which underwent tremendous deindustrialization in the wake of the collapse of the Soviet system, saw a fall in emissions by one third between 1990 and 2005, China and India have more than doubled their emissions since 1990. Conversely, total greenhouse gas emissions appear to have dropped in 2009 due to the global financial crisis (Allison et al. 2009).

Atmospheric carbon dioxide reportedly has a "removal time of more than 100 years, perhaps as long as 1000 years" (Richter 2010: 21). Removal time, according to Richter (2010: 20), refers to "how long it would take for something to come out of the atmosphere if we stopped adding to it." Although methane (CH_4) has a removal time of about ten years, it is sixty-four times more powerful than CO_2 in terms of climate change potential, more than twenty years and twenty-three times over 100 years. Methane comes from biomass decomposition, coal mining, natural gas and oil system leakages, livestock production, waste water treatment, landfills, rice cultivation, burning of savannah, and to a degree from the burning of fossil fuels. Given problems with measuring methane levels in the atmosphere, some scientists contend that its impact generally has been underestimated. With rising temperatures and melting tundra, there is the danger that the methane locked up in permafrost and as hydrates in the oceans will be released into the atmosphere and significantly increase the current warming trend.

Nitrous oxide (N_2O) comes from the heavy use of nitrogen fertilizers in industrial agriculture, the production of synthetic materials, and the burning of fossil fuels. It is 296 times more powerful than CO_2 over a 100-year period and remains for 120 to 150 years.

The F-gas family consists of chlorofluorocarbons (CFCs), hydrofluorocarbons (HFCs), perfluorocarbons (PFCs), and sulphur hexafluoride (SF_6). Most of these gases come from refrigeration and air-conditioning, including in cars. They are used as solvents; as blowing agents in foams, aerosols, or propellants; and in fire extinguishers. The F-gases were developed by the chemical industry. The fluorocarbons have a lifetime of approximately 1,000 years (Richter 2010: 24).

Numerous climate scientists have attempted to define a "safe temperature" limit. *The Copenhagen Diagnosis* asserts that global greenhouse gas emissions need to peak between 2015 and 2020 and then to decline rapidly if global warming is to be limited to a maximum of 2°C above preindustrial values (Allison et al. 2009). Stabilizing CO_2 at 445 ppm would require a drop of 89 percent in global emissions. At 445 ppm, global temperature would still rise by 2°C (relative to preindustrial times) (Li 2008). Christopher Shaw (2010) queries the two-degree limit that numerous governments, corporations, the European Union, and even many nongovernmental organizations have adopted as the safe temperature limit. He argues that this arbitrarily designated limit "makes climate change a problem for the future which allows humanity to continue with 'business as usual' whilst the search for a techno-fix continues," an argument that anticipates our critique of existing climate regimes and green capitalism with its emphasis on ecological modernization that we discuss later in this book.

The IPCC distinguishes between Type I climate change, which is gradual, and Type II, which is much more abrupt and results in crossing *critical tipping points*. Pearce (2006: 346) asserts that both humanity and planet may be entering a "terra incognita climatically," which is manifesting itself in melting Arctic ice, the possible collapse of the West Antarctic ice sheet, the contraction and demise of the Amazonian rain forest, the acidification of the ocean, and the increasing emission of methane from a number of sources, including peat bogs.

Another profound danger from reaching tipping points includes the risk of a complete shutdown of circulation of the major Atlantic Ocean currents, resulting in a drastic cooling of Europe. The thermohaline circulation, which results from the interaction of temperature, salinity, and prevailing wind, constitutes the major driving force underlying the movement of water between the different oceans of the world is endangered as cold, fresh water from melting ice from the Arctic and Greenland icecaps hit the Atlantic Ocean. James Hansen, the Director of NASA's Goddard Institute of Space Studies based at Columbia University, and his colleagues argued in a 2007 paper for seeking to achieve of a limit of 1.7°C increase on the basis that potential changes above this level—including irreversible loss of Greenland and Antarctic ice sheets and species extinction—would be "highly disruptive" (Hare 2009: 19). Hansen maintains that humanity needs to reduce atmospheric carbon level below the present 390 ppm, to 350 ppm or less to avoid irrevocable damage to human societies and the planet. If a tipping point is passed, then a subsequent cooling of the climate system would not necessarily reverse the change.

GLOBAL CAPITALISM AS A GENERATOR OF CLIMATE CHANGE

Climate change perhaps more than any other environmental crisis illustrates the contradictions and unsustainability of global capitalism. Table 4.1

Table 4.1
Average Total CO_2 Emissions and CO_2/Unit GDP for Income Groups of Countries, 2000

Category of Countries	Average Total Emissions (million tons CO_2)	Average Cumulative CO_2/ Unit GDP
High-income countries (24)	120,162	0.1479
High-middle income (20)	5,917	0.2710
Middle income (33)	18,161	0.2960
Low income (54)	20,155	0.5262
Low income (61)	28,834	0.4066

Source: Adapted from Roberts and Parks (2007: 147).

indicates that while the total CO_2 emissions in the high-income countries greatly exceeds the total CO_2 dioxide emissions in the high-middle, middle-income, and low-income countries combined, the production efficiency in all of the latter countries is worse than that for the high-income countries. As Roberts et al. (2003: 288) observe, developing countries have "enough fossil-fuel dependent technology to compete in the world market, but not enough sophisticated infrastructure to do so efficiently."

Although production efficiency has tended to improve over time in developed countries, there has also been a tendency for total CO_2 emissions and per capita emissions to increase, as occurred in most developed countries, including the United States, Canada, the Netherlands, Japan, Austria, and Australia between 1975 and 1996 (Clark and York 2005: 412). Such a trend is consistent with the need of global capitalism to continually grow. Roberts, Grimes, and Manale (2003) identify various social factors underlying the intensity of production of CO_2 within countries, as defined by quantity of CO_2 released for each unit of GDP/capita. Advanced capitalist (i.e., developed countries) are both economically able to and politically pressured by their respective citizen environmental movements to reduce pollution (Roberts, Grimes, and Manale 2003). In 2005, the top ten emitters of greenhouse gases were either specific developed countries, such as the United States, Japan, and Canada, as well as the European Union, or the "large emerging market economies" (e.g., China, India, Brazil, Mexico, and Indonesia; Barbier 2010: 35). Altogether, already developed and emerging developed countries accounted for more than 70 percent of the world's greenhouse gas emissions in 2010.

In terms of historical responsibility in global carbon emissions in the years between 1750 and 2006, the United States accounted for 28 percent, the United Kingdom 6 percent, Japan 4 percent, Russia 8 percent, Germany 7 percent, the remainder of Europe 18 percent, and China 8 percent

(Schor 2010). Conversely, "Per resident, the UK, the US, Russia, Belgium and Germany [in that order] have the largest historical responsibility for CO_2 emissions, at around 1,000 tonnes per person living today" in contrast to India and China which "don't even make it into the top 20" (Chivers 2009: 89). In 2008, the single largest producer of CO_2 was the small Arabian Peninsula country of Qatar (which also has the world's highest GDP) at 53.5 metric tons per capita, compared with the United States at 17.5. The Qatar population, however, is under 2 million (including 1.5 million expatriate workers from other countries), whereas the U.S. population is approximately 313 million people.

Ward (2010: 63) reports that the work of climate scientists associated with RealClimate.org suggested that "2008 promised to have the highest rate ever" of CO_2 entering the atmosphere, despite the economic downturn of 2007 and 2008 as well as efforts to lower emissions. According to Ward (2010: 63), the "published figures for 2007 showed a 3 percent increase in the amount of carbon put into the atmosphere compared to the year before" (Ward 2010: 63). The Global Carbon Project, a collaborative initiative of several environmental and environmental research organizations, reports:

The annual growth rate of atmospheric CO_2 was 1.6 ppm in 2009, below the average for the period 2000–2009 of 1.9 ppm per year (ppm = parts per million). The mean growth rate for the previous 20 years was about 1.5 ppm per year. (Global Carbon Project 2010: 1)

CO_2 emissions in various developed countries declined appreciatively in 2009: the United States by 6.9 percent; United Kingdom by 8.6 percent; Germany by 7 percent, Japan by 11.8 percent, and Russia by 8.4 percent (Global Carbon Project 2010: 3). The Global Carbon Project (2010: 5) estimated there would be at least a 3 percent increase in CO_2 emissions during 2010.

Much of the economic growth in developing countries, including China and India but also the oil-producing countries like Qatar, results from the production of luxury goods for the wealthy and "new middle class" in those countries. In China many of these people can be found in the eastern provinces where the individual purchasing power now exceeds $US 7,000 annually (P. G. Harris 2010: 126). The Netherlands Environment Assessment Agency calculated that in 2006 China had surpassed the United States in total CO_2 emissions (Camilleri and Falk 2010). China builds a new coal power plant approximately every four days and appears to have become the single largest emitter of CO_2 in the world due to rapid growth in fossil fuel consumption and cement manufacturing.

Roberts and Bradley (2007) delineate four factors contributing to differences in national responsibility for climate change: (1) national wealth (per capita GDP or total GDP), (2) CO_2 emissions per unit of GDP (called "carbon intensity"), (3) per capita CO_2 emissions, and (4) cumulative emissions over fifty years starting in 1950. Various studies indicate a curvilinear relationship exists in which intensity first rises as one moves from poorer to wealthier nations status but then declines among the wealthiest nations. International trade and globalization shunt off greatest the ecological impacts of production from developed societies to developing societies as heavy industrial manufacturing has been outsourced from the former to the latter (Roberts and Bradley 2007: 161). In terms of historical responsibility, China and India combined hold 37 percent of the world's population but contributed only 9 percent of the total quantity of accumulated anthropogenic greenhouse gas emissions, whereas the United States, with 22 percent of the world's population, has contributed more than 30 percent.

THE HEAVY RELIANCE OF GLOBAL CAPITALISM ON FOSSIL FUELS FOR VARIOUS PRODUCTION ACTIVITIES

Oil was the principal source of economic growth during most of the twentieth century and continues to be so in the twenty-first century (Heinberg 2006). It is a substance with multiple uses. Besides fueling transportation of various forms, oil is an essential ingredient in the production of plastics and various chemicals. In many locations, oil has replaced coal in the heating of dwelling units, offices, and factories. Oil also serves as an important energy source in the production of asphalt, and in industrial agriculture, it is the primary fuel for mechanized farm equipment as well as critical to the production of pesticides. It is estimated that nearly half of global oil consumption is devoted to the products of the global auto industry. Oil presently supplies about 40 percent of the world's energy and 96 percent of its transportation energy (Forest and Sousa 2006: 1). The Institute for the Analysis of Global Security projects that world oil consumption will increase by about 60 percent between 2006 and 2020. Energy Intelligence Administration projects an increase of more than 50 percent between 2006 and 2025.

Natural gas was used as early as 1821 to heat homes in Fredonia, New York (White 2008: 120). It began to take off as a major source of fuel in the 1880s, starting with its use for lighting and industrial heat in Pittsburgh, Pennsylvania. As easily acquired oil approaches depletion, the oil industry is exploring other sources of oil, such as oil derived from shale, tar sand pits in Alberta, and the Arctic region as the retreating Arctic cap exposes new potential sites. Furthermore, many parties are looking to natural gas as a cleaner energy resource because it produces lower emissions than either oil or coal. Also, it can be converted into many other products, such as liquid fuels, artificial fertilizers, and hydrogen for use in fuel cells.

Natural gas is used primarily to generate electricity, heat homes and commercial buildings, and for various industrial and agricultural purposes. The European Union and Japan have been shifting from coal to natural gas in electricity generation to comply with the Kyoto Protocol, a United Nations agreement ratified by 162 countries in which developed nations committed to a CO_2 reduction of 5.2 percent of 1990 levels by 2012 (Klare 2008: 44). The only developed country that has not ratified the Protocol is the United States, despite the fact that the Clinton administration was a signatory to it. The Kyoto targets were designed to be only a "first step" for developed countries to reduce their greenhouse gas emissions but have not even been met by many of the countries that ratified them. Canada is on track to increase its emissions by about 30 percent since 1990 and instead of facing the threat of penalties has opted to repudiate its obligations and withdrawn from the Protocol.

Metz reports that transport accounted for 20 percent of total energy use in 2006, almost all of it in the form of oil products (Metz 2010). Of this, motor vehicles accounted for more than 75 percent, with automobiles accounting for 45 percent, trucks 25 percent, and buses eight percent. Airplanes, shipping, and rail transport accounted for 20 percent of the transport energy consumption. According to Metz (2010), greenhouse gas emissions from the transport sector accounted for about 13 percent of the total global emissions in 2004. The products of the global automobile industry account for nearly half of the global oil consumption (Dauvergne 2005). The car consumes up to 63 percent of the oil consumed in the United States and about 35 percent of the oil consumed in Japan, a country with a vastly superior public transportation system to that of the United States. Oil is also a major resource utilized in road construction (Patterson 2007).

Although motor vehicles are a major contributor to greenhouse gas emissions, various sources indicate that air travel alone may be contributing from 3 to 8 percent of greenhouse gas emissions (Spence 2005; www.chooseclimate.org/flying). Whereas in 1950, there were 31 million air passengers who traveled 28 billion kilometers, by 2005, there were 2,022,000 air passengers who traveled 3,720 billion kilometers (Chafe 2008: 71). Unfortunately, the Kyoto Protocol exempts emissions from aviation and marine shipping. Airplane travel presently represents 12 percent of CO_2 emissions from transport (Gautier 2008:118). Airplanes also emit nitrous oxide and other contrail or exhaust fumes meaning that a "factor between two and three is normally applied to the CO_2 emissions from aviation to account for the additional warming impact" (Tickell 2008).

Marine transport has sometimes been posited as a reasonably sustainable sector for moving freight compared with airplanes, trucks, and railways. In terms of CO_2 emissions (in grams/ton kilometer), freight transport by road creates 98.301 (grams/ton kilometer), rail 28.338 grams/ton kilometer), and short-distance sea shipping (15.450 grams/ton kilometer; W. R. Black 2007). Unfortunately, shipping emits high levels of sulphur dioxide and the shipping of oil in tankers has resulted in numerous oil spills.

The contribution of military operations to global warming remains an underresearched topic. However, the Pentagon's activities reportedly resulted in about 46 million tons or 3.5 percent of U.S. CO_2 emissions in 1988 (Renner 1997: 121). More recent figures indicate that CO_2 emissions came to 60 million tons from U.S. military operations in 2005 and 5 million tons from UK military operations in the same year (Parkinson 2007: 4).

Militaries with their heavy reliance on airplanes (ranging from jet fighters to planes carrying troops and cargo to Air Force One), battleships, aircraft carriers, tanks, and other military equipment rely heavily on oil. The 2007 *Energy Bulletin* reported that the Pentagon is the single largest consumer of oil in the world, with an official figure of 320,000 barrels of oil per day being used for vehicle transport and facility maintenance. The official figure does not include "energy for the manufacture of vehicles, energy for building and dismantling military facilities, energy for construction of roads, and energy consumed while rebuilding whatever the military blows up" (Fitz 2007). Klare (2007) maintains that the Pentagon consumed 134 million barrels of oil in 2005, as much as the entire country of Sweden. One-third or more of U.S. military oil consumption reportedly occurs outside of the United States (G. Smith 1990–1991). Sanders (2009) asserts that the "military—that voracious vampire—produces enough greenhouse gases, by itself, to place the entire globe, with all its inhabitants large and small, in the most imminent danger of extinction." In the War on Iraq, the U.S. military used 1.5 million gallons of fuel every day to power its tanks, fighter jets, Black Hawks, Humvees, hospitals, and base camps (Little 2009).

The manufacture of products obviously too numerous to list contributes to greenhouse gas emissions, particularly of CO_2. Steel and aluminum are the most common metals that are utilized in the manufacture of numerous products, including motor vehicles, trains, airplanes, ships, along with factories, office and residential buildings, appliances, and electronic equipment. In 2006, China was the leading steel producer, with 419 million tons or over one-third of the world total (Liu 2008). The number two and three steel producers in 2006 were Japan, with 116 million tons, and the United States, with 99 million tons. Russia came in at number four and South Korea at number five in terms of steel production in 2006. Recycled iron and steel scrap has become an important raw material. In 2006, China accounted for 26 percent of the primary world aluminium production and China, Russia, Canada, the United States, and Australia for 59 percent of primary world production (Gardner 2008). Cement and concrete are important components of many building materials and road construction and result in large amounts of CO_2 emissions. According to

Little (2009: 319), "Buildings alone account for nearly 40 percent of all energy use and contribute nearly 40 percent of the world's annual greenhouse gas emissions." Dwelling units in developed societies, particularly in North America, Australia, and New Zealand, have become larger and larger over time. Needless to say, these larger dwelling units generally require more and more energy to heat or cool and encourage their occupants to purchase more and more consumer items, such as wide-screen television sets, computers, huge BBQ grills, and so on.

To survive, capitalism must generate artificial needs, including the need to endlessly consume a wide array of commodities, even potentially dangerous and lethal ones. As Panayotakis (2006: 265) observes, "As capitalist consumer culture continues to liquidate non-commercialized local cultures, the migration of meanings and values from relationships with people to relationships with market goods and spectacles channels people's consumption preferences and conceptions of the 'good life' in a consumerist direction."

Consumer capitalism began to take off in a profound way beginning in the 1950s when households in developed societies were flooded with energy-intensive appliances and devices, including electric cookers, washing and drying machines, refrigerators, toasters, electric irons, microwave ovens, electric toothbrushes, electric razors, televisions sets, record players, cassette players, video-recorders, computers, printers, electric tools, power lawnmowers, hedge cutters, leaf blowers, elaborate lighting systems, and so on. Capitalism, with its predilection for in-built obsolescence, encourages people to update older models of appliance and entertainment devices with new ones, such as regularly occurs with new models of plasma televisions, CD and DVD players, mobile phones, computers, and many other items. Although developed societies constitute the leading cultures of consumption, various developing countries, such as China and India, are quickly joining the pack. Although many of the refrigerators, air-conditioners, washing machines, televisions, and computers manufactured in China are exported, many are sold to the members of the new Chinese middle-class as well as elites. Klare (2008: 69) reports most of the apartments and shopping malls in Shanghai are "cooled in summer by air-conditioning; most house computers and other advanced electronic devices as well as a wide variety of modern appliances, [are] all powered by a vast electrical grid."

GREENHOUSE GAS EMISSIONS FROM AGRICULTURE AND DEFORESTATION

The Green Revolution (the effort to move food production in developing countries to an industrial model based on petrochemical fertilizers, pesticides, and herbicides) and industrial agriculture in developed countries are heavily reliant upon fossil fuels, extending from the production of fertilizers, the operation of farm machinery, to transportation and storage of agricultural products. An estimated three calories of fossil fuel energy are required to produce one calorie of food energy (Bello 2009). Reportedly four hundred gallons of oil equivalents were needed in 1994 to feed each American (Ruppert 2009).

Meat production requires 7 kilograms of grain for 1 kilogram of beef, 3.5 kilograms of grain for 1 kilogram of pork, 2 kilograms of grain for 1 kilogram of poultry and 1.2 kilograms of grain for 1 kilogram of fish (Metz 2010). Much of the soybean production around the world is devoted to feeding livestock (Dauvergene and Lister 2011). In 2002, the regional meat per capita production came to 271 pounds in North America, 154 pounds in South America, 62 pounds in Asia, 163 pounds in Europe, 103 pounds in Central America, and 57 pounds in North Africa (P. Murphy 2008). The UN Food and Agriculture Organization has indicated that meat production alone may be contributing to 18 percent of total global greenhouse gas emissions, largely due to the fact that livestock emit huge amounts of methane (Hertsgaard 2011: 180). A vegetarian diet reportedly requires about 80 percent less land than what is needed to feed a person on a meat-based diet. According to Metz (2010), "changing to a vegetarian diet can avoid N_2O emissions from grasslands, CH_4 emissions from livestock and manure, CO_2 emissions from fossil fuel use, and free land for other purposes."

Deforestation, intensive tillage, and overgrazing release CO_2 from living or recently live plants and organic matter in soil. Growing plants can sequester huge amounts of CO_2 from the atmosphere and store it in vegetation and soils. Conversely, land changes contribute to the release of CO_2, nitrous oxide, and methane. Deforestation reportedly "increased Brazil's total carbon emissions fivefold in 2002, moving it from the ninth-largest emitter to the fourth-largest after the United States, China, and Russia" (Bodley 2008a: 46). According to Gore (2009: 175), "[W]hile Brazil is destroying twice as much forestland each year as Indonesia, Indonesia is emitting twice as much CO_2 from deforestation as Brazil—primarily because the carbon-rich peatlands from which the Indonesian forests are being cleared dry up when the tree cover is gone and burn much longer when set ablaze, emitting far larger quantities of CO_2 into the atmosphere."

More than half of the world's paper is consumed by the wealthiest 20 percent of people, yet much of the deforestation that produces this paper is concentrated in the semiperiphery and periphery (Synott 2004). Americans constitute the largest global per capita paper consumers, much of which is used for advertisements in newspapers and magazines and "junk mail" (Dauvergne and Lister 2011: 116). The Amazon rain forest experienced widespread drought in 2005, which transformed the region from a sink to atmospheric source of carbon (Allison et al. 2009: 41). Global warming is a likely cause of the drought, an example of a feedback loop driving the buildup of greenhouse gases.

THE IMPACT OF CLIMATE CHANGE ON HUMAN SETTLEMENT PATTERN, SUBSISTENCE AND FOOD SECURITY

Climate change endangers people's cultures as a result of rising temperature, sea levels, droughts, and heavy rains, hurricanes, and cyclones. A sea level rise of 0.2 to 0.7 meters could result in increased beach erosion and coastal flooding, and the loss of various coastal ecosystems (such as mangroves, wetlands, the Great Barrier Reef, formations that protect land areas from flooding during extreme weather) as well as the displacement of millions of people from low-lying areas, and the intrusion of saltwater into coastal aquifer water supplies, thus posing a danger to farming and human habitation. Rising sea levels threaten entire populations of islands, particularly in the South Pacific and the approximately 1,200 islands of the Maldives in the Indian Ocean. Tuvalu in the South Pacific, following an old mining practice, is often depicted as one of the "canaries in the coal mine" of climate change. New Zealand, although not officially recognizing the category of "environmental refugee" or "climate refugee," has increased its intake of Tuvaluan migrants—however, only if they are employable and under age forty-five. In the words of David Stanley, "as ocean levels continue to rise, the entire population of Tuvalu may have to evacuate, third world victims of first world affluence." More than 300 million people live within three feet of sea level (National Geographic 2004), many of them at risk from sea rise. Coastal megacities in danger of flooding include Shanghai, Calcutta, Lagos, Bangkok, Dhaka, London, Rotterdam, New York, Miami, and New Orleans. Populations under threat from a rise in sea level also include many people living in Vietnam, Bangladesh, eastern China, India, Thailand, the Philippines, Indonesia, and Egypt. The Native Alaskan village of Shishmaeref, home to some six hundred Native Alaskans living at the far western edge of the state and about sixty miles north of Nome, has been eroding into the Bering Sea due to rising seas and increased storm surges (Johansen 2006). Already there are some 10 million environmental refugees in the world, and it has been estimated that there could be 150 million by 2050 (Cowie 1998). Environmental refugees are individuals who must flee their homelands because of the development of inhospitable environmental conditions.

The Arctic Climate Impact Assessment report sponsored by nations with an interest in the region pays special attention to species important to the Arctic's indigenous peoples (Symond, Arris, and Heal 2005).

Indigenous Arctic peoples will have to cope with the loss of sea ice for hunting and fishing, changed animal migration patterns, loss of perma- frost, and changes in the availability of traditional food sources. The Inuit who hunt Peary caribou during the summer months on Arctic Island have experienced a decline in these herds from 26,000 in 1961 to 1,000 in 1997 due to climate change (Flannery 2005). Other mammals, including polar bears, seals, and walruses, on which the Inuit have relied, have also be- come endangered species due to climate change. Huslia, an Athabaskan village some 300 kilometers (186 miles) west of Fairbanks, has experi- enced the disappearance of nearby lakes, which provided valuable food resources for villagers (Lynas 2004).

The Swiss village of Sas Balen consists of 423 inhabitants who reside three kilometers (1.8 miles) below the Gruben Glacier, which has been melting for more than a century and has been losing sixty to seventy centimeters in height annually (Cowie 1998). The village was flooded in 1968 and again in 1970, eventually prompting its residents to drain one of the melt water lakes in 1995 to prevent further flooding. Wilfried Haebrli, the Director of the UN's Glacier Monitoring Service, linked the threat of the village being flooded by mud and water to climate change (cited in Cowie 1998). Montana in the northwestern United States had been adversely affected by climate change in that this state that has historically experienced marginal rainfall has become even drier. Drought has resulted in the abandonment of many farms in eastern Montana (J. Diamond 2005).

According to UN figures, about half of the world's population relies on mountain-produced water for agriculture, electricity, industrial produc- tion, and drinking purposes (Lynas 2004: 235). Andean mountain villages and towns in Peru, Ecuador, Bolivia, and Colombia are losing water for both irrigation and drinking. La Paz and Quito both derive their water supply from glacial runoff, which may eventually diminish. Mountains in humid regions supply an estimated 30 to 60 percent of downstream fresh- water. Melting of the Sierra icepack will increase the likelihood of water shortages in Los Angeles (J. Diamond 2005).

As Flannery (2005: 204) observes, cities "constitute fragile entities vul- nerable to stress brought about by climate change." Major cities in the developed world already suffering from water shortages, possibly related to climate change, include New York, Los Angeles, Chicago, Washington, DC, Tucson, Sydney, and Melbourne (Glantz 2003).

Case Study: Climate Change Experience of the Inuit

One of the important contributions that anthropology can make to the understanding of climate change and its impacts on human populations is through on-the-ground ethnographic studies of the lived-experience of climate change, its impacts on people's lives and attitudes, and their varying efforts to cope with their changing environment. The Inuit peoples of Alaska, Canada, and Greenland have been studied over the years by a number of anthropologists. Traditionally hunting, trapping, and fishing peoples (a way of life already changed by contacts with the wider world and incorporation within nation-states and the capitalist market economy), they have a long history of successfully coping with harsh environmental conditions. Unfortunately, they live in a part of the world that is experiencing some of the most rapid changes due to global warming. The Inuit have been closely attuned to the changes going on around them in recent years, changes many Inuit view with considerable uneasiness. These changes are challenging aspects of their traditional way of life, subsistence strategies, and cultural identity. In the words of a local Inuit leader, as a consequence of global warming, "Arctic . . . peoples are threatened with the extinction or catastrophic decline of entire bird, fish and wildlife populations, including species of caribou, seals and fish critical to . . . food security" (quoted by Bodley 2008b: 221).

A team of climate change educators that visited numerous Inuit settlements early into the twenty-first century, found that the Inuit they encountered talked about fast-melting ice causing unexpected decreases in hunting days each year, and greater difficulty constructing ice-block igloos with lower-than-usual amounts of snow and ice. They discussed changes that they felt were without precedent in Inuit memory. Three experienced Inuit hunters traveled with the educational team and along the way pointed out examples of the environmental effects of climate change, such as the way shifting winds were reshaping ice formations that had been used for generations as critical directional landmarks in an otherwise hard to navigate terrain. Similarly, anthropologist Mark Nuttall (2009: 292) notes

on recent travels in Greenland, I hear people say with increasing frequency "Sila kiagukkalattunnarpog"—"the weather is getting warmer and warmer." Hunters in communities along the northwest coast talk of having to travel further in search of seals and fish, of the sea ice forming late and breaking up earlier, and of not being able to live as they once did.

As a result of these environmental changes, the Inuit express concern about hunters falling through melted ice, homes slipping from their perch on melting tundra into the ocean, and people switching from a diet high in wild-caught protein to one based on store-bought junk food. According to Barry Smit, a researcher at the University of Guelph, Canada (quoted in Davies 2010), "The stores only have food that's easy to transport and doesn't perish, so there are no vegetables. The young people are increasingly eating highly processed junk food, so we are seeing more teeth problems and obesity."

In 2005, the former international chair of the Inuit Circumpolar Council, Shiela Watt-Cloutier, accompanied by sixty Inuit hunters, submitted a petition to the Inter-American Commission on Human Rights. The petition asserted that the mass emission of greenhouse gases by the United States was, because of its effects on the environment, a violation of Inuit human rights. Specifically, the petition stated "the subsistence culture central to Inuit cultural identity has been damaged by climate change" (Watt-Cloutier 2005: 5). Although this kind of activist response is not shared by all Inuit, some of whom are hopeful that climate change will open up new resources (e.g., fishing sites), it does reflect an important aspect of varied Inuit attitudes about climate change. On the basis of a study in a Inuit community called Sach's Harbour in Canada's Western Artic, Berkes and Jolly (2001) concluded that local ability to successfully cope with and adjust to the health and social challenges of climate change will be determined by people's resilience, including their ability to adopt a flexible seasonal hunting pattern, commitment to passing down across generations detailed traditional knowledge about the environment, and maintenance of inter- and intracommunity sharing relationships in harsh times. The challenges of "adapting" to climate change now being faced by the Inuit, may well foretell dramatic changes (and losses) that will occur in societies around the world as temperatures continue to rise over the coming decades.

CLIMATE CHANGE AND HEALTH

Various scholars have recognized the impact of climate change on health. In his now-classic *Planetary Overload*, Tony McMichael (1993), an epidemiologist at the Australian National University, discusses the direct effects of global warming on health in the form of heat stress and respiratory ailments, and the indirect effects in terms of the spread of vector-borne and waterborne diseases. Paul R. Epstein (2002, 2005), a biomedical physician trained in tropical public health and the associate director of the Center for Health and the Global Environment at Harvard University, has also published extensively on the impact of climate change on health. The paucity of attention that medical anthropologists had devoted to the impact of climate change on global health prompted Baer and Singer (2009) to co-author *Global Warming and the Political Ecology of Health*, an examination of the range of diseases and other threats to health internationally introduced or exacerbated by a warming planet. Since then Singer, in particular, has published additional materials on the relationship between climate change and health, relying particularly on the concepts of *ecosyndemic* (examined in Chapter 10) and *pluralea* (examined later in this chapter).

We can speak of the *diseases of climate change* as a varied cluster of threats to health including nutritional deficits, temperature effects on the body, allergies, and infectious diseases. These diseases include any "tropical disease" that spreads to new places and peoples because of rising temperature but also inadequate nutrition and lost access to fresh, unpolluted, water supplies because of desertification or flooding of farmed areas. The UN Food and Agriculture Organization has warned that in some 40 percent of the poorest developing societies with some two billion people, climate change could dramatically increase the numbers of malnourished people (Changchui 2012). The growing tendency to power motor vehicles with biofuels such as corn and sugarcane, which are seen by many as producing less greenhouse gas emissions, has already contributed to a global food crisis. In referring to developments in India, Vandana Shiva observes:

Today, cars eat men [as well as women and children]. Land is diverted for parking, roads, highways, overpasses, and car factories. The mining of the iron ore and bauxite that makes the steel and aluminum is destroying the land and ecosystems. The atmosphere is being eaten up with fossil fuel emissions. (Shiva 2008: 50)

The full range of known health-threats of climate change are discussed in the subsections that follow.

Heat Exhaustion and Stroke

More frequent heat waves, particularly in urban areas, threaten the health and lives of especially vulnerable populations, such as the elderly, the sick, and infants. The estimated mortality of some 35,000 people during the European summer heat wave of 2003 were not only a consequence of high temperatures during the day but also the fact that nighttime low temperatures had risen at a rate nearly twice as high as the rise in daytime temperatures. The lingering nighttime warmth deprived people of normal relief from blistering daytime temperatures and the opportunity to recuperate from heat stress. Indeed, cities act as "heat islands" because of the presence of heat-retaining concrete roads, buildings, factories, and motor vehicle exhaust fumes. A U-shaped relationship exists between temperature and mortality, resulting in more deaths at the extremes of hottest and coldest weather (Drake 2000). Air pollution linked to longer, warmer summers particularly affects those suffering from respiratory ailments, such as asthma, as well as cardiovascular problems. Temperature increases also contribute to an increase of ozone in the atmosphere. According to Epstein and Rogers (2004: 6),

Heat waves take a disproportionate toll on those living in poor housing lacking air conditioning, and those with inadequate social supports. The majority of those affected during the 1995 heat wave in Chicago, for example, were African-Americans living in substandard housing.

The Spread of Vector-Borne Diseases

Currently, infectious diseases contribute to approximately 37 percent of all deaths in the world, a percentage that is expected to go up as a result of climate change. Various human disease vectors that previously were restricted in their distribution by seasonal cool temperatures have begun invading new areas in response to climate changes. Moreover, a temperature rise of only 2°C will more than double the metabolism rate of mosquitoes, including species that spread deadly human diseases. Warming at this level could also expand malaria's domain of active infection from 42 percent to 60 percent of the planet.

Climate change has been implicated in the resurgence of numerous infectious epidemics, including malaria, cholera, dengue, West Nile, and yellow fever, in environments north and south of the equator and at higher elevations. For example, higher temperatures in South Asia have caused elevated rainfall levels and contributed to greater breeding opportunities for mosquitoes. Berger provides the following overview of the impact of climate change on the prevalence of certain diseases:

Milder temperatures have contributed to the spread of mosquito-borne diseases in Africa. Richards Bay, South Africa, for example, which was once malaria-free, had 22,000 cases in 1999. Malaria has also reached the highland areas of Kenya and Tanzania where it was previously unknown. In the Andes of Colombia, disease-carrying mosquitoes that once lived in altitude no higher than 3,200 feet have now appeared at the 7,200-foot level. (Berger 2000: 36–37)

Although climate change is not the only factor involved, today it is estimated that there are 300 to 500 million cases of malaria each year in Africa, resulting in between 1.5 and 2.7 million deaths, more than 90 percent occurring among children under five years of age. Climate change appears to have contributed to the various other epidemics, including a major cholera outbreak in Latin America in 1991, pneumonia plague in India in 1994, and the eruption of the hantavirus epidemic in the U.S. Southwest in 1994. Tony McMichael presents the following sobering observations:

The main anticipated impact of climate change on the potential transmission of vector-borne would be in tropical areas. In general, populations on the margins of endemic areas in tropical and subtropical countries would be most likely to experience an increase in transmission. . . . This appears to reflect a combination of increasing population mobility, urbanization, poverty and regional warming, along with a slackening of mosquito control programmes. Meanwhile, in temperate zones, climate change may also affect diseases such as tick-borne viral encephalitis (which occurs in parts of Western Europe, Russia, and Scandinavia) and Lyme disease. (McMichael 2001:302)

Waterborne Diseases

Waterborne diseases, those acquired through contact with a body of water, currently are the source of 90 percent of deaths from infectious disease in developing countries, and, with further global warming, their impact is likely to grow in developed nations as well. The effect of global warming on water-borne diseases is seen in the case of shellfish poisoning caused by the bacterium *Vibrio vulnificus,* a member of the family of bacteria responsible for cholera. *V. vulnificus* is a not yet well-known organism found in oysters, clams, and crabs. It was only discovered to be a source of human disease in 1979. Warming ocean waters are expanding its range. The cause of a growing number of seafood-related deaths, it also can infect wounds, as well as trigger gastroenteritis and septicemia, producing a mortality rate of between 20 and 50 percent of infected individuals, depending on the nature of the infection and the prior health status of the sufferer.

More than half of all waterborne disease outbreaks in the United States occur after a heavy storm, like the kinds of extreme storms made more common by global warming. The Environmental Protection Agency (2012) estimates that heavy rains cause more than 850 billion gallons of raw sewage and storm water—the equivalent of one million Olympic-size swimming pools—to spill into U.S. waterways each year.

Climate Change Denial

Not everyone accepts that climate change is occurring, that a changing climate represents a serious threat to human health, or that humans are having much impact on climate or the environment generally. There are many factors that contribute to climate change skepticism. These include the complexities of the issues involved, most notably the multiple factors that shape climate and the unfamiliarity of the general public with the multiple disciplinary scientific languages and types of data at play; the admitted existence of many arenas of scientific uncertainty; confusion about the differences between weather (current conditions) versus climate (long-term weather trends); and the sheer terrifying nature of the implications of climate change once you recognize it is happening. Also there are many other competing or confusing issues, including the state of the economy, the threats of war and terrorism (which may seem like a more immediate danger than something that supposedly will not be too bad until later in the century), personal dreams of achieving material wealth and its benefits, the leak of e-mail messages from prominent British climate scientists at the University of East Anglia that admitted overstating the evidence for global warming, and the discovery of small errors in the United Nations climate report.

Beyond these issues, however, is that of *planned doubt*—that is, intentional efforts to promote public uncertainty about and denial of climate change. What is the source of planned confusion about climate change? Not surprisingly, it involves those who benefit most from the status quo, especially sectors of the fossil fuel industry. In 1998, in one of the first attempts to confuse the public on climate change, a proposal was circulated among U.S. opponents, including both the fuel industry and conservative political groups. Written by a public relations specialist for the American Petroleum Institute, the proposal discussed a plan "to recruit a cadre of scientists who share the industry's views of climate science and to train them in public relations so they can help convince journalists, politicians and the public that the risk of global warming is too uncertain to justify controls on greenhouse gases" (Cushman 1998). The *Guardian* newspaper reported that after the IPCC released its 2007 report on climate change, the American Enterprise Institute offered British, American, and other scientists $10,000 each, plus travel expenses, to publish articles critical of the IPCC assessment. The American Enterprise Institute, which has received more than $1.6 million from ExxonMobil, sent letters that "attack the UN's panel as 'resistant to reasonable criticism and dissent and prone to summary conclusions that are poorly supported by the analytical work' and asked for essays that 'thoughtfully explore the limitations of climate model outputs'" (Sample 2007). ExxonMobil has given about $3 million to U.S. groups that "misinformed the public about climate change," thirty-nine of which "misrepresented the science of climate change by outright denial of the evidence" according to the Royal Society, the premier science institute in the United Kingdom.

Several environmentalists have drawn up lists of the top global warming deniers. Senator James Inhofe, a Republican from Oklahoma, asserts that global warming is "the greatest hoax ever perpetrated on the American people" (quoted in Stephanie Rogers 2011). Where does Inhofe get his information of climate issues? A key source is the writings of Michael Crichton, the fiction author of books such as *Jurassic Park*. Crichton claims that the environmental and scientific communities completely invented the climate change threat. Other well-known deniers are news commentator Steve Milloy, a former lobbyist for the fossil fuel and nuclear energy industries, as well as for the National Mining Association, and radio host Glenn Beck, who has likened Al Gore's effort to educate people about climate change to Hitler's effort to exterminate Jews. Many prominent deniers are themselves scientists (although not necessarily climate scientists), including Ross McKitrick, Richard Lindzen, Willie Soon, and Sallie Baliunas. All of these individuals have strong ties to ExxonMobile (e.g., working for ExxonMobile-funded institutes). Notable among the most prominent deniers are oil billionaires David and

Charles Koch, owners of Koch Industries, the second largest privately owned company in the United States. The Koch brothers have given more than $60 million to fund denier organizations. Charles Lewis, the founder of the Center for Public Integrity, a nonpartisan watchdog group, asserts, "The Kochs are on a whole different level. There's no one else who has spent this much money. The sheer dimension of it is what sets them apart. They have a pattern of lawbreaking, political manipulation, and obfuscation. I've been in Washington since Watergate, and I've never seen anything like it. They are the Standard Oil of our times" (quoted in Mayer 2010). Adds Jane Mayer (2010), "In a study released this spring, the University of Massachusetts at Amherst's Political Economy Research Institute named Koch Industries one of the top ten air polluters in the United States. And Greenpeace issued a report identifying the company as a 'kingpin of climate science denial.' The report showed that, from 2005 to 2008, the Kochs vastly outdid ExxonMobil in giving money to organizations fighting legislation related to climate change, underwriting a huge network of foundations, think tanks, and political front groups." In late 2000, Koch Industries was charged with covering up the illegal releases of ninety-one tons of the known carcinogen benzene from its refinery in Corpus Christi. Initially facing a ninety-seven-count indictment and potential fines of $350 million, Koch cut a deal with then–Attorney General John Ashcroft to drop all major charges in exchange for a guilty plea for falsifying documents, and a $20 million settlement. In everyday usage, the word *uncertainty* means not knowing. In science, however, uncertainty refers to how well something is known. In science, there is often not absolute certainty, but research reduces uncertainty, making it possible to talk about degrees of certainty. Climate scientists know with high confidence (90 percent) that

- human-induced warming significantly influences physical and biological systems throughout the world;
- cold days and nights are becoming less frequent and hot days and nights more frequent over most land areas;
- sea levels are rising;
- glaciers and permafrost are shrinking;
- oceans are becoming more acidic; and
- ranges of plants and animals (and pathogens) are shifting.

Despite the extensively broad agreement among scientists that global warming is a reality and that human activity is the primary cause (Oreskes 2004), deniers remain adamant that the science is unsettled and that therefore there is no reason to regulate the production of greenhouse gases. Why this stance? Science historians Naomi Oreskes and Erik Conway

(2010), in their book *Merchants of Doubt: How a Handful of Scientists Obscured the Truth on Issues from Tobacco Smoke to Global Warming*, offer the following answer: there is a lot of money at stake for industrial polluters and those they fund to deny global warming.

Winners and Losers

An important debate concerning climate change is the issue of "winners and losers"—namely, the idea that while some parts of the planet will suffer grave consequences, others will benefit from the changes global warming ushers in. As Arthur Caplan and coworkers note (1999): "Simulations carried out using general circulation models . . . frequently predict that a 'win-lose' scenario may occur, whereby a group of nations, or regions within nations, actually benefit from global warming while others are hurt. Typically, the sector driving this result is agriculture." Some of the commonly cited losers, include countries in Africa that are prone to drought under current conditions; these will face much more severe conditions as the planet warms, as will parts of central Asia, where temperatures already regularly exceed 40°C (104°F). These regions will face even hotter temperatures with painful consequences in food production. Increases of more than 5°C in countries from Kazakhstan to Saudi Arabia could lead to widespread famine. A commonly cited winner is Luxembourg and the surrounding region. Also Minnesota and contiguous U.S. states and parts of Canada (the so-called corn/soybean and wheat belts) are said by some analyses to be likely winners, with increased food production. Countries that some analysts say will have only limited climate change are the United Kingdom and Ireland in the Northern Hemisphere and Argentina, Uruguay, Chile, and New Zealand in the Southern Hemisphere.

What is wrong with this kind of "silver-lining" picture of the future and with the "winners and losers" scenario? The "winners and losers" thinking suggests that wealthy countries will do OK or even do better under conditions of rising temperature, while poorer countries will not be able to adapt and will face the most severe weather and other temperature-related changes. There are at least four primary shortcomings of this approach.

First, climate change is not one-dimensional; it entails multiple changes of diverse sorts, including health impacts. Water is a critical component of global warming changes. Snowmelt runoff will decrease in many places, so significantly that we lose winter, and snowfall increasingly turns into to rain. This will mean more runoff in "winter" and less in the spring when it is more likely to be needed for irrigation and other agricultural purposes. And, as seen in the U.S. Midwest in the summer of 2008, more flooding of so-called winner regions. Similarly, one consequence of global warming is disease vector movement: new diseases will present challenges for so-called winner regions. Also forested areas, like those in northern North America, are increasingly susceptible to bark beetle attacks because warming climates speed their metabolism. Hence forests across an alleged winner area are in increasingly worse condition. Furthermore, songbirds are a major form of insect control. If the birds move farther north, as has already begun, forests may be even more susceptible to insect attacks, which means more dead wood, which means more fire and more air pollution.

Second, in a globalized and heavily interconnected world (as seen in the impact of economic problems in one country on the state of health of many economies), disaster in one place has impacts in many places. As David Rind of the Goddard Institute for Space Studies points out: "We may say that we're more technologically able than earlier societies. But one thing about climate change is it's potentially geopolitically destabilizing" (quoted in Kolbert 2006: 111). Countries or regions that appear to be "winners" climatically may find themselves inundated by migrants from so-called loser areas because of the rise in sea-level and associated disasters, flooding, droughts and agricultural devastation ushered in by climate change. If there is rampant starvation in many parts of the world, will milder winters in Minnesota feel like winning?

Third, while we have learned an enormous amount about climate change over the past twenty-five years, we still do not understand global warming sufficiently to fully anticipate all of its consequences, including secondary and tertiary consequences, and consequences further down the line. Thus, will Minnesota actually be a winner climatically? One model, developed by David Rind, of the Goddard Institute for Space Studies says no. It suggests that Minnesota and indeed most of the continental United States will experience increasingly frequent and prolonged droughts. This conclusion is based on the interpretation that current climate change models underestimate the intensification of drought because they do not use detailed enough models of land surfaces. Consequently, Minnesota may be more like Missouri and Arkansas by the end of the twenty-first century, or it may be more like the Mohave Desert.

Finally, countries and peoples of the world are not just facing climate change, as discussed in greater detail later in the chapter, they are encountering many (often interacting) anthropogenic threats to the environment. The U.S. corn belt, for example, might have some growing-season gains from global warming that are lost to other kinds of environmental degradation and destruction, such as the elimination of flood-containing wetlands, the intentional straightening of rivers, which, in a storm, promotes flooding, and the replacement of deep-rooted grasses and other plants with shallow-rooted crops that cannot withstand flooding. These factors, acting in interaction with climate change, probably contributed to the extensive flooding of the corn belt during the summer of 2008. In short, as freelance writer Kurt Cobb (2006) asserts, "To imagine that global warming is a game with 'winners' and 'losers' may be the surest way to make losers of us all."

Other Health Ecocrises

Nuclear Threat

In the first scholarly attempt to calculate numbers of cancer cases in the general public (and excluding workers at the plant) and deaths resulting from the Fukushima Dai-ichi nuclear accident in Japan in March 2011, M. Jacobson and Hoever (2012) report that the total deaths will lie in the range 1,300, and the total number of accident-caused cancer cases will number approximately 2,500. The nuclear disaster at the Fukushima plant, located 135 miles (220 kilometers) north of Tokyo, caused the worst nuclear accident since Chernobyl (in the former Soviet Union) in 1986. The Fukushima accident forced the evacuation of 160,000 people (approximately 600 people died because of the evacuation, mostly due to fatigue and exposure among the elderly and chronically ill). Radiation from the plant produced a 132 square kilometer "no-go zone" that will remain in force for decades. This challenges statements made by the Japanese government that the explosion would probably not produce a single radiation-linked fatality in the general public. In fact, Jacobson and Hoever maintain that fatalities would have been ten times greater if most of the radiation had not fallen into the ocean. Only about one-fifth of the radioactive material vented into the air and fell onto land; more fallout on land would have caused a much higher casualty figure. Overall, more than 350,000 Japanese die each year of cancer, and many of these deaths too are products of various forms of environmental pollution.

In a nuclear accident, radioactive isotopes—including iodine-131 and cesium-137—contained inside a nuclear power plant's fuel rods, may be released into the atmosphere as gases or particulates. These can be inhaled or ingested through contaminated food or water. It is estimated that the Fukushima Dai-ichi plant emitted about 900,000 terabecquerels (a unit of measurement for level radioactivity) of the iodine equivalent of radioactive iodine 131 and cesium 137 into the air. This amount is about two times more than the 480,000 terabecquerels estimated originally by the Nuclear and Industrial Safety Agency. In the Chernobyl accident, the total radiation release at the plant was estimated to be about 5.2 million terabecquerels.

In the case of Chernobyl, four hundred times more radioactive material was released than the U.S. atomic bombing of Hiroshima during the Second World War. Radioactive fallout hit over a dozen countries, especially

Russia, Ukraine, and Belarus. Thyroid cancer among children was one of the primary health impacts of Chernobyl, with more than four thousand cases being reported. Regarding the death toll from the accident, it is known that twenty-eight emergency workers died from acute radiation poisoning, and it is estimated that cancer deaths caused by Chernobyl may reach four thousand. Fred Mettler (2004), a radiation expert at the University of New Mexico, estimates the number of worldwide cancer deaths outside the highly contaminated zone at approximately five thousand, for a total of nine thousand Chernobyl-related fatal cancers. Importantly, more than twenty-five years after Chernobyl, accident-associated deaths continue to accumulate, and the catastrophic legacy of the accident, and of all nuclear accidents, lives on. The accident in Fukushima, as well as the near-disaster at the Three Mile Island nuclear power plant in Pennsylvania in 1979, and many other smaller accidents, leaks, and malfunctions at nuclear plants around the world, confirm the ongoing health threat of nuclear energy production. Because of the Fukushima nuclear disaster Germany decided to shut down all nuclear plants by 2022 and has already begun dismantling some of them. Fifty other nations, however, continue to build and operate nuclear facilities. As a result, past experience suggests that it is only a matter of time until the next significant nuclear catastrophe. Moreover, the industry remains highly resistant to regulatory efforts. Dave Lochbaum, who served as a technology instructor for the U.S. Nuclear Regulatory Commission, points out "the nuclear industry practices ethical cleansing. Raising safety concerns in the industry is the surest ticket out of it" (quoted in Tuttle 2011: 13).

Overfishing the Oceans

In the second half of the twentieth century, the marine food industry increased its catch of edible fish by 400 percent by doubling the number of boats and using more effective fishing technology. One result has been intense overfishing, which means catching fish faster than they can reproduce. The scale of the change is seen in what is called the "global marine capture" (i.e., seafood caught). In 1950, 16.7 million metric tons (mmt) of fish were harvested from the oceans; in 2006, this had risen to 77.9 mmt (i.e., 170 billion pounds), which is about three times the combined weight of every person in the United States. This level of harvest is unsustainable. Overfishing pushes the fish population ever lower, until fish of a desired species are so few that fishermen cannot make a living off of them anymore and fisherman move on to another, previously less desirable species, and the pattern is repeated. This pattern is called serial depletion. Many fisheries have already collapsed. An analysis (Myers and Worm 2003) of almost eight thousand species of seafood found that

29 percent of species are now 90 percent below the averages of fifty years ago. Large predatory fish (cod, flounder, marlin, swordfish, and tuna) have suffered a 90 percent population decline over the last half century. According to Ransom Myers (quoted in Melville 2003), fisheries biologist at Dalhousie University, "From giant blue marlin to mighty bluefin tuna, and from tropical groupers to Antarctic cod, industrial fishing has scoured the global ocean. There is no blue frontier left. Since 1950, with the onset of industrialized fisheries, we have rapidly reduced the resource base to less than 10%—not just in some areas, not just for some stocks, but for entire communities of these large fish species from the tropics to the poles." In short, notes Montaigne (2007), "the number of fish swimming the seas is a fraction of what it was a century ago."

A total collapse of commercial wild seafood is projected for 2050 if current patterns of industrial fish harvesting continue. Moreover, notes Daniel Pauly (quoted in Greenberg 2010), a fisheries scientist at the University of British Columbia, "A country can acquire [seafood] by fishing, or it can acquire it by trade. It is the sheer power of wealthy nations to acquire primary production that is important." Hence a key issue in terms of responsibility is not just who owns the ships but also who eats the catch.

Growth in the world's fishing fleet size has been driven by several pressures, including the fact that wealthy countries have been subsidizing their commercial fishing sector in the amount of about $30 billion a year. Such policies boost the number of working boats; their technology to find, catch, and process fish; and, while fish stocks last, increase the global catch. Consequently, a vast flotilla of industrial trawlers from the European Union, China, Russia, and elsewhere search the world for fish. One place they find them is northwest Africa, off the coast of countries such as Senegal. European trawlers have now so thoroughly scoured northwest Africa's ocean floor that major fish populations are collapsing. Increasingly, people in developing nations who live near the oceans of the world, and who depend on fish for much of the protein in their diet, are finding it harder and harder to both catch and eat the fish that once lived along their shores (but were fished out by trawlers from wealthy nations).

Another product of overfishing is a phenomenon called *trophic cascades*. This refers to a kind of domino effect that occurs when one component of an ocean ecosystem is eliminated. For example, overfishing of sharks off of the eastern coast of the United States resulted in an explosion in the population of the cow-nosed rays, a primary food source of sharks in the region. The rays, in turn, with their greater numbers, ravaged their own primary food source, scallops, essentially destroying the local scallop fishery (Myers et al. 2007). Another example of this phenomenon occurred off of the coast of Namibia, a traditionally plankton-rich area that provides food to many fish including sardines. During the 1970s, European trawlers overfished the area, and the sardine population collapsed. The result was a buildup on the ocean floor of decaying plankton, which released hydrogen sulfide and methane in great quantities. These toxins, in turn, interacting with oxygen to create sulfur, turned the ocean white and killed other fish in the area. At the same time, methane was released into the atmosphere, contributing to the greenhouse gas blanket that continues to build around Earth.

Water Pollution

Waste-water release and water pollution comprise substantial threats to global health and well-being. Although Earth is a wet planet, less than 1 percent of available water is drinkable. Not only do agriculture and industrial production consume most readily accessible freshwater, they are primary sources of water pollution. Every day, at least two million tons of sewage and industrial and agricultural waste are discharged into the world's waterways, which is equivalent to the weight of the entire human population on the planet. Moreover, it is estimated by the United Nations World Water Assessment Program (2009) that the amount of wastewater produced annually is about 1,500 km^3 or about six times more water than exists in all the rivers of the world. In developing countries, 70 percent of industrial waste is disposed of untreated in local water systems. The World Health Organization estimates that only one-sixth of the world's population, including four of five children in developing countries, currently drinks safe water. According to UNICEF (2005), lack of safe water results in 1.4 million child deaths each year, one every fifteen seconds.

Water pollution is also an issue for highly developed nations. A 2008 Centers for Disease Control study found a link between industrial pollution in the Clinton and St. Clair Rivers and high disease rates among the people of Macomb County, Michigan (pop. 800,000, 97 percent urban). According to Howard Frumkin (2008: v), "[C]areless practices over many years have resulted in contamination of the Great Lakes ecosystem. Countless chemical products and byproducts of modern life—solvents, metals, pesticides, persistent organic pollutants, and more—have found their way into the air, water, land, and biota, and even into people's bodies." In Macomb County, the report concluded that a "vulnerable population" of 348,000 people is at risk due to chemical contaminants released into the air or water by local industry. Compared to similar counties, the study found high rates of infant mortality and deaths from breast cancer, colon cancer, coronary heart disease, lung cancer, and stroke in the Macomb population living near the water. Lake St. Clair, the drinking water source for the southern half of the county, is fed by the Clinton and St. Clair Rivers—two areas of concern long plagued by industrial pollutants. The report cited discharges of lead, mercury, PCBs and other manufacturing byproducts. The St. Clair River is home to Sarnia's "Chemical Valley," which contains numerous industrial facilities that handle hazardous materials.

Mining is another massive source of water pollution. Most of the material exhumed from mines is waste—much of it quite toxic—which is discarded in tailing ponds or other depositories. These sites are under growing threat from extreme storms produced by global warming. In 2010, for example, acidic waste escaped from a copper mine in Fujan Province, China, poisoning the Ting River and killing enough fish to have fed 72,000 people, but the mining company waited nine days to report the spill (Sun 2010). In 2008, another runoff at a Chinese gold mine contaminated the drinking water of more than 200,000 people. The U.S. Environmental Protection Agency (2000) estimates that 40 percent of all watersheds in the western United States are negatively affected by mining pollution, including mercury and acid mine drainage—an acidic water that leaks from both active and abandoned mines. The impact on water-related resources from mining is also illustrated by what happened to the Tsolum River in British Columbia, Canada. Historically the river ran clear from its source near Mount Washington and was home to large runs of coho, pink, chum, and cutthroat salmon as well as steelhead trout. In 1964, the Mount Washington Cooper Mining Company opened a small open-pit mine on the upper Tsolum watershed and extracted 360,000 tons of ore along with 940,000 tons of waste rock before the mine was abandoned in 1966. Left behind was a toxic legacy. Virtually all salmon and trout disappeared from the river due to acid mine drainage.

What of the impacts on human health? A case in point is Central Appalachia, a place with a long mining history. There is little disputing that a health crisis exists in the area. West Virginia, for example, ranks last among the states in terms of the physical health of residents based on the 2011 Gallup Healthways Well-Being Index. West Virginia's 3rd District ranks next to the bottom at No. 435 among America's 436. Kentucky's 5th Congressional District, an area that is mined using mountaintop-removal methods, ranks No. 436. A number of studies, including more than a dozen carried out by Michael Hendryx of West Virginia University and colleagues between 2007 to 2011, have found severe health problems in central Appalachia. In a study of age-adjust mortality for the years 2000 through 2004 relative to tons of coal mined in a person's area or residence, Hendryx (2009: 243) found that "counties with the highest level of coal mining were significantly higher relative to non-mining areas for chronic heart, respiratory and kidney disease." Additionally, people living near mountaintop mining sites have been found to have cancer rates 50 percent greater than people living in nonmining areas. Mortality rates also have been found to be significantly greater, even after researchers adjusted for reported rates of smoking, alcohol use, and access to health care. Concludes Hendryx et al. (2008: 1), "Higher mortality may be the result of exposure to environmental contaminates associated with the coal-mining industry, although smoking and poverty are also contributing factors."

Air Pollution

Air pollution has been defined as a condition of the air that endangers the health, safety, or welfare of persons; interferes with normal enjoyment of life or property; endangers the health of animal life; or causes damage to plant life or property. Outdoor air pollution is estimated by the World Health Organization (2011) to be a direct cause of at least 1.34 million premature deaths annually. Within the United States, which is a major producer of global air pollution, as many as half a million people die annually from cardiopulmonary disease, which is linked to breathing fine particle matter pollution in the air. In a study of the association between air pollution and mortality in six U.S. cities, Dockery et al. (1993) found that while smoking had the highest levels of association with mortality, after adjusting for smoking, there were statistically and robust associations between city air pollution and mortality. In Dhaka, the capital city of Bangladesh (which is projected to be the world's third largest city by 2020), it is estimated that local air pollution is the cause of 15,000 deaths a year (Mahmood 2011). During the period of December through March 2006–2007, the density of airborne particulate matter in Dhaka reached 463 mcm, the highest level in the world. A country environment analysis conducted jointly by the government of Bangladesh and the World Bank identified air pollution as the leading cause of both morbidity and mortality related environmental risk in the country, with PM10, PM2.5 (particulate matter equal to or less than 10 and 2.5 micrometers, respectively), black smoke, and sulfates showing the most consistent association with pollution-related mortality (World Bank 2006). Vehicular, construction, and industrial waste production are the primary sources of this killer pollutant. In its effort to develop following the Western industrial model, Bangladesh, like other countries in similar circumstances, is adding an enormous new health burden for its population, especially among the poor, children, the elderly, and pregnant women.

Hazardous Waste

One potent way human activities affect the environment is the production and dispersal of hazardous waste as a by-product of industrial manufacture and other production. Defined as anthropogenic substances that are harmful to life and the environment, hazardous waste includes various solids, liquids, gases and sludges that are poisonous, flammable, explosive, corrosive, radioactive, disease-causing, mutagenic (damaging to genetic material), teratogenic (causing defects in utero) or bioaccumulative (collecting in living organisms and in food chains). Its creation, where its goes, and why (including who has voice in decisions about waste) raise critical issues for anthropology in the domains of morality, human rights, environmental justice, structural violence, sustainability, social suffering, and the political ecology of health.

Pluralea

Unfortunately, not only are there multiple anthropogenic environmental threats to human health; many of these ecocrises threats are interactive resulting in even greater health risk for the people of Earth. Singer (2009e, 2010a) has labeled these interacting anthropogenic ecocrises *pluralea*. This term is derived from the Latin words *plur,* meaning "many" and *alea,* meaning risks or hazards. *Pluralea,* then, are two or more human-caused environmental crises, that interact and magnify the intensity of human risk. Of central importance in the study of *pluralea* are their proximate and ultimate causes, and especially, from the anthropological standpoint, the precise role of human social and economic systems in generating health damaging environmental conditions and the intertwined ecocrises that result. Similarly, the pathways and mechanisms through which two or more ecocrises interact to produce synergistic, magnified environmental and health impacts is a central concern of *pluralea* research.

Global health currently is threatened by *pluralea* interactions on land, in the air, and at sea. One of the most notable *pluralea* interactions occurring in marine environments is the entwined processes of overfishing and global warming. As summarized by S. Feldman (2008), because of overfishing and global warming, we are approaching a world by the middle of the twenty-first century of rising seas empty of fish and devoid of ice. Similarly, the United Nations Environmental Programme (Nellemann, Hain, and Adler 2008) warns of the food availability impacts of the merging of climate change, water pollution, overharvesting of fishing stocks, and invasive species infestations in the world's fishing zones. One of the ways climate change adversely affects sea life is through a process known as ocean acidification. The source of this change is increasing carbon emissions that are landing in the ocean and changing the pH balance therein. Coral, which serves as a nursery area and home base for many commercial fish are damaged by acidification. So too are shellfish, which have a difficult time building their shells in acidic water. Ocean acidification and ocean warming may interact to limit the areas habitable by species like crabs. In addition to harvesting too many fish, industrial trawlers destroy seabeds and fish habitats. Moreover, fishing boats are contributing to ocean pollution. Maritime traffic generates more than 20 million tons of harmful hydrocarbon waste in Europe as well. The Mediterranean is in even worse shape from hydrocarbon contamination. These multiple and mutually enhancing pressures have created a *pluralea* that threatens the nutritional status of millions of people around the world.

Another *pluralea* example involves air pollution. The burning of fossil fuels produces nitrogen oxides. Volatile organic compounds are given off by paint and solvents. Mixed together in the air in the presence of solar heat and sunlight, these two substances combine to form ground-level ozone. With each degree of atmospheric warming caused by greenhouse gases, ground-level ozone rises by two parts per billion above current levels. This is a sufficient increase in breathable ozone to cause 2.8 million respiratory diseases such as asthma (Perera 2011). Those at special risk for this harmful *pluralea:* infants and children, seniors, low-income individuals and families, and people who work outdoors.

CONCLUSION

In this chapter, we have catalogued, described, and analyzed the health and related risks of global climate change, other threats to the environmental health, and the damaging intersection of these environmental hazards known as *pluralea*. The take-home messages of this chapter are as follows:

- Environmental health is of critical importance in human well-being.
- Climate change constitutes an environmental health risk on a magnitude unparalleled in human history.
- The primary driver of climate change is the nature of the dominant economic system because of its emphasis on ever-increasing production and consumption, activities that are outstripping the capacity of nature to rebound with replenished resources while filling the environment with the health-threatening by-products and waste from production.
- The health risks of climate change are not standalone risks but rather are magnified by other degradations and damages done to the environment by the world economic system.
- Although all nations and regions of the world are suffering the ill effects of climate change, pollution, overharvesting of resources and other ecocrises, poor nations and poor people in all nations (those usually least responsible for pushing the planet toward even more drastic changes) are burdened disproportionately with the consequences.

CHAPTER 5

Poverty, Injustice, and Health in the World System

We know that both class and the uneven development of capitalism are reflected in unequal morbidity and mortality (Wilkinson 1986; Wilkinson and Pickett 2010). Societies with less income inequality have populations in better health than those with wider income gaps between rich and poor (M. Susser and Stein 2009). In the United States, increasing wealth inequities have been associated with increasing inequalities in health (Pappas et al 1993). In addition, a strong welfare state contributes to a healthier population (Judt 2010). Thus, there is little doubt that contemporary policies, which have cut back the welfare state, have a negative impact on the health of populations, but we need to consider the actual processes that lead to such ill health and those that protect people.

Because global inequalities are crucial to health disparities, anthropologists have explored the ways World Trade Organization policies about food tariffs and agriculture (Edelman and Haugerud 2005) as well as intellectual property rights to medicine (I. Susser 2009b) seeds (Gupta 1998) and medicinal herbs (A. Escobar 1998) frame the experiences of poverty in both the centers of capital and the periphery. In addition, we need to explore the interaction between the precipitous growth in cities of the capitalist periphery over the past three decades and the shocking disparities in health found in such new urban formations as well as the increasing disparities in the centers of capital (Khan and Pappas 2011). This chapter begins with a discussion of poverty and health as it has emerged historically in the centers of capital and then considers the history of poverty, injustice, and health in the periphery and particularly in the growing cities of displaced peoples. We discuss ways in which anthropologists have conducted research with respect to the crises and disasters exacerbated by contemporary capitalist processes and critically assess questions of intervention and engagement. Overall, this chapter understands critical medical anthropology not only in terms of identifying unjust processes but in terms of searching for the appropriate interventions or social movements that may tilt the scale in favor of promoting justice and specifically better health for the populations with whom we work (Singer 1995a; S. Schensul 2011; I. Susser 2011).

The concept of *wounded cities* (J. Schneider and Susser 2003) was developed to address the destruction and reconstruction of cities that has taken place under global policies of neoliberalism since the 1980s (Harvey 2005). *Wounded Cities* (J. Schneider and Susser 2003) provides an outline of key aspects of the globalization process that seem particularly destructive of contemporary urban life: redirected public investment away from social services and toward the commoditization of urban space, the marginalization of the urban middle-class and poor, increasing or concretizing of ethnic and racial divisions, increasing subordination of women in new ways, and a burgeoning criminal economy resting heavily on drug traffic. Each of these changes has particular implications for health. The widespread reductions in social services and access to health care can be traced throughout the United States, Europe, and the capitalist periphery and have specifically reduced the resources available to women and children. The undermining of women's access to reproductive health is outlined in our chapter in this volume on reproduction and inequality. We also discuss elsewhere in this volume the issues of substance abuse in the global criminal economy. Here, we focus more centrally on the reorganization of cities in the centers of capital and the new invisibility of the poor and homeless.

Cities bring together large numbers of people leading to different challenges in terms of housing, clean water, sanitation, garbage collection, and the containment of infection. We know that, in a dense population, a virus can thrive and that bacterial infections can easily spread from person to person. Such issues have been recognized and tackled at least since the times of the Romans. However, the ways in which such health challenges are addressed in cities are crucially political, cultural, and social. Starting in the fifteenth-century European cities—London quintessentially— were breeding grounds for cholera, typhoid, and other diseases, carried through water, fleas, and rats. In London, after the last massive plague epidemic in 1665 and the great fire in 1666, as the bourgeoisie achieved political representation in government, they began to rebuild the city with space and better sanitation for the new middle classes. In the early nineteenth century, after the unsuccessful urban rebellions of 1848, Paris was rebuilt with wide boulevards for the bourgeoisie to enjoy and under-ground water and sanitation systems. As has been much described, this reconstruction of the city facilitated a separation of rich urban dwellers from the poor and was seen at the time as a protection for the better-off from the diseases of the poor (Harvey 2003).

By the early 1800s, European cities were inhabited by a poor working class where the children worked in factories, caught their fingers in the machinery, and often went blind as they did fine needlework and other jobs by candlelight. Rickets and other diseases, related to specific vitamin deficiencies, were endemic. Women scavenged for food to support their families and often died in childbirth. Malnutrition was a major killer for men, women, and children. By the late nineteenth century, in both Europe and the United States, overcrowding and damp housing among the working class had led to tuberculosis as the major killer. In places such as New York City, cholera epidemics occurred up until the twentieth century because garbage collection and sanitation were neglected. It was not bet-ter medical treatment that led to the eradication of cholera and tuberculo-sis in Europe and the United States by the 1930s; it was improved housing and nutrition for the working class as well as a commitment to municipal services. Treatment for tuberculosis and other infectious diseases were not invented until ten years after the diseases abated.

As discussed in the edited volume *Wounded Cities* (J. Schneider and Susser 2003), although some destructive processes, such as earthquakes or hurricanes, are not directly caused by global policies, "the necessity or opportunity for reconstruction exposes a city immediately and powerfully to neo-liberal capitalist pressures." *Neoliberal* has come to be used as shorthand to cover the ideas that were first discussed in the 1930s by Friedrich Hayek and then developed by the Chicago School economist Milton Friedman in the 1970s (Harvey 2005; Naomi Klein 2007; Robotham 2009). Generally, neoliberalism refers to the deregulation of business and the fostering of a privatized market model to replace services, such as health, education, and welfare, that were previously performed by the state. This has been accompanied by a reduction in the funding for many services and increasing gap between rich and poor. It has also resulted in what might be seen as the re-regulation and increased policing of the poor (Peck and Tickell 2002). In the United States, this is reflected in the tightening of regulations for public assistance as well as the massive increase in incarceration (for example, see Mullings 2003; Rhodes 2004; Gilmore 2007; Fine and Ruglis 2009).

As many have documented, the neoliberal turn precipitated increas-ing inequality and accompanying health challenges at the same time as, in some global cities, the overall economy appears stronger (Harvey 2005; Khan and Pappas 2011). For example, in India today, the GNP has increased, and the wealthy middle class has grown dramatically, yet the rates of infant death in the first year of life have risen instead of dropping, reflecting the conditions of the majority of the population who are still poor. In the United States, we now have convincing data showing that the health of a significant proportion of the population has actually declined for the first time in a century. In fact, a recent study showed that the life expectancy of white women who did not complete high school actually dropped by five years between 1990 and 2008 and is now less than the life expectancy for black women, which was never good, in the same situation (Oshansky et al. 2012). As the data indicate, the general deterioration in health of the poor white population in the United States is not simply a result of the 2008 market crash but can be traced back to the reversals of government policies and cutbacks in the welfare state since the 1980s.

We see examples of such deterioration in Mexico City following the 1992 market crash, which heralded the imposition of neoliberal policies as well as the earthquake of the early 1990s. Claudio Lomnitz (2003) connects these events to a growing sense of alienation and corruption in Mexico City, which he illuminates with reference to the prevalent symbols and ironic metaphors of the dead. We can see the escalation in violence and drug feuds of the following decade in the light of these arguments. Over the same years, the issue of access to drinking water also became critical among poor people in Mexico and elsewhere as public funding and distribution declined (Meyers 2003).

In socialist or postsocialist societies such as China and Vietnam, since the 1990s, there have also been cutbacks in state funding for health care and social services and new participation in the capitalist market. Capitalist enterprises have rushed to such regions in the effort to benefit from the new reservoirs of labor. In the wake of the massive rapid industrialization of such places as the Mekong Delta and China, the health of workers in Southeast Asia has emerged as a pressing issue (Castells 2002; Chae 2003; Khan and Pappas 2011). As Apple has become the most successful corporation in the world, American students, particularly, have been shocked to learn of the poor conditions and environmental hazards of work among Apple laborers in China. Many workers in these regions are viewed as rural migrants and denied access to the social and health services they would supposedly be entitled to if they had stayed in the poverty-stricken rural villages. Critical medical anthropologists have long been concerned with occupational hazards and worker organizing (I. Susser 1985, 1988), and these emerging labor patterns are becoming important arenas for international research.

Another area of global inequality that at first glance seems unrelated directly to health is the increase in tourism that has been regarded as a major source of capital, although, as many have shown, again, it barely improves the economic opportunities of local residents (Appadurai 2001; Babb 2011). As Dennis Altman (2001) points out in *Global Sex*, sexual tourism is a major aspect of globalization and the accompanying neoliberal policies have had predictable consequences in the worldwide escalation of sexually transmitted diseases, and specifically HIV/AIDS (Kreniske 1997; Hirsch 2010. Less widely discussed has been the commodification of blood and plasma and its sale from poor to rich countries, which has also been strongly implicated in the global exacerbation of HIV/AIDS and other diseases (Pepin 2012).

In the United States, we can understand the processes leading up to and following Hurricane Katrina in 2005 in terms of the history of New Orleans and the incomes and race of the people who were displaced. First, historically, as a southern city with a large Black population, some of whom had arrived from Haiti in the nineteenth century, New Orleans had been a disadvantaged city receiving less than its share of federal funding. The levees built to contain the water had broken and flooded the poorest housing, belonging to African Americans in 1911. In the past decades, local newspapers and urban planners had known that the barriers were not sufficient to prevent flooding and that the poorest housing was built in the district most at risk for this flooding. The actual 2005 hurricane was most likely made more extreme as a result of global warming, and, as we might expect, the people who suffered the first dramatic impact of this global warming in the United States were African American and poor. Their suffering was overdetermined by the fact that they did not have cars to get out of the city, and when they did manage to leave on buses, many did not have the resources to return. Critical medical anthropologist Ann Lovell has been conducting path-breaking research on the ways in which the timing of rescue and the value placed on time for saving research as opposed to saving poor hospital patients may have affected mortality during Katrina (Lovell 2011).

Others have shown the difficulties homeowners and renters encountered in finding their way back to the city. Financing was easier for those whose houses were originally worth more, which severely disadvantaged lower-income homeowners. Return for renters, particularly the poor and people of color, was that much harder because landlords, looking to charge higher rents for the new buildings, did not rebuild affordable housing (Queeley 2011). In fact, the declines in the availability of public housing had begun a decade before Hurricane Katrina, and the disaster dramatically sped up this process. The flooding followed by the failure to rebuild or refinance public housing also doubled the number of homeless in New Orleans (B. Wright 2011) and led to the closure of the major hospital for the uninsured, Charity Hospital. Even before the flood, New Orleans had one of the highest rates of uninsured people of any city in the United States, and after the flood, it was estimated that about 200,000 people in Louisiana lost health insurance (Rudowitz et al. 2006). Those entitled to Medicaid could not access it in private hospitals in nearby towns to which they had been evacuated (Rudowitz et al 2006). Poor women of color were the most vulnerable during the disaster and also the least likely to return to New Orleans (Helmuth and Henrici 2010). We see the importance of under-standing the pressures of both race and gender in an intersectional analy-sis when we learn that "The U.S. Census and ACS data reveal that significantly fewer single mothers live in New Orleans than did so pre-Katrina; in fact, the number of single mothers has decreased by 40.6 percent" (Helmuth and Henrici 2010: 1) As Helmut and Henrici dem-onstrate, "Women and girls in poverty, as well as single mothers and sin-gle mothers in poverty, were already vulnerable groups in New Orleans prior to the disasters of Hurricane Katrina and the levees breaking in August 2005. To escape the flooded city, along with everyone else in New Orleans, poor women and girls had to leave their homes. As the city and surround-ing area continue to rebuild, perhaps more of those with fewer resources will be able to return" (Helmuth and Henrici 2010: 1).

Although there have been strong neighborhood movements trying to re-create old communities and affordable housing, the first areas to recover were the tourist hotels and the musical venues and upscale restaurants of the French Quarter. With the departure of many working-class residents, the workers imported to rebuild the city in its gentrified form were undocumented, nonunion Mexican immigrants who worked at below minimum wage. It was estimated that approximately 54 percent of the new construction workforce were undocumented and therefore without any form of health insurance (Rudowitz et al. 2006). Thus, we see the process of gentrification of a "wounded city" being accelerated by Hurricane Katrina and the workers hired to build that city replace the previous poor citizens of color, but this time without citizenship rights and with even less access to health care. Interestingly, during Hurricane Isaac, the major storm of 2012, the new levees of New Orleans held, but the nearby surrounding poor areas of Louisiana, Missouri, and Mississippi were hit with devastating floods—another measure of the effects of inequality, this time after the partial gentrification of New Orleans.

Cities in crisis have become a familiar theme in these early decades of the twenty-first century. The 2010 earthquake in Haiti killed thousands of people as the buildings and shanty towns of Port au Prince collapsed around them. Women again were particularly vulnerable, as they lived in poorly built housing and were subject to violence even before the earth-quake (Henrici 2010). Three years later, despite millions donated to help the residents, hundreds of thousands of people were still living in tent camps, having been subjected meanwhile to a cholera epidemic from pol-luted water. The problems of housing sound similar to New Orleans after

Katrina. According to the *New York Times*, "Haiti's shelter problem has been tackled unsystematically, in a way that has favored rural over urban victims and homeowners over renters because their needs were more easily met. Many families with the least resources have been neglected unless they happened to belong to a tent camp, neighborhood or vulnerable population targeted by a particular program" (Sontag 2012: A1). The money had been earmarked to "rebuild" Port au Prince as a major global city, but the majority of the original poor residents were living in shacks and temporary homeless shelters. This disaster, like Katrina, destroyed the lives of the poorest and also left them suffering in the following years in the face of alternate agendas to create a modern global city without a focus on the original poor urban dwellers.

In 2009 in China, thousands of children died when their school buildings collapsed during an earthquake; in total, 70,000 people perished, 10,000 of whom were children in their schools. As the documentary produced by Peter Kwong (2010) demonstrates, in the village where the documentary was filmed, all the other buildings were left standing—only the school buildings collapsed, killing three hundred children. Even before the earthquake, parents saw that the school was poorly constructed and suspected corruption. Later, as the parents protested in the streets, it became evident that, had the schools been built to code, the deaths would not have occurred. In 2010, a nuclear plant in Fukushima, Japan, the hazards of which had been documented, erupted. The unthinkable happened as radiation spewed out across the surrounding towns and villages, nearly threatening to engulf the city of Tokyo, with its 15 million people (Tabuchi 2012). These disasters, like Katrina, were exacerbated by the lack of attention to environmental regulation.

As societies change, cities are transformed and the health needs of urban populations take on different dimensions. Often these changes in health reflect chronic conditions and do not appear as dramatic as the crises outlined earlier, although they may kill as many people in the long run (Khan and Pappas 2011). Homelessness in the globalized cities of the United States provides a searing example of increasing poverty and disease occurring in the face of increasing wealth and overall economic growth (I. Susser 1996; Goode and Maskovsky 2001; Morgen and Maskovsky 2003). We can begin to see the way urban processes and stages of capitalism define the health problems of different populations. In the 1990s, homelessness in the U.S. appeared to be a widespread and perhaps unchanging condition. However, in most cities, as we shall see, homelessness reemerged as part of the American experience only in the late 1970s and early 1980s (Dehavenon 1996; I. Susser 1996). In fact, in New York City in 1975, the Governor's Task Force counted only thirty homeless families, whereas by the 1980s, this figure had risen to ten thousand. The number of families seeking emergency shelter did not begin to drop until the late 1990s. By 2001, homelessness had risen once again to the high levels of the 1980s. In the same period, estimates of the number of homeless individuals in New York City have varied from thirty-five thousand to one hundred thousand (I. Susser 1991a).

In 2012, although the numbers of homeless in New York City increased after the economic crash of 2008, few homeless people could be identified on the streets of Manhattan. Certainly, the media portrayed the 1990s as the period of epidemic homelessness and poverty in New York City (Marcus 2006). In 2012, as a result of social movements that demanded housing for the mentally ill, disabled, and homeless as well as movements for affordable housing, we do see fewer homeless people in the streets. However, the restructuring of cities has also led to the invisibility of the poor rather than a decrease in the proportion of the people in poverty (I. Susser 1996).

Surprisingly Ida Susser's (2012) updated study of a previously working-class community, in the now-trendy, Greenpoint-Williamsburg, Brooklyn, demonstrated that the proportion of poor people had not decreased since 1975. Within the same census blocks, the difference in incomes between the rich and the poor had widened. In 2010, the proportion of people receiving public assistance had declined with the 1996 Personal Responsibility and Work Opportunity Reconciliation Act (PRWORA) "welfare reform" measures. Nevertheless, in 2010; fully 40 percent of the population of the upscale neighborhood of Williamsburg qualified for some form of government assistance such as food stamps or disability pensions. At the same time, the municipal government had rezoned the area to allow high-rise luxury condominium apartments to be built, only marketed to families with incomes over $200,000. Such municipal policies have edged the poor out of Manhattan and made it harder for middle-income households to survive throughout the boroughs, but they have not addressed the problems of poverty, homelessness, and health. In fact, whereas in 1975 there were almost no homeless people in Greenpoint-Williamsburg, in 2012, there were a wide diversity of homeless people, including Latinos and Polish immigrants. Since the late 1970s and the implementation of neoliberal policies, municipal hospitals and community clinics have been cut back, and food and shelter have become more expensive. These are the processes that help to explain the increasing disparities in health in the United States. As we have seen, in the United States, people without homes, either doubling up with relatives, sleeping in cars, or seeking shelter in churches, warehouses, and municipal institutions have become less visible but not less numerous in the gentrified city. In addition, in the 1990s, when homeless people were more visible and when an epidemic of homelessness seemed to be occurring throughout the United States, many anthropologists were recruited to conduct ethnographic research in coordination with medical projects concerned with mental illness, tuberculosis, HIV, and other health issues. Homelessness and its representation became crucial issues for medical anthropology. A fundamental question concerned the causes of homelessness. Frequently, there exists an underlying assumption that people may be homeless because of problems with mental health or learned behavior. In the course of their research, anthropologists and other social scientists have consistently found that homelessness is best explained in relation to housing and poverty rather than specific mental problems (Hopper, Susser, Conover 1986). Many health problems stem from deprivation or can be found among homeless people, but such problems are not confined to the homeless. In contrast to much media representation and popular assumptions, mental illness and substance abuse do not define this population, nor do such issues alone account for homelessness.

To understand homelessness, we need to see how it has been created in different historical contexts and in different societies. A brief consideration of the word homeless already shows us some of the issues to be addressed. There are poor people without shelter all over the world. Mexico City, Rio de Janeiro, and many other major cities in Latin America are surrounded by shantytowns or informal settlements outside the formal municipal districts. *Favelas*, informal settlements in Brazil, have been the subject of much anthropological research in Latin America since the 1960s and recently the most famous of these *favelas* in Rio has been threatened with gentrification. Many cities in Africa have been circled by growing informal settlements for the past thirty years. In Durban, South Africa, hundreds of thousands of Africans moved into informal settlements surrounding the city after apartheid laws restricting the movements of Africans were repealed. None of these populations is usually referred to as homeless. However, in the past decade, an internationally connected "shack dwellers" movement has emerged linking social movements against displacement for gentrification from Latin America, to India to Southern Africa.

In the United States, the term *homeless* came into popular use in the late 1970s as a way to describe the growing numbers of poor people who were sleeping in the streets and public places. The advent of visible poor people without shelter was a direct product of the shift to neoliberal policies first implemented in New York City after the fiscal crisis of 1975 (Susser 2012) and later implemented nationwide after Ronald Reagan became president in 1980. In the 1980s, as many people temporarily found overnight shelter in churches, warehouses, and armories, municipalities began to count homeless populations. The 1990 census contained an institutional recognition of the new homeless population, and anthropologists were called on to define and count street people for the national statistics (Hopper 1992, 2003). Homelessness had become a predictable aspect of life in American cities, and the fact that the phenomenon was qualitatively new and different from experiences of poverty in the 1950s, 1960s, and 1970s had been quickly forgotten (I. Susser 1996). With the restructuring of New York City since the 1990s, the bankrupt hotels in Times Square and other central locations in Manhattan that had housed the homeless with municipal subsidies in the 1990s were closed down. Major financial investment through a public-private partnership in Times Square and nearby Bryant Park turned these areas into exciting tourist spots subsidized by municipal funds, while homeless people were bused to shelters in the outer boroughs or, increasingly, to upstate New York (I. Susser 1993; Fainstein 2001). The center of the city was rebuilt for the better-off. Except for high-end escort settings, the old pornographic sites and other bars that had characterized Times Square for decades migrated to dark warehouse districts in Queens (Maia 2012). Thus, along with the poor and indigent, the sex workers and drug users were also edged out of sight or sometimes incarcerated to create the New York City of 2012. These changes represent what urban researchers have come to understand as the policing of urban space and the re-regulation of the poor.

In fact, it would seem, the sudden visibility of poverty and homelessness that occurred in the United States and western Europe in the 1980s and 1990s signaled the brutal transition to neoliberalism. Once that transition had been effected, cities were restructured to relegate the poor to the hidden margins of the centers of capital. One stark measure of the transfer of the poor and homeless out of the visible gentrifying cities in the United States can be traced in the shift in homelessness from 2007 to 2010 (U.S. Government Annual Report on Homelessness 2010: ii): "Since 2007, the annual number of people using homeless shelters in principal cities has decreased 17 percent (from 1.22 million to 1.02 million), and the annual number of people using homeless shelters in suburban and rural areas has increased 57 percent (from 367,000 to 576,000)." Two recent ethnographies of poor people (Lawinski 2010) and shelters for battered women (Davis 2006) in previously well-off suburbs and towns in upstate New York document the lives of the poor in these outlying regions. Since the 1980s, there has been manifest progress in response to social movements and political mobilization in general to house the long-term homeless, and specifically the single homeless who have disabilities, whose numbers decreased as a consequence of permanent supportive housing programs. However, with the recession that started in 2008, there has been a dramatic increase in U.S. homeless families, headed largely by black and white women, who have no history of disability:

the proportion of family households has increased, as has the percentage of White, non-Hispanic shelter users. The number of homeless persons in families has increased by 20 percent from 2007 to 2010, and families currently represent a much larger share of the total sheltered population than ever before. The proportion of homeless people who are using emergency shelter and transitional housing as part of a family has increased from 30 percent to 35 percent during this same period. The majority of homeless families consist of a single mother with young children. (U.S. Government Annual Report on Homelessness 2010)

Despite this dramatic increase in families needing emergency shelter, as homeless and poor people have been displaced from the central cities and relegated to the suburbs, the image of homelessness that led one activist group to call itself "Picture the Homeless," and indeed the term *homelessness*, have practically disappeared from the media or indeed from much anthropological literature (see Marcus 2006 for a discussion of the changing media representation of the homeless). Nevertheless, as ethnographers (Lyon-Callo 2004; Gowan 2010) continue to remind us, people still live and strategize for survival in the streets of major U.S. cities.

Here, we briefly examine experiences of vagrancy and poverty and their treatment by governments during the emergence of capitalism in Europe and later in the United States. This will give us some background for understanding poverty today and putting homelessness in historical and geographic perspective. Because Britain was the first country to develop industrial capitalism, we begin there in looking for the roots of modern poverty and homelessness. Vagrants and wandering poor people began streaming into London in the sixteenth and seventeenth centuries. As feudal lords entering commercial wool production found it more profitable to keep sheep on wide areas of land, Enclosure Laws were introduced to allow the displacement of serfs from their ancestral cottages and farm plots. As people flocked to towns looking for work and for new ways to survive in an emerging capitalist economy, they were separated from their hereditary ties with the rural villages of Britain.

As many people were freed from agricultural serfdom, the creation of wage labor was accompanied by a new form of insecurity in the form of unemployment. The British government had to introduce a way of coping with the poor, who had previously been tied to and supported by the land of feudal lords. Throughout the sixteenth century in Britain, the number of beggars grew; the British government started first to register, license, and count beggars and later to punish and enslave those without licenses. Later, laws were passed that taxed local villages to provide funds to support the poor of their own districts (Piven and Cloward 1971).

In the nineteenth century, with the expansion of agriculture, the taking over of common lands, and the introduction of machinery, many more people found themselves out of work. The poor relief system was greatly expanded to address this issue. In the United States as well as in Britain, poorhouses were created, where people lived and were also forced to work for their living, as the government authorities saw fit. Clearly, under current usage, we would have called such people homeless. It was not until the twentieth century that methods of controlling the destitute through poorhouse residences and work requirements were abandoned and other forms of public assistance were implemented in most industrialized countries.

Given this brief history, let us now return to consideration of the United States during the twentieth century. New institutions are usually initiated in times of crisis, and the Great Depression was one such period. After the financial crash of 1929, the population of the United States experienced unemployment rates through the 1930s of around 40 percent. New words became popular, such as *hobos*, for individuals who crossed the country looking for work, and *Hoovervilles*, for makeshift settlements set up by families evicted from their homes because unemployment had made it impossible to pay the rent or mortgage. These settlements around the country, like the one in Central Park in New York, were named after President Herbert Hoover, who in the depth of the Great Depression did not believe the government was responsible for solving the unemployment situation. As a consequence, he lost the presidency to Franklin Delano Roosevelt.

Anthropologists and sociologists have published studies of the hobos, conceived of consistently as men (N. Anderson 1923). Surprisingly little attention was paid to the squatter settlements known as Hoovervilles, where women and children were also to be found. In 1934, President Roosevelt initiated the Social Security Act to provide the first federal public assistance program for widows and orphans: Aid to Dependent Children. No specific provision was outlined for homeless people, but public assistance did include a calculation of the cost of rent and housing. However, having a home was not made into a socially guaranteed right, which might have prevented future homelessness. It was not until the new homelessness of the 1980s that the constitutional right to shelter began to be established in some courts (Hopper and Cox 1982).

From the 1940s to the 1970s, high employment rates and the increasing employment of women combined with entitlement programs and Social Security to keep families in homes and most people from sleeping in the streets. Even Michael Harrington's (1962) famous study *The Other America,* which reminded Americans that the poor existed, does not mention the word *homelessness*. Anthropologists studied the poor of Appalachia or the minority populations of the inner cities, but homeless people did not yet exist as a distinct cultural category.

Homelessness again emerged as a public issue in New York City at the end of the 1970s (Baxter and Hopper 1981). In 1975, New York City was declared bankrupt. In response, social services were cut, and tax benefits were allotted for real estate development (I. Susser 1982). Housing costs rose, and poor people began to lose their homes. By 1978, homelessness had begun to emerge as a visible phenomenon in New York City, as individuals sought shelter in railroad stations and other public spaces (Baxter and Hopper 1981). By 1982, homeless families were being housed in rundown hotels around the city (I. Susser 1989). Throughout the 1980s, federal services were reduced, real estate prices rose, and the departure of industry reduced available work; homelessness became a widespread phenomenon across the United States (Dehavenon 1996). Between 1985 and 1987, most cities in the United States reported annual increases of between 15 percent and 50 percent in their homeless populations (U.S. Conference of Mayors 1987).

From 1980 to the present, homelessness has been described by anthropologists and sociologists in a variety of settings (for a review see, I. Susser 1996). For example, in *Checkerboard Square,* David Wagner (1993) describes in detail the lives of street people in a northern New England city in the 1980s. *Checkerboard Square* challenges stereotypes, in that the homeless population is found in a small New England town and most of the homeless people are white, although the homeless population resembles that of large U.S. cities in proportionate size, income, and joblessness.

In contrast to many studies that rely on interviews with individual homeless people, Wagner's is a community study. He describes the social interactions among the people he studies, their shared values and evaluation of U.S. society, and their efforts at collective action. Through the voices of the homeless he convinces us that many people have a clear and rational perception of deindustrialization and the shortage of work. On the basis of their own experiences, homeless people in North City have constructed a critical view of U.S. society. They do not accept explanations of their homelessness put forward by members of the wider society, which blame individuals for their problems without considering the changing economic context.

In the early 1980s, the Coalition for the Homeless was formed in New York City and fought through the courts for the legal right to shelter (Hopper and Cox 1982). New York City was required by law to provide housing for men, women, and families without shelter. Armories were opened up as temporary shelter for homeless men and women; families were housed in a variety of rundown hotels. Since that time, many legal battles have been fought over the lack of provisions for housing homeless people, and an entire bureaucracy has been created to address the issue (Gounis 1992; I. Susser 1999). As a result of the ongoing activism of the homeless and their advocates New York funded permanent supportive housing. This was of great benefit to people with disabilities who had previously found shelter in the single room occupancy hotels now demolished or upgraded. However, it did not address the needs of homeless families who needed stable affordable housing. Periodically, with each recession, 2001, 2008, and in between, lawsuits have been filed against the mayor of New York for the lack of housing as the growing numbers of families with children overwhelm the emergency housing facilities. Such pressures that force the Mayor to take action are based on the important victory of the Coalition for the Homeless that residents of New York State have a right to shelter.

However, the basic problem of the increasing gap between rich and poor and the difficulty for the poor to find homes or to retain their footing in working-class neighborhoods remains (Sharff 1998; Susser 2012). In the 1990s, people became homeless when the economy failed to provide work for the growing population of poor people. In 1996, after the welfare laws introduced in the 1930s were replaced by Temporary Assistance to Needy Families, which required welfare recipients to find paid work, many people found themselves working in such low-paid jobs that they could not afford rent (Morgen and Maskovsky 2003). We can see the health effects of poverty in cities manifest in studies of Harlem (Mullings and Wali 2001) Overall, we see the concept of syndemics (as developed by Merrill Singer) most useful to this approach.

The U.S. media and much of the social science literature have focused on the individual problems of homeless people. Homeless people suffer from many health problems, including mental illness and substance abuse. Some researchers have suggested that the increase in homelessness was precipitated by the closing of state institutions for the mentally ill, which was mandated by the Kennedy administration in the late 1950s. However, large numbers of homeless people did not appear on the streets until twenty years later. Increasing homelessness corresponds directly to changes in the United States such as deindustrialization in the 1980s and globalization since the 1990s, which have resulted in the loss of jobs combined with a shift in public expenditure away from health care, social services, and public housing. Reductions in the federal budget for social services, changes in real estate regulation and taxes, and the increasing cost of housing, rather than individual issues such as mental illness and substance abuse, make people most vulnerable to homelessness in a worsening economic situation (Hopper, Susser, and Conover 1987; Dehavenon 1996; I. Susser 1996).

Since the 1980s, homelessness has become one aspect of life frequently experienced by poor working-class people in the United States (I. Susser 2002). For example, it has been estimated that in the 1990s about 5 percent of New York City's poor population experienced homelessness every year, including about 10,000 families with children. People found themselves doubling up in apartments with relatives long before they ended up in public shelters. Later they had to pass through the shelter system before they could find an affordable apartment. Many people living in homeless shelters have children living in homes with friends and relatives. In 2010, the estimates remained the same as in the 1990s— about 10,000 families with children, comprising over 30,000 people, were still in emergency shelter or transitional housing (Coalition for the Homeless 2010). In 2012 in New York City, twenty thousand children slept in homeless shelters every night, possibly the highest number since the Great Depression (*New York Times*, 2012). In addressing the health problems of the homeless, researchers have found that they must address the problems of access and continuity of care throughout the growing poor population of the United States.

HEALTH ISSUES AMONG U.S. HOMELESS POPULATIONS

Although homeless people in the United States suffer from the same health problems as other Americans, the problems are magnified many times by lack of social support, lack of housing, poor nutrition, lack of economic support, and lack of access to medical services. Death rates and rates of disease are all higher among the homeless population, even in comparison to poor people with homes. Studies of the health of homeless adults and children find more health problems in general than among a poor population that has housing (for a review of these issues, see Schanzer et al. 2007). However, as people become homeless and enter the shelter system in New York City, research suggests that they often become connected with health care services that they have not been able to access previously. In fact, it seems many poor people have been passing intermittently through emergency rooms without any continuity of care for major health problems. Once they enter homelessness, they finally receive attention from a variety of social services that help them to sort out their medical needs. It seems that many poor people had to go through homelessness before they were connected with Medicaid and other forms of assistance to which they were previously entitled.

Two of the increasingly serious health problems confronted by the poor and homeless population in the United States of the 1990s were tuberculosis and HIV infection. The two conditions are directly related, because HIV infection undermines the immune system and leaves individuals particularly vulnerable to contracting tuberculosis. In the 1990s, it was estimated that one-half of those individuals with active tuberculosis in New York City were also HIV-positive (Landesman 1993). Tuberculosis, which is spread through respiratory secretions, has historically been associated with poor housing conditions and poor nutrition. It should come as no surprise that the problem resurfaced among people deprived of homes and surviving on the margins of the U.S. economy. Crowded conditions, such as those found in shelters and prisons, provide excellent breeding grounds for the tuberculosis bacterium. Exacerbating this situation was the dramatic cutback in clinics and preventive services addressing the problem of tuberculosis in U.S. cities. Between 1960 and 1980, most of the preventive network of clinics and community services constructed over the previous sixty years to combat the tuberculosis epidemics of the nineteenth and early twentieth centuries were dismantled. As a result, between 1979 and 1986, the incidence of tuberculosis in New York City increased by 83 percent. Twenty to 30 percent of the people with tuberculosis were homeless (Lerner 1993). As tuberculosis resurfaced, cities had to attempt to rebuild lacerated community prevention networks. New York City implemented monitoring programs to make sure people took their medications. The implications in the media and some of the health literature was that the reason tuberculosis was spreading was that people, particularly poor people like the homeless population, were not taking their medications. This blaming of the victim ignored the systematic causes of the spread of tuberculosis in relation to poor housing conditions and the dismantling of the preventive public health system, which had in previous decades set up clinics in poor areas that provided free X-ray screenings, free medications, and ongoing treatment and evaluation for community residents.

HIV infection (AIDS) is still increasing among poor and minority populations and also among those who have lost their homes. For poor homeless men and women, the sale of sexual services is one avenue through which to earn money. The need for money may also be exacerbated by addiction to many and diverse substances from cocaine to prescription drugs. Among many poor people, beset by violence and hopelessness, attention to the prevention of HIV infection may appear too distant a concern. Many may not envision themselves as living long enough to die of AIDS. Epidemiological research in the shelters of New York City suggests a high rate of HIV infection. Because people usually have sexual relations and share needles and drugs with people in their networks, this puts shelter residents at even higher risk. A team approach involving anthropologists with psychiatrists, caseworkers, and epidemiologists proved extremely effective in implementing and evaluating an intervention for mentally ill homeless men in a shelter in New York City (E. Susser et al. 1993). The purpose of the intervention was to assist homeless men in finding appropriate housing and to continue to maintain contact with and provide assistance to them in accessing social services for nine months after they had relocated. The aim was to reconnect the men with social services in the community to which they relocated so that they would not be left without supports in the new setting. The men were divided into two groups of approximately one hundred men each. Those who were assigned housing with no follow-up intervention formed the controls. The experimental group received nine months of follow-up transitional services. Working with the research team, two anthropologists were given the task of tracking all the men, from both groups. They were required to meet with each man on a monthly basis to document his housing situation, whether he was taking his medication for mental illness, and other problems.

Working with mentally ill men as they left the shelter system was not easy. To be recruited for the study, the men had to have a diagnosis of schizophrenia, schizophrenic personality disorder, or manic depression. Many of the men were not communicative in general and were suspicious of health workers and questionnaires. Because they lived in an environment where illegal activities such as drug dealing took place, they were suspicious of people who were trying to track down lost individuals. Few people had access to telephones or addresses where they received mail. Mentally ill homeless men were often cut off from their families either by their choice or their family's. Frequently, calling a family member would not help in finding them. Men also circulated between mental health institutions, shelters, and prison; visiting them or accessing information from these institutions was extremely difficult. Bureaucracies often have strict regulations about not providing information about clients, which, while important for reasons of confidentiality, makes it difficult to keep in touch with people.

The anthropologists began the study by spending time with the men in the large armory where they originally found shelter. They spent several months sitting in the room provided for mentally ill homeless men to socialize and organize group-counseling sessions. They became familiar figures around the shelter and explained to many people that they were conducting an anthropological study of the shelter and the lives of mentally ill homeless men. As men began to be recruited to the study and assigned housing, the anthropologists followed them to their new locales. They visited the men on a monthly basis or arranged for them to come back to the shelter and discuss their situation there. Because the men already knew the anthropologists and had established informal relationships with them, such interviews were not usually regarded as onerous. Because interviews were also paid for (at the rate of $15 per interview), the anthropologists encountered requests for unnecessary repeat interviews by men in need of cash.

Over the course of two years, the anthropologists established credibility and trust with mentally ill homeless men and their friends and relatives. Despite shifting locations from the streets to various sectors of the shelter *unsystem*, institutionalization, and frequent disappearance of clients, the anthropologists were able to maintain a 95 percent follow-up rate over a period of two years. This was higher than the usually acceptable 80 percent follow-up rates common to research conducted among educated middle-income populations with permanent addresses and telephones (Conover et al 1997; Marcus 2006). This study clearly shows the significance of an anthropological approach, even in a quantitative epidemiological experimental study. Because of the financial and theoretical support for anthropology in this research, the anthropologists were able to gather important material for an ethnographic description of the lives of mentally ill homeless men, documenting the constantly shifting population as it moved from shelters to hospitals to prisons and back again. At the same time, the anthropological connections provided an excellent research setting for psychiatric epidemiologists.

In a related research project, anthropological researchers in a homeless shelter for men in New York City were involved in a project to assist in the prevention of HIV infection among mentally ill homeless men. They initiated the production of a video to be made by the homeless men themselves for the shelter. Planning this project and filming it in the shelter proved an important experience for the staff and the homeless men in education concerning HIV infection. In addition, the video provided material for anthropological analysis of the perceptions of homeless men concerning sexuality, drugs, and the residents and staff of the shelter (I. Susser and González 1992). The video demonstrated the close connections in the lives of the staff and the homeless men, their experiences with drugs and AIDS, and the conflicts between the two groups around these issues. In addition, it documented a problematic perception of women as evil and as purveyors of disease, a further example of arguments that "blame the victim" rather than comprehend the overall situation. In general, the making of the video provided a forum for homeless men to work out conflicts and attitudes concerning sexual orientation, HIV infection, and other issues and to construct ways of addressing one another with respect to AIDS prevention. Anthropologists have been particularly involved in interdisciplinary collaboration in such programs as the development of HIV prevention programs (Susser and González 1992) and in evaluating interventions in community psychiatry. As in the approach to HIV, most anthropologists working with homeless populations have seen themselves both as researchers and as activists concerned with the improvement of conditions faced by the population they serve (M. Singer 1995a).

Many critical medical anthropologists have found Foucault's ideas useful in discussing neoliberal policies and the disciplining of populations. Lyon-Callo's (2004) ethnography of a homeless shelter in Northampton, Massachusetts, a town where 40 percent of the jobs disappeared with deindustrialization, considers the ways in which homeless people come to be categorized by staff and consent to be described as deviant individuals with specific problems rather than seeing themselves as part of a disenfranchised working class. As Alfredo Gonzalez (2008) pointed out in his review of Lyon-Callo's study, this powerful ethnography was published after the media and funding interests in "homelessness" had declined and would benefit from being placed in the context of the previous literature on class, social movements, and homelessness (Abu-Lughod 1994; I. Susser 1996; Hopper 2003; Marcus 2006). Catherine Kingfisher (2007), also following Foucault, on the basis of her research in a small town in Canada, has discussed the ways in which the "Discursive constructions of homelessness, categorizations of homeless persons as Native addicted men and of homelessness as a property of individuals [are] produced." She asks, "Moreover, how are they produced in such a way as to be taken as common sense?" Again, how do the day-to-day practices of neoliberalism lead homeless people and social service workers to understand homelessness in terms of individualized "blaming" categories rather than as a product of the low pay for work and the high costs of rent, as Lyon-Callo also asks? We need to remember here that Marcus and Neil Smith (1996) both describe the occupation of Tompkins Square Park in the 1990s where homeless people joined with youth and other groups to protest the ongoing gentrification of the Lower East Side in New York City. At that time, and in the urban movements such as "Parents on the Move" many homeless people perceived their situation as a product of changing real estate and deindustrialization rather than in terms of the individual deviance and medicalization fostered by the shelter as an institution.

In an ethnography, based on a decade of participant observation, Philippe Bourgois (Bourgois and Schonberg 2009) described the lives of drug users on the streets of San Francisco. He and his coauthor and photographer Jeff Schonberg documented the ways in which their lives were constrained and constructed by what Bourgois, following Foucault, perceived as biopolitics. In other words, the lives of street drug users were framed by the policies of the state. To quote Bourgois, "Foucault's term biopower refers to the ways historically entrenched institutionalized forms of social control discipline bodies. The bio-politics of substance abuse include a wide range of laws, medical interventions, social institutions, ideologies, and even structures of feeling." As Bourgois stresses, "The state and medical authorities have created distinctions between heroin and methadone that revolve primarily around moral categories concerned with controlling pleasure and productivity: legal versus illegal; medicine versus drug" (2009: 167). Thus, even street people are never outside society; their lives are framed by societies' institutions and the way they experience poverty, homeless or housed, is produced by the laws of society. However, here again we need to remember the social movements that have emerged, among street people, homeless people, and unemployed workers at different historical movements. We might ask whether such movements might be connected with broader questions that emerged recently in the "Occupy Wall Street" events where, in fact, the issues of youth and college students collaborating with homeless and street people did become a complicating question. We still need to ask what conditions might lead to changes in the direction of justice for the poor and homeless today and whether they were included in the 99 percent that was demanding recognition in the Occupy movement of 2011.

POVERTY AND HEALTH IN THIRD WORLD CITIES

In parts of Africa and other colonial territories of the twentieth century, critical medical anthropology has illuminated the political economy of disease. Populations were decimated not only by direct brutality through forced labor and other measures but also by the increase in disease. Viruses and bacteria, which probably lay dormant for centuries, were suddenly able to multiply through urban overcrowding, poor sanitation, and malnutrition. Meanwhile, the clearance of forest and the reduction of animal hosts led to sleeping sickness and malaria as the tsetse fly and the mosquito preyed on humans. As men, forced to raise cash for taxes, left their rural villages to work in the mining towns, the skewed sex ratio in the growing colonial cities set the scene for migrant women to find informal employment on the margins of industrial development as beer brewers and sex workers. Rates of syphilis, a major scourge among rich and poor in European cities, rose precipitously in the colonial towns as the need for African men to migrate for work and the brutal conditions of colonialism destroyed previous household and marriage patterns. As many effective public health measures were introduced, they brought with them iatrogenic infections through less than sterile needles and blood transfusions. It has been convincingly argued that these same colonial migrant cities of the 1930s were the crucible for the AIDS epidemic (Pepin 2012).

Post–World War II, as colonized countries won liberation, the pattern of diseases shifted once again. In the first years of liberation, the 1960s and 1970s, new states attempted to build approximations of the welfare states that had emerged in Europe and the West in the early twentieth century. However, after the Washington consensus that adopted the neoliberal policies of 1980, which cut back the funding for poor countries and required them to invest in business before they could budget for health, education, or other services, cities in the periphery were seeing an increase in inequality, accompanied again by malnutrition and infectious diseases. By the close of the twentieth century, the postcolonial cities of the world had expanded far beyond any cities in the centers of capital and with the influx of industrial investment through globalization, the diseases began to reflect the environmental pollution of the new industries as well as the lack of administrative investment in the densely populated informal settlements. As noted earlier, rises of water, sanitation, radiation, and other forms of pollution devastated urban populations. Chronic diseases such as cancer, respiratory diseases, diabetes, and obesity began to escalate in Third World settings. However, even though peripheral regions were manifesting more of the diseases of the industrialized centers, famine, drought, and floods still affected the countries of the periphery more drastically than those in the centers of capital. With the famine in the Sahel in the early 1970s, a new era of crises exacerbated by the density and poverty of the new urban populations became widespread. Although such crises, which have become more frequent and visible in the twenty-first century appear natural, we can see, as discussed in *Wounded Cities*, that they are directly related to the political and economic policies of globalization.

Over the past thirty years, population increases have combined with the development of agribusiness in many poor rural areas to create a population of unemployed wage laborers who are forced to move to the cities in search of work. The development of expensive agricultural technology combined with international corporate investment in agriculture has made it increasingly difficult for small peasants to retain their land. Only peasants with large enough landholdings to withstand the large debts accumulated in bad harvest years and to produce enough to compete with foreign investors had any hope of surviving. World Trade Agreements, such as NAFTA, have undone domestic tariffs that protect local producers and opened the markets of poor countries such as Mexico to the products of major corporations. So, for example, as the last stages of the NAFTA agreements between the United States and Mexico went into effect, farmers growing rice and beans in Mexico led a million-person march through Mexico City because they could no longer make a living in competition with imported food from the United States. As a result of breaking down of such protections and the "unfettered markets" advocated by global neoliberal policies, there has been a progressive loss of landholdings among the poorer peasantry and a consolidation of income among corporate investors. The increasing inequality found in many rural areas has contributed to the creation of a population of landless laborers. In contrast to peasants who own their own land and may scrape a living from the sale of produce, such people have lost their land and have to work for wages like industrial workers. However, increasing agricultural technology has reduced the need for rural wage laborers. Along with the undermining of local agriculture, there has been an increase in food insecurity among the poor populations of the periphery. To quote Marc Edelman who has studied peasant farmers since the 1980s,

"Beginning in the 1980s, deregulation of agricultural trade led many developing countries to rely on imports of cheap subsidized grain from the US and EU, glutting markets and undermining livelihoods for the nearly two billion people who still live on small farms. The free-market juggernaut also dismantled or downsized institutions key to rural people's survival: state development banks that made loans, agriculture ministries that provided technical assistance and purchasing agencies that paid farmers adequate prices for crops. Peasants and small farmers are losing control of their seeds to a handful of biotech giants. In the face of these onslaughts, rural people worldwide abandoned the countryside and flooded into urban slums or migrated abroad. (Edelman 2012)

This in turn has precipitated the waves of poverty-stricken populations that have migrated to Third World cities over past decades and continue to flow into unserviced areas of major municipalities.

Since the early 2000s, more than half of the world's population has lived in cities, many in such poor cities that it led Mike Davis (2007) to title his book, *Planet of the Slums*. As Sidney Mintz (1985) documented for the urban workers in industrial Europe, the exigencies and long hours of factory work changed not only the time and labor patterns of Europe's former peasantry but also their diets and leisure pursuits. Mintz shows that industrial workers in Great Britain were forced to reduce their daily meals to such fast foods as bread and jam and tea and sugar, which also carried with them stimulants to get through the long laboring days. Mintz relates these new forms of consumption to the capitalist merchants and traders who brought the sugar and tea from slave plantations in the Caribbean and elsewhere in the British Empire and sold them to the impoverished urban dwellers who no longer had the land or the access to firewood to grow and cook their own food. In the contemporary global era, we also see changing diets as rural laborers mass in cities, no longer able to supplement their meals by picking breadfruit, mangoes, bananas, or avocados from the local trees. Instead, we find the new proletariat spending their minimal incomes on soda pop, potato chips, and fast foods, sending the rates of obesity and diabetes soaring. We find people in the periphery buying more and more cigarettes from multinational corporations as regulations against smoking proliferate in the centers of capital.

As an aspect of industrialization and, its corollary in the hiring of low paid women in rural and urban areas, we find new health challenges that have been studied by medical anthropologists. For example, we find women giving up the healthiest form of baby food, breastfeeding, which is known to provide immunity and contribute to brain development, for baby formula. Women adopt formula partly because they have to work long hours and sometimes because they have been led mistakenly to believe that formula is more modern and better for their offspring. In the 1970s, an early global movement led to the regulation of the sale and advertising of baby formula among populations where neither clean water nor the funds to buy sufficient formula were available. In the 1990s, some of these worldwide gains were undermined as researchers became concerned that breastfeeding was a conduit for the AIDS virus. After much debate and continued research, it has been established that for babies in poor countries with limited access to clean water, breastfeeding saves more infant lives than formula, despite the AIDS virus. In spite of the recommendations of the American Academy of Pediatrics for six months exclusive breastfeeding (http://pediatrics.aappublications.org/content/129/3/e827.full), we find in 2012, U.S. hospitals, in the face of previous bans and regulations, donate free baby formula to all mothers, encouraging American mothers to believe that formula is a desirable replacement for mother's milk (Belluck 2012). In each of these cases, as with the mobilization around the price of food and the privatization of water, grassroots populations combined with community health advocates and global human rights activists continue to struggle to adequately address problems taking into account the perspective and rights of local populations.

Many critical medical anthropologists studying social ills outside the United States have pursued aspects of a Foucauldian approach to develop important arguments. Adriana Petryna, in her ethnographic research with respect to the aftermath of the 1986 nuclear disaster at Chernobyl, talks about citizenship based on claims to disease as another aspect of biopolitics as outlined by Foucault. Social movements demand entitlement on the basis of their suffering. As Petryna argues, "one can describe biological citizenship as a massive demand for but selective access to a form of social welfare based on medical, scientific and legal criteria that both acknowledge biological injury and compensate for it" (Petryna 2002: 6). She shows the way bureaucratic compensation and scientific research around Chernobyl is used in the Ukraine in the construction of a postrevolutionary democratic legitimacy on a global scale. As she describes, in postsocialist Ukraine in the face of "fundamental losses" in employment and legal securities, "A stark order of social and economic exclusion now coexists with a generalized discourse of human rights" (Petryna 2002: 6). Jonathan Stillo has similarly described poor tuberculosis sufferers in Romania. Under the social cutbacks of postsocialist Romania, a TB diagnosis might be one of the few remaining ways to protect people from destitution (Stillo 2012).

In countries on the periphery, the concept of exclusion and "letting them die" as discussed by Foucault has been found most explanatory by several authors. Joao Biehl, in his description of the treatment of poor people labeled as mentally ill in urban Brazil sees the government as simply abandoning the population and "letting them die." In coming to this conclusion, Biehl traces the life story of a destitute woman named Catherina living in a practically abandoned institution, Vita. He shows that her poverty has even prevented her from receiving the correct diagnosis for her genetic disorder, which is not in fact mental illness. Similarly, in South

Africa in the early 2000s, a study of women sex workers living with AIDS in the vicinity of major mining works led Catherine Campbell (a social psychologist) to go so far as to call her book *Letting Them Die* (2003).

Informal settlements lacking major public health foundations have characterized the massive growth of cities in the periphery. Such settlements lack sewage facilities and electricity, paved roads, and transportation as well as running water and drinking water. In addition, they are not easily covered by regulations and make the registration of births and deaths or the tracking of health problems virtually impossible. Even when residents of informal settlements find work and pay taxes, their needs are often ignored in the spending of municipal funds. Because of the frequent lack of running water and sewage facilities, informal settlements are at risk for cholera and other infectious diseases. Mass vaccination campaigns, where the local community workers occupied in thankless, frustrating street visits are frequently underpaid, have proved difficult to sustain (Closser 2010).

Focusing on domestic grassroots organizing, Gregory Pappas has documented the battle for a sewage facility in a poor community in Karachi, Pakistan (Pappas 2010). In 2007, the community at the grassroots level worked with a local politician to penetrate the bureaucracy and inertia of the state to build a sewage pipe. Sadly, in 2012, demonstrating how difficult such changes are to maintain, the same politician, along with the mayor who supported him, was murdered in urban rioting. Similarly, in the 1980s, a key public health activist who was organizing against violent drug murders in Medellin, Colombia, was murdered during a campaign for human rights. As people continue to fight for social justice, we as anthropologists have to recognize the stakes involved and how important such changes are for leaders and local residents who, time and again, risk their lives to improve the living conditions for all.

Because of the lack of industrial and environmental regulation, informal settlements have been the sites of some of the world's most tragic industrial disasters in recent history as well as ongoing industrial hazards (Susser 1985, 1988, 1991b). In Bhopal in 1984, most of the people who died when poisonous gas escaped from the Union Carbide plant that manufactured fertilizers for Indian agriculture were living in an informal settlement between the plant and the city limits. Although regulations stated that the plant could not operate near the resident population, the thousands of people housed in the informal settlements on the outskirts of the city had not been considered by the plant managers or the city government in evaluating safety concerns for the continued operation of the plant. Kim Fortun (2001) has analyzed the different perceptions of advocates and professionals, both from India and the United States, in addressing the reparations and clean up of this disaster. Seeing herself as an anthropologist concerned to address injustice, she has pointed to the contradictory decisions that environmental justice activists in India had to confront. For example, it was clear that since Union Carbide was a U.S. company, the trial should take place in the United States, placing responsibility in that country. Nevertheless, there was also a strong argument for the trial to take place in India, to demonstrate that the Indian government had the power and the resources to try a U.S. company. Thus, Fortun, beginning her fieldwork in 1990, six years after the disaster occurred, explores the difficult questions of global justice and grassroots negotiations in the assigning of responsibility and reparations for the deaths of close to fifteen thousand people.

POLITICAL CHANGE AND HEALTH IN SOUTH AFRICA

As noted earlier, in informal settlements in both poor and wealthy countries, public health measures such as immunizations and medical care follow-up are difficult to implement. For example, in 1992, the clinic that served Alexandra Township in Johannesburg, South Africa, introduced a program in which a van drove mothers and their newborn babies home after childbirth. In a township without street addresses and where people often had to build their housing from cardboard and scrap metal, the clinic devised this method to help keep in contact with mothers and newborn babies. The reduction of infant mortality depends partly on follow-up care and well-baby visits, which could not easily be implemented in the shifting situations of South African shantytowns.

Beginning in the early 1990s, during the transition in South Africa from a racist white oppressive regime to a democratic nonracial democracy, here we outline the experiences of poor grassroots women struggling to protect the health of their communities and the many challenges they confronted over time. Among a shifting population with no fixed addresses, in which political violence made it difficult for outside health workers to visit or for people to stay in one place, Ida Susser worked with a group of researchers and local women to develop an AIDS prevention strategy. They found that the most effective way to reach the population was to rely on the grassroots women who communicated through already-structured routes of political mobilization (I. Susser 2009a). In a situation in which telephones did not exist and shacks were reached by narrow, winding, uphill mud paths, people familiar with the community were the only ones who could contact the residents. The public health situation was made particularly difficult by the fact that this area was the center of the Kingdom of Kwazulu, where, at that time, political officials supporting the Zulu king were in competition for power with the African National Congress (ANC), which was not associated with a particular ethnic group. In one part of the settlements that

Ida Susser visited in 1992, there were eleven political funerals in one week. For this reason, many people moved quickly from place to place, to escape political reprisals and murder. Shacks were frequently burned down as residents were suspected of being members of opposing political factions. It was virtually impossible for an outside health worker to maintain direct contact with large numbers of people.

In 1992, the researchers met with the local representatives of the ANC, who organized regular meetings in the informal settlements. At that time, the ANC was still struggling for political power in South Africa, and Africans had not yet been permitted to vote. An important woman leader and member of the research team, Dr. Nkosazane Zuma, had mobilized a grassroots women's marketing cooperative in the informal settlement. Through her introductions the HIV prevention team was able to attend meetings and recruit a local community health worker. This local woman, an active and respected leader in her own right, learned about the threat of HIV infection, safe sex, condoms, and female condoms. Using a bullhorn and arranging for space in the back of a local store, she organized meetings where women could learn about HIV infection and discuss methods of prevention.

Three years later, when Ida Susser returned to the informal settlement, many women were clearly informed about HIV and asking to be trained as community health workers. By that time, the ANC, with Nelson Mandela as its leader, had been elected to form a transitional government in South Africa, and Dr. Zuma had by 1995 become minister of health for South Africa. The ANC had built a large, well-designed meeting hall in the center of the informal settlement. In 1995, meetings were still called together by bullhorn, but the government had paved the mud paths, and the meetings were held in the new hall. At the meetings in 1995, local women were demanding housing and employment. They also demanded free distribution of the female condom, which they themselves had decided would be the most effective HIV prevention method for their community. Indeed, partially as a consequence of the previous community work, the national AIDS director, Quarraisha Abdool Karim, who had also been a researcher on the study just described, had ordered female condoms to be distributed free among poor women in South Africa.

One of the most important findings from this anthropological study of HIV prevention in an informal settlement was that it was possible to implement public health education and keep in contact with people over time in a politically violent and shifting community. Despite the lack of permanent addresses, telephones, and roads, people in the local population were well able to use their own forms of political mobilization to implement health measures when they understood their importance to their own survival. It is also significant that three years later, women's access to information and ability to mobilize around health issues had increased. Public health awareness had also increased, despite the fact that the health team had not visited the site in the intervening period, political violence continued intermittently, the population was still shifting, and people still had no permanent housing.

By 2000, the new South African government had built new housing and provided adequate sanitation, community clinics, and clean water in the Durban neighborhoods described above. In this case, we can see clearly the basic political issues underlying health. With the improvements in democracy in the new South Africa, the potential for a poor population to be healthier also increased. Unfortunately, also by 2000, Thabo Mbeki, the newly elected president, was beginning to implement cuts in funding for social policies in line with a global turn toward neoliberalism. He had, in addition, initiated a decade of denial that AIDS was a virus. Thus, health measures did not improve, nor did inequality. Social movements in South Africa and globally emerged to combat these new policies, and after another decade of struggle, a new plan to treat AIDS as well as some improvement in social assistance was again in place in South Africa (for a review of these issues see Susser, 2009a, 2010, 2011).

CONCLUSIONS: ENGAGEMENT AND SOCIAL JUSTICE

As noted at the start of this chapter, public health research demonstrates that the greatest predictor of poor health indicators in any country is the degree of income inequality documented for that country. Absolute poverty is not as accurate an indicator of poor health statistics as is inequality. Thus, we can see why poverty in the United States leads to high levels of mortality, although the per capita income and GNP figures in the United States might lead us to expect better results. Increasing income inequality in the United States has been accompanied by the neglect of public health standards for immunization, adequate nutrition, and access to health care for the poor and uninsured. In 2013, the Affordable Care Act, introduced by President Barack Obama, was in the process of being implemented and in the next decade we may see a massive reduction in Americans without health insurance and possibly an increase in life expectancy for the poorest. Nevertheless, the new act excluded the undocumented immigrants such as those described by Steve Striffler in *Chicken* (2005) who labor throughout the country. For them and their families, we may in fact see life expectancy drop to more tragic levels. The development of powerful social movements for immigrant rights may yet lead to this crucial expansion of health care for all. Fortunately, policies are never written in stone, and, as we have seen with homelessness, poor Americans have continually contested their conditions. Although based on a privatized market model, the Affordable Care Act, introduced under the Obama administration in 2009, is one step toward improving health coverage in the United States. If implemented as passed into law, it will remedy the lack of health care insurance that has accompanied the loss of employment for millions of Americans since the 2008 economic crash.

In many poor countries with a small population of increasing wealth and a large population living in worsening poverty—many without adequate housing—we find the breakdown of basic measures of public health and the resurgence of the threat of epidemics of cholera and other more terrifying diseases, high rates of infant mortality, and shortened life expectancies. As we have seen, critical medical anthropologists have explored the ways in which statistics of health and mortality are related to global policies, national politics, social organization at the grassroots, and political mobilization from the local to the global.

Social science research has made important contributions to understanding the lives of the poor and homeless in many parts of the world. From both a theoretical and a practical perspective, critical medical anthropology, which as we have seen takes into account the political and economic circumstances of health and disease as well as ideas of discipline, citizenship, and governmentality, is essential to a clear understanding and documentation of the needs and voices of the majority of the world's population. In addition, in the face of the continuing and increasing inequality we currently confront, the significance of fieldwork with the people in power as well as those who do not have direct access to public institutions and an activist approach to this fieldwork, which may assist in addressing their needs, becomes more central all the time.

Critical medical anthropologists have always taken engagement seriously (M. Singer 1995a; G. A. Smith 1999; Merry and Low 2010; Susser, 2010; Maskovsky 2013). In some forms of engagement, such as the documentation of "letting them die," medical anthropologists have developed searing critiques of the systematic injustices reflected in patterns of disease, lack of access to health care, or lack of appropriate culturally relevant services that would contribute to the health of a population. As Stephen Schensul (2011) wrote in his acceptance speech for a Career Achievement Award from the Society for Medical Anthropology, intervention is a crucial aspect of medical anthropology. However, he notes that "we find that individual behavior change represents the most common approach in seeking positive change through intervention projects. This individual focus fails to take into account social and economic challenges in peoples' lives, the shortcomings of systems of care, the fit with local knowledge, and the presence of natural support systems within communities." As he points out, anthropologists can help to develop societal interventions in which the anthropologist works with the local people to develop appropriate interventions taking into account the historical and political constraints. James Pfeiffer and Mark Nichter (2008: 413) noted,

By illuminating the social processes, power relations, development culture, and discourses that drive the global health enterprise, medical anthropologists can contribute in valuable ways to health diplomacy and advocacy efforts, as well as on-the-ground transdisciplinary problem solving. We can help ensure that the evidence base that frames global health debates is inclusive and represents multiple dimensions of the human experience, including the voices of those whose lives are affected by global processes.

Ida Susser (2010, 2011) has conducted research that follows interventions and social movements to explore the ways in which grassroots leaders act as a lynch pin with wider interests at the national and global level. Such grassroots leadership imagines and initiates change in an interactive process with people at the local level. From this perspective, engaged anthropology involves documenting, analyzing and possibly facilitating the processes that contribute to social justice. All such forms of engagement have important effects, and the way medical anthropologists see their contributions will vary with the context; however, critical medical anthropologists working in conditions of poverty and inequality understand their research as one small, certainly insufficient effort in the long-term struggle for social justice.

CHAPTER 6

Reproduction, Biotechnologies, and Inequality

REPRODUCTION AND HEALTH: AN OVERVIEW

This chapter considers issues of reproduction and health that have been a central concern for medical anthropologists from many perspectives. Questions about population growth led to studies of fertility and abortion in nonstate societies before practices of childbirth and women's experience in pregnancy were explored. With the reinvigoration of the feminist movement in the 1970s, we see anthropological studies that take the agency of women and their experience into account. We learn about menstruation ceremonies, childbirth, and women's life cycles. In the following decades, we find studies of women, reproductive health and choice, and childbirth in both wealthy and poor countries around the world.

Initiated by Emily Martin (1987) with *The Woman in the Body*, among others (Scheper-Hughes 1987), we have seen a theorization of the body with respect to such concepts as the disciplining of the body (Foucault 1979, 1980), the suffering of the body (Kleinman, Das, and Lock 1997), and the medicalization of the body (Lindenbaum and Lock 1993). Such theorization has led to an extrapolation from the person to the body politic and concepts of embodiment (Csordas 1994) as well as ideas of bodily dissent and the protests of the body (Ong 1987; Lock 1993). Since the 1990s, as biotechnology has widened the horizons of reproduction, anthropologists have been in the forefront of discussions of the new age in all its many respects (M. Strathern 1992; Rapp 2000; Franklin 2003; Stolcke 2012). In this chapter, we follow these trends in the anthropology of reproduction.

Throughout we explore the complex relationship among cultural paradigms of kinship, gender, and the politics of reproduction. In the last section, we highlight the impact of dramatic changes in reproductive possibility and its interaction with globalization and patterns of income inequality and gender hierarchies.

A chapter on reproduction is clearly a context in which the issue of gender and women must be considered. Here we are using gender as the term that describes the characteristics of masculine and feminine that are culturally recognized and women as a gendered category. Sex, for example, as used in medical research, refers to the particular biological characteristics of an individual. As Marcia Inhorn (2006) has pointed out, the vast majority of articles by medical anthropologists on women's health are concentrated in discussions of reproduction. Clearly this is a crucial issue for women but hardly the only one. We believe it is essential to discuss women's experiences throughout the different topics reviewed, and so we have endeavored not to ghettoize women or questions of gender. Researchers have also noted that even when reproduction is discussed, the woman is often seen as the conduit for the child and, as we shall discuss later in the chapter, in some circumstances, the woman is only treated as much as is necessary to produce a healthy child.

We want to note that here, following the tenets of feminist theory, we understand women as agents who endeavor to shape their own situations and frequently struggle to promote their family's health, sometimes to the detriment of their own. Hierarchy, inequality, and control over one's life are all strong predictors of health outcomes, such as heart disease and mortality. As the women's health movement, in the United States and elsewhere, demonstrated unequivocally, when women began to take control over their own health and demand knowledge and the decision-making power with respect to their own needs, the entire way we understand health care was transformed (Morgen 2002). Thus, in this chapter, we take care to reflect women as actors and consider women's perspective on reproduction centrally, as an area in which they are fundamentally involved.

REPRODUCTION AND INEQUALITY

Reproduction and the health of mothers and infants cannot be understood separately from the gendered distribution of resources and the division of labor in any society. Women's access to education and employment has a direct effect on patterns of family size and the health of the mother and child. Despite many improvements, women continue to be disadvantaged with respect to men in employment and health, and, in general, poorer and minority women suffer poorer health with a direct relationship between degree of disadvantage and the extent of health problems

(World Health Organization [WHO] Women and Health 2009). In fact, many women and children are dying, especially in low-income countries, from their experience of gendered discrimination (WHO 2009). Girls are less likely to be taken for treatment should they fall ill and more likely to suffer from malnutrition, which particularly affects their childbearing years (WHO 2009). Even female fetuses are less valued; for example, when amniocentesis was introduced in India, most of the fetuses aborted were female (B. Miller 2000). Among poor households, the health effects of gender, as measured in the morbidity and mortality statistics for women in relation to men, are frequently magnified by lifelong nutritional deprivation combined with lack of care in pregnancy and childbirth. Institutional discrimination against women combined with household inequality is also manifest in the high maternal mortality rates and infant mortality rates common in many poor regions. In 1990, WHO (L. Freedman and Maine 1993) estimated that about 500,000 women died every year in childbirth and pregnancy, mostly from preventable causes. In 2010, the numbers had been reduced by half: 270,000 women died in childbirth (UNFPA 2012). Clearly the global focus on this problem has saved hundreds of thousands of lives over the past two decades, but the problem of maternal mortality is still immense and challenging.

Patterns of reproduction represent one of the most dramatic indicators of the differences in life conditions of rich and poor populations in the world today. In countries on the periphery of the world system, both maternal and infant mortality have remained much higher than in the core capitalist countries. Maternal mortality, most effectively prevented by the availability of emergency obstetric facilities, remains much greater in countries where women still do not have immediate access to blood transfusions, antibiotics, and cesarean section (WHO 2010). In fact, today, 99 percent of maternal mortality occurs in low-income countries. For example, in sub-Saharan Africa, one mother dies for every thirty-one children born. In Northern Europe, approximately one mother dies for every fifteen thousand infant births.

However, as we shall see later in the chapter, in the section on biotechnologies and changing patterns of reproduction, we cannot understand these inequalities alone. They have to be understood in the context of global processes as well as the ongoing interactions between the wealthy and the poor both transnationally and internally within each nation-state.

Poverty and inequality also affect the health of women in the centers of the capitalist system. Within the United States, one of the world's wealthiest nations, poor and minority women face dilemmas concerning pregnancy that are different from the higher income populations (Mullings and Wali 2001). The ongoing daily stresses of poorly paid work combined with the long waits for impersonal prenatal care in municipal hospitals, the lack of funds for shelter and good nutrition during pregnancy, and the lack of access to well-baby care for infants are associated with a higher frequency of low birth weight, premature infants with less chance of survival in the first year, and lower life expectancies than babies born in middle-income communities (Hogue 2000). Sadly and somewhat shockingly for a wealthy nation that spends more on health care than any other country, the situation for women in the United States has been getting worse rather than better with respect to maternal mortality. According to Amnesty International, "Women in the United States have a higher risk of dying from pregnancy-related complications than women in 40 other countries. . . . Estimated maternal mortality ratios have doubled in the past 20 years, from 6.6 deaths per 100,000 live births in 1987 to 13.3 deaths per 100,000 live births in 2006. . . . Each year, 1.7 million women suffer serious complications" (2010: 1).

ANTHROPOLOGICAL PERSPECTIVES ON REPRODUCTION

As reproduction is central to human existence, so it has been to the development of anthropology. Beginning with the publication of the *Vindication of the Rights of Women* by Mary Wollstonecraft in 1792, Western social theorists hotly debated values, rites, and regulations around sexuality and virginity, marriage, and childrearing practices. In 1877, one of the founders of American anthropology, Lewis Henry Morgan, contributed to this discussion in his effort to organize his collected data about rules of kinship and marriage in different societies in relation to the means of subsistence. Karl Marx and Friedrich Engels used Morgan's research to connect women's subordination to the development of capitalism. Inspired by the notion that women were not universally dominated by men, nineteenth-century feminists from many parts of the world, such as Olive Schreiner from southern Africa and Alexandra Kollontai in Russia, delineated women's rights to work and love with greater freedom.

In the early twentieth century, another American anthropologist, Margaret Mead, a student of Franz Boas, entered the fierce public debate concerning the place of women by documenting the flexibility of human sexual behavior and the malleable definitions of masculinity and femininity through her pioneering ethnographies in Samoa and New Guinea. Mead was among a number of independent-thinking women anthropologists of her time, including researchers such as Elsie Clewes Parsons and Ruth Landes, who were critically exploring the roles of men and women and rethinking gender and reproduction.

Nevertheless, for the first half of the twentieth century, despite the internationally renowned writings of such eminent theorists as the anarchist leader and Russian immigrant to the United States Emma Goldman and the French existential philosopher Simone de Beauvoir, most ethnographies although they might well include descriptions of rituals of betrothal and childbirth did not set such discussions squarely within a broader analysis of sexuality and power relations. Indeed, kinship and marriage, or the constitution of the rules for the reproduction of a society, were generally analyzed without attention to the controversial issues of power and autonomy between men and women (Rubin 1975). Later feminist anthropologists insisted that reproduction must be analyzed in the context of varying power relations as well as changing expectations of maleness and femaleness (Lamphere and Rosaldo 1974; Reiter 1975). Rather than interpreting sexual difference simply in terms of biological characteristics, analysts began to see people and societies making or performing masculinity and femininity, fatherhood, and motherhood. Rules of marriage and reproduction were recognized as intertwined with such issues as colonialism, nationalism, and state power as well as family and community expectations. Later research has deconstructed the notion of gender even further, drawing attention to the experience of transgendered and third genders. Recognizing that the situation and power of the researcher affects their work, feminists emphasized the significance of the analyst's position as well as that of informants. As Christine Gailey (1998) has noted, feminist methods in anthropology, require a recognition of the researcher's own position and an understanding of the social construction of gender but also involve a commitment to working for the empowerment of women (see also Behar 1996; Lamphere, Ragone, and Zavella 1997). Because women suffer inequality in most of the world, it seems particularly important to examine reproductive health within this context. As we shall see, ethnographic analysis has been making significant contributions to our understanding of reproduction in the changing world system, the impact of historical shifts in gender and class relations, government regulations, nationalism, and globalization.

Because reproduction is so crucial to social continuity, both symbolically and biologically, decisions about sexuality, fertility, pregnancy, childbirth, and even childrearing have seldom been left solely to the parents involved. Societies have generated rituals, rules, and regulations designating the responsibilities for the bearing and rearing of children and the continuation of populations. Frequently, such expectations are deeply embedded in the symbols of kinship as well as perceptions of gender roles (Lindenbaum 1987).

In modern states, political concerns expressed in terms of overpopulation, underpopulation, nationality, ethnicity, and religious precepts have been translated by governments into regulations about reproduction. We find varying legal restrictions with respect to contraception, abortion, and reproductive technologies. Such laws crucially affect men's and women's strategies and options with respect to family size and childrearing (Ginsburg and Rapp 1995). Values or laws that do not directly address reproduction, for example, with respect to men and women's inheritance of land, employment, nutrition, or public health, may also constrain the sexual and fertility decisions of men and women or affect the mortality of infants in unexpected ways.

Sexuality, marriage and fertility, labor, and childbirth will be fundamentally shaped by the class position of a man or woman's family in society and his or her access to resources and power (Schneider and Schneider 1996; Whiteford 1996; Lamphere et al. 1997). Within these contours, contemporary medical anthropologists have looked at reproduction from the point of view of rituals of the life cycle, changing perceptions of the body, negotiations over sexuality, marriage and parental roles between men and women, and the cultural perceptions surrounding men and women's practices (Martin 1987; Ginsburg and Rapp 1995; Browner 2001).

In recent decades, reproduction has become a contested issue in global regulation and struggles around international human rights. In world forums and regulatory bodies, such as the United Nations and the 1995 Beijing NGO Forum on Women (Friedlander 1996), people have called for reproductive rights and freedom of sexual orientation to be included in human rights and for rape to be understood as a violation of human rights. Even as many people have organized to promote human rights, religious fundamentalism, incorporating patriarchal values and the subordination of women, has undermined the recognition of sexual and reproductive freedoms (Petchesky 2000). For example, although the U.S. Supreme Court has supported the right of women in the United States to choose to terminate a pregnancy, the U.S. government now denies that right to women served by U.S. funded agencies outside the country, and, under the presidency of G.W. Bush, severely limited their access to education about contraception and reproductive strategies (see Susser 2009).

In this chapter, to highlight different possibilities in the social organization of reproduction, we look first at childbirth and childrearing patterns in some indigenous societies, such as the San people of southern Africa, and the ways in which the lives of men and women changed as their communities were incorporated into the world system. Then we consider the changing patterns of reproduction in state societies and the impact of colonization. Finally, we return to an examination of the contrasting contemporary experiences of reproduction and the biotechnology of reproduction in the world system among populations in peripheral and core nations as well as the commodification of reproduction at the global level.

REPRODUCTION IN INDIGENOUS SOCIETIES

In the late 1950s, many of the San peoples of the Kalahari Desert still maintained a foraging way of life, wandering in small bands in search of fruits, nuts, berries, and other plants and hunting game (Lee 2012). The

San speak many languages and live in many areas; the group we refer to most often are, in fact, the Ju'/hoansi (Lee 2012), among whom Ida Susser conducted fieldwork with Richard Lee with respect to HIV/AIDS prevention (I. Susser 2009a). For simplicity we have chosen to use the more general term *San* throughout this book.

The San knew where to find water from hidden springs scattered over the dry land, and when the trickles dried up, they knew where to dig for roots that stored liquid. They built groupings of shelters from branches or caked mud and shifted these temporary villages as they sought to renew their sources of food. Over centuries, the San peoples interacted with the surrounding cattle herding populations, living and working with them from time to time and exchanging goods and services. As Dutch, British, and German colonial powers established their territories, the San intermittently worked for encroaching farm settlements, raided the encroachers, and were shot and imprisoned for their wanderings (Gordon 1992).

Under these conditions, ethnographers of the San in the 1950s and 1960s described such societies as more or less egalitarian. Women were seen as autonomous, in that they made their own decisions about subsistence activities and the tasks for which they were responsible (Draper 1975; Leacock and Lee 1982; Lee 1979, 2012). Anthropological descriptions of the autonomous San woman have been criticized as romanticized representations of the colonial other and certainly egregious stereotypes of the San woman were common in colonial discourse (di Leonardo 1998). Nevertheless, the situational differences Lee and Susser identified between San women and women in the surrounding populations suggest that the availability of foraging, collaborative child care, and the ease with which women could construct their own new dwellings continued to facilitate or led to the reinvention of some forms of women's autonomy even into the 2000s (I. Susser 2002a, 2009a). We must make clear here that we are discussing San gender relations at a particular moment and under specific historical conditions and do not mean to suggest that their way of life represents all foraging societies nor that the San themselves have no agency or variation in their own history.

As observed by anthropologists since the 1960s, although San men predominated as folk healers, both men and women could learn to become practitioners and lead curing rituals. The propensity to trance was often passed down from mother to daughter, and there was a specific drum dance performed by women. Men did most of the hunting. However, contrary to common Western stereotypes, a number of women knew how to set traps and hunt small animals. Women also made poisoned hunting arrows used by the men, although they did not often accompany the men on long hunting trips.

San women gathered food together, usually trailed by young children. Sometimes mothers carried their infants on such daylong expeditions, but on other occasions they would leave them behind in the village under the supervision of other women in the band. Sometimes women breastfed each other's children.

Childrearing, shared by both men and women, was an easier task than in many industrialized societies, as, from infancy, children, like adults, were allowed a high degree of independence and autonomy. Children of one band grew up together, almost as brothers and sisters. The young were not forced early into adult labor, and children often mimicked adults in their days of play, including games of hunting as well as sexual experimentation (Draper 1975; Lee 1979, 2012)

Among the San at this time, kin often arranged marriage for prepubescent girls to boys a few years older. One incentive for a family to arrange an early marriage for their daughter was that the groom's family was expected to provide gifts for the family of the bride and her new husband would hunt for her family as bride service. To indicate betrothal, a young girl was ritually carried to her future husband's hut, but, in fact, for several years after this ceremony, she might stay with her own family.

Despite what appears to be a somewhat subordinated or constrained initiation to marriage, a young girl actually had a variety of options. Without being subject to force or other negative repercussions, although certainly subject to teasing by privileged joking members among her kin, she could decide when, or even if, she wanted to interact sexually with her new husband. Indeed, because work and resources were substantially shared with other band members, if a woman wished, she could leave her husband without punishment or much loss of economic resources, and he could leave her without subjecting his family to destitution. Much flexibility and freedom for women and men continued through the life cycle. In *Nisa: The Diary of a !Kung Woman* (Shostak 1981), which records one woman's story as a wife, mother, and lover in a foraging society, we see that even after many years of marriage, a woman could leave her husband, taking her children with her to another village, without fear of loss of resources or the physical abuse and social ostracism common in many other societies.

Among the nomadic San, girls tended to begin menstruation in their late teens, in contrast to the earlier onset of menarche in modern industrialized societies (Howell 2000). One reason for this may have been their low fat diet. Meat was not plentiful, and because the foragers of that period did not keep cattle or goats, dairy foods were practically nonexistent. In addition, San women were physically active on a daily basis and often walked twenty miles a day with their bands. Among such active women with little excess fat, ovulation might start late and be irregular even among adult women (Lee 1979; Howell 2000).

There was little dairy produce to substitute for mother's milk and, because the San did not grow cereals, there were few soft foods or alternate sources of protein; thus many foraging women breastfed their babies for four or more years. This too contributed to a lack of excess fat and a reduced likelihood that a woman with a young child would ovulate regularly. In fact, demographic research demonstrated that nomadic women spaced their pregnancies, on average, about four years apart. However, this was not simply a biological or natural consequence of diet, exercise, and breastfeeding. The San adopted a variety of rules and practices that prevented a new child from being an insupportable burden as the small band wandered many miles on foot seeking food and water.

If the cultural strategies that limit fertility failed, foraging mothers faced a tragic dilemma in which their options were limited and shaped by their environment and access to resources. Under conditions of famine and starvation, a San woman had the autonomy to decide how to cope. If a mother did become pregnant again, before her last child could travel long distances without being carried, she might try to abort the pregnancy or not allow the infant to survive.

Nisa (Shostak 1981) tells a story of a pregnant mother, wishing to save the life of her youngest child, whom she sees as mortally threatened by the future infant in competition for nutrition and resources. The mother gives birth outside the village, accompanied only by her small daughter, and then abandons the new baby.

From the 1960s, as vast stretches of foraging land were taken over by cattle ranches and roads built through the desert, the San settled near bore holes built by the local governments (advocated by the filmmaker John Marshall and others), raised a few cattle and goats, and received free supplements of grain. As people kept dairy animals and more soft food was available for infants, women did not exclusively breastfeed their babies as long and were more likely to ovulate and become pregnant sooner and more often (Howell 2000). In addition, young girls and women were expected to be more subordinate to men, and the learning of gendered sex roles by girls was more obvious, as young girls played with dolls and young women were expected to obey their husbands (Draper 1975).

For the first seventy thousand years of human existence, societies survived by foraging, and populations remained relatively stable. Because population size is more directly limited by the number of women, anthropologists have suggested that female infanticide was among the strategies used by foragers to maintain small populations in order not to strain the resources available (Harris and Ross 1987). A man can father any number of children at one time, whereas a woman can only carry a finite number of pregnancies to term.

Populations began to increase with settled agriculture. It is not clear whether settlements came first or the population increase precipitated settlement. Possibly, as some researchers have argued, people resorted to horticulture or herding animals, because they had to feed growing populations. Because farming for subsistence required more intensive labor than foraging, kin groups and lineages valued children as future workers. However, as among foraging societies, farming societies still sought to culturally define household and population size. Spacing strategies, such as the separation of the mother and child from the father immediately after birth, and local abortion practices were common in horticultural and pastoral populations.

In many societies, women established power in their descent group by bearing children, and particularly sons, who would represent their interests later (Kabeer 1985; Gammeltoft 1999). In contrast to the customary requirements in Mediterranean states for a bride to be a virgin (Schneider and Schneider 1996), women among many other peoples such as the Kadar of Nigeria were highly valued if they had a child before marriage, for this demonstrated their fertility to their future husband and his kin, and when the young girl married, the children joined her husband's patrilineage (M. G. Smith 1968: 113).

Barren wives, or women who did not have children, were often penalized in such lineage societies. However, biological fertility does not always limit women's access to influence through children. Mona Etienne (2001) described the way in which barren women among the Baule in Ivory Coast enhanced their political status by migrating to urban areas and adopting children to maintain and later inherit their property in their rural village. Only such connections insured a woman influence while she was alive and a respectable funeral at her death.

Francis Nyamnjoh (2002), a sociologist from Cameroon, describes his own upbringing and adoption by two social mothers besides his biological mother and two men who regarded him as a social son, contributing toward the cost of his education and providing him with land. His social mothers and fathers (his biological mother had passed away and he did not know well or like his biological father) attended his wedding. Nyamnjoh notes that in the grassfields of Cameroon, among a vibrant, changing population trying to negotiate the opportunities of the global marketplace without losing their collective rights, migrants adopt children in an effort to negotiate continuity in their native regions while traveling far afield in their entrepreneurial activities.

Thus, in many pastoral and horticultural societies, in contrast to foragers like the San who had to carry their infants long distances, both men and women had reasons to want a large number of children. As we noted earlier, when the San settled more permanently around government dug boreholes, they also had more children, spaced closer in age (Howell 2000).

Because children were highly valued, kin groups carefully defined through marriage to which lineage or household they belonged. However, although marriage defined a child's status, sexuality and biological kinship were not necessarily limited by these rules. Among the Nuer, for example, a pastoral society in which people inherited cattle through their patrilineal connections, a woman who had many cattle and whose husband had died could marry another woman (Evans-Pritchard 1940). This strategy allowed the new wife to find her own partner to bear children for her "ghost" husband's patrilineage. Such offspring would help herd the cattle and generally bolster the position of the first woman. Clearly, the new children would have a biological father, but his status was irrelevant to the status of the children, who would belong to the lineage of the "woman-husband" and her wife. Kathleen Gough (1971) demonstrated further that, in the 1930s, a Nuer woman from a high-status patrilineage, rather than marrying into another Nuer descent group as prescribed by patrilineal rules, might find a partner among ostensible "strangers" from the nearby Dinka population and thus keep her children attached to her own patrilineage.

Sharon Hutchinson and Jok Madut Jok (2002) have described the tragic contemporary transformations of Nuer and Dinka gender relations in the militarization of an independent state in the Sudan. As the Nuer and Dinka have been drawn into ethnic conflicts over land, tribal allegiance is no longer as flexible as it was, and, sadly, women and children, previously interrelated through marriage and off-limits in battle, have become the targets for greater and more brutal assault and killing (Hutchinson and Jok 2002).

In many indigenous societies, although marriage clearly defined the status and lineage of their children, both men and women were allowed a degree of sexual freedom. In other societies, men but not women were allowed such freedoms, and in some societies, sexuality outside marriage was heavily sanctioned for both men and women (Scheffler 1991). The relationship between kin terms and customary practice has to be examined rather than assumed (Scheffler 1991). As noted earlier, rules about gender, social reproduction, or the rearing of children may not necessarily correspond with biological reproduction, or sexuality (Collier and Yanagasako 1987). Indeed, some anthropologists have suggested that they correspond more closely to rules about the division of labor (Leacock 1972). Frequently, the claims of family, motherhood, and fatherhood are negotiated to accommodate patterns of migration, investment, and other changes, such as wars and militarization. Differences between rules of marriage and kinship and patterns of sexual behavior and biological links become extremely important in understanding the transmission of genetic traits or sexually transmitted diseases such as HIV/AIDS.

In Richard Lee's (2012) and Ida Susser's (2009a) research in Botswana and Namibia from the 1990s, they found that, although much has changed among the San and foraging is no longer their fundamental form of subsistence, women still maintained unusual sexual autonomy. In addressing questions about HIV/AIDS, San women said they were able to refuse sexual advances from their San partners or else ask them to use condoms. They were less confident in discussing their sexual relationships with men from other groups. In contrast, Ovambo women, living in farming settlements in Northern Namibia, were more likely to be afraid that they might be beaten if they refused to have sex with their partners or asked them to use condoms (I. Susser and Stein 2000; I. Susser 2009a). But, despite the San women's history of autonomy, at least in relation to San men, as ecotourism was developing and more roads constructed into the San villages, many road builders, guards, construction workers, and other men from the surrounding groups found their way to the villages, and, along with these new sexual partners, the risk of HIV/AIDS was increasing among the San along with their growing interactions with the global economy (I. Susser 2009a). As we have seen, all populations have been incorporated into the world-system under capitalism. Contemporary global changes have led to oil and mineral speculation, tourism, safaris, and conservation policies penetrating the remotest areas, whether ice, rainforest, or desert. For this reason, the next sections of this chapter consider the relations among state policies, gender, and reproductive health.

State Societies: Inequality, Men and Women, Sexual Rights, and Children

For more than five thousand years, human populations have lived in various forms of state societies, characterized by different patterns of inequality and class stratification. Rules of marriage and kinship under these unequal state societies often delineated hierarchical relations between men and women. In fact, some anthropologists have suggested that early state societies, in the effort to centrally control households and kin groups, stressed men's rights over women and their children. Women's competing influence over their own children was restricted in this way, and men were also given license to control women's sexuality (Gailey 1987). Others have argued that women's historical subordination represents a Western image of the state and that in other circumstances elite women ruled in parallel to elite men (for a discussion of debates concerning women's inequality in state societies, see Silverblatt 1991). Only historical research will disentangle the particular struggles around gender, power, and resistance fought by men and women in any specific state.

In settled agricultural states with urban centers, epidemic disease was a frequent occurrence and, under such conditions, infants were then, as now, the most susceptible to infectious diseases. Thus infant mortality rates were high, often one in four died in the first year of life. Maternal mortality was also very high. Many women died in childbirth, and for this reason, women had a shorter life expectancy than men all over the world. A man frequently outlived several wives, as each wife might bear a number of children but not live to see them grow up (M. Susser, Watson, and Hopper 1985). Under these conditions, a man might marry again to find a partner to care for the children, or the oldest child might be expected to care for his or her siblings, or, in fact, children might be reared by adoptive parents.

With the advent of capitalist societies and later industrialization, populations increased dramatically, but for several hundred years, health and life expectancy decreased. In London, in the 1800s, for example, infant mortality rates and the general death rates from disease were surpassing the birth rate. The population would have declined dramatically if thousands of migrants had not streamed into the city. Later, as wages increased and sanitation improved in the new industrial cities, infant mortality rates decreased and epidemics of the plague, cholera, and other diseases became less frequent (M. Susser, Watson, and Hopper 1985; see also Chapter 5, this volume). However, even as general conditions improved, women continued to die at younger ages than men until the twentieth century (Hogue 2000).

From antiquity, states, like later governments in industrial societies, were much involved in regulating women's sexuality, controlling patterns of reproduction and defining the status of children. In the 1960s, Jane Schneider traced the virgin complex through North Africa and the Mediterranean to the changing relationship between pastoral societies and the state (J. Schneider 1971). Many anthropologists have tried to understand the strength of this honor and shame complex and the varying significance of the enforcement of virginity before marriage. The Eurasian complex of virginity, dowry, and patrilineality also has been associated with a class system and the control of property as men seek to control women's reproductive capacity in order to ensure inheritance in the men's family group (Goody 1976). In addition, Jack Goody (1983) develops an important argument about the role of the church in structuring European inheritance patterns, family, and kinship. Many of those who have studied the dowry in India have noted that inheritance is completely controlled by men, and the value of the dowry assures only that the woman marry a man of rank as the property passes from the bride's family to the groom (B. Miller 2000). The low value of women's paid work and the reduced value of her domestic role in the rearing of children in recent years has contributed to the importance of the dowry in defining the economic value of the woman and in some instances has led to murder, as men wish to get rid of one wife to collect a new dowry from another woman (B. Miller 2000).

Colonial governments, also, regulated marriage and sexual relations (Leacock and Etienne 1980). In Indonesia, after one hundred years of colonial rule, the Dutch administration legally forbade European settlers to marry members of the local population in their efforts to institutionalize racial divisions and control the colonized (Stoler 1991). In addition, the transformation of societies under colonization often undermined cooperative organization among women and decreased their political influence while increasing their workload in agriculture and domestic responsibilities (Guyer 1991). From this early period, although there was much variation in the local strategies of men and women and the specific histories of resistance to colonialism, unequal employment opportunities, segregated living conditions, unequal health care provisions, and the institutionalized discrimination and regulation of women among colonized populations set the scene for the differences between the maternal and infant survival rates documented between Third World countries, often previously colonized, and core capitalist countries to this day. From the 1940s, in the industrialized Western countries, with improved housing, education, and nutrition; the discovery and generalized distribution of penicillin, vaccines, and other medical interventions; and the implementation of hospitalized childbirth in sterile conditions, many more women survived labor and childbirth. In fact, World War II had an interesting impact on women in the United States, as it represented the first time the majority of women gave birth in hospital settings, funded by the health insurance payments of soldiers. This shift, represented in the high levels of access to medical care, also contributed to a nationwide lowering of maternal mortality rates. While infant mortality rates dropped dramatically and life expectancy increased for everyone, women actually began to live longer than men (Goldman and Hatch 2000).

Throughout the twentieth century, maternal and infant mortality rates have been decreasing in Western industrialized countries. This was a gradual process, and the survival rates for women and children of different age groups varied over the time period. But the health of poor men and women and infant mortality rates for poor and minority populations did not improve at the same rate as those with more wealth. In the past three decades, there has been an increasing gap in the United States among the income, living conditions, and health of the poor, minorities, and that of the better-off (I. Susser 1996, 2009b; Pappas et al. 1993; see also Chapter 5, this volume). From 2000 to 2010, shockingly, for the first time in a century, the life expectancy of poor men and women in the United States actually decreased. The biggest drop in life expectancy involved white women who did not complete high school. They had life expectancies five years less in 2008 than in 1990, and by 2008, white women who did not complete high school had lower life expectancies than black women in the same situation (Olshansky et al. 2012).

CLASS AND REPRODUCTION

Although Malthus once argued that the poor have more children and therefore are responsible for overpopulation and subsequent reduction of available resources, the relationship among income, fertility, and resources is much more situationally determined than such an argument suggests. Reproductive decisions are made at the household level, or even simply between a man and a woman, but inheritance patterns, labor patterns of men and women, state policies including taxes, and many other factors promote the size and shape of families. In a historical analysis of fertility shifts in Sicily, Jane Schneider and Peter Schneider (1996) documented the changing demographic patterns among different classes that accompanied one hundred years of modernization. Their study, as an anthropological contribution to demography, undermines age-old modernization arguments that rely on ideas that poor people "have less self-control" or fail to plan for the future and so have more children. In contrast, in the nineteenth century, the Sicilian aristocracy, healthier and more affluent, reared more children while the impoverished peasants, due to higher rates of mortality, had fewer children surviving to maturity. Later, to preserve their wealth, the landed gentry reduced the number of children per family, and, during the Great Depression, the merchant class began to change their household strategies to limit conception and childbirth to rear fewer children with more opportunities. Lastly, in the 1950s and 1960s, again as a strategy for upward mobility, poor Sicilian landless laborers began to implement their own methods to reduce fertility. In a Mexican village in the 1980s, Frances Rothstein (1982, 2007) documented similar historical contingencies among working-class households whose members cycled between agricultural labor and factory employment; as possibilities for mobility through education seemed to emerge, families changed their reproductive strategies and fewer children were born.

Household members strategize to achieve culturally defined goals within the constraints of the situation in which they find themselves. We cannot define laws of reproduction, such as to argue that working women always have fewer children or that poor people have more babies. In the Western industrialized states of the twentieth century, as women entered the workforce in greater numbers, the average number of children per household decreased. However, this was also accompanied not only by the invention of new methods of contraception, which could for the first time in history be controlled by women, but also by increasing levels of education for women of all incomes and, as noted earlier, improved housing and health and a dramatic decrease in both infant and maternal mortality (M. Susser, Watson, and Hopper 1985).

In Western societies, images of motherhood and fatherhood changed dramatically over the twentieth century. In Providence, Rhode Island (Lamphere 1987), in the early 1900s, daughters went out to work while mothers worked at home, taking in boarders, sewing or baking or preserving fruits for extra income. By the 1970s, mothers were working outside the home in increasing numbers. In the second millennium, as reflected in the U.S. federal policy, which has dismantled public assistance, women are expected to earn money at paid work whether or not they have to care for infants or young children (I. Susser 1996). Changing government policies also structure family relations. In the 1980s and 1990s, as the alterations in tax laws precipitated a rising cost of housing and the eviction of poor New Yorkers, this process of gentrification led to increased periods of homelessness. When families lost housing, children were often separated from their parents by government officials seeking to put them in institutional housing. Institutional policies also varied by gender, as women were more likely to be able to keep their children than men. Boys were often separated from their mothers at age nine, whereas most girls were allowed to stay with their mothers through their teenage years (Susser 1993).

These family transformations are not a predictable or one-way process. Ruth Milkman (1987), in her historic analysis of American women during World War II, shows how they were encouraged to work outside the home: day care was provided and the work was glorified in images of the hard-working patriotic "Rosie the Riveter." Dolores Hayden has described the ways in which housing estates were remodeled for Rosie to make women's household tasks easier while they worked as welders on the nation's ships. Vanport City was built in 1943 with six day-care centers built along the bus line that the women took home from work (Hayden 2002). This "was the most ambitious attempt ever made in the United States to shape space for employed women and their babies" (19). It was subsidized with $11 million from the U.S. government and extremely profitable for Henry Kaiser who built it. It offered energy-efficient, rental houses planned for single-parent households, mostly women alone with their children. As servicemen returned after the war, women lost their jobs. As Hayden describes, in contrast, Levittown, on Long Island, opened six years later than Vanport City, after the war, and was also government subsidized. Levittown was built exclusively for two-parent households with no consideration for public transportation, day care, or energy efficiency. In addition, Levittown, which was an instant commercial success, offered homes for sale, not rent, to the returning GIs who bought their houses with the newly insured government mortgages. Women and African Americans were rarely eligible for such mortgages. Levittown became the new image of the American family home. Simultaneously, images of motherhood and home dominated the media. Women's magazines showed the perfect baby with the mother in the kitchen baking cookies or driving her children to school with the dog in the back of the car. Such images were hardly brought into play in the 1980s when the New York City administration was making decisions about homeless children (I. Susser 1991a, 1993). In contrast, in 1996, through the Personal Responsibility and Work Opportunity Act, known as "welfare reform," poor women were mandated to work whether or not they were responsible for infants or young children. Thus, as we can see from these historical shifts in the United States, both individual goals and culturally approved roles for women change at different historical moments, and patterns of reproduction and childrearing reflect these changes.

THE SOCIAL CONTEXT OF REPRODUCTION TODAY

Reproduction today takes place within a global capitalist economy, which affects people in different places at different points in interconnected ways. In the following section, we discuss first the changing ways states have framed and regulated reproduction and sexuality within the world system and globalization; next we explore the different interests and control that members of a household may have with respect to the birth and rearing of children. Lastly, we outline the contrasting experiences of reproduction and the contrasting approaches of anthropologists as they examine reproduction in wealthy and poor countries of the world system.

The Consequences of State Regulation of Population

As we have seen from the experiences of Rosie in World War II and later, images of women, family, and reproduction have been shaped by projects of nationalism. Many nations have made efforts to limit their populations partly as a symbol of progress and modernization and also as a way to be able to invest in the education and skills of the population. The state may not necessarily implement the policies in the interests of fulfilling the potential of all women as productive human beings. But, as a component of this modernist project, family planning resources allow women some choice about the responsibilities of motherhood. Women's option to control their own fertility is one step toward greater autonomy in their ongoing struggle against a long history of gendered discrimination in their own homes, education, and the workplace.

Other national projects emphasize images of women as mothers, confined to their role in procreation, as powerful symbols of national or religious continuity and also as a way to keep women out of the skilled workforce. Such an idealization of motherhood in the effort to reinforce nationalist sentiments has not generally resulted in the empowerment of women. To the contrary, an emphasis on women's role as mothers has historically been associated with the subordination of women to their fathers, husbands, and other male kin and to oppressive constraints on women's work, travel, and sexual and reproductive rights as enforced by religious institutions or the government (Das 1995; Aretxaga 1997; Kligman 1995; Freedman 2000; Petchesky 2000).

There are also well-documented instances in which population control policies were introduced in a government assault on "undesirable populations" whether in terms of "race" or other supposed characteristics. The Eugenics movement in the United States, from the late 1890s to the 1930s, was supported among others by anti-immigration groups and white supremacists and precipitated discriminatory legislation. The movement also singled out the physically and mentally disabled for sterilization and implemented state laws that allowed forced sterilization and prohibited marriage among targeted groups. Hitler's government in Nazi Germany used the Eugenics movement in the United States as one justification for their plans for the deaths of the disabled, Jews, Romani, and gays and lesbians. Contemporary examples such as the apartheid government of South Africa, which tried to limit the black population in the 1980s, and the communist regime in Romania, which tried to reduce births among the stigmatized Romani group while forcing population growth among other Romanians (Kligman 1995), remind us that state intervention in population growth or reduction can have destructive rather than liberationist intent.

In the 1960s, international policymakers raised the specter of population growth and connected it to world poverty. Although other explanations for world poverty pointed to the history of colonialism and the unequal distribution of resources within the world system, U.S. foundations began to fund family planning programs internationally. In many poor countries governments may have been seeking to reduce the population, but it became evident that households were strategizing with different aims. In a classic evaluation of a Harvard School of Public Health birth control project, funded by the Rockefeller Foundation, Mahmood Mamdani (1972), conducting research in one of the Indian villages where the program was in operation, found that only those families who were already limiting their fertility actually made use of the pills they were given. At each income level, families had pressing economic reasons for wanting more children. Among poor peasants, more children meant more laborers to work the land, and among the middle classes, more children meant that the family could train doctors, lawyers, and businessmen and thus hope this diversity allowed them security and financial gains in the future. In each situation, girls were less desirable, because they could not hope to earn as much as men. The subordination of women in every sphere led to corresponding poor health, less food, less education, and less employment opportunities. Women's continuing inequality undermined efforts to introduce birth control as mothers who might have welcomed contraceptive methods for the purposes of spacing their children and taking control of their own fertility had little power over family planning.

A contrasting set of problems occurred as European industrialized countries began to face declining birthrates and aging populations (M. Susser, Watson, and Hopper 1985). In the 1980s in Romania, the communist government banned abortion in their effort to increase the population and build their idea of a successful and powerful nation (Kligman 1995). As a result, many women died from attempting illegal abortions in unsafe circumstances. Many of those who did not risk this dangerous option carried their pregnancy to term but did not have the resources to raise the child. As a result, thousands of children were put into state orphanages, where they suffered from malnutrition and disease. In 1989, when the Romanian government was overthrown, the conditions in these orphanages came to international attention, and it was discovered that many of the children had contracted HIV/AIDS through the sharing of needles for vaccination and the blood transfusions that were apparently given for anemia caused by malnutrition. Thus, the government's efforts to foster population growth had, instead, led to the death of hundreds of mothers from illegal abortions, the mistreatment of infants, and the death of thousands of children from disease (Kligman 1995).

The Romanian experience introduces adoption as another kind of window into the different ways states institutionalize rules of the family in a changing world. The adoption of a child by a middle-class American family generally reflects the patterns of class stratification in the United States, such that the child may be most easily legally adopted from a poor household and reared in a household with access to wealth and education (Gailey 2010). However, as in the case of Romania, the child may be adopted from a poorer country or a country in political turmoil and the source of such adopted children, as well as their health and the legal regulations binding the adoption, will depend on the particular historical moment and the uneven access to resources between core and periphery in the world system (Ginsburg and Rapp 1995; Kligman 1995; Gailey 2010).

As in India and Romania, ethnographic research has revealed that government policies that attempt to directly control household reproductive decisions and family structure can have unforeseen and sometimes tragic consequences, often differentiated by gender. However, making options available to men and women to control family spacing and size can also increase the possibilities for women's autonomy. In the next section, we explore the complex interaction among government policies, changing societal conditions, and household strategies.

Men, Women, and Children: Decisions in the Household

Carole Browner (2001) tells of contrasting interests among men and women in a rural Mexican household. Women, already exhausted by their multiple responsibilities of housework and agriculture and often suffering from malnutrition and vitamin deficiencies, insisted that more children make more work and that they did not wish for further pregnancies. Men were more likely to want their wives to rear another child. Meanwhile, government concern for population growth precipitated family planning policies, which had little impact on the village households.

A similar case study in Bangladesh notes that in poor households, men and women may have different perspectives on reproductive decisions: "Women have the responsibility for feeding children, particularly in the early, less productive years of their lives. They cannot walk away from them in times of crisis, the way men can and do" (Kabeer 1985: 105). Frequently women had less mobility and fewer options than the men in poor households. Once children were grown, however, such poor landless women maintained little authority over their offspring. Under these conditions, most women still expressed a preference for sons, because in the long run, the main position from which a woman could exert power was as a mother-in-law to her adult married son. Nevertheless, as they perceived much drudgery and little advantage from rearing many children a number of "women from landless and near-landless households took advantage of the family planning services offered by the local women's project, often without their husband's knowledge" (Kabeer 1985: 104).

The struggle among the different interests of men and women, daughters and mothers-in-law within the context of shifting state and national policies, will be expressed in family planning choices. As a result, unless gendered inequality is considered and addressed in the local arrangements, the outcome may not necessarily be in the best interests of the health of the women and children.

Labor and Childbirth

In addition to looking at family-planning strategies, anthropologists have described the different ways in which women have experienced childbirth and contributed to our understanding that women can participate in decisions about childbirth and labor (Michaelson 1988; Davis-Floyd 2001).

In preindustrial Europe and the United States, labor and childbirth were managed and controlled by women in the household, often with the assistance of midwives or their equivalent. In the late nineteenth century, as Western doctors were beginning to conduct scientific experiments and to establish the medical profession, women were still active as midwives. However, in the early-twentieth-century United States, as the medical profession became more rigorously licensed and depended on an extensive education, women were excluded from such training. Childbirth became less the sphere of midwives and more an arena of professional male doctors. This process, sometimes called the medicalization of childbirth, involved the introduction of anesthetics to reduce the pain of labor, which, also, as the woman lost consciousness, placed labor further under the control of medical authority (Wertz and Wertz 1979).

The conflicting issues related to the medicalization of pregnancy and labor were recently highlighted in controversies among Inuit women in Canada, as they continued to insist on their rights to home births supervised by local women. They resisted being flown to a well-equipped hospital for labor and childbirth, far away from their community support (P. Kaufert and O'Neil 1993). Although science and technology have clearly prolonged the lives of women dramatically, women have lost some of the responsibility and autonomy previously associated with the process of childbirth.

THE ANTHROPOLOGY OF REPRODUCTION AMONG POOR POPULATIONS

In poor and especially the vast majority of poor rural populations, medical anthropologists have to consider reproduction within the context of the lack of prenatal care, the distance to the nearest clinic, the expense and consequent unavailability of antibiotics and other medications fundamental to public health, the shortage of immunizations, poor nutrition of the mother and infant, and the lack of clean water to wash food or dilute formula. Anthropologists and public health researchers have noted that, throughout the world, women's health is often neglected in favor of children's health, to the detriment of both.

As in the core countries, we find women on the periphery of capitalism trying all available methods, those of Western science as well as those of other healers. However, in poor countries, the lack of doctors, trained nurses, and medical provisions leads to greater dependence on alternative medical models, indigenous knowledge of herbal treatments, and communal rituals of healing. Many ethnographies document folk practices in childbirth and pregnancy, as well as the communal aspects of childbirth in the domestic setting. In such settings, critical medical anthropologists are careful to understand reproduction within the context of the availability of care and resources and also to include both the men's and women's points of view. What strategies are available to men and women to assure the health and welfare of their families? How do men and women make decisions about family size, the timing of births, the survival of the newborn and the access to resources of boys and girls? (Scheper-Hughes 1992; Gammeltoft 1999; Browner 2001).

Tine Gammeltoft's (1999) study, *Women's Bodies, Women's Worries*, of rural women in Vietnam, provides us with a clear sense of women struggling to maintain their own and their children's health in the context of patriarchal rules and their own recognition of the need for a unified family to build strong economic resources. As one woman says, "Women know how to put up [with situations], to endure. Men often flare up so it is mostly women who endure" (Gammeltoft 1999: 201).

However, this does not mean that women do nothing. On the contrary, as another rural Vietnamese woman makes clear, "If you go to a hospital in secret, who will know? If your husband wants more children and you don't, he can't force you. You decide for yourself first. The husband's opinion is only a small part. For women, if you want a child, you have a child. You don't have to say anything to your husband until your stomach is big, and then what can he do? . . . It's all up to you" (Gammeltoft 1999: 187).

Since the 1980s, HIV/AIDS has emerged as a central concern in reproduction. Women worldwide have been contracting the virus earlier and at a greater rate than men (Piot 2001). HIV-positive mothers can transmit the virus both through pregnancy and labor (perinatally) and through breastfeeding.

Since the end of the 1990s such transmission has become preventable. In Western societies, as well as in Brazil, Argentina, and Uruguay, mothers may opt for testing prenatally and also be entitled to treatment for themselves. Mothers in poorer countries who would not go for testing for themselves, because almost always treatment is available for the baby but not necessarily for the mother herself, will take the risk of testing for HIV/AIDS knowing that it may save the baby. If the mother tests positive, she often faces ostracism and stigma from her husband and family and knowledge of certain death. Nevertheless, she will be offered medications in the last few months of pregnancy to take during labor. The baby will be given the medications for a short period after birth. If the baby is exclusively breastfed or formula-fed, these simple procedures will reduce the perinatal transmission of HIV. Sometimes the mother will continue to receive medications for her own continued health, but in some situations in poor countries, the baby may live but less attention will be paid to the courageous mother's survival (for a review of these issues, see I. Susser 2009a).

Many poor mothers in southern Africa and other parts of the world do not yet have access to such preventive measures for their babies, nor treatment for themselves, although there are ongoing efforts to improve this situation. For example, postexposure prophylaxis that protects a woman who has been raped from infection with the AIDS virus is often not available in high-conflict, high-risk areas. As a response to worldwide social movements that demand that pharmaceutical companies provide affordable options for poor countries and that wealthy countries contribute resources for public health in poorer countries, medications have slowly become available for free or at lower prices (Farmer, Connors, and Simmons 1996; I. Susser 2009a). However, government policies that neglect HIV/AIDS, combined with the domestic subordination of women and the fact that many people do not live near clinics, or cannot afford the transportation, or the clinics do not provide testing or treatment still present challenges to prevention and care (I. Susser 2009a).

BIOTECHNOLOGIES AND THE ANTHROPOLOGY OF REPRODUCTION IN THE CENTERS OF CAPITAL

In wealthy, mostly urban, populations, medical anthropologists have to confront the challenges of high-level technologies that can offer mothers a painless, generally safe, birth. The women's health movement in United States questioned the shift to high-technology births and the accompanying reduction in women's control and community supports, as well as the class and racial inequalities in access to reproductive health care (Morgen 1987, 2002). Betty Levin (1990) has studied the dilemmas of doctors, health care workers, and parents faced with medical interventions that can, in fact, save the lives of extremely low birth-weight premature infants, but with no guarantee of their future physical and mental abilities. How are decisions made about extraordinary measures that prolong invasive and expensive procedures when the infant may not benefit from the interventions and the parents may suffer inordinately without saving their child? Others have analyzed the changing perceptions of parents and the commoditization of motherhood as couples who might not otherwise have children are offered assisted conception through in vitro fertilization and surrogate motherhood (Franklin and Ragone 1998). As Rayna Rapp (2000) has clearly delineated in her discussion of women as moral pioneers, in the United States, questions arise after amniocentesis results demonstrate that the fetus has the genetic mutation for Down syndrome. Such a diagnosis indicates that if the child were to be born, it might never have full mental capacities. Nevertheless, Rapp's research indicates that the decision to terminate a pregnancy is embedded in the class and institutional realities of the historical moment, including the available services for the parents of Down syndrome children and people with disabilities.

Other researchers, such as Lynn Morgan (1998) and Sarah Franklin (Franklin and Ragone 1998), have taught us how U.S. perceptions differ from other cultural constructs of life and the fetus and how Western perceptions have changed as sonograms and video technology have catapulted representations of conception in the uterus and the developing fetus into our consciousness. In the nineteenth century, quickening, or the first flutter of movement felt by the pregnant woman, generally in the eighteenth week of pregnancy, represented the entry of the soul into the womb. Nowadays, technology and genetic engineering, combined with fundamentalist religious beliefs, have precipitated debate about the life of the embryo. Powerful scientific developments with respect to conception and pregnancy have not only made conception more predictable and childbirth safer but also made the fetus more visible.

Such technologies have obviously broadened choices available to women in core capitalist countries. The morning-after pill, which acts to prevent conception and addresses some of the U.S. cultural constructions concerned with the life of the fetus, is now available in most Western countries. Women, informed through sonograms and laboratory testing that their pregnancy may lead to a mentally disabled child, have the option to terminate the pregnancy. At the same time, the invasion of science into the domain of the woman and her body has in some ways reduced the woman's own decision-making power. Representing the fetus and even the embryo, as a separate legal entity, even though it is still completely engulfed in the uterine environment and completely dependent on the woman's body for survival reduces the control of women over their own conception.

Scientists have understood since the mid-twentieth century that certain substances such as benzene, radiation, and nitrous oxide may affect the developing fetus. Women who may be exposed to such substances in the workplace can protect their future child by requesting to be moved to a safer environment, and in the United States, legal regulations allow her to move at work without losing her job. However, now that we know that alcohol, smoking, and drugs may affect a fetus, women can be limited by state policy in what they do during pregnancy, and, in the extreme, a mother can be jailed for putting the fetus at risk (Whiteford 1996). In fact, recent findings have shown that a father's exposure to environmental hazards may also affect a future infant and may, in time, come to affect men's decisions or autonomy in the legal sphere.

As medical anthropologists have noted, violence in the household is one problem that First World women share with poorer countries where battering, murder, and sexual violence, frequently directly associated with a male partner's unemployment, also reach epidemic proportions (Heise 1993; Jewkes 2002). However, violence against women has to be understood within the context of the world system and the impact of globalization, as men have lost jobs, women have been increasingly employed long hours in low-wage sweatshop conditions, and resources available to poor families have been reduced (Susser 2009a). To quote Lynn Freedman from the Center for Population and Health, Columbia University, "Even domestic violence can not be delinked from the growing impoverishment experienced in vast portions of the world since the 1980s. For example, studies conducted as early as 1988 documented an explicit connection between the implementation of International Monetary Fund and World Bank structural adjustment programs, the upheaval that the resulting impoverishment caused and an upsurge in domestic violence" (2000: 436).

The research of medical anthropologists in countries on the periphery, as opposed to the centers of capitalism, asks fundamentally different questions, but in their very difference, they raise basic questions of their own. As earlier in history, reproduction in 2012 was still intimately interconnected with the rights of women to autonomy, education, and employment (Freedman 2000; Farmer, Connors, and Simmons 1996; I. Susser 2009a). Reproductive health is also crucially determined by the histories of colonialism, the uneven development of the world system, and the current impact of globalization. Globalization, which has involved massive privatization of public resources, has contributed to the increasing gap between rich and poor, as well as to the undermining of women's autonomy with respect to reproductive options, as resources for reproductive choice and education are increasingly limited. Nevertheless, there have been global and national movements contesting the limitations on women's reproductive choice (Petchesky 2003; I. Susser 2009a).

Thus, any movement for the reproductive health rights of women must incorporate recognition of women's own abilities to strategize in any historical situation (Freedman 2000; I. Susser 2002). International agencies or movements can assist local women in creating spaces of autonomy, in countering fundamentalist assumptions that limit access to reproductive choice, and in providing the resources for education, the technologies of birth control, the funds for medications, and employment opportunities. As we have seen from the historical record, with access to funds, health facilities, employment, and education, men and women themselves adapt their reproductive strategies to the changing situations in which they find themselves.

"A Closer Look"

U.S. MORALITIES AND WOMEN'S REPRODUCTIVE HEALTH

We can see the politics of reproduction as they have been contested over the past thirty years in the United States.[1] Under President George W. Bush, from 2001 through 2008, the U.S. government changed laws with respect to gender and sexuality on a domestic and on the global level, cutting funding for science and technology, women's reproductive health, and studies that mentioned sexuality—but also funding faith-based groups world-wide (Girard 2004; National Council of Research on Women 2004). At the same time, $50 million a year in federal funds was mandated for abstinence-only programs in the United States.

It turned out the programs had no significant effect in persuading teens to abstain from sex, and teens who had been trained in the programs had no less unprotected sex than those who did not ("Impacts to Four Title V, Section 510 Abstinence Education Programs," available at: www.mathematica.org). A general review of abstinence-only programs throughout the United States found that they were "undermining comprehensive sexuality education and other government-sponsored programs . . . by withholding information and promoting questionable and inaccurate opinions" (Santelli et al. 2006).

In addition, from 2001 to 2008, much information about birth control, condoms, and abortion disappeared from federal websites (National Council for Research on Women 2004). Department of Health websites actually changed to say that condoms can cause infection and do not prevent AIDS. Notices appeared claiming that abortion causes breast cancer. Some of the worst cases of misinformation, such as the two noted here, were toned down after an outcry from public health professionals (National Council for Research on Women 2004).

Thus, policies of the Bush administration undermined the freedom of women in their access to reproductive choice and even "morning-after" pills (National Council for Research on Women 2004). As was evident in the rhetoric concerning gay marriage in the 2004 U.S. elections, sexual orientation also became a related arena of battle (Girard 2004).

Lack of comprehensive sexual education and reproductive health programs had a particularly deleterious impact on poor women and women of color. To quote an article discussing the challenges facing women and girls in South Carolina and Florida:

The politicization of pregnancy, sexuality and women's reproductive rights [has] created a uniquely contradictory situation in many states. Policymakers are

---

1. This section is largely drawn from Ida Susser's work on imperial moralities (2009b).

working to control women's reproductive choices and sexuality, and restricting sex education, but doing little to address the overall lack of access to quality reproductive health care. (McGovern 2007: 119)

The regime of President George W. Bush reoriented both national and international funding in the direction of ever more constricting moral imperatives. Through U.S. contributions to the World Health Organization and the United Nations, which constrains UNAIDS, UN Population and Family Health, and UNIFEM (the United Nations Development Fund for Women), the United States influenced policy worldwide with respect to comprehensive sex education, sexuality, abortion, gender-based violence, substance use, and women's reproductive health. Agencies were denied funding because of association with reproductive education. In 2004, the U.S. government withdrew $34 million from the United Nations Population Administration because they were accused of funding Marie Stopes Programs in China. Marie Stopes organized other services where abortion information was available. This decision had an immediate and intimidating effect on all UN agencies.

As Ida Susser (2009b) has argued, there were three main precipitants of what might be termed the new imperial morality under President G.W. Bush: increasing domestic inequalities associated with globalization and cutbacks in government services, the alliance of the U.S. Republican Party with the religious right, and the nationalism and neoconservative policies associated with the war in Iraq. Each of these processes contributed to a heightened emphasis on sin and morality as well as gender subordination. Such imperial moralities were reflected in constraints on sexuality, sexual orientation, and women's reproductive choice and health. They contributed to stigmatizing vulnerable groups and damaged AIDS prevention possibilities worldwide.

The abstinence-only programs were ended in 2008 when Barack Obama became president and, over the next four years, the Agency for International Development changed the emphases for programs outside the United States. Rules that had restricted AIDS prevention programs to exclude people by sexual orientation or to neglect sex workers and drug users were modified. However, the United States and the ongoing congressional and presidential battles over family planning and abortion remain an important lesson in the politicization and struggles for control of women's bodies.

THE BODY

Much of what has been discussed in this chapter could be rephrased in terms of theories of the body and the embodiment of social and cultural issues. As Margaret Lock has noted, "Historicized, grounded ethnography, stimulated by the close attention paid for the first time to the everyday lives of women, children, and other "peripheral" peoples has led to a reformulation of theory. The body, imbued with social meaning, is now historically situated, and becomes not only a signifier of belonging and order but also an active forum for the expression of dissent and loss, thus ascribing it individual agency. These dual modes of bodily expression—belonging and dissent—are conceptualized as culturally produced and in dialectical exchange with the externalized ongoing performance of social life" (1993 : 140). Thus, we can talk about the processes of reproduction in terms of the expectations and experiences of the *Woman in the Body* (Martin 1987). The battles over women's access to contraception and reproductive choice are, primarily, battles over women's control of their own bodies. They are also, as we have seen, tightly bound with the ongoing politics of class and race at any historical moment.

The focus on the body has opened up important arenas of discussion and helped to illuminate the dialectical interactions between gender and biological sexual characteristics as well as the powerful significations of the body in society. From the point of view of critical medical anthropology, it remains crucial to analyze the body within a systematic understanding of the processes of the state and global processes within capitalism. One of the dangers of starting with the body, rather than the nation-state, is that although the body itself has become a site of anthropological analysis that breaks down some of the Western Cartesian dualisms of the mind and the body, questions of inequality and justice, even if often alluded to, cannot be fully analyzed in this framework. To work for social justice, we need to know the historical conditions which have precipitated the sufferings of the body. We need to understand the processes that lead to "exclusion" or "abandonment." Although it is crucial to recognize the protests of the body, it is also crucial, as Ong (1987) showed in her description of Malaysian women workers, to place these protests within a clearly delineated moment in the domination of global capital.

As Lock (1993) also points out, "Foucault's discussion of biopower has had a profound effect on anthropological representations of the body. Central to this theory is the concept of 'surveillance,' institutionalized through disciplinary techniques, resulting in the production of docile bodies (Foucault 1979, 1980)."

Following Foucault (1998), we might see modern states as developing demography, statistics, and the implementation of public health as part of an overall method of governance, which he termed *biopower*. Foucault discussed neoliberal regimes as leading even further toward a governance through biopower and a number of anthropologists have followed this lead, analyzing biological citizenship as being one claim that carries legitimacy under these conditions (for example, Petryna 2002). As the feminist theorist Susan Bordo (1999) has noted, although much of Foucault's writing precludes any possibility for transformative social changes, his later works, importantly, recognize heterogeneous forms of resistance. However, if we start with a generalized discussion of biopolitics and neoliberalism, we lose the historical specificity and analyses of the use of moralities as powerful political symbols in the building of power-blocks within particular nation-states.

The increasing inequality between rich and poor that has characterized global relations since the 1980s has led not only to increasing inequality in health but also increasing exploitation of the bodies of the poor for the benefit of the wealthy. With the growing sophistication of medical technology, under the current policies of unfettered capital, socialized debt, and privatized wealth, we see the escalating commodification of body parts. In the global marketplace, the poor have been reduced to the selling of blood, plasma, organs, sperm, eggs, and the use of the uterus. As modern technology has allowed for the farming of organs from the poor to the wealthy, within both the global South and the global North as well as from the global South to the Global North (Sharp 2006), reproduction itself has become further commodified. Reproductive tourism has been added to transnational adoption and sex tourism as a new form of exploitation of the poor by the wealthy, within one country and also transnationally. For all these new or further developed commodifications, major health centers with the best of global facilities have been developed in emerging middle-income countries such as India, Pakistan, Brazil, and elsewhere, so that with other aspects of the new global inequality, reproductive farming and other forms of organ buying can be efficiently and safely organized for those who can pay.

We find global policy addressing different aspects of reproduction, from laws and funding for abortion, to decisions to farm eggs, to ideas of childbirth. We also find that this commodification of bodies has led to the transmission of multiple diseases across the world from hepatitis to AIDS (for example, Pepin 2012) although the better-off may be somewhat less likely to become infected when the diseases are easily detectable and prevention is possible.

We have also seen a continuation of an old practice that involves using the global South as a laboratory. Historically, many diseases that were chronic in colonial countries had largely disappeared or were not manifest in the centers of capital. With colonialism, populations were decimated both through disease and brutal treatment (Vincent 1982; Pepin 2012). Laboratories were set up in the Belgian Congo, Kenya, Uganda, Nigeria, and elsewhere to study the tsetse fly (sleeping sickness), malaria, and mosquitoes and their possible treatments for the benefit of the colonizers and also to maintain the health of the colonial workforce (Pepin 2012). Over the past decades, with both birth control and later HIV, poor women of the global South served as the experimental populations for new drugs and technologies. In many cases, these were drugs or new technologies that would be useful to the North as well as the South and sometimes were more crucial for the global South, as with AIDS treatment in southern Africa. However, as a medical doctor from Malawi noted at the International AIDS Society in Washington, DC (July 2012), if such treatments are tested on poor African women, they should also be made affordable and accessible to them when the drugs prove successful.

As biotechnologies of reproduction have become ever more widespread and complex, the relationship between biology and the ideologies of kinship has become a rich area for anthropological research. In the United States, research in the 1970s demonstrated that the practical experience of kinship was very different from the ideology of the nuclear family (Stack 1974; D. Schneider and Smith 1982; I. Susser 2012). Schneider and Smith (1982) argued that the ideology or cultural template for the American family was universally the nuclear family. However, their data showed dramatic variation both in family forms and in kin terms among the working class and the middle class of their era. They argued that poor people adapted kinship to suit their situations but still adhered to the ideal of the nuclear American family. There was no room for other visions of the family in their theory—ideas such as the importance of grandparents in the household, different visions of family expressed by immigrant groups or black families, the mother who chose to live with other women to rear her children, or any other arrangements. None of these were theorized as valued in American families; they were simply viewed as strategies designed to address exigent circumstances.

Historically, same-sex relationships led to the creation of new kinds of kinship, particularly as women living together formed communities tied together by the responsibilities of childrearing. However, as the mobilization of gay social movements has led to the increasing recognition of same-sex marriage, many same-sex families have, like adoptive families and families facilitated by biotechnology, worked to create the accepted ideological boundaries of the nuclear family template described by David Schneider (1968) in *American Kinship*. Although the cultural bonds that Schneider saw as symbolized by blood and sex are no longer, and possibly never were, actually tied to blood or sex, such new families, at least among the middle class, have striven to be recognized as the nuclear family in the image of middle America. Although many families do not correspond to the bounded nuclear family image of two parents and (biological or not) children, the image that biotechnology and adoption, whether domestic or international, or same-sex families have tried to create has remained surprisingly uniform.

Just as with international adoption, the biotechnologies of reproduction have so far been set in place by families with the resources to re-create the image of the nuclear family. Christine Gailey (2010) argues that adoption, both domestic and international, might be seen as enlarging the family to include kin from the birth family and social background of the child. However, she suggests that this is seldom the case because many middle-class families are committed to re-creating the limits and boundaries of kinship that fit with childrearing and inheritance expectations in the United States. She argues that working-class families who generally have negotiated domestic adoptions are more likely to extend kinship expectations more widely, as in fact, Stack (1974) showed for black working-class women who were rearing their children in the 1970s.

Verena Stolcke (2012) makes some similar points in her discussion of the biotechnological revolution in kinship. She suggests that, for the most part, new parents who have arranged the birth of their legal children through surrogates, in vitro fertilization or other procedures do not include all the players in their creation of kinship for their infants. In fact, many families have been protective of the image of the nuclear family, no matter what the source of the original egg or gametes of the newborn infant. However, Stolcke argues that as such technologies become even more commonplace, children would often benefit from wider kin networks that would include the recognition of the connections of the different people who may have contributed to their birth.

CONCLUSIONS

Over the past decade, anthropological analyses of reproduction have been analyzed in terms of three approaches: political economy, theories of the body, and the challenges of the new biotechnologies. These approaches, or perhaps entry points, are not necessarily contradictory and can be overlapping, but they represent different research priorities within the field. Critical medical anthropology prioritizes questions of inequality and political economy, and we began this chapter from that perspective. We then progressed to a discussion of theories of the body with an emphasis on how these productively inform political economic analyses. Finally, we outlined the ways in which current debates with respect to biotechnology and kinship are essential to an analysis of the global inequality of reproduction.

PART III

Social Diseases
and Social Suffering

CHAPTER 7

Violence and War

ENCOUNTERING VIOLENCE

There is a long history recognizing the multiple ways that war, other forms of violence, and disease are not only intimately linked casually but constitute alternative expressions of common underlying forces. More than 150 years ago, activist physician leader Rudolph Virchow (1985: 122) made the observation that "War, pestilence and starvation mutually engender one another; we do not know of any great period in world history when these did not occur to a greater or lesser extent, simultaneously or in short succession." More recently, the Nobel Peace Laureates' Charter for a World without Violence (World March for Peace and Nonviolence 2009) emphasized: "Violence is a preventable disease" and that "those most harmed by violence are the weakest and vulnerable" (Permanent Secretariat of Nobel Peace Laureates Summits 2009). As these comments suggest, war and human conflict are health issues and hence are of concern to medical anthropology. Moreover, war and violence emerge as critical contexts in which the interface of power and health are indisputably interlocked (Panter-Brick 2010).

Especially since the War in Vietnam (1959–1975), a war that produced almost 60,000 U.S. causalities and well over a million Vietnamese causalities, cultural anthropologists have studied "modern" violence, including domestic, intimate partner and community violence, as well as war at the local and global levels within broader frameworks produced by culture and the political-economic forces of state, power, and finance. At the same time, medical anthropologists, seeking to assess the varied health implications of human conflict, have also begun to work ethnographically in war zones. On the basis of the growing body of anthropological work on the intersection of health and war, this chapter examines social conflict as a prevalent source of human suffering, disease, and death. This chapter considers the human capacity for violence, the devastating toll taken by conflict on human health and survival, the overt and hidden injuries of war, the significance of human resilience in the face of atrocity, trauma, and unspeakable aggression, and the lessons of studies of war and health for medical anthropology.

A VIOLENT SPECIES?

Are we inherently a violent species, and are war and other forms of human physical conflict, bullying, and abuse of others merely natural expressions of our genetically rooted aggressiveness? Certainly this idea has had its backers. Some even point to the high levels of intercommunity and intracommunity lethal aggression of our nearest animal relatives, the chimpanzees, as evidence of our aggressive biological heritage (DeWall and Anderson 2011). Findings from ethnographic research on human foraging societies, however, have found low rates of physical aggression (Boehm 1999). Based on more than seventeen months of field work with two groups of Nyae Nyae !Kung in Namibia, for example, Marshall (1998) observed only loud arguments, and heard about only three others in a neighboring group. By contrast, in his many years of research among the related Dobe Ju/'hoansi of Botswana, Lee (2012) identified twenty-two cases of homicides (fifteen of which were products of feuds between family groups) in the period between 1920 and 1955, and fifteen additional nonfatal fights between individuals. He also found that the Ju/'hoansi "had many [cultural] mechanisms for controlling aggression and preventing serious fights from breaking out" (Lee 2012: 126). One of these, the *hxaro*, a form of trading partnership, diminished conflict by "circulating useful goods and spreading the risk of ecological disaster so that everyone may live with an adequate, if not luxurious, food supply" (Lee 2012: 135). In short, although humans, as a species that evolved under conditions in which fending off carnivores and protecting resources from other groups, have the capacity to engage in violence if needed, we are biocultural beings by nature, and both our biology and our cultural heritages must be considered in assessing human nature.

This point is supported by multiple ethnographic accounts of societies with limited evidence of interpersonal violence and the absence of intergroup warfare (Dentan 1968, 2008; Bonta 1996; Fry 2006; Sponsel 2009). Further, as Sponsel (2009: 36) notes, looked at historically the "overwhelming majority of [individual] humans [across societies] have not been involved directly in any kind of killing" throughout their lives, further challenging the notion that humans are characterized by powerful and uncontrollable biological tendencies toward violence. Additionally, moving from interpersonal fighting to intergroup warfare is a significant shift, because wars are sociopolitical events that are not fought because of individual characteristics, inclinations, or motives. Soldiers go to war for many reasons (they are forced by society; they want to uphold family traditions; they do not want to appear to be cowardly; they want to defend their country/group and its values; they have been convinced by propaganda that the enemy is evil and threatening; their friends are going to war; they seek the financial, health care, and educational benefits of military service; they have no other economic options), but none of these explain why wars occur. Likewise, over time, as the capacity for devastation increases, even the prevailing rationales for engaging in warfare seem much more convincing at the start of armed conflicts than they do later as the grim toll of modern warfare is once again revealed, leading to the rise of antiwar social movements in combatant countries.

WAR CAUSALITIES IN THE TWENTIETH CENTURY

Although humans are not innately inclined toward war, wars certainly have a telling impact on human life and well-being. As we push deeper into the twenty-first century, it seems appropriate to go back and assess the health toll of war by looking back at the entire prior century and determining what were the human costs during the one hundred years from 1900 through 1999.

It is estimated that 160 million people died in the wars of the twentieth century (Scaruffi 2009) or the equivalent of the densely populated country of Nigeria. The century was ushered in by the Chinese Boxer Rebellion against the imperial designs of the U.S., Britain, France, Russia, and Japan against China. Thirty-thousand people were killed in the rebellion, which, notably, set the stage for a legacy of conflict related to the colonial ambitions of various countries. Thus, in 1904, Germany went to war with Namibia to gain advantage in Africa, followed by Italy's invasion of Ethiopia in 1936, the Japanese assault on China in 1937, the French-Vietnam war of 1946–1954, and the French-Algerian war of 1954–1962. Early in the century, the Ottoman Empire's slaughter of more than a million Armenians signaled the significant role genocide would play in the conflicts of the twentieth century. It is estimated that twenty million soldiers and civilians died in World War I, a figure that was surpassed by the estimated fifty-five million deaths in World War II. In the aftermath of World War II, there followed a series of armed anticolonial wars for independence and multiple civil wars. The civil war in Mozambique alone, which raged for a decade and a half, is believed to have led to a million deaths and five million refugees. One of the last conflicts of the century was the Kosovo War, which was fought from early 1998 to mid-1999. A war that pitted ethnic Albanians and Serbians in Yugoslavia and included an extensive bombing campaign by NATO against the Serbians, produced more than thirteen thousand fatalities, many of which were civilians (Spiegel and Salama 2000). The war introduced the term *ethnic cleansing* into the language of human social life and underscored the fundamental role played by genocide in the wars of the twentieth century. Additionally, although wars have long produced civilian losses, a social shift occurred in the latter half of the twentieth century toward forms of warfare in which civilians—especially women and children—comprise the majority of war's casualties. In today's wars "civilians [are killed] more callously and systematically than ever before (United Nations Population Fund 2002: 3).

The conflicts noted here are just a few of the wars fought in local or broader contexts around the globe during the twentieth century, making it, no doubt, one of the bloodiest centuries in human history. In the last half of the century alone, there were more than 160 wars, with more than twenty-four million people killed (mostly civilians), and tens of millions more displaced from their homes by internal conflict (Pedersen 2002). Although many of these wars lasted several years, others "persisted for two, three, or even four decades or more, spanning the entire lifetimes of multiple generations and fundamentally shaping the social realities of many tens of millions" of people (Lubkemann 2008: 1). Under such conditions, war is not a time-limited event, nor even a sudden breach that temporarily disrupts everyday life; instead it becomes a way of life. Observes anthropologist Veena Das (2008: 95) "the reality of violence includes . . . its potential to both disrupt the ordinary and become part of the ordinary." Violent conditions and the constant slide into war during the twentieth century led some anthropologists to talk about a *global culture of war*. Observes Carolyn Nordstrom (1997: 123), "Violence becomes a cultural fact, a persistent enduring dynamic. This cultural force of violence maintains the reality of violence beyond its mere physical expression." In short, as Nordstrom points out, hostilities may end but the impacts of war often are enduring in the minds and bodies of soldiers and civilians, as well as in crumbling health and social infrastructures, and in health-threatening damage done to the physical environment. Additionally, as Pederson (2006: 299) accentuates,

Modern warfare is concerned not only to annihilate life, but also to destroy "ways of life," trying to eliminate entire ethnic groups and eradicate entire cultures and social systems, thus undermining the critical means whereby people endure and recover from suffering and loss.

"A Closer Look"

WARS OF THE TWENTY-FIRST CENTURY

As noted, from the perspective of war, the twentieth century, an era of natural resource depletion and struggles for vital resources, sharp "ethnic" antagonisms, and two hot wars and one cold war on a global scale, was particularly brutal and deadly. What can we say about the twenty-first century so far? Certainly, in its first decade, the twenty-first century was not a time of global peace but rather in many ways an extension of patterns seen in the previous century, while adding some new dimensions to its blood-stained warscapes around the planet. An example of the continuation of patterns is seen in the conflict that has raged in the western Sudanese region of Darfur since 2003 pitting several rebel groups against the Sudanese government. The rebel's maintain that they were forced to pick up arms because of the government's oppression of non-Arab Sudanese in Darfur. In response to the rebellion, the government has quietly sponsored paramilitary forces known as the Janjaweed militias, which have carried out a vicious campaign of slaughter against the civilian population of Darfur. Observes Morse (2005),

this war is being fought with Kalashnikovs, clubs and knives. . . . [T]he preferred tactics are burning and pillaging, castration and rape—carried out by Arab militias riding on camels and horses. The most sophisticated technologies deployed are, on the one hand, the helicopters used by the Sudanese government to support the militias when they attack black African villages, and on the other hand, quite a different weapon: the seismographs used by foreign oil companies to map oil deposits hundreds of feet below the surface.

In other words, the war in Darfur combines the features of a resource war (a fight among powerful nations for the resources of poor and weaker nations), a war of proxies (Sudanese fighting Sudanese to the advantage of foreign oil companies), a war waged on a civilian population (who occupy land that sits over oil deposits), and an invisible war (because it has received limited mainstream media coverage, perhaps because of the role of the powerful oil industry). Comments Morse (2005), "When Darfur does occasionally make the news—photographs of burned villages, charred corpses, malnourished children—it is presented without context."

In a number of its features the war in Darfur resembles civil wars of the twentieth century. But there are some new features in other twenty-first-century wars. One of these is the growing presence of asymmetrical wars, such as the U.S. war against Iraq or the U.S. against Afghanistan. Whereas the United States is a world superpower with an enormous nuclear arsenal, its opponents in these two wars are groups of insurgents with fabricated weapons and irregular armies. Another feature of some twenty-first-century wars is the use of private armies and support personnel. Private contractors play an ever-greater role in U.S. wars in the Middle East, for example. War, in essence, has become a commodity that can be bought and sold in the marketplace along with potato chips and underwear.

WAR AS A COMPLEX BIOSOCIAL DISEASE

Singer and Hodge (2010: 4) use the term *war machine* to draw attention to the whole complex of contemporary war, including "the varied forms of direct armed hostility, . . . their heavy toll on environments and workers, the international weapons trade that reaps great profit while helping to fuel new conflicts, the saber-rattling ideologies and policies that justify and encourage war, and war budgets that rob public treasuries of funds needed for pressing health and social needs." All of these constitute what war is; they are part and parcel of contemporary warfare and indivorceable from it. War is also disease and malnutrition. Thus, the damage done to human lives in contemporary warfare is caused as much or more by the spread of disease and hunger as by being exposed to the use of deadly armaments (Human Security Research Group 2009). The Global Burden of Armed Violence report issued by the Geneva Declaration Secretariat (2008), for example, estimates that for every one of the six hundred thousand individuals who died violently in the wars fought around the globe during the years 2004 to 2007, four more were victims of war-related disease and malnutrition.

Consequently, war can be described as not just something that causes disease but as a complex form of biosocial disease (Rylko-Bauer and Singer 2011). Central to this understanding is recognition that as conceived within critical medical anthropology, disease is never a simple biological fact. To say that a community is suffering an outbreak of intestinal worms, for example, says far more than that a particular parasite that causes specific harm to the human body has spread within a group of people. It is also a statement about social conditions locally, and structures of social relationship that extend from the local to the global that have facilitated disease outbreak. In this sense, disease is a *biosocial fact*, and this is true of war as well. War incorporates both complex political economic and physical conflicts as well as a wide set of deleterious psychobiosocial factors. In other words, war is not just "similar to a disease" in that it is a source of human injury, suffering, and death, but rather disease and hunger are among the most potent weapons of war, as is the intentional use of trauma and terrorization among civilians (Nordstrom 1998). All of these are part of what war is and not merely what has been called the *collateral damage* (or unplanned consequences) of war.

Figure 7.1
Health Impacts of War

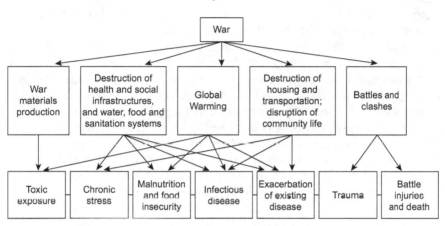

The Overt and Hidden Injuries of War

The health impacts of war are both overt and hidden. Moreover, they are multiple, enduring, and interactive, with both general and subgroup specific features as discussed in this section. The health-related and inter-related impacts of war are depicted in Figure 7.1. As this figure reveals, actual battlefield clashes and attacks account for only a small portion of the health burdens of war.

Overt causalities of war are those individuals who are killed or injured during battles, bombings, attacks, or other military clashes and assaults. Even here there often is considerable controversy as to the actual numbers involved, for several reasons. War can be waged over a wide area; injured individuals may flee and never be identified as a war casualty; bodies are buried, sometimes in mass graves and never counted; combatants may undercount their own losses and exaggerate the number of enemy that have fallen; enemy civilian deaths may be counted as combatant losses or ignored; and deaths (and how they died) may be intentionally hidden to keep the world from knowing heinous plots and acts of brutality. The latter include people who die or are intentionally murdered in prisoner-of-war camps, civilian concentration camps, or torture rooms or who "disappear" by way of paramilitary action.

Notable among hidden casualties of war were the thousands who disappeared in Argentina after the overthrow of the government by a military junta in 1976. In what even the junta labeled its "dirty war," civil liberties were suspended, the country's congress was shut down, judges were fired, and universities were purged of many of their students. The military then initiated a highly organized campaign of brutal violence against civilians that included abduction, torture, and disappearances. The exact number of people who were never heard from again is unknown, but human rights organizations estimate that approximately thirty-thousand people disappeared or were known to have been killed by the government during the period of military rule. Included on the list of the *Desaparecidos* (disappeared) were high school students who protested government abuses (Armed Conflict Events Data 2003). Additionally, young children of progressive or antimilitary parents were kidnapped, and pregnant women were taken and kept alive only until giving birth. With changed identities, these children were appropriated by the families of military personnel and raised as their own children (Jelin 2004). It is only in recent years that some of these children, now grown, are beginning to find out who they really are and how their lives were radically altered by the dirty war. This practice is reminiscent of the removal of Native American, Native Canadian (First Nation), and Australian Aboriginal children from their families to be placed with white foster families (see Robbins 2002) in earlier eras. Civilian opposition to these attacks on the young are symbolized by the courageous work of the Mothers of the Plaza de Mayo, an Argentine organization (named for the plaza in central Buenos Aires where bereaved mothers and grandmothers first congregated to challenge the government and publicize their plight) composed of human rights activist women who, for more than three decades, have fought for the right to be reunited with their abducted children or otherwise learn the truth about them.

The many controversies concerning the scale of civilian war losses and the degree of intentional hiding of war's victims are illustrated by Iraqi civilian deaths in the U.S. War on Iraq. As Harding and Libal (2008: 65) note, "U.S. forces in Iraq never provided data on civilian causalities and deaths, a deliberate effort to deflect attention from the human cost of the war and maintain domestic support for military operations." Efforts by various organizations to establish civilian losses for the war have produced (through 2008) widely varying findings ranging from 34,353 (by the United Nations) to 1 million (by the British polling company Opinion Research Business). One consequence of the significant scale of war-related deaths in Iraq is that life expectancy has fallen dramatically (to only forty-eight years for males).

The public secrets of war "tend to coalesce around matters of power and abuse" (Nordstrom 1996: 147). It is fair to say that all wars have their secrets, some far worse than others. Part of the social function of secret keeping about horrendous things is "normalizing the unthinkable" (Peattie 1984). After World War II and the ghastly Holocaust inflicted on Jews and other targeted groups by the Nazis, many Germans claimed not to know about the mass slaughter that occurred during this period in their country. Indeed, psychologically, while they certainly noticed their neighbors disappearing or other signs of the Holocaust, not "seeing" the atrocities around them was emotionally protective, life could go on as usual; birthdays could be celebrated, new babies welcomed, and romance initiated. Most people, including those who realized something was terribly amiss "did not want to know." Indeed, until 1944, both the British and U.S. governments, as well as the Western mass media, downplayed the Holocaust, often treating reports of mass killings as communist propaganda (Leff 1999). Some would argue more or less the same pattern has occurred with the U.S. War in Iraq, with Americans not wanting to know, and the mass media rarely reporting the staggering size of the civilian casualty list.

Enduring Health Consequences

Wars eventually end, but the misery they cause remains. This occurs through several pathways, including long-term damage to the environment, destruction of health and social infrastructure, and the spread of malnutrition and disease.

Environmental War

First, war and war materials production cause extensive and enduring damage to physical environments, creating danger zones for local populations. Minefields, for example, continue to cause death and injury in considerable numbers for decades after hostilities have ceased (Sirkin et al. 2008). In this sense, antipersonnel mines are not time bombs but timeless bombs that prolong the agony of war indefinitely. Mines produced in South Africa before the fall of apartheid have been found on the ground in Angola, Mozambique, Namibia, Zambia, Zimbabwe, Rwanda, and Cambodia. As Vine (1995) notes, "[L]andmines are blind weapons that cannot distinguish between the footfall of a soldier and that of an old women gathering firewood. Casualty rates due to landmines show that they recognize no cease-fire and, long after the fighting has stopped, they can maim or kill the children and grandchildren of the soldiers who laid them."

A case of unfortunate landmine discovery, in this case by two young boys tending their families' cowherds, has been described by Farmer (2009a) for Rwanda. The landmine in question, which exploded in 2006 and significantly injured one of the boys, had been laid during the early 1990s as part of the Rwanda civil war, a conflict triggered when the Tutsi-led Rwanda Patriotic Front invaded northern Rwanda from Uganda in an attempt to depose their rival Hutus from state dominance. In 1994, following the assassination of the president, a deadly new phase of the civil war began. During the course of the one hundred days following the president's death, between half a million and a million people (or 20 percent of the total population), most of whom were Tutsi (but included pro-peace Hutus), were systematically murdered in well-planned and often grisly attacks. Nonetheless, the Tutsi-led Rwanda Patriotic Front took control of the country, and two million rival Hutus fled to neighboring countries. The genocide was planned by elements within the Hutu government who subscribed to the nationalist and ethnocentric philosophy known as Hutu Power. With the aid of France, those who had planned and managed the genocide, were airlifted to safety in neighboring Zaire, where they tried to rally refugee Hutus for a counterattack and a (failed) prolongation of the war.

Although distinctions between Hutu and Tutsi predate the colonial era, Belgium, the European colonial power in the region, had played on and enhanced tension between these two groups (which are not historic ethnic or tribal groups) as a "divide-and-conquer" means of remaining in control. In other words, the ultimate origin of the landmine being discussed was the colonial legacy in Africa, the self-serving effort by European powers to divide up, control, and exploit indigenous peoples and their local environments for the benefit of wealthy classes in colonial European nations.

In 1992, the Rwanda government had purchased two thousand plastic MAT-79 antipersonnel mines as part of a much larger arms acquisition from weapons dealers. It is estimated that 150,000 landmines were planted in Rwanda during the Civil War. After the war, antimine experts uncovered thirty-nine types of mines in the country, some of which were designed to attract children because they looked like toys. They had come from many countries, including Belgium, the United States, Pakistan, China, the former Soviet Union, and Egypt, that were more than willing to sell massive quantities of weapons to the emergent nations of the world. As this example suggests, the turning of Rwanda's environment into a deadly zone of waiting landmines was far from a local affair.

Another expression of the way war affects environments is seen in the mining of uranium to both fuel nuclear power plants and to make the fissile core of nuclear warheads. Government focus on uranium as a weapon of war escalated during the Cold War era after the Second World War. In the United States, an important deposit of uranium was found on the lands of the Navajo Nation in the Colorado Plateau in the area where Colorado, Utah, Arizona, and New Mexico meet to form Four Corners. Although the desired ore is on Indian land, the Bureau of Indian Affairs awarded the mining rights to Kerr-McGee Corporation, which presented uranium mining as a "jobs creation" program to the Navajo Tribal Council. The significant health risks associated with uranium mining, including lung cancer, were well known and had been published many years before the opening of the Kerr-McGee facility in Shiprock, New Mexico.

During several decades the facility was in operation, approximately 150 Navajo miners found employment there. Of these, 38 had died of radiation-induced cancer by 1980 and an additional 95 were suffering from serious respiratory diseases and cancers. Other health consequences for these miners and their families (as workers did not receive showers or a change of clothes before returning home each day) included high rates of miscarriages, cleft palates, and other birth defects. A medical records review for more than thirteen thousand Navajo born in Shiprock from 1964 to 1981 found statistically significant associations between exposure to uranium (because of living near mine tailings or dumps or because of family mine employment or employment in the Shiprock electronics assembly plant) and unhealthy birth outcomes (Dawson 1992; Johnston, Dawson and Madsen 2007).

Another expression of the radioactive legacy of the Cold War is found in anthropologist Paula Garb's (2008) study of the environmental and health catastrophe wrought by radioactive accidents at Soviet nuclear facilities in the Russian Urals that released into the atmosphere approximately twice the number of curies released by the meltdown of the Chernobyl nuclear power plant in 1986. Dating to the Cold War period, the Soviet Union operated a nuclear weapons production facility in the city of Chelyabinski (now called Ozersk), which suffered several accidents releasing strontium-90 and cesium-137 into the environment, radioactive chemicals that can survive for hundreds of years before breaking down. Both chemicals are readily taken up by living organisms (as they mimic organic chemicals) and become part of the food chain. In the early 1950s, doctors in the area began seeing a marked increase in disease and death in their patients but did not understand the cause. Local residents called their strange illness, which had symptoms of numbness of the limbs, pain in the joints, frequent severe headaches, nosebleeds, and fatigue, the "river disease." Indeed the local Techa River had been a dumping ground for radioactive materials from the nuclear factories. Ultimately the cause of these symptoms became clear when the Soviet Union finally admitted that many accidents had occurred at the factories, a fact that the U.S. government knew but chose not to make public (perhaps to protect its own nuclear industry from questions about safety; Garb 2008). Since the 1950s, the incidence of diseases like leukemia among the population exposed to radiation had increased by 41 percent, all cancers have risen by 21 percent, and circulatory system diseases have increased by 31 percent.

Ecosystems are also decimated by the construction of military sites and fortifications, by factories that produce arsenals and other war equipment, and military attacks that amplify their impact by the release of stored energy or pollutants. Westing (2008) thus typologizes the environmental consequences of the war into three categories: (1) unintentional, (2) intentional, and (3) intentional for amplification (i.e., explicitly to release energy stored in the environment to cause harm to civilians, such a bombing dams). Unintentional damage results from the direct use of weapons, especially high-explosive munitions. Use of uranium-bearing hardened military shells, for example, has affected the environments of Kosovo and Iraq in recent twentieth-century wars, although environmental damage was not the motivation for their use. Armies also use the intentional destruction of environments and environmental resources as a means of pressuring the enemy population. "Ecocide" (such as forest clearing) is an intentional use of weapons to damage the environment, as seen in the slaughter of entire herds of bison by the U.S. Army during the nineteenth-century campaign to deprive Native Americans of food sources (see Robbins 2002) or the more recent cutting down of olive trees in Palestine by the Israeli army (Avram Bornstein, personal communication, 2009). Amplification involves the intentional release of potentially dangerous pent-up forces (man-made or in nature). An example would be bombing an enemy nuclear energy plant to release deadly radioactive material on the local environment. Short of this, attacks on industrial facilities can also release dangerous toxins that spread as clouds over a wide expanse of enemy territory.

The environmental stakes of war are actually much higher than has been described thus far. In recent years, there has been growing realization of the significant role played by war, war preparation, and war production on one of the most threatening environmental issues of the twenty-first century: global warming. As Baer (2010: 157) stresses, war

generates a considerable level of greenhouse gas emission, which, in turn, contributes to global warming and resulting impacts on health. At the same time, global warming contributes to armed conflict, creating a vicious cycle for the planet and its inhabitants.

Here Baer is arguing that there is an active feedback loop linking war and global warming that magnifies the undesirable health consequence both from war and from global warming. War's contribution to greenhouse gas buildup comes especially by way of the massive size of the fossil fuel–powered vehicular stock of the world's armies—from fighter planes to automobiles, trucks, and other vehicles—and from military buildings and other facilities. As a result, the U.S. Department of Defense (DoD), the administrative center of one the largest and most powerful militaries on Earth, is the single largest consumer of oil in the world (360,000 barrels of oil each day). In fiscal year 2009, the DoD guzzled almost 1,000 trillion

British thermal units of site-delivered energy at a cost of $13.3 billion, or about the same as the African nation of Nigeria, which has a population of more than 140 million people (Karbuz 2011). Energy consumed per active duty military and military-related civilian personal is 35 percent higher than nonmilitary civilians. In turn, in 2009 the DoD emitted 73 million metric tons of the CO_2, or just over 4 percent of the total emissions of this increasingly menacing greenhouse gas. It is primarily CO_2 that has contributed to the steady warming of the planet, and the health-related consequence of this trend from extreme storms, increased wildfires, and the spread of vectors that transmit various infectious diseases (e.g., the mosquitos that transmit black Nile disease and malaria, the sandflies that transmit leishmaniasis, and the ticks and mice that transmit Lyme disease). Oil lies at the heart of the military power of the United States, and hence access to the dwindling stocks of accessible oil on the planet is a critical issue for the DoD and for U.S. foreign policy.

The contribution of global warming to armed conflict arises from the changes wrought on the plant as the temperature rises. Water immediately emerges as an ever more precious element—something worth fighting over—as global warming causes drought to spread to new areas. Declining agricultural productivity in some areas and improved productivity in others, further increases the likelihood of armed conflict over this precious resource. The creation of environmental refugee populations could also become an issue of conflict between neighboring countries. In short, global warming is intimately entwined with conflict, a connection that is likely to grow stronger as projected climate changes become everyday realities.

Infrastructure Destruction

War also affects health by destroying or significantly degrading social infrastructure, including housing; health care facilities (and personnel); roads, bridges, and transportation; school and education systems; sewage and potable water systems; social welfare institutions; energy grids; food distribution; and related institutions of civil society. This kind of destruction and outright fear of abuse often produced large numbers of both cross-border refugees (now totaling some twelve million worldwide) and internally displaced persons (twenty million to twenty-five million internally). Both of these groups of refugees suffer long-term poor health outcomes as a result of displacement and destruction of infrastructure.

Analyses conducted by the United Nations concluded that by the end of the U.S.-Indochina wars in 1991, Cambodia had only thirty doctors left (Machel 1996). As a result of the U.S.-funded Contra War against the Sandinista government in Nicaragua from 1982 to 1987, almost a quarter of the country's health centers were partially or fully demolished or forced to close because of frequent attacks by the right-wing Contras. Although the infectious disease of smallpox had been all but eliminated in Bangladesh before its 1971–1972 war of independence, an outbreak of the disease began in the midst of the fighting resulting in more than eighteen thousand deaths. Similarly, during the early 1970s, Uganda, which had achieved immunization coverage of 75 percent of all children witnessed a steady decline in vaccine coverage resulting in fewer than 10 percent of eligible children being immunized with antituberculosis vaccine (BCG), and fewer than 5 percent against diphtheria, pertussis, and tetanus (DPT), measles, and poliomyelitis at the end of the civil war (Machel 1996). Losses of this sort extend the impacts of war into the future and constrain the return to peace and civil stability.

Infectious Disease and Malnutrition

War also leaves a lasting impact through its contribution to malnutrition (including outright starvation) and the spread of infectious diseases. This intertwined toll of war is illustrated by the cases of the internal war in Somalia that raged through the end of the twentieth and into the twenty-first century. War (and drought) have driven hundreds of thousands of people from their homes throughout south and central Somalia. Between July and mid-October 2011, it is estimated that as many as two hundred thousand displaced people were forced to settle in overcrowded camps in the country's capital of Mogadishu (Cabrol 2011). An additional 110,000 people fled to Kenya, bringing the total number of Somalis refugees in that country to 440,000. Because the established camps were already full and overcrowded, the new wave of refugees had to settle in out-of-the-way areas characterized by limited access to water, sanitation, food, and meaningful shelter. The same has occurred in Ethiopia, where almost 100,000 Somalis have fled to similarly overcrowded camps with inadequate aid to meet basic human needs. Between mid-May and mid-October 2011, medical teams from Doctors without Borders/Médecins sans Frontières (MSF) treated more than 20,000 severely malnourished people in Somalia, 18,000 in Ethiopia, and 11,000 in Kenya. Some projects in Mogadishu were seeing high rates of severe acute malnutrition, and at the Hilaweyn refugee camp in Liben, Ethiopia, medical teams found that a staggering 20 to 30 percent of refugees were suffering from severe malnutrition. Approximately one-third of severely malnourished children admitted to MSF's intensive care units were diagnosed with kwashiorkor (an acute form of malnutrition characterized by edema).

Arriving refugees, especially children, suffer from severe malnutrition and are at significant risk of contracting measles, cholera, and other infectious diseases. Additionally, Kenyan security forces have been accused of abusing Somali refugees, a not uncommon fate for a highly vulnerable population. A study by Dunbar (2007) conducted among Somalis living in a refugee camp that had been considered to be well stabilized found a rising prevalence of protein-energy malnutrition. In the study, more than 17 percent of children were found to be at 80 percent of healthy weight/height levels, and almost 2 percent were found to be at 70 percent. Further, there was a high prevalence of anemia among children. Stool examination found that almost 30 percent of these children suffer from giardia infection from tainted water.

Impacts of War on Children

Ostensibly wars are not fought against children, although in some cases, they are, in fact, intentionally targeted (as a means of demoralizing the opposing side); in all cases they are negatively affected. The ways in which war affects children are varied. Damage to social and physical infrastructures and family disruption caused by war have been found to be associated with high-risk drug use and sexual behavior among youth. In war zones, soldiers and even peacekeepers are known to prey on young people in the surrounding civilian population for sex or other services. Armies also are known to force children into military service or to openly recruit them into joining the military effort. Often there are long-term consequences for children of their war experiences. Studies suggest that in war, a child's level of exposure to atrocity (i.e., being raped, seeing parents killed, being forced to be a combatant, displacement) predicts resulting levels of trauma and associated mental health problems. Based on a review of existing literature, Werner (2012: 553) concludes that "[t]he more recent the exposure to war, and the older the child, the higher was the likelihood of reported post-traumatic stress disorder symptoms. Especially vulnerable to long-term emotional distress were child soldiers, children who were raped, and children who had been forcibly displaced." Such effects may be enduring over lifetimes, as adults who suffered war trauma as children continue to report a significant number of health and mental health problems, including cardiovascular diseases (Santa Barbara 2008). Various factors were found to moderate the health impacts of war on children, including having a strong positive bond with primary care providers, supportive teachers, and friends. Beyond these impacts, anthropologists Jason Hart and Bex Tyrer (2006: 9–10) stress the need to expand our understanding of the impacts of war on children: "Without denying the existence of trauma and without refuting the idea that the young may be victimised, we should learn more about the strategies children employ to deal with their adverse circumstances and maintain material, psychological, emotional and physical wellbeing." These researchers urge the development of participatory approaches to research that are designed to explore the lives of war-exposed children from their own (emic) perspective.

Women and War

Armed conflicts are never gender-neutral and increasingly bear unique risks for women and girls. According to UNICEF (1996), during the civil war that ripped apart Rwanda (leaving almost a million people dead) virtually every adolescent girl who had survived the genocide of 1994 was subsequently raped. As anthropologist Cheryl Magnant (2011) observes, "[A]s long as there is war, there will be crimes against women." Summarizing some of the special impacts of modern war on noncombatant women and children, the United Nations Population Fund (2002: iii) maintains:

The impact of conflicts on women and girls' reproductive and sexual health can never be underestimated. Their psychological, reproductive and overall well-being is often severely compromised in times of conflict. Conflicts tend to increase the incidence of sexual violence; rape; sexually transmitted infections (STIs), including HIV/AIDS; and unwanted pregnancies.

Moreover, as many as 80 percent of war-related internally displaced individuals and refugees in the world are women and children.

Research among women in Afghanistan, for example, where war has continued for decades, documents high levels of depression, anxiety, and trauma among women, levels that are far above those that spark clinical concern. Women use several culturally meaningful idioms of distress to express their lived experiences of losing husbands and other family members, daily threat, and worry about their children's well-being, including *jigar khan* (grief tied to painful life events), *asabi* (a mixture of nervousness and anger), *fishar-e-bala* (feeling completely overwhelmed), and *fishar-e-payin* (loss of motivation) (Omidian and Miller 2006).

Of course, women are not only frequently present among the casualties of war. Increasingly anthropologists have sought to stress that women worldwide are taking an increasingly central role in both peacekeeping and healing the many wounds of war. These efforts, discussed toward the end of this chapter, unexpectedly are often seen in countries where women traditionally have had limited access to public leadership, highlighting both human resiliency in the face of unspeakable atrocity and the ultimate malleability of culture in responding to changing circumstance and evolving need.

Traumas of War

War produces both physical and emotional trauma. The U.S. wars in Afghanistan and Iraq showcase the kinds of trauma found in contemporary warfare. One lesson of these wars is that in the modern era, the battlefield has become increasingly brutal, with high numbers of single and multiple amputations, genital injuries, and head injuries. In recent years, combat-related traumatic brain injury, in particular, has garnered considerable attention as the insidiousness of this kind of wound has become better understood. Research now shows that even when a soldier caught in an explosion suffers no outward signs of injury, microscopic alterations may occur deep in the brain that have an impact on metabolism and cause cell death, leading to headaches, lethargy, memory loss, and anxiety. In U.S. wars in Afghanistan and Iraq, roadside bombs, known as improvised explosive devices, are the cause of most cases of brain injury that have been diagnosed and account for almost 80 percent of all wounds suffered by U.S. troops. Soldiers caught near these blasts often suffer from perforated eardrums, blurred vision, memory lapses, and headaches, but deeper brain traumas are another consequence.

Awareness of emotional trauma (a concept that dates to the end of the nineteenth century), and how extensive this problem is among veterans has grown significantly since the U.S. War in Vietnam. Indeed, in recent years "traumas research has erupted as a major field of enquiry" (Pederson 2006: 299). Various factors are associated with the emotional traumas of war including the still somewhat controversial diagnosis of post-traumatic stress disorder (PTSD), a complex of symptoms (varying by patient) including lingering fear, a sense of helplessness, feeling haunted by recurrent memories, avoidance behavior, and hyperarousal. Specific outward signs of this disease (American Psychological Association 2012) include a long list of items:

- Expressed guilt about actions or shame over some failure
- Excessive drinking or drug use
- Uncontrolled or frequent crying and other extreme reactions to events that normally would be handled more calmly
- Sleep problems (too little, too much)
- Expressed depression, anxiety, or anger
- High level of dependence on others
- Verbal or physical family violence
- Complaint of specific physical conditions (headache, backache, gastrointestinal problems, poor stamina)
- Reported inability to escape from horror scenes remembered from the war
- Difficulty concentrating
- Suicidal thoughts or plans

One factor associated with suffering from PTSD is age (Harmless 1990). Young adults exposed to military combat may be at greater risk than their older peers. During the War in Vietnam, veterans who during the war were aged nineteen years or younger were found to be significantly more likely than older veterans to suffer drug abuse, be engaged in other criminal activity, have difficulty finding or sustaining employment, and report problems with social relationships. Witnessing the injury or death of fellow soldiers is also associated with higher rates of postconflict trauma (J. Escobar et al. 1983). Other research from the War in Vietnam (King et al. 1996) has found that there is a gendered set of salient prewar factors that have an impact on the onset of war-related PTSD. For women, instability within the individual's family of origin was shown to have the greatest impact on PTSD. Also of importance for women is suffering from an early history of prewar trauma, including experiencing accidents, assaults, and natural disaster. For men, important prewar impacts on war-related PTSD included family instability and childhood antisocial behavior. In this study, suffering an early trauma history was found to interact with war zone stress, which, in turn, exacerbated PTSD symptoms for high combat-exposed male veterans. Research also shows a link between suffering war trauma and the development of physical health problems, including the development of chronic diseases and premature death (Wagner et al. 2000).

Anthropologist Erin Finley (2012) has written an award-winning study of emotional trauma among veterans of U.S. wars in Iraq and Afghanistan, interconnected wars in which more than 30,000 U.S. soldiers have been wounded in action (20 percent of whom have suffered serious brain or spinal injuries), and more than 120,000 returned home with symptoms of PTSD. The goal of her study was to examine the cultural, political, and historical factors that have shaped combat PTSD among male American soldiers. Based on her twenty months of ethnographic research, Finley (2011: 9) concluded that PTSD means "many different things to many different people" and that "the myriad ways in which combat PTSD is understood in American life have a profound effect on how veterans with PTSD understand their own symptoms, feel about their diagnosis, and make what may be life-changing decisions about coping and care seeking." Moreover, she argues that the nature and severity of PTSD symptoms are not merely a product of combat trauma, they have as much to do with the expectations society and family members put on veterans, and veterans put on themselves (e.g., to effectively fill social roles as fathers, husbands, workers, family members, and friends). As this interpretation suggests, PTSD is very much a biosocial disease.

Syndemics of War

The impacts of war are multiplied through their adverse involvement in disease syndemics. Syndemics (Singer 2009a) involve the deleterious interaction of diseases that tend to cluster within population and increase the disease burden of that population because of unhealthy social conditions. War is certainly an unhealthy social condition (promoting, as we have seen, malnutrition, intense and prolonged stress and emotional trauma, open wounds, pollution of the environment, and a breakdown of health prevention and treatment systems), and its occurrence, as noted, promotes the occurrence of disease, especially the occurrence and spread of infectious diseases. This is especially noteworthy in the case of children because of their vital dietary needs and the premature state of their immune systems even under ideal conditions. Consequently, negative interaction between war-related malnutrition (which weakens the immune system) and the spread and severity of opportunistic and nonopportunistic infectious disease takes its toll on children in war zones (Barker and Osmond 1986). Further studies show that children who suffer from malnutrition as infants, a common outcome of prolonged warfare, are likely to experience immunosuppression that may persist into their adult life. Moreover, Hogan and Burstein (2002: 41) point out that diseases such as "Human immunodeficiency virus (HIV) [infection] spreads faster during emergencies when conditions such as poverty, powerlessness, social instability, and violence against women are most extreme," and this can certainly be the case during war.

The operation of a syndemic in a war zone is illustrated by the U.S. War in Afghanistan. During the war, there has been a significant rise in cases of a potentially disfiguring disease known as cutaneous leishmaniasis, named for William Leishman who identified its pathogenic cause. This protozoal disease is spread by small sandflies that tend to live in unhygienic pockets of severe poverty, with poor sanitation and waste removal, poor housing, and a weak public health infrastructure. Like malaria, leishmaniasis is spread through a bite from the host insect. When the lesions caused by leishmaniasis appear on the face, they can cause permanent scars and disfigurement including partial or even total destruction of the mucous membranes of the nose, mouth, and throat cavities and surrounding tissues. This can be especially harmful for young women who are stigmatized by those around them and often left unmarriageable. Young mothers with leishmania scars may be blocked by their kin from even holding their own babies.

War readily promotes the conditions in which sandflies thrive and in which early access to treatment is blocked. Leishmaniasis is one of a group of what have been called neglected tropical diseases, including lymphatic filariasis, onchocerciasis, ascariasis, hookworm, whipworm, dracunculiasis, schistosomiasis, oriental liver fluke, cysticercosis, trachoma, leprosy, Buruli ulcer, human African trypanosomiasis, and Chagas's disease, conditions that are all facilitated by the disruptive conditions of war.

Moreover, leishmaniasis is known to interact adversely with other diseases, including HIV. HIV and leishmaniasis coinfection has been reported in more than thirty countries in Africa, Asia, Europe, and South America. Moreover, monitoring by the World Health Organization indicates that more than 70 percent of HIV cases in southern Europe are coinfected with leishmania (Molina, Gradoni, and Alvar, 2003). In particular, the countries of Spain, Italy, and France are seeing growing incidence of coinfection among youth. People with HIV who are coinfected have both a reduced immune capacity to contain the initial infection by the leishmania protozoa or block it from progressing to the most severe expression of the disease. As HIV infection progresses, immune capacity is further diminished, allowing latent leishmanial infection to become active, propagate, and spread within the body. In coinfected individuals, leishmaniasis has been found to "be particularly severe and unresponsive to treatment" (Olivier et al. 2003: S85). At the same time, leishmaniasis has been found to enhance HIV infection through several complex biochemical pathways. Consequently, the interaction of these two diseases promotes the progression of each, thereby both increasing the illness state of sufferers and the often additionally damaging social consequences (e.g., stigmatization) that accompany these infectious diseases.

Human Resilience in the Face of Atrocity, Trauma, and Unspeakable Aggression

In the 1984 John Carpenter movie *Starman*, actor Jeff Bridges, playing an alien, tells an Earthling what he likes about humans, saying: "You are at your very best when things are worst." Although not all responses to the tragedies and cruelty of war live up to this standard (indeed the occurrence of war often unleashes other forms of interpersonal violence including the nonmilitary harassment and abuse of women), there are notable responses from around the world that certainly qualify. This capacity to do well or even unusually well under extreme conditions, or to bounce back after initial distress is variously termed *hardiness*, *sense of coherence*, and, increasingly, *resilience*. Resilience exists at both the individual and group levels, with the former referring to individual capacity to rebound and the latter referring to group efforts to pull together and rebuild in the context of extreme duress. Notably, at the individual level, resilience capacity appears to be relatively equally shared among males and females (Vogt et al. 2011), but at the group level, women often play the lead in organizations designed to halt a war or rebuild in its aftermath. Notes Pederson (2006: 300):

in every village or small scale community, there are endogenous, protective or ameliorative influences which are largely derived from resilient structures, as well as survival and conflict resolution strategies followed by communities in post-conflict. Some of these include: community-based strategies for reconciliation, ideological shifts (for instance, conversion into other religions or political conversions), spontaneous forms of enhancing social support (e.g., community festivals, religious and public ceremonies, social gathering around significant events, etc.), self-support groups (i.e., widows and women's community organizations), and also belief systems which provide the basis for constructing meaning for experienced trauma.

In the following, "A Closer Look," we further explore the concept of resilience through the examination of an outstanding case

"A Closer Look"

WOMEN AND RESILIENCE IN A WAR ZONE

An exemplary case of intersection between personal and group resilience is Liberian peace activist and Nobel Peace Prize winner Leymah Roberta Gbowee, a leader of the Liberian women's peace movement who helped to end the Second Liberian Civil War in 2003. This conflict saw all of the worst features of modern warfare, including ethnic hatred, child soldiers armed with Kalashnikovs, a ruthless warlord, attacks on civilian populations, and far-reaching destruction of national infrastructure. Gbowee rose as a peace activist in 1998 when she volunteered with the Trauma Healing and Reconciliation Program operated by St. Peter's Lutheran Church in Monrovia, the capital of Liberia. She put her prior training in art to use as she worked with traumatized child ex-soldiers. During this period, Gbowee, who had four children at the time, concluded that if peace were to come to Liberia, the mothers of the country would have to lead the way. She began to read literature on peace building, following attendance of a training conference in Ghana organized by the Women in Peacebuilding Network (WIPNET). Gbowee returned to Liberia having been appointed as the head of the WIPNET's new Liberian Women's Initiative. From this small group sprang a mass women's movement against the war in Liberia that included thousands of women, both Christian and Muslim. Using classic nonviolent tactics, the group (now called the Women of Liberia Mass Action for Peace) engaged in marches, sit-ins, and rallies outside of the executive mansion. The woman proclaimed that they were

tired of war. We are tired of running. We are tired of begging for bulgur wheat. We are tired of our children being raped. We are now taking this stand, to secure the future of our children. Because we believe, as custodians of society, tomorrow our children will ask us, "Mama, what was your role during the crisis?" (Gbowee 2011: 141)

In an innovative step, Gbowee called for a sex strike, in which women refused to have sex with their husbands unless the now fourteen-year-old civil war ended. The movement won a promise from President Charles Taylor to negotiate a peace treaty with the two rebel groups fighting for his overthrow. Gbowee led a women's peace delegation to the negotiations to pressure the combatants to lay down arms. As talks dragged on, she led a sit-in in the hotel where the peace talks were occurring. The women threatened to take off their clothes if the men could not reach an agreement, a culturally striking symbolic gesture that would have been highly embarrassing for all concerned. The end result was the signing the Accra Comprehensive Peace Agreement on August 18, 2003, leading in 2005 to the election of Ellen Johnson Shirleaf as president of Liberia, the first women elected the leader of an African country. As the dust of the war settled, its toll became clear:

Two hundred and fifty thousand people were dead, a quarter of them children. One in three were displaced, with 350,000 living in internally displaced persons camps and the rest anywhere they could find shelter. One million people, mostly women and children, were at risk of malnutrition, diarrhea, measles and cholera because of contamination in the wells. More than 75 percent of the country's physical infrastructure, our roads, hospitals and schools, had been destroyed. (Gbowee 2011: 167)

Moreover, Gbowee (2011: 168) observed,

A whole generation of young men had no idea who they were without a gun in their hands. Several generations of women were widowed, had been raped, seen their daughters and mothers raped, and their children kill and be killed. Neighbors had turned against neighbors; young people had lost hope, and old people, everything they had painstakingly earned. To a person, we were traumatized.

Charles Taylor was subsequently sentenced to fifty years in prison for murder, rape, sexual slavery, and other inhumane acts, and Liberia continues slowly to recovery from its destructive civil war.

Lessons for Medical Anthropology

What lessons does medical anthropology learn from its increasingly robust study of war and health? The most sweeping lesson, we believe, is that the better we come to understand war and its varied arsenal against human health and well-being, the better we will be armed to avoid war or, at least, to be prepared to intervene appropriately in responding to the health needs war produces. In other words, studying war is a strategy of preparedness and recovery. Rylko-Bauer and Singer (2012) have called for the building of a "medical anthropology against war," a goal we share without any expectations that war will end any time soon. One way that medical anthropology can contribute toward this goal, however, is by carrying out research that seeks to achieve the following:

- Provide real-life examples in which conflict did not lead to war, how this happened, and how might it be replicated in other contexts, including using such cases to call into question the inevitability of war.
- Make the true, prolonged, and hidden dimensions of war and its extreme toll on human life and well-being issues of public discourse.
- Counter with vivid ethnographic examples, as public intellectuals, the well-rehearsed and oft-repeated "buildup to war" by serving as a countervoice when national leaders begin to repeat (long-discredited) cultural and emotionally laden platitudes about the tragic but necessary of war in any particular instance.
- Promote a public image of war as a disease, a pathology of power and social inequality.
- Develop evidence-based ethnographic accounts that unveil nonstereotyped portrayals of vilified ethnic, religious, or other social groups.
- Work with local and broader social movements in support of the development of protective or ameliorative values and activities, conflict-resolution strategies, peace organizing training, community-based initiatives for reconciliation, local forms of enhancing cross-ethnic solidarity (e.g., community-wide festivals, unifying public ceremonies, celebratory social gathering around the value of cultural diversity), trauma healing programs, and antiwar movements.

CHAPTER 8

Legal and Illegal Drugs: Experience, Behavior, and Society

ALTERED MINDS

The term *myrmecomany*, from the ancient Greek words for ant (*myrmex*) and obsession (*mania*), refers to a behavior that has been observed among some birds, including ravens, jays, thrushes, blackbirds, and parrots. When performing this behavior, birds sit on the ground on or near an ant nest, spread their wings, and curl their tails up toward their stomachs. The birds let themselves be covered by swarming ants and sometimes, they pick ants one by one and push them into their feathers. Once covered by ants, the birds contort their bodies, and spin. This step lasts roughly thirty minutes. Afterward, birds shake themselves to get rid of the ants. Scientists believe that the birds use the formic acid secreted by ants to clean their plumage out of lice or other parasites. However, some believe that the birds also use the acid as a drug to alter their state of consciousness. Birds have been observed using other substances such as caterpillar secretions, flour larvae, and plant juices in the same way. Birds are not alone in this kind of behavior. It is well known that cats are attracted by the valerian plant (*Valeriana officinalis*) and catnip (*Nepeta cataria*), the sniffing and eating of which seem to provoke them into a state of high satisfaction. Cattle have been observed ingesting plants with certain alkaloids that appear to have a narcotic effect (Dudley 2002). Birds and other animals have been recorded eating highly fermented fruit and afterward appearing to be drunk, stumbling and acting as if under the influence. All of these behaviors suggest that many species—including, of course, humans—have long evolutionary histories of seeking to alter their state of consciousness through the consumption or exposure to some form of psychoactive compound. In the view of ethnopharmacologist Ronald Siegel (2005: 10), "ethnological and laboratory studies . . . and analyses of social and biological history, suggest that the pursuit of intoxication with drugs is a primary motivational force in the behavior of organisms." Siegel calls this behavior "the fourth drive" after the biologically based drives of hunger, thirst, and sex.

Among humans, there is a long documented history of using mindaltering and potentially addictive drugs dating to at least eight thousand to ten thousand years ago. Despite this lengthy history and broad distribution of human and nonhuman animal use of mind-altering drugs, anthropology as a field of behavioral study was slow to pay close attention to drug use. Up to the early 1970s, "anthropology had not yet developed an explicit drug research tradition, especially with respect to the abuse of drugs" (L. Bennett and Cook 1996: 236). Until this time, the study of drug consumption was not "treated as a highly venerated arena of anthropological research" (Singer 2001: 210). The reason for this inattention was that anthropology was seeking to understand "normative behaviors" across cultural settings rather than what came, initially in sociology, to be called deviant behavior. Additionally, early in its history, anthropology was oriented toward a functionalist perspective that directed researchers' attention to the ways parts of a culture were integrated and mutually reinforcing. One consequence, as Bourgois (2003: 14) maintains, is that historically, anthropologists "avoided tackling taboo subjects such as personal violence, sexual abuse, addiction, alienation, and self-destruction." The scattered initial anthropological approach to drug use and abuse (involving individual researchers recording observable local use patterns of locally available drugs), lack of a systematic approach to drugs and society or a guiding theoretical framework continued until the later part of the twentieth century.

During the 1970s, this pattern began to change, influenced by what has been called the youth drug revolution and the significant expansion in the number of people reporting using drugs in the West, as well as by the growing anthropological focus on Western societies and the application of anthropology to addressing pressing social problems (Rylko-Bauer, Singer, and van Willigen 2006). Another factor in this shift was the significant growth in student interest in anthropology at this time, a time when drug use became widespread on college campuses. Also critical to the rise of the contemporary anthropological concern with drug use was the role of this behavior in the HIV pandemic. A few years into the pandemic, the potential contribution of anthropology to the study of connections between drug consumption and both the initiation of HIV infection and disease progression were recognized, and ethnographic methods gained new value in public health efforts (Carlson et al. 2009). As a result, although in the past anthropological researchers often "fell into" careers in drug research, recent research by Page and Singer (2010) suggests that anthropologists increasingly are choosing to study drug use and to explore the concepts of addiction and drug treatment. This work has focused on traditional, indigenous drug use, such as the consumption of *ayahusasca*, a drug derived from tree vines, among New World peoples, illicit drug use and its impact in complex societies, including the diversion of pharmaceutically produced medicines for nonmedical, mind-altering purposes, alcohol consumption in its many forms, and the smoking or other use of tobacco.

Indeed, wherever anthropologists have traveled, they have almost always encountered the use of psychoactive compounds to alter consciousness, sometimes alone and sometimes in combination (i.e., drug mixing), sometimes as socially accepted and integrated components of broader social systems and sometimes as behaviors viewed, at least by those holding the reins of power, as problematic, unhealthy, and a threat to society. However, there is no agreed-on scientific or anthropological definition of the word *drug*. Some illegal drugs, like heroin, are addictive (i.e., the body builds up a physical dependence on them and suffers withdrawal symptoms upon discontinuance of their use) and others, like LSD and marijuana, are not. The same can be said of legal drugs. Nicotine (in cigarettes) and caffeine (in coffee) are quite addictive. Some illegal drugs, such as cocaine, stimulate the central nervous system, whereas others, like heroin, depress it. This is also true of legal drugs. Amphetamines are stimulants, and barbiturates and alcohol are depressants, and all of these can be purchased legally (although not without restrictions). In the end, it appears that what drugs have in common is their classification by society. Yet as Matveychuk argues:

That the only commonality among drugs is their label implies that the category "drugs" is an arbitrary definition, a linguistic category that changes overtime. Yet this is not to suggest that this linguistic category of drugs naturally emanates from the voice of the people. We do not equally share in the task of making social definitions. . . . What becomes truth and gets accepted as reality benefits some individuals and social groups more than others. (Matveychuk 1986: 9)

In other words, to understand why a particular substance is classified as an illicit drug or a legal commodity, it is important to understand the political and economic interests of various groups in society and the power they are able to exert relative to the drug in question. From a straightforward public health standpoint, it would seem that the harmfulness of a drug to human users might be the basis for establishing drug control policies. But this does not seem to be the case. Overall, the World Health Organization

(2010) estimates that drugs of all kinds are involved in approximately 14 percent of all deaths in the world each year. Comparing alcohol and illicit drugs, globally, approximately thirty-nine deaths per 100,000 population are attributable to alcohol and illicit drug use, out of which thirty-five deaths are attributable to alcohol use and only four deaths to illicit drug use. It is further estimated that there are 185 million illicit drug users, 2 billion alcohol users, and 1.3 billion tobacco smokers in the world's 7 billion people. In other words, it is the legal drugs, alcohol and tobacco, that are responsible for most drug-related mortality. This is also true of morbidity.

In this chapter, we examine all forms of drug use and anthropological approaches, theories, and studies of illicit drug, alcohol, and tobacco use cross-culturally. Our conception of drugs is sufficiently broad to include topical ointments, pills, teas, and powders, as well as smokeable, chewable, or inhalable plant (or some animal) products, and injectable and drinkable liquids that have psychoactive properties and alter states of consciousness, or, as in the case of steroids, bodily states and performance. Although different drugs have somewhat different biochemical effects on the brain, most alter the brain's intercellular communication systems. Furthermore, all drugs, directly or indirectly, target the brain's internal reward or pleasure system by flooding the area with the brain neurotransmitter chemical dopamine. The overstimulation of the reward system produces the euphoric effects sought by people who use drugs, reinforcing the experiential benefits of repeat drug use behavior. With addiction, pleasure recedes as the goal of use and is replaced by seeking to feel normal.

One characterization of drugs that is widely used but remains controversial (and hence merits addressing) is the idea of "recreational drugs." When some pharmaceutical preparations (including over-the-counter products) or other drugs are consumed in contexts in which the shared intention of the consumers is to "party," "get high," "get wasted," or "have fun," this behavior has been called recreational drug use. Most important, this term is used when identified consumers are not perceived as being "impaired" by or "addicted" to the drug(s) in question but instead are seen as pursuing a temporary (and from the user's perspective, enjoyable) if potent altered state of consciousness. The subtext of this term is that, because of their socioeconomic status and their status as occasional users of their drugs of choice, "recreational" users are somehow exempt from the risk that their drug use may lead to regular, impaired, or addictive use (i.e., misuse). In other words, recreational drug users are not seen as being on the margins of society or as members of socially threatening subgroups. The important distinction here is one's place in the prevailing social structure not the actual behavior involved (as "recreational" drug use certainly can lead to undesirable outcomes). At the same time, contrary to prevailing assertions, the use of illegal, socially disapproved drugs, such as heroin and cocaine, does not inevitably lead to conditions of impairment and dependence.

In light of this discussion, it is best to call *all* drug use by a common name and sort out the consequences as they emerge from the study of specific drug using populations. Additionally, some drug use occurs in a religious or spiritual context, as part of the ritual complex of a particular tradition (e.g., peyote use among members of the Native American Church) and in that sense is neither recreational nor deviant. As this discussion reveals, there are many complexities in the study of humankind's interaction with psychoactive compounds, from understanding what may be a biologically rooted drive among most or all animal species for altering consciousness, to the meanings human societies invest in drug-related experiences, to significant health risks stemming from this behavior (for human and non-human animals), and, further, that among humans the consequences of drug use are significantly tied to how any particular drug is viewed by the dominant society as well as by sectors of society that have a vested interest in drug availability (e.g., the alcohol or tobacco industries).

"A Closer Look"

EMERGENT DRUG USE

One of the lessons of the anthropology of drug use is that drug use patterns are dynamic, ever-shifting, and responsive to changing circumstances. Moreover, these changes have potentially significant health implications. Over time, the popularity of a drug may diminish as people come to see its negative aspects; meanwhile, a different drug may be spreading among existing drug users as well as individuals who are just testing and exploring drug use. Another factor is availability. Because of a variety of issues, from the conditions of production and distribution to the War on Drugs, drug availability is uncertain, as is—from the user's perspective— drug quality. Over time, new drugs are "discovered" or created and introduced to drug markets. New drugs may catch on and develop a following, or they may disappear for lack of user interest. Moreover, drug users are inventive and are routinely trying new ways to improve a drug's effect, leading to changes in modes of consumption. Examples of changing patterns in the world of drug use include the following:

- Appearance of new behaviors linked to drug use (e.g., development of "crack house" sex-for-drugs transactions during the 1980s)
- New risks inherent in old practices (e.g., appearance of HIV and syringe transfer/ sharing of a deadly virus)

- Development of new populations of drug users (e.g., elderly residents of senior housing have been found to be involved in the use of drugs introduced by commercial sex workers; Schensul et al. 2003)
- Shifts to new polydrug use mixing patterns (e.g., combining heroin and Xanax)
- The introduction and spread of new drugs and drug combinations (e.g., diffusion of methamphetamine, diversion of pharmaceuticals like Oxycontin)
- The marketing of new forms of older drugs (e.g., crack cocaine, high THC marijuana)
- Use of new adulterates (e.g., the many alternative chemicals in ecstasy)
- Appearance of new drug use equipment (e.g., gas masks among ecstasy users)
- Emergence of new drug-use settings (e.g., clubs and raves among club-drug users)

DRUG USE, ABUSE, AND ADDICTION

As the foregoing discussion indicates, one of the controversies in the multidisciplinary field of drug studies is the relationship of drug use to drug abuse to the concept of addiction. For some people, all drug use (at least of certain drugs) is defined as abuse. Rarely, however, do individuals or organizations who take this stand include tea and coffee as drugs, although they clearly are psychoactive compounds and should be included in the family of substances that we recognize as drugs. A critical question in this discourse therefore is the following: When does drug use (or "recreational" drug use) become drug abuse? Oftentimes, the emergence of personal and social problems (e.g., with one's health, family, employment, the legal system) is used to distinguish drug use from drug abuse. In fact, considerable effort has been invested in "finding" the harm that drug use, especially illicit drug use, is presumed (to always) cause. Indeed, early anthropological work on marijuana studies was funded by the U.S. federal government with this intent, although the researchers could not actually find harm being caused to users except by the legal penalties imposed on arrested users.

Anthropologists who have addressed the issue of use versus abuse have focused on the perspectives of users. Geoffrey Hunt and coworkers (2007), for example, collected in-depth qualitative data from three hundred attendees at a youth dance event (a rave) in San Francisco. Although the federal government, through the 2003 law called the Illicit Drug Anti-Proliferation Act (originally known as the Reducing Americans' Vulnerability to Ecstasy Act or RAVE Act) criminalized the owning and operating of any place for the purpose of using, distributing, or manufacturing a controlled substance, rave participants viewed the law as an "attack on their leisure activities . . . [and] as largely unjustified [representing] yet another example of the authorities' unwillingness to understand the meaning of these events for the participants or to see these events as anything other than drug-infested hedonistic gatherings" (Hunt et al. 2007: 74). Furthermore, these researchers found that, contrary to the idea that people use drugs because they are ignorant of the harms involved, participants routinely researched drugs to assess potential risk. Rather than ignoring or not knowing about the risks of ecstasy use, study participants recognized contradictions between official pronouncements about drug risk and their own and their friends' lived experiences with using specific drugs. Moreover, from the user's perspective, the benefits of drug use—as they experienced them—outweighed the risks involved. Thus, "[w]hile they may have disagreed about the nature or severity of the risks, or how to deal with those risks, the majority of the respondents engaged in a process of negotiation balancing risk with pleasure" (Hunt et al. 2007: 86). In a parallel study in Hartford, Connecticut, Singer and Schensul (2011: 1685) found that young ecstasy users not only recognize risk but

are able to creatively assert agency and control over their drug use habits by taking steps to help manage the risks of use in order to ensure a pleasurable drug use experience both immediately and in terms of continued use. Notably, for certain participants . . . making the decision to use Ecstasy in order to cope with mental health issues is in and of itself a way of managing the risks associated with structural oppression and limited access to mental health services.

The idea of addiction has gained new popularity in the drug field in recent years as a result of brain research. This began with neurophysiological research at the Addiction Research Center in the U.S. Public Health Service Narcotics Hospital (nicknamed "The Narcotic Farm" or "Narco") in Lexington, Kentucky, during the mid-twentieth century. During the 1940s, researchers there became interested in understanding what was happening in the brains of people who appeared to be emotionally and physiologically dependent on drug use. Also contributing to this trend was research during the 1940s and 1950s by Abraham Wikler on the underlying neurophysiological mechanisms of addiction with special focus on conditioned cues. Most recently, addiction has come to be defined as a "chronic, relapsing brain disease" characterized by compulsive drug seeking and use, despite suffering harmful consequences. This perspective has been strongly promoted by both Alan Leshner and Nora Volkow in their respective tenures as the director of the National Institute on Drug Abuse. Undergirding this view has been the use of powerful imaging technologies that reveal what happens electronically inside brains under the influence of drugs and the restructuring of the brain's neuropathways among regular users (Leshner 2003). Of note, important corollaries of this view are that compulsive drug use is not a moral failing or a lack of willpower; it is a consequence of observable alteration of the brain. Also raised is the rationale for criminalizing a disease, as has been the case with many types of drug use.

While recognizing the value of reframing drug use as a health issue, anthropologists have tended to be somewhat hesitant about fully embracing this perspective, in that many "addicts" recover on their own without treatment, including those whose interest in drugs wanes with age; many regular users of drugs such as heroin and cocaine or heavy alcohol consumers maintain controlled usage with limited consequences in their daily lives; drug use patterns change as people's social situation changes; and the recognition that how people react to drug use is not narrowly determined by drug chemistry but rather is strongly influenced by learning and social reinforcement of particular culturally constituted expectations.

ALTERNATIVE ANTHROPOLOGICAL MODELS OF DRUG USE

In developing their understanding of drug use and drug addiction, anthropologists have embraced several explanatory frameworks. The core component of the anthropological approach to human interaction with psychotropic drugs is known as the *cultural model*. To this anthropological researchers have added several additional analytic approaches designed to address specific issues. Reflecting a general tendency in the broader multidisciplinary drug field, anthropological research has been somewhat fragmented into separate streams concerned with individual drugs. Only recently has there been an effort to unite the study of alcohol with that of other drugs, including tobacco, and the study of street drug use and addiction with patterns of consumption in the wider society (Singer et al. 2006; Page 2011).

The Cultural Model

The emergence of a distinct anthropological perspective on drug use and abuse has its deepest roots in the study of drinking behavior. In the 1950s, anthropologist Dwight Heath (1991) conducted focused ethnographic research among the Camba, a mestizo population in eastern Bolivia, who, when he first encountered them, were involved in horticultural production in a forested area. His experience with the Camba led Heath to question the view that heavy drinking is inherently disruptive and that continued heavy use is inevitably both addicting and damaging to health. Heath observed that most adult Camba drank notable quantities of 178-proof rum and became intoxicated for several days in a row at least twice a month. These heavy drinking events were organized around annual community festivals. Furthermore, he found that among the Camba intoxication was socially valued and was the sought after goal of festive drinking. Yet alcoholism, as that form of addiction has been defined in the drug literature, was not identifiable among the Camba, nor were there any signs of antisocial behaviors such as failure to live up to social responsibilities, incidents of interpersonal aggression, or evidence of alcohol-related sexual disinhibition. Among the Camba, argues Health (2000: 162), "it was unthinkable that anyone would drink in any other context [than weekend group drinking parties and] . . . it was also unthinkable that anyone would have negative consequences from drinking. Drunkenness was a quiet affair of simply staring into space or passing out for a while. Aggression, whether verbal, physical, sexual, or other, was virtually unknown among the Camba, drunk or sober. Similarly absent were boisterousness, clowning, maudlin sentimentality, or other exaggerated comportments such as tends to be associated with intoxication in other cultures." Instead, consuming high doses of alcohol, even to the point of unconsciousness, contributed to Camba social solidarity and group health, including facilitating rapport among individuals who otherwise tend to be isolated and introverted. These findings threw into question the common belief that heavy drinking is inherently disruptive and that continued use is inexorably addictive and damaging to the consumer's health. In response to this unexpected finding, and based on the subsequent examination of the cross-cultural alcohol literature, Heath proposed a cultural model of alcohol use.

According to this model (Heath 1987), which achieved broad acceptance among anthropologists, the association of drinking with any specific "problem," be it physical, economic, psychological, or interpersonal is quite unusual among cultures through history. Further, most consequences of alcohol consumption are mediated by cultural factors rather than being narrowly determined by pharmacobiological factors (MacAndrew and Edgerton 1969). Although not denying that alcohol is a potent chemical, from the perspective of the cultural model, what is most important in determining the effects of heavy drinking are culturally constituted understandings about what will happen to you when you drink in quantity (Butler 2006). Of equal importance is the issue of meaning. As a culturally constructed social practice, drinking (and the type and context of consumption in any social setting) evokes emotionally charged cultural meanings about quite diverse issues, including (potentially) social solidarity, ethnic or personal identity, recognition of new social statuses and accomplishment, nostalgic remembrances, the honoring of loved ones, hospitality, mourning, initiation of work efforts, transitions between activities and statuses (e.g., getting married), celebration of cultural heroes, intimacy, fun, health, improving one's mood or drowning one's sorrows, religious experience, and anticipated futures. This is an admittedly long list that reveals the multiple ways alcohol plays an important role in human society. For example, palm-wine drinking among the Lele of the Cameroon, according to Ngokwey (1987), served historically to reaffirm cultural values and categories of social organization such as those between males and females, the well and the sick, and the young and the elderly. Indeed the role of drinking in affirmation of social solidarity has been a regular theme in the anthropology of drinking literature (Ames et al. 2007). At the same time, the cultural model has guided studies of how people think about and define alcohol. Strunin (2001), for example, probed a group of Haitian youth about what is and what is not an alcoholic beverage. She found that two favorite drinks among Haitians in her study, *kremas* and *likay*, that are made from a mixture of coconut, condensed milk, and rum, are not considered to be alcoholic drinks.

Another component of the cultural model grows from the observation by MacAndrew and Edgerton (1969: 16) that "[t]he way people comport themselves when they are drunk is determined not by alcohol's toxic assault upon the seat of moral judgment, conscience, or the like, but by what their society makes of and imparts to them concerning the state of drunkenness." Adds Mac Marshall (1979: 100), "The most important contribution anthropology . . . made to the alcohol [and wider drug] field was in demonstrating to non-anthropologists the importance of sociocultural factors for understanding the relationship between alcohol and human behavior."

In sum, at its core, the cultural model stresses that human interaction with alcohol is largely determined by cultural expectations and understanding (sometimes called *local knowledge*) about the expectable effects of this drug on the human mind and body. These cultural constructs are products of the social history of a cultural group, their contact with neighboring peoples, and the configuration of opportunities and challenges presented in their social and physical environment. Many of the effects of abusive drinking in Western societies, this model suggests, are not products of the chemical composition of ethanol but rather of beliefs about alcoholic drinks.

The cultural model of drinking has been sharply criticized by sociologist Robin Room (1984) among others. Room asserted that the various health and social problems associated with drinking are "systematically underestimated in the ethnographic literature," a pattern he terms "problem deflation." Listening to speakers at a conference on alcohol consumption, Room noticed that unlike researchers from other disciplines anthropologists "tended to downgrade the severity of the problems" associated with heavy drinking. In fact, they tended to emphasize the positive aspects for cultural functioning of this behavior. Room attributed the problem deflation tendencies he found in anthropological studies of drinking to inadequate familiarity with the multidisciplinary alcohol literature, the vague and unclear nature of the concept of addiction in cross-cultural contexts, and the fact that many ethnographers of drinking were the products of a "wet generation" (i.e., a drinking generation) socialized as they were growing up to view alcohol consumption as normal.

Notably, over time, even Heath came to recognize that among the Camba, patterns of drinking began to change as their traditional way of life became untenable when the local forests were cut down to gain profit by lumber companies. As a result, many Camba were dispossessed of their land and, with it, their customary way of life. At the same time, the Camba horticultural economy was "displaced by the illegal trade in coca and cocaine paste" (Heath 2004: 132). In other words, Heath's work, and that of other anthropological contributors to the cultural model, suggests that although routine heavy drinking without signs of addiction still occurs, it tends to be found in settings in which traditional community social life has not been fully penetrated and disrupted by the forces of capitalist globalization. In short, the relation of a cultural group to the world system is a significant influence on the role and impact of alcohol consumption. Traditional, communally oriented groups, socially organized around what are conceived of as traditional practices and ways of life that have not been significantly penetrated by the global market or other expressions of globalism may not face alcohol-related problems despite episodic heavy drinking. In complex societies, with (overtly or covertly) antagonistic social classes or other stressful social divisions in which ideas about alcohol are themselves conflicted (e.g., the tensions between seeing alcohol as a threat to society but also as an important source of income or as a way of celebrating the good life), drinking may be an immediate cause of significant health and social problems. These points find expression in other aspects of Heath's work including ethnohistoric research on the changing patterns of consumption through time and across societies and examination of the impact of globalization on consumption and consequences of use, two important themes in the contemporary anthropology of drug use generally (Gamburd 2008; Pine 2008).

Despite the position of the cultural model at the core of anthropological thinking, and Room's criticism notwithstanding, anthropologists were never blind to disruptive, dysfunctional, and debilitating effects of alcohol consumption in nontraditional, industrial, and post-contact indigenous societies, as seen in the following two early studies. On the basis of research among the Inuit of Frobisher Bay, John Honigmann and Irma Honigmann (1965) present heavy drinking as a substantial personal, health, and social problem. Likewise, based on interviews with thirty-five self-described Native American problem drinkers living off-reservation in urban settings, Paul Spicer (1997) emphasizes that his study participants were deeply ambivalent about their drinking, seeing it as both profoundly embedded in significant social relationships and at the same time an obstruction to the fulfillment of key social obligations. Drawing on these findings, Spicer proposed the development of a clinically sophisticated anthropology of alcohol.

The cultural model informs a growing body of anthropological literature including book-length accounts of drug use, addiction, and the behavioral strategies of drug addicts (e.g., Spradley 1970). An especially useful aspect of this work has been its revealing accounts of previously less studied subgroups, such as female drug addicts. Thus, in her book *Tricking and Tripping: Prostitution in the Era of AIDS*, Sterk (2000:70) reports the case of a research participant who told her:

The guys think about us as their fucking property. Like they own us because they give us some smoke. . . . You see this black eye? . . . I got beat up because he couldn't get it up. I had been rubbing and sucking him for a long time. He was bleeding, and he wanted to go on. . . . Finally he gave up and made me have sex with this other girl.

Another important contribution of the cultural model has been promoting the systematic study of *hidden populations* of drug users (Singer 2012). This term refers to populations that live somewhat outside the boundaries of mainstream society (and mainstream acceptability) and, as a result, are less understood and, when in need of health care or other services, less connected to available programs. During its development, the ethnography of street drug use focused on the public health need to find and characterize patterns of drug consumption (and related health risk) that operated outside of the public view in complex societies. Ethnography has given anthropologists access to the social settings in which drugs are acquired and consumed and where drug-related behaviors and risk activities take place, such as drug injection sites, crack houses, the homes of drug addicts, user encampments, dance clubs, bars, private parties, and even prisons. This body of research helped to reveal some of the complexities of modern urban life as it is lived in alleyways, cars, "abandoned" buildings, rooftops, and forested patches in the city. In other words, it contributed to the study of the secluded, the unnoticed, and those who disguise their presence by staying in the shadows of the urban environment.

In more recent years, without abandoning the cultural model, anthropologist have framed drinking behavior in terms of broader processes of globalism and the effects of neoliberal restructuring, labor migration, the worldwide flow of alcoholic commodities, contextualized time/space/social group configurations, and the role of drinking in disease risk behavior (e.g., Gezon 2012; S. Liu 2011).

Lifestyle Model

Beyond alcohol research, the cultural model found expression in anthropological research on other drug use using a lifestyle or a distinctive subculture tradition model (B. Johnson et al. 1985). This approach reflects the two ways in which anthropologists use the term *culture*. As used by Heath, culture refers to the distinctive way in which all human communities engage the world through a socially generated and shared set of understandings, meanings, and values. In addition, as reflected in the lifestyle model, anthropologists speak of specific cultures and subcultures that have their own (more or less) unique configuration of evolving knowledge, attitudes, norms, and behaviors, as seen in usages such as *inner-city street culture* and *street cultures of drug use*.

The lifestyle model first appeared in a series of publications during the 1960s and 1970s (Sutter 1966; Hanson et al. 1985). One paper that played an especially important role in ushering in the lifestyle or subculture of drug use model was Preble and Casey's (1969) notable "Taking Care of Business: The Heroin User's Life on the Streets," which was based on street ethnographic research in New York City. The primary aim of the subculture approach is the development of a holistic description of the people for whom drug use has become a central organizing mechanism in their lives. In an effort to counter simplistic stereotypes and narrow pathological portrayals of drug users, Preble and Casey (1969: 2) argued, "Their behavior is anything but an escape from life. They are actively engaged in meaningful activities and relationships seven days a week." In constructing their description of drug users, anthropologists and related ethnographic researchers of other disciplines use participant-observation ethnography to better understand and represent the world as it was actually seen and experienced by drug users themselves (to the degree that that is possible by an outsider). As Friedman, Des Jarlais, and Sothern (1986: 385) comment:

In contrast to views that see drug use as simply a matter of individual pathology, it is more fruitful to describe drug users as constituting a "subculture". . . . This calls our attention to the structured sets of values, roles, and status allocations that exist among drug users. . . . From the perspective of its members, participating in the subculture is a meaningful activity that provides desired rewards, rather than psychopathology, an "escape from reality," or an "illness."

Although varying in specific focus, the literature produced by this approach is comprised of accounts of multiple issues, including (1) the survival strategies used to sustain a drug-focused lifestyle in light of drug laws and law enforcement; (2) the components and organization of the underground drug economy; (3) processes and routines of socialization into drug use social networks and the street drug use subculture; (4) the social settings and key locations, such as places to "cop" (acquire) drugs and shooting galleries, that comprise drug users' social environments; (5) the cultural frameworks used by drug users to classify various social statuses within the subculture (e.g., "a righteous dope fiend"); (6) risk behaviors and risk environments; (7) the street jargon that developed to communicate issues of concern to drug users as well as a sense of in-group membership; and (8) the daily routines and experiences of active drug users.

Michael Agar (1973) is noted for having initiated an ethnography that involved the collection and analysis of the cultural categories that guided the everyday events in the lives of street drug addicts. Agar began this work during two years of fieldwork with patients at the Addiction Research Center in Lexington, Kentucky, which had been renamed the National Institute of Mental Health Clinical Research Center. His approach was guided by the then-emergent view of culture as a shared cognitive template for enacting socially appropriate behavior and for interpreting the behavior of others. His goal was to understand the world, to the degree possible, from the perspective of street drug users. Using this approach, Agar was able to construct an "experience-like" account of key scenes, concepts, relationships, artifacts, activities, and understandings that comprise and are activated in the street drug user's everyday life. Later, Agar was able to test the ethnographic validity of his understanding of this lifestyle with drug users on the streets of New York City (Agar 1977), and he became a pioneering proponent of intense street ethnography as the best method for understanding the culture of drug users. One of the notable insights of Agar's work was his realization that some of the very behaviors (e.g., strong skepticism, constant suspicion, and testing of dependability) that drug treatment staff see as evidence that drug-using patients are maladapted, resistant to treatment, and have not internalized appropriate values, goals, and rules of proper social behavior are in fact quite appropriate to and useful for survival on the streets where there are many threats, threats that often come in human form.

In short, the ethnographic literature on street drug use from the 1960s onward emphasized the lived-worlds, social and cultural patterns, and self-identities of drug users as purposeful and meaningful constructions for participants. Through their lens on culture and lived-experience within the frameworks of daily lifestyles, anthropologists and their colleagues in related disciplines developed practical insights into the emic or insider perspective of street drug users, their experience and daily routines, the nature of their social relationships, and the culturally constituted emotions attached to actions, actors, and social contexts.

In attempting to counter popular and academic images of the urban drug user framed by the paradigms of psychopathology and the sociology of deviance, however, anthropologists initially ignored the wider social context that fosters drug use and addiction, the phenomenon Wolf (1982) has called the "wider field of force," a core issue among critical medical anthropologists studying drug use.

The Critical Medical Anthropology Model

The critical medical anthropology model emerged in the early 1980s and was quickly applied to the analysis of drug use (Singer 1986; Stebbins 1987). Its development reflected a recognition that whatever its strengths, the cultural model falls short in failing to consider the importance in drug use of macrolevel structures (e.g., significant economic inequalities, institutions of social control), social processes and dominant institutions (such as corporate activities, the dominant media, and systems of discrimination), and relations of power (e.g., social classes, unequal relations among nations and the development of underdevelopment). Across all of these dimensions, unequal distribution of power enforces disparity directly and hegemonically through domination of the major institutions involved in the production and dissemination of prevailing ideas in society.

Within the domain of drug use, the critical medical anthropology model has emphasized three issues: the social production of suffering, the use of drugs to self-medicate the emotional injuries of injustice and mistreatment, and the political economy of the licit and illicit drug markets, including their parallels and entwinements. For example, the crack cocaine users Bourgois (2003) came to know through his fieldwork in New York City live in abject poverty but are daily exposed (at a distance) to the great and even unimaginable wealth of other residents of the city. This social disparity is maintained through numerous social practices, such as public policies (e.g., the weakening of social welfare, tax policies that disproportionately burden the poor) that favor urban gentrification and the needs of the wealthy while producing mounting despair among the poor.

In the context of structurally imposed distress, the term *social suffering* (Singer 2006) has been used by anthropologists to refer to the immediate personal experience of broad human problems caused by the exercise of political and economic power. In other words, social suffering refers the misery among those on the weaker end of power relations in terms of physical health, mental health, and lived-experience. As Chopp (1986: 2) comments:

Knowledge of suffering cannot be conveyed in pure facts and figures, reportings that objectify the suffering of countless persons. The horror of suffering is not only in its immensity but in the faces of the anonymous victims who have little voice, let alone rights, in history.

From the perspective of critical medical anthropology, inequality as it is experienced by people who must endure its consequence is a major force driving heavy drug use. Life for a drug addict often is a vicious cycle of felt stress followed by self-medicating drug consumption and resulting social stigmatization and a sense of damaged self-worth (which, in turn, triggers the desire for comfort through drugs). Moreover, because of the damaging effects of drug use (e.g., hepatitis, HIV infection, overdose), addiction contributes to health disparities. Whatever the harm wrought by legal and illegal drug use, at the moment of craving and desire they are seen as relief temporarily removing the sufferer from their prison of personal misery. The consequences of such "relief" always comes back to haunt users as craving returns and they are confronted with the fact that there are always more drugs available to those in need of being "fixed."

Experiential Model

Anthropologists influenced by phenomenology, the study of subjectivities, meaning-centered approaches within medical anthropology, and the questioning of objectivity found in postmodernist perspectives recently have added what they have termed a new *experiential orientation* (Rheinberger 1997) to the cultural and critical medical models. This refers to the idea that in addition to causing suffering, drug abuse and even addiction have other experiential dimensions, including creating opportunities for novel experiences and the development of new social relationships, some of which provide positive, self-affirming experiences for drug users (Pine 2008), as noted earlier by Friedman and coworkers (1986). Addiction, these researchers argue plays a role in the making of personal identities and is thus more than suffering and social rejection, and more than just self-medication of distress. In addition, those who embrace the new experimental model believe, as French philosopher Gilles Deleuze (2007) argued, that some addictions or aspects of addictions can be affirmative, creative, and sustainable, at least at the individual level.

Moreover, within this perspective is a focus on drug therapies and the subjective experiences of being in treatment. This approach to drug use and addiction was first presented at a workshop titled the "Anthropologies of Addiction" held at McGill University in 2009. Subsequently, one of the participants in that gathering, Angela Garcia (2010), wrote a book-length account of her study of addiction, dispossession, and treatment among rural Latino drug users in New Mexico. In addition to showing how addiction in this context is interwoven with cultural and political history, and hence with political economy (involving the historic dispossession of Latino land holdings in the Southwest and emotional responses to this process of losing one's physical heritage; Garcia 2008), Garcia reveals how prevailing drug treatment models force patients to relive their personal and social histories, further enhancing their addiction-propelling melancholy. Additionally, Garcia (2010) is concerned with forms of addictive experience, such as "getting high, overdose, suicide," that are at once social and yet, in the end, are individual and highly internal and subjective As such, they are seemingly closed even to the anthropological researcher. One bridge across this interpersonal divide, according to Garcia, that reflects the special nature of ethnography as a field-based, researcher-embedded method, is "common vulnerability," by which she means it is through his or her own vulnerability (including personal suffering and moments of intimacy in the field) that the ethnographer can, to some degree, connect emotionally with the melancholy subjectivity of the addict.

Another advocate of the experiential approach, Raikhel (2009) studied drug treatment in two institutional settings in contemporary Russia. He notes:

To put it in overly simplified terms, at the Addiction Hospital the identification of alcoholism was an act of diagnosis carried out by physicians. At the House of Recovery, it was an act of self-identification carried out by participants. (226)

At the second of these two institutions, Raikhel observed how drinkers come into an identity as an alcoholic, a personal developmental process that is socially conditioned and culturally informed.

SPECIFIC ANTHROPOLOGICAL RESEARCH ON DRUG USE

Although the ethnography of drug use is concerned with all categories of drugs, it is important to recognize differences brought to light by ethnography in behaviors, users, contexts, and consequences of tobacco, alcohol, and illicit drug use. Also, there are differences in the quantity of ethnographic research carried out by ethnographers on these different kinds of drugs. Individually, anthropologists have tended to focus their work exclusively on the study of tobacco, alcohol, or illicit drugs, creating somewhat siloed bodies of literature. In recent years, there has been a movement to break down these barriers, in part driven by the realization that people who use drugs are often not single-drug users: smokers drink, drinkers use illicit drugs, illicit drug users smoke and drink. Often times these behaviors occur in tandem or in sequence (e.g., smoking while drinking, lighting a cigarette after injecting heroin). In the following subsections, we present overviews of the major bodies of anthropological research by drug category.

Human Use of Tobacco

The English word *tobacco* was derived from the Spanish *tabaco*, which in turn was taken directly from the Arawak word for cigar. The Arawak were the indigenous people that Christopher Columbus encountered in the Caribbean on his first and subsequent voyages to the New World. In his log, Columbus recorded his impressions of the Arawak: "They . . . brought us parrots and balls of cotton and spears and many other things, which they exchanged for the glass beads and hawks bells. They willingly traded everything they owned. . . . They were well-built, with good bodies and handsome features" (quoted in Zinn 1980: 1). Among the items that the Arawak brought to Columbus were the dried leaves of a cultivated plant that the Europeans had never seen before. Members of Columbus's crew observed the Arawak people smoking huge cigars made from this plant. The Arawak told the Europeans that smoking tobacco soothed their limbs, helped them not to feel weary, and eased the passage into sleep. Columbus and his crew brought tobacco back with them to Portugal. From there it diffused, first to France in 1560 and to Italy in 1561. By the turn of the century, it was being grown in Europe and had become a widely used substance on the European continent. Europeans, in turn, carried tobacco to much of the rest of the world, even to areas of the New World where it was unknown before Columbus's voyage (e.g., the subarctic and artic regions). Among Indian peoples, tobacco had both religious and secular uses. Shamans, or indigenous healers, used tobacco to enter into a trance state and communicate with spirit beings to diagnose the nature of a health or social problem. It also was commonly used in rites of passage to mark changes in an individual's social status. Smoking tobacco communally was often done to mark the beginning or continuation of an alliance between tribes or to make binding an agreement or contract.

As this description suggests, tobacco was deeply rooted in the indigenous cultures of many peoples of the New World. Given the ceremonial controls on the frequency of consumption and the diluted form in which tobacco was consumed (compared with modern cigarettes whose addictive nicotine level is artificially enhanced by tobacco manufacturers), as well as the fact that inhalation of tobacco smoke into the lungs was not emphasized, tobacco may not have been a significant source of health problems among Indian people before European contact. However, with the diffusion of tobacco to Europe and with the rise of industrial capitalism, tobacco was transformed from a sacred object and culturally controlled medicament into a commodity sold for profit. With the emergence and development of the tobacco industry and the intensive promotion of cigarettes, the per capita consumption of tobacco increased dramatically (especially in the early and middle decades of the twentieth century), with significant health consequences. As Barnet and Cavanagh (1994: 184) observe, "The cigarette is the most widely distributed global consumer product on earth, the most profitable, and the most deadly."

Indeed, tobacco, it has been said, is the one product that if used as directed by the manufacturer will lead to certain disease and death. The significant negative health consequences of smoking are now widely known. Three commonly lethal diseases, in particular, have been closely linked to the use of tobacco: coronary heart disease, lung cancer, and chronic obstructive pulmonary disease. Other fatal or disabling diseases known to be caused by or made worse by smoking include peripheral vascular disease, hypertension, and myocardial infarction. Smoking also causes cancer of the mouth, throat, bladder, and other organs.

The World Lung Foundation (WLF) estimates that if current trends continue, one billion people around the world will die from tobacco use and exposure during the twenty-first century, as tobacco-related deaths have almost tripled since 2002 (Ericksen, Makay, and Ross 2012). Tobacco is already the number one killer in China, causing more than a million deaths a year. The WLF estimates that about 80 percent of people who die from tobacco-related illnesses live in low- to middle-income countries. Furthermore, an estimated 600,000 individuals died from exposure to secondhand smoke in 2011; the majority of secondhand smoking deaths occurred in women and children. There is no safe level of exposure to secondhand smoke. Globally, about 40 percent of children and a third of nonsmoking adults were exposed to secondhand smoke in 2004 according to the WLF.

Why this terrible toll on human health? The WLF and many other organizations and antitobacco activists point a finger at giant transnational tobacco corporations, accusing them of undermining efforts to assist people to stop smoking and actively seeking to addict new smokers each year. Producing about six trillion cigarettes and large quantities of other tobacco products, Big Tobacco reaps almost half a trillion dollars in revenues and 35 billion dollars in profits a year. In 2010, the tobacco industry's profit was equivalent to US$6,000 for every death caused by tobacco.

The exact origin of tobacco use is still unknown. However, botanical study has demonstrated that the cultivated forms of the tobacco plant (several different species have been domesticated) all have their origin in South America. The wild ancestors of domesticated tobacco species are not indigenous to the Caribbean area but are found in Peru, Bolivia, Ecuador, and Argentina. The tobacco plant and the knowledge for both cultivating and consuming it likely diffused from South America to the Caribbean (perhaps through Mexico) along with various cultivated food plants many years before the arrival of Columbus. Other species of tobacco were indigenous to North America, and these came to be among the most widely cultivated plants grown by the Indians of what was to become the United States. Commonly, North American Indian peoples mixed tobacco with other plants such as sumac leaves and the inner bark of dogwood trees. In fact, the Indians of the Eastern United States and Canada referred to the substance they smoked in their pipes as *kinnikinnik,* an Algonquian word meaning "that which is mixed" (Driver 1969). Different tribal groups consumed tobacco in different ways. Among the Indians of the Northwest coast, tobacco was chewed with lime but not smoked. Among the Creek, it was one of the ingredients of an emetic drink. The Aztecs ate tobacco leaves and also used it as snuff. Distinct cigarettes with cornhusk wrappings were smoked in the Southwest (although this may not have been an indigenous means of consumption). Smoking tobacco in pipes also was widespread.

Anthropology of Tobacco Use

Systematic study of tobacco use was relatively limited in anthropological texts historically, with the use of tobacco usually only gaining passing mentions in most ethnographic accounts of day-to-day social life in various communities. Peter Black (1984) maintains that tobacco use has been understudied by anthropologists because of its place in the Western cultures in which most anthropologists traditionally have been socialized. As a commonly individualized act with limited ritual elaboration and symbolic content in the West (although, as Mark Nichter [2003] stresses, these certainly are not absent), the smoking of cigarettes, in particular, is more expressive of internal mood states (e.g., a time-out from daily routine) than shared cultural content. As such, the behavior did not attract extensive ethnographic attention as anthropologists examined the social worlds of diverse societies, although, in recent years, with growing awareness of the health risks of tobacco use, this has changed (Nichter et al. 2002;).

At the same time, there has been increased attention to the heretofore understudied Western cultural context of smoking. One ritualization of smoking that has been described ethnographically involves tobacco use as an anticipatory rite of passage for subordinated social groups, including youth, women, and ethnic minorities (Robb 1986). Smoking can also sometimes serve as a badge of group membership (Eckert 1983); ironically, the antismoking movement may have contributed to heightened sharing of "resistance themes" among smokers (Rhodes et al. 2008). In their ethnographic study of smoking among Puerto Rican adolescents, for example, Sarah McGraw and colleagues (1991) emphasize the ways in which this behavior is used to establish or affirm social connections among peers. Alternately, Quintero and Davis (2002) discuss the role of smoking as a means of mood management or to provide a "cool identity" among Hispanic youth.

In his study of smoking in a small Pacific island community, Marshall (2005) maintains that anthropologists have an obligation to pay particular attention to tobacco because, much more so than in complex Western societies, in more traditionally oriented communities tobacco use—even though a behavior introduced by contact with complex societies—is embedded in and encoded with cultural meanings; in addition, it is a "learned, patterned and typically social behaviour" (M. Marshall 2005: 367).

One of the earliest ethnographic descriptions of tobacco use was Alfred Louis Kroeber's (1941) account of the roles of tobacco, salt, and dogs among several western U.S. Native American groups. He observed that tobacco was an important ritual offering in religious rites among tobacco cultivators. Among groups that gathered wild tobacco but did not grow the crop, he found that tobacco did not serve this religious function. He also noted that the use of tobacco in shamanic healing only occurred in groups that smoked tobacco and not in those that chewed the drug.

It is in Oceania that the most extensive ethnographic studies of tobacco use have been conducted. In this context, Peter Black (1984) carried out his ethnographic study on tobacco use in the Tobian Islands, tracing the ethnohistorical development of tobacco consumption after its introduction by European explorers and traders. Ultimately, tobacco came to be highly valued among the people of the Tobian Islands as a marker of social status. In a related study, Mac Marshall (1979, 1990) assessed the social role of tobacco on Truk, noting that by age nineteen all young men in the village he studied had begun smoking, whereas girls were less likely to smoke. Marshall analyzed both tobacco and alcohol consumption on Truk as key cultural symbols of masculinity, a pattern also seen elsewhere in Micronesia. As contrasted with the gender patterning noted by Marshall, pipe smoking in Melanesia has been found to be a common practice among women (Keesing 1983).

Among the Trobriand Islanders, who live near Australia, tobacco was seen as a something used by sorcerers to attack their victims (Weiner 1988). In contrast, in some circum-Caribbean spiritist religions, such as *espiritismo*, adherents believe that tobacco smoke passed over the body has a cleansing effect, and it is thus used in this fashion in the ethnomedical treatment of alcoholism and other personal problems (Singer and Borrero 1984). Gilbert Herdt's (1987) ethnographic work among the Sambia of New Guinea led to observations of the role of tobacco's role in relaxation and multigenerational socializing following work in the food gardens.

In recent years, a number of anthropologists have taken up studies of tobacco use in light of globalization and the worldwide marketing of tobacco products as commodities sold for a profit. Part and parcel of this trend is the transition to studying the health consequences of tobacco consumption in relation to the mass marketing of tobacco products. As Kenyon Stebbins (2001: 148) stresses, many traditional smoking behaviors around the world, including limitations on the frequency and quantity of consumption, have generally been overwhelmed "by aggressive marketing by transnational tobacco companies." In his own studies of smoking, Stebbins has shown how the tobacco industry has turned to markets in the developing world to make up for a loss in sales first in the United States and subsequently in parts of the European market. Governments in developing nations often do not have the ability to limit tobacco marketing and, being usually in need of financial help, they are open to introducing taxable commodities to their citizens. As a result of extensive advertising in developing nations, Stebbins (1990) notes that worldwide tobacco consumption has increased at the rate of 1 percent a year, with countries such as Brazil, India, and Kenya exhibiting the greatest increases. The result has been rising rates of cancer and other adverse health outcomes of tobacco consumption. As Stebbins (2001: 164) puts it, the tobacco companies "have been making a killing (in more ways than one)." Related research by Nichter and Cartwright (1991) describes the complicity of the U.S. government in promoting cigarette use in developing countries. They argue that the U.S. support of public health focused on improving child health in the world diverts attention from the health consequences of expanded tobacco production and consumption in developing nations and ponder whether health promotion efforts are saving children from infections only to allow them to fall prey to the multinational tobacco industry (Nichter and Cartwright 1991).

In a study designed to show how structural factors like inequality, poverty, and exploitation, as well as cultural understandings of relief, combine to create social patterns of tobacco use, Roy (2012) studied the use of *bidis,* or hand-rolled, filter-less cigarettes in Bangladesh. Roy found that among the poor of Bangladesh, smoking a few *bidis* with several cups of tea (also a drug) in the morning was looked at positively as a way of saving poor people the expense of breakfast. The hunger suppression provided by *bidis,* a coping strategy not uncommon among marginalized groups, allowed poor people to make it to lunchtime before having to invest their limited resources in food acquisition. In that the people studied by Roy struggle to feed their families every day, this is no small issue. People also use *bidis* to self-medicate various symptoms. *Bidis* are seen as a much cheaper strategy than seeing a doctor. Additionally, people reported that smoking several *bidis* in rapid succession is an effective means of achieving a calming sensation when feeling upset or under pressure. For example, people who whose work involves heavy physical labor complained to Roy about being underpaid by their employers, including not being given the amount they had originally been promised. *Bidi* smoking was seen as a way of living with feeling cheated and abused. Indeed, it is to the poor that *bidis* are marketed in Bangladesh, providing profit for wealthier individuals and a cheap, legal "opiate for the masses."

In other research, Nichter, Nichter, and Van Sickle (2004) examined the perceptions of tobacco use among male college students in India. They found that these students believe that smoking a cigarette enhances one's manliness, relieves boredom, and eases tension. Moreover, their informants indicated that the more expensive a cigarette was, the less dangerous it was to one's health. Recognizing that physicians can be important in role-modeling smoking cessation, Mark and Mimi Nichter and coworkers (Mohan et al. 2006) subsequently examined tobacco use among doctors in Kerala, India. They found that a substantial proportion of physicians and medical students continue to be smokers despite the global promotion of smoking cessation.

This work indicates the growing involvement of ethnographers using their findings in the analysis of tobacco-related health risks and risk promoters, including risks tied to the marketing of tobacco products such as flavored cigars to underage populations, as found by the research teams of Page and Singer (e.g., Page and Evans 2003; Singer et al. 2007, 2010), and secondhand smoking (Singer et al. 2010), as well as in the development of ethnographically informed, culturally targeted, and socially appropriate tobacco interventions (Nichter 2006) and policy change initiatives (Skeer et al. 2004). As Glasser (2012) notes, the recent inclusion of anthropologists on drug treatment outcome teams allows the collection of emic data on program operation, client appeal, and effectiveness, "which includes discovering which approaches are in need of change and determining the viability of new treatment techniques." Overall, from a public health standpoint, as Nichter (2003: 140) points out, the contemporary ethnography of tobacco consumption allows closer examination of "the role that cultural institutions, values, and processes play in: (1) protecting against smoking . . . , (2) fostering smoking as a normative behavior within particular gender and age cohorts, and (3) affecting the distribution of particular smoking trajectories" in society.

The cascading revelations of tobacco consumption's immense health risks has, to a degree, overwhelmed consideration of tobacco use as anything other than a bane of human existence. The ethnographic handling of tobacco use in recent years has tended to begin with assumptions of addiction and damage. Yet, as the review in this subsection suggests, to understand and effectively intervene to avert the grave threat of tobacco use it is necessary to understand smoking as a social behavior that is meaningful and socially valuable to users.

Also, it is necessary to understand the supply side of the tobacco industry to be able to implement structural interventions to restrict tobacco promotion. Increasingly, anthropologists have begun to write book-length accounts of this aspect of human interaction with tobacco, creating a body of literature that raises an important issue of moral responsibility.

In the oldest of these books, *Tobacco Culture: Farming Kentucky's Burley Belt*, John van Willigen and Susan Eastwood (1998) use oral histories of farmers involved in white burley tobacco production in central Kentucky to tell the story of tobacco farming as a way of life in a changing world. Although not concerned with the health consequences of tobacco per se, the book provides a useful account of "tobacco farmer culture." The authors note, "We were struck by the ironic contrast between what we saw as vilification of tobacco and tobacco producers in the media and the grace and dignity of these hardworking craftsman" (Willigen and Eastwood 1980: viii). A second book, Ann Kingsolver's (2011) *Tobacco Town Futures: Global Encounters in Rural Kentucky*, has many parallels to Willigen and Eastwood's book, including its focus on tobacco farmers in Kentucky, but moves beyond the lives and experiences of individual farmers to show how people in dispersed communities collectively participate in a global economic system of tobacco production that is driven by a globalizing capitalist logic and practice. Like van Willigen and Eastwood, Kingsolver (2011: 25) observes, "In communities around the world, [tobacco] both feeds the people who produce it and kills those who consume its smoked and 'smokeless' products." Finally, there is *Tobacco Capitalism: Growers, Migrant Workers, and the Changing Face of a Global Industry* by Peter Benson (2012). This work, based on ethnographic research with tobacco farmers and farm workers in North Carolina, examines the growing tensions between Big Tobacco manufacturers and tobacco family farmers in light of globalization and the ever-greater control cigarette makers have over tobacco growers. Additionally, like the other authors cited earlier, Benson addresses the seeming contradiction in the life experience of those working in tobacco production—namely, that their livelihood depends on the production of a substance that kills enormous numbers of people. Reports Benson (2012: 146), "Growers are often quick to insist they make an agricultural product. 'I grow tobacco,' they say, 'not cigarettes.'" For them, this thin factual distinction—which may not be accepted as valid by others who emphasize agency and personal responsibility—provides the foundation for justifying their contribution to the tobacco industry.

In a recent paper, David Griffith (2009), based on his own research with tobacco farmers, employed the concept of *moral economy* to elaborate on this point. A moral economy is the cultural side of the economic coin, the set of culturally constituted and shared beliefs, values, and logics that affirm the social correctness of particular economic behaviors in a given social context. For example, mugging people for money may be profitable from a narrow economic standpoint, but is it morally acceptable? According to Griffith, in any community, social morality (e.g., it is wrong to harm others) is balanced against moral economy. Thus he quotes one of the farmers he interviewed, who told him (Griffith 2009: 438): "I know they say tobacco's bad for people, that it kills people. But four generations of my family were raised on tobacco money. Tobacco money sent my brother to medical school. Tobacco money is paying for my son's education and buying my daughter goats and a steer to show in the county fair." In other words, to this typical farmer, growing tobacco supports proper and socially valuable outcomes (providing for your family, supporting the filling of socially useful roles). Farmers also stress that growing tobacco allows them to employ people (often the same people year after year). Another component of this moral economy Griffith found was the accepted practice of tobacco buyers offering higher purchase prices to the widows of long-time tobacco producers, thereby contributing to the welfare of the tobacco-growing community and affirming the morality of that community. Tobacco growing, in short, is justified as a moral behavior that affirms established multigeneration cultural traditions, supports families, and contributes to community welfare. Government restrictions on smoking, in fact, are seen as immoral and a threat to the growers' way of life and livelihood. Despite the embrace of these values, Benson (2008: 140) found that some farmers "admit to feeling moral ambivalence about their crop." By contrast, the transnational corporations that buy up tobacco and produce, advertise, and market an ever-widening array of tobacco products would appear, based on a constant history of deceiving the public about the dangers of their products, the constant search for new ways to get young people to adopt smoking, and the vigorous (sometimes legal, sometimes illegal, often coercive) effort to get their products sold everywhere in the world), would seem to have no such ambivalence (Singer 2008). As Jeffrey Wigand (2007), a former senior executive at the tobacco giant Brown and Williams (B&W) testified before the House Subcommittee on Workforce Protections,

As I continued to work at B&W, I realized that the company was not interested in making safer products, but only in finding new adolescent consumers and maximizing profits. Disturbingly, I learned that the culture of the tobacco industry was one in which great importance was placed on keeping the public ignorant about the addictive and lethal nature of tobacco products. The industry most wanted to protect its fundamental legal and PR platform that tobacco use was not addictive, that tobacco use was a free, consumer choice, and that tobacco use was not the source of the scientifically linked morbidity and mortality.

Human Use of Alcohol

Drinking alcoholic beverages is a behavior that we see every day in Western society and, increasingly, globally. Until the health campaigns of recent years, this behavior had become so commonplace that it was hardly noticeable. Like swinging our arms when we walk, it seemed to be a natural part of life. Indeed, through a nonstop barrage of TV, radio, billboard, magazine, newspaper, and other advertisements, as well as their frequent presence in movies and online, drinking came to be seen as part of the good life, a symbol of personal success and achievement. As a result, many adults became drinkers and, in turn, directly or indirectly (by setting an example) taught this behavior to their children.

The health consequences of being a drinking society can be significant. Drinking is a major contributor to morbidity (i.e., disease) and mortality (i.e., death). The liver is the body organ most significantly damaged by extensive alcohol consumption. Because the liver oxidizes alcohol and helps eliminate it from the body, it remains longer in contact with ingested alcohol than other body organs. The increased activity in the liver needed to breakdown alcohol causes cell death and hardening of the tissue, producing the disease called liver cirrhosis. Cirrhosis is one of the most common diseases associated with alcohol consumption. As of 2010, chronic liver disease and cirrhosis were the twelfth leading cause of death in the United States.

Eventually, some people in public health began to argue that, although legal, alcohol should be classified as a drug on the basis of its association, in various contexts, with health and social problems. Others (not the least of which are those involved in the alcohol industry) have had difficulty lumping alcohol with cocaine and heroin, because the first is legal to possess and use and the latter two are banned. Also, cocaine and heroin commonly are seen as being especially dangerous and a threat to society. As Matveychuk (1986: 8) stresses,

if I were to say that I used drugs this afternoon, most people would be either disappointed or amused to find that what I meant is that I drank a glass of beer, smoked a cigarette, and took two aspirin. Though alcohol, nicotine, and aspirin are all psychoactive, they do not fit our stereotype of what a drug is.

Alcohol, in fact, is the most widely used psychoactive drug in the world. Moreover, it is probably the drug with the longest history of use by humans. Fermentation is a relatively simple and quite natural process that occurs fairly quickly in many fruits, vegetables, and grains with adequate concentrations of sugar. Additionally, alcohol is undoubtedly the most versatile drug available, serving at various times and places as a food (providing two hundred calories per ounce, although no vitamins, minerals, or other nutrients), medicine (e.g., for symptomatic relief of pain and insomnia), aphrodisiac, energizer, liquid refreshment, payment for labor, and narcotic. Human use of alcohol is probably as old as agriculture itself; even before the rise of Europe as a global world power, alcohol had spread to or had been independently discovered in most parts of the world (except in much of indigenous North America and in Oceania). Some historic researchers have suggested that the oldest intentionally produced alcoholic beverages were made from the fruit of the date palms of the eastern Mediterranean and Mesopotamia areas. Dates and the sap of date palms have one of the most concentrated levels of naturally occurring sugar. Humans have been drinking wine and getting drunk while consuming it for all of recorded history and, with little doubt, previous to the emergence of writing. Archaeologists have identified wine residues in ancient pottery, confirming human consumption of wine as much as eight thousand years ago. Beer use is documented from as early as five thousand years ago in early Sumerian and Akkadia texts, and alcohol production is depicted in Egyptian murals from the Predynastic period.

Anthropology of Alcohol Use

Cross-culturally, anthropologists have described hundreds of patterns of alcohol consumption, from palm wine to pulque, from gin to aguardiente (Page 2011). In all societies in which it is consumed, alcohol is invested with special cultural meanings and emotions, although sometimes, as in the case of the United States, ambiguous and conflicted ones. It is probably not a coincidence that according to the *Random House Dictionary*, the word *drunk* has more synonyms than any other word in the English language; indeed, most students are capable of reciting quite a list of such terms. Societal understandings of alcohol are culturally conditioned. Thus, wine is not just a certain type of alcohol made from fruit. The Eucharist wine, the very expensive bottle of imported French wine, cooking sherry, and the cheap bottle of rotgut passed around a group of huddled men on skid row may be quite similar chemically but mean very different things culturally. Similarly, in Islam, drinking alcohol is sacrilegious, yet in Catholicism it can be a sacramental act. Even within a single broad religion like Christianity, attitudes vary. As anthropologist Genevieve Ames (1985: 439–440), who has spent much of her career as an alcohol researcher, indicates,

Although the American branches of some large church groups of Europe, such as the Lutherans and Episcopalians, have not opposed moderate drinking, other religious groups, such as Baptists, Methodists, Presbyterians, Congregationalists, and members of small and fundamentalist groups, have a history of strongly opposing alcohol use and drunkenness as sinful.

That alcohol can be dangerous "has been widely described for as long as we have written records, and elaborate sets of legal, religious, and other norms have been developed to regulate who drinks how much of what, where, and when, in the company of whom, and with what outcomes"

(Heath 1990b: 265). Alcohol, wherever and in whatever form it is consumed, has been subject to cultural rules and regulations that do not apply to other kinds of consumable liquids. In other words, there almost always is a cultural awareness that alcohol has unique properties, although just what they are varies across cultural systems.

A unique and somewhat insulated research tradition has developed in the ethnography of alcohol use. Despite the fact that alcohol is the only drug in the pharmacopoeia that has a dedicated institute among the National Institutes of Health focused on the study and control of its use and health consequences, it has received much less attention in ethnographic and other research than illegal drug use, both in terms of overall expenditures on scientific study and in terms of grant-supported efforts. Unlike the case of tobacco, however, many ethnographers who have written about alcohol consumption have done so based on ethnographic research that set out intentionally to focus on patterns of alcohol use cross-culturally, especially in attempts to characterize problematic patterns of consumption.

One important genre within this larger body of work is the study of the ways alcohol has played a role in the control and oppression of marginalized populations. In her book *Drinking and Sobriety among the Lakota Sioux,* Beatrice Medicine (2007: 11) comments,

The term "alcohol," as used in reference to American Indians of all tribes, is an exceedingly value-laden and emotion-evoking one. . . . It is [critical to] the widespread image of the drunken Indian. This descriptive gloss is commonly used in any area where natives of any tribal affiliation reside. It is an all-encompassing and convenient stereotype for all natives—American Indians and Alaska Natives.

Beginning in the 1960s, there emerged a conscious revitalization movement among American Indians in response to a long history of brutalization, encroachment, dispossession, and forced acculturation. Part and parcel of this effort is that "belief that alcohol is an introduced evil that was part of the genocide and ethnocide policies of the conquerors" (Medicine 2007: 81).

Part of the struggle against alcohol as an imposed evil in American Indian communities involves gaining access to alcohol treatment and the achievement of sobriety, also issues of concern to Medicine and other anthropologists. At issue here is the degree to which available treatment options are culturally appropriate (which among American Indians may mean including traditional spiritual components and behaviors) and are community controlled, as opposed to being imposed from without using one-size-fits-all treatment modalities (Prussing 2011). Thus, Paul Spicer (2001), based on interviews with American Indian heavy drinkers in

Minnesota, argues that his participants view Alcoholics Anonymous as a process constructed within the cultural values and goals of non-Indians and hence as unsuitable for people with traditional Indian identity and values. While recognizing that drinking can lead to health and social problems, for many Indians, Spicer argues, drinking is an assertion of Indian identity in a world of alien cultural discourses.

Whether focused on negative effects of alcohol use, ambivalent attitudes toward drinking, or cycles of recovery from alcohol impairment, common assumptions of this body of work is the likelihood of finding a certain rate of impairment in the populations under study and that intoxication or drunkenness brings about erratic, often embarrassing, and sometimes dangerous behavior that affects drinkers, their significant others, and the wider community. Thus, in a review of the anthropological literature on drinking from the 1970s through the 1990s, Mac Marshall, Ames, and Bennett (2001: 156–157) comment that "anthropologists working in the alcohol field have been concerned with the application of their findings to such domains as public health . . . , clinical intervention . . . , and international assessments of drinking problems." The dominance of this orientation has troubled some anthropologists, such as Geoffrey Hunt and Judith Baker (2001), who complain that the ascendancy of a public health models puts anthropological alcohol and other drug researchers in danger of being controlled by other disciplines through the adoption of nonanthropological, noncultural, social-problem modes of viewing human behavior. Heath's work in Latin America, discussed earlier, represents a notable exception to this tendency in the literature. Furthermore, much of anthropological study of drinking only infrequently addresses the fact that often it occurs in contexts in which people use and mix various drugs. In the United States, for example, the most frequently found patterns of polydrug consumption involve at least three or four of the "big five" drugs (Page 1999), which have extensive histories of use and are the most widely distributed in the world (heroin, cocaine, tobacco, alcohol, and marijuana).

Considerably less frequent than studies addressing problematic alcohol use are studies of routine drinking in establishments where people congregate to drink and (often) to interact with other drinkers, such as described in Sherri Cavan's book *Liquor License: An Ethnography of Bar Behavior* (1966). Ethnographies like this have demonstrated the importance of drinking sites in the making of social lives, social relations, and personal identities that extend far beyond their immediate settings. They also succeed in avoiding assumptions about the nature and impact of drinking. Still, until recently, studies of this kind were somewhat rare in the literature on alcohol. Fortunately, this pattern has begun to change, and ethnographers have in recent years produced a spate of new book-length ethnographies organized around examinations of the place of alcohol consumption in diverse societies (e.g., Butler 2006; Pine 2008). These newer works, which affirm the value of drug ethnography, seek to understand drinking within the intertwined and unsettled arena of local cultural traditions and fast-paced globalizing changes.

A good example of how global transformations are affecting alcohol use is provided by Michele Gamburd (2008). Writing about illicit liquor consumption in Sri Lanka, she notes that, traditionally, women worked in the domestic sphere and provided economically critical but unpaid household services for their families. The significant economic challenges that now face poor families, including the inability to make enough money to buy land and build a home, have led to the decision, at the family level, to respond to the demand for housemaids in countries such as Kuwait, Saudi Arabia, and the United Arab Emirates, countries with oil-rich families that can afford maids. In 2005, for example, Gamburd reports that more than a million Sri Lankans participated in international labor migration, two-thirds of them women. Often, these women are hired on two-year contracts and leave behind their husbands and children. In this way, women—for the first time—have become household breadwinners and men homemakers. Consequently, older gendered divisions of labor and social roles have been thrown into severe question and doubt. As a result, Gamburd notes, many men turned to alcohol consumption to self-medicate their damaged identities and diminished sense of self-worth. As explained by one of Gamburd's key informants: "I was home while my wife worked in the Middle East as a housemaid. I was drinking then. . . . [Men drink] because they have no job. They can't help their kids. While their wives are abroad, the husband is doing the housework. Then this goes to his head and he gets confused and upset. . . . Then men drink and forget [their sense of failure as a man as they culturally understand it]" (Gamburd 2008: 116).

Human Use of Illicit Drugs

Illicit substances are those that society (or at least those in society with the power to make and enforce such decisions) has come to define as being unacceptable for use and, within the context of the modern state structure, made illegal (recognizing that to a degree which drugs these are varies over time and place, as seen historically in the Western acceptance of imposed opium exports to China by Britain, France, Portugal, Holland, and the United States during the 1800s, or more recently in the level of societal acceptance of medical marijuana). Today, the term *drug*, which probably gained acceptance because of its brevity from the perspective of the mass media, is used widely to refer explicitly to illicit consumables, although this was not always the case. Before the First World War, and before the United States and other countries began defining drug use as a problem, the term generally was not linked with the notion of illicit consumption, nor with the concepts of abuse or addiction. The original edition of the *Oxford English Dictionary* (published in 1897) defined the noun *drug* as a "simple medicinal substance" without any reference (as is now found in all dictionaries) to narcotics. In fact, after the First World War, pharmacists (who in time stopped calling themselves druggists) fought a losing battle to convince newspapers to not use the term *drugs* in referring to nonmedicinal substances consumed without medical approval for their mind-altering effects. The 1930 annual meeting of the American Pharmaceutical Association (APA), in fact, passed a resolution urging the press to use the term *narcotic* (a term derived from the Greek word *narke*, which means stiffness) to refer to drugs such as marijuana, heroin, and cocaine. Ultimately, pharmacists gave up this struggle, and in 1987 the APA urged its members to use the terms *medicine* and *medication* and to avoid the term *drug* to label pharmaceutical products. Of course, the earlier medical meaning of the term drug did not go out of existence, contributing to the broader terminological/conceptual jungle that surrounds this topic (e.g., use vs. abuse, addiction vs. dependence, recreational vs. ritual use). More recently, there have been public health efforts to expand the term drug to include legal substances like alcohol, creating increasing use of the acronym ATOD (alcohol, tobacco, and other drugs) in public health discourse and practice.

All regions of the world have their own particular histories with mind-altering substances. In Europe, for example, unlike many other parts of the world, mind-altering drug ingestion did not develop as a central part of religious ritual. Beginning at least as early as the Middle Ages, many such drugs were banned, and the herbalists who created and used them were punished. Today, illicit drug abuse is commonly seen as a significant health and social issue throughout Europe as well as many other countries around the world. Indeed, drug abuse is known to be an international phenomenon, with the plants that produce most mood-altering chemicals being grown in one country, processed into useable form in another, and consumed primarily in a third country. With the development of an extensive international system of illicit drug production, smuggling, and sales, many forms of use have become internationalized.

Globalization, the term used to describe an ever-more-intertwined world economy, is nothing new in the realm of drugs. The reason for this is that drug use is and has been for a long time big business, and, in fact, many big businesses, from illicit drug smuggling organizations to legal financial institutions are involved in the action. In recent years, for example, a number of otherwise austere and seemingly proper banking firms have been exposed as important sources for the laundering of illicit drug dollars (i.e., hiding the source of great sums of money to avoid taxation through outright seizure by legal authorities). In 1985, money laundering was found to be an $80 billion-a-year industry, with the majority of the money coming from illegal drug sales and involving major banks and brokerage houses throughout the United States. For example, a federal probe into Los Zetas, a so-called Mexican drug cartel, found that this illicit drug group had been laundering some of its illicit profits ($1 million a month) through accounts at the Bank of America, one of the world's largest financial institutions (Eichler 2012). Curiously, as the result of the extensive money-laundering operations and with the widespread use and trafficking of cocaine, virtually every piece of. U.S. currency is contaminated with microscopic traces of cocaine (Dell'Amore 2009).

Anthropology of Illicit Drugs

Although the use of ethnographic methods in the study of illicit drug use dates to the 1930s and began to pick up steam after the emergence of what has been called the youth drug revolution beginning in the 1960s, it was the HIV disease pandemic, dating to the mid- to late 1980s, that really awakened the field, as evidenced by the sudden involvement of a significant number of anthropologists (Page and Singer 2008). Since then, the ethnography of drug use has been strongly influenced by the pandemic and by public health, driven by the availability of research funding on HIV risk and prevention and related topics (e.g., HCV risk, drug overdose). Changes flowing from this development include the following:

- A rapid expansion of the anthropology of illicit drug use literature
- Emergence of fine-grained observational studies of drug-related practices and risk behaviors
- Exploration of the health impacts of drug use
- Examination of the social contexts and physical locations of use ("drug scenes" or "risk environments"), as well as drug and resource acquisition sites as social locations
- Study of "drug culture" in diverse locations, including jargons, socialization processes, daily routines, key events, and social interaction
- Tracking of emergent drug use and drug use behaviors, including the diversion of legal pharmaceutical drugs for nonmedical illegal uses
- Documentation of the life histories of drug users in social context
- Research on the social networks of out-of-treatment drug users and their impacts on behavior
- Consideration of local and broader drug distribution networks and practices

- Study of drug treatment, recovery, and relapse
- The use of multidisciplinary and multisited (i.e., collaborative research in multiple places) team research.
- Situating local drug use within the wider political economy of drug flows and drug control efforts

Beyond HIV-related studies, drug ethnographers in recent years have extended their focus to include a variety of new issues, including the spread, in the late 1990s, of heroin to suburban youth; the use of so-called club drugs such as ecstasy, GHB, ketamine, and Rohypnol, in and out of youth-oriented dance clubs and raves, and increasingly on the street; the geographic spread and social and health impacts of methamphetamine; the mixing of drug cocktails (e.g., crack with marijuana, cocaine with club drugs) to form new polydrug use patterns; the emergence and diffusion of new street drugs such as "illy" (embalming fluid) or new consumption methods like crack cocaine injection; the nature and ideologies of drug treatment; and the spread of injection drug use to developing countries where this practice previously was rare or unknown. This new wave of studies, to a fair degree, represents the products of anthropologists adopting drug research careers beginning with HIV disease and expanded to include a growing range of other drug-related health and behavioral topics. The result has been the full emergence of a broadly focused drug research tradition within anthropology.

In response to the HIV pandemic, and the recognized role of drug injection in this disease crisis (as well as the role of pipe-sharing among crack users as a route of HIV infection), a number of anthropologists initiated ethnographic studies of so-called risk behaviors such as needle sharing. One of these researchers, Stephen Koester, began studying injection drug users in Denver, Colorado, in 1988 through a National Institute of Drug Abuse–funded research project. He describes his research methodology as follows: "Direct observation was carried out in the neighborhoods targeted for intervention, and open-ended interviews were conducted with a sub-sample of injectors who were also recruited as subjects for the survey instrument designed to assess HIV risk behavior" (Koester 1994: 288).

Like other ethnographers working in the HIV pandemic, Koester (1994: 289) found that the notion of "sharing" is a misnomer because it "implied that the exchange of a syringe between users is conscious and deliberate, and that it occurs as an act of reciprocity." In fact, long-term injectors have several motivations not to share needles. Many have contracted hepatitis B from previously used needles and are aware that there are health risks involved in this behavior. Moreover, the needle on a standard diabetic syringe loses its sharpness with each subsequent use, making it harder and more painful to penetrate a vein. Additionally, used needles clog up (because of blood coagulation), which slows the relief that drugs offer the addicted individual. Also, because using a previously used needle means possibly injecting the blood of another individual into your body, there is a potential for "an unpleasant experience called a 'bone-crusher'" (Page, Smith, and Kane 1991: 71) if the two blood types are not compatible. Despite these multiple disincentives, Koester (1994: 292–293) argues that drug injectors still use previously used syringes because

Sharing syringes and injecting in high-risk environs like shooting galleries are not maladaptive rituals of a vast drug subculture, and they do not necessarily occur because of poor planning on the part of street-based injectors. On the contrary, these high-risk activities often continue as deliberate responses to what drug injectors perceive as a more immediate threat than HIV infection. Laws criminalizing syringe possession have made drug injectors hesitant about carrying them, especially during the times they are trying to obtain drugs. As a result, users are frequently without syringes when they are ready and eager to inject.

In other words, syringe reuse is, in part, a product of a set of laws and a set of practices among law enforcement agencies. As long as laws against purchasing syringes or possessing syringes without a prescription exist and are enforced by the police, drug injectors are forced to make use of previously used syringes if they are the only injection equipment they can get their hands on at a time of addictive drug craving. There is no evidence that laws that regulate injection equipment prevent drug abuse. However, they do, Koester maintains, promote the spread of HIV disease. Exemplary is a Scottish study that found that in Glasgow in Scotland, where the police were not enforcing needle possession laws, the rate of HIV infection among drug injectors was 5 percent. In nearby Edinburgh, where needle possession laws were strictly enforced, the rate of infection among injectors was 50 percent (Convisier and Rutledge 1989).

Why do ineffective and even counterproductive laws stay on the books, and why are laws that promote disease and death in one sector of the population enforced, often intensely so? Why do societies have unhealthy health policies (Castro and Singer 2004)? As Michael Parenti (1980: 120–121), a critical political scientist, has written,

Since we have been taught to think of the law as an institution serving the entire community and to view its representatives—from the traffic cop to the Supreme Court justice—as guardians of our rights, it is discomforting to discover that laws are often written and enforced in the most tawdry racist, classist and sexist ways.... Far from being a neutral instrument, the law belongs to those who write it and use it—primarily those who control the resources of society. It is no accident that in most conflicts between the propertied and the propertyless, the law intervenes on the side of the former.

Although there are doctors and lawyers who are drug addicts (indeed, those in demanding, stressful professions tend to have comparatively high rates of drug abuse), the individuals who are most subject to syringe prescription and possession laws tend to be poor and African American or Hispanic. These individuals have little in the way of status, wealth, or power and hence little influence on lawmakers. Dorie Klein (1983: 33), a criminologist with a long-standing interest in drug policy, in fact, argues that a review of the enactment of drug policies shows that they are "part of a larger state project of social control." Similarly, the enforcement of possession and prescription laws is not automatic. Indeed, "[n]onenforcement of the law is common in such areas as price fixing, restraint of trade, tax evasion, environmental and consumer protection, child labor and minimum wage" (Parenti 1980: 123). A study by the New York court system (reported in Parenti 1980) found that individuals arrested for small-time drug dealing receive harsher sentences than those convicted of big-time security fraud, kickbacks, bribery, and embezzlement, so-called white-collar crimes that tend to be committed by comparatively wealthy white males. As these examples suggest, risk behavior among drug users unfolds within a sociopolitical context; the nature of class, race, and other relations that comprise this context may be of far greater importance in determining risk than the rituals or values of the subculture of drug users.

In addition to looking at on the ground observable behaviors, ethnographers have looked beyond the local level of illicit drug acquisition, consumption patterns, and health effects to the place of drug use and drug users in the wider political economy and in light of sweeping globalization even among previously remote peoples (S. Lin 2011). One of the most extensive efforts to develop a critical approach to illicit substance abuse is Allise Waterston's (1993) book, *Street Addicts in the Political Economy*. In this volume, which is based on the analysis of an extensive set of interviews conducted with active street drug users in New York City, Waterston disputes many of the conventional truisms about street drug users and the causes of their behavior. While recognizing the achievements of earlier ethnographic studies of the daily life and system of cultural meanings embraced by street users begun during the 1960s, Waterston (1993: 27) ultimately is critical of the tendency in these studies to portray their subjects as if they constituted "distinct and autonomous social phenomena." By exoticizing street drug users as a distinct group with their own unique and insulated subcultural system of behaviors and beliefs, the early studies, she believes, failed to examine the "basic social forces, such as economic activities, class conflict, and labor-market composition" (Waterston 1993: 29) that drive behavioral patterns as well as the web of meanings and beliefs said to be part of the drug subculture. It is Waterston's critical anthropology argument that the "drug scene" described by earlier ethnographers is, in fact, not an independent cultural development at all but rather is a product of a particular stage in the evolution of a particular type of political economic system, one that many writers have referred to as "late capitalism." In this political economy, street drug users serve identifiable roles and functions. First, they form a pool of cheap, expendable, and highly disorganized laborers, taking odd jobs as they can for minimal pay and without health benefits or occupational safety protection. Second, they serve an ideological role as a "scapegoat of the bourgeoisie, always ready to feed the fires of xenophobia and racism" (Castells 1975: 33). Street drug users, in other words, represent an example of what sociologists call a "negative reference group," a group that can be pointed to as an example of what happens to those who reject conventional values and behavior. Moreover, by having drug users to point to as a primary source of social problems and community fear (up to and including, in some federal antidrug commercials, terrorism), the larger system of extreme social inequality and unequal distribution of wealth is shielded from public scrutiny or concern. Finally, she argues, drug addiction pacifies unrest in the most oppressed sectors of society. Illustrating this point, Waterston (1993: 233) cites the following comment by a drug addict she called Carl: "I was willing, able, and ready to fight anyone. I felt powerful, and I wouldn't allow anyone to put a damper on that." But once he discovered tranquilizer, narcotic-type drugs, [Waterston observed] Carl's violence ended, and he was back in the womb—warm, protected—and numb to the world emotionally. Any resistance by street drug users to the structures of dominance in society is "highly individualistic, privatized and self-destructive" (Waterston 1993: 244). Although many of drug user activities are illegal, and participants, to some degree, enjoy being outside of the law, ultimately drug subculture accommodates rather than challenges the status quo. It could also be argued that because many street drug users engage in various property crimes, including shoplifting, burglary, and mugging, and because some of what they steal is taken from the middle class and sold at below market value to poor and working people, they serve to control social unrest by redistributing social wealth. Following Leeds, Waterston concludes that Leeds is correct in asserting that the so-called drug subculture should not be viewed as a "bounded and self-perpetuating design for living" but rather as a set of social "responses to adversity as it is structured within a particular social system" (Leeds 1971: 15–16).

An effort to situate drug use within its encompassing historic and political economic contexts can also be found in the work of Merrill

Singer, who was involved in the study of drug use in the Puerto Rican and African American communities of Hartford, Connecticut, between 1988 and 2008. One of the goals of this research program was the development of an understanding of the sociopolitical origin and spread of injection drug use among Puerto Ricans, and the particular pattern that marks Puerto Rican drug injection. According to Singer (1995b), Puerto Rican illicit drug use dates to the late 1940s and early 1950s, as large numbers of Puerto Ricans were migrating to the United States from the island. As U.S. citizens, a status conferred on them in 1917 so that they could be drafted to fight in the U.S. armed forces during World War I, Puerto Ricans were free to travel and relocate to the mainland. After the war, many were attracted to the United States by the loss of jobs brought on by industrialization of agriculture on the island and the appeal of U.S. agribusiness seeking cheap labor. What they encountered upon arrival in the United States was a society that did not understand or respect them. Trapped by racism, a shifting economy, and other structural forces plaguing the American underclasses, Puerto Ricans found themselves "limited to the poorest-paying jobs and to the most dilapidated housing and with only limited access to education and other public services" (Meier and Rivera 1972: 257). These conditions created sharp tensions that were multiplied by overcrowding; being forced by low income to dwell in high-crime, inner-city areas; and facing daily rebuke from the dominant society. In addition to the trauma born of severe economic disadvantage, Puerto Ricans endured a number of other stressful life experiences, including pressure to learn a new language; cultural differences with the dominant society; intergenerational conflict as parents and children come to have differing values and beliefs; and a sense of failure produced by an inability to fulfill traditional role obligations (such as being good family providers for men and protective, nurturing mothers and wives for women).

In addition, they encountered heroin, a wonder drug that appeared to offer relief from their daily misery. Singer (1995b) reports that during the nine-year period between 1941 and 1950, only twenty adolescents were admitted to Bellevue Hospital in New York as drug addicts (six of them in 1950). However, in January and February of 1951, sixty-five boys and nineteen girls were admitted with this diagnosis. A study conducted in the early 1950s of twenty-two of these youth, most of whom were Puerto Rican or African American, found that they "suffered psychologically from the discriminatory practices and attitudes directed against their racial groups. They feel more keenly than other national minorities that they live in an alien, hostile culture. . . . They suffer almost continuous injuries to their self-esteem" (Zimmering et al. 1951).

These youth were similar to Ramon Colon (pseudonym), a Puerto Rican man interviewed by Singer in the late 1980s in Hartford, Connecticut. Born in East Harlem in 1939, Ramon recalled that he first began to hear about heroin from his friends in about 1947. He stated,

When heroin came into our neighborhood, we were 13 or 14 years old, in middle school. Latinos, African Americans, and Italians all started using at the same time. We would play stick ball in the street and pass a bag around to get loaded. We didn't know anything about addiction. Heroin was as easy to get as candy then, it was everywhere and it was pure. One time the baseball player, Frankie Robinson, came to our school to talk and I bet every kid in that room had a bag of dope in his pocket. I learned about it first from a neighbor who lived upstairs in our building. I began to dip into his stuff. We frowned on guys that were shooting up then. For the first six months it was just snorting. My brother put it up his nose for four years before he started shooting. My cousin snorted for seven years. But I told them they were wasting their dope and got them into shooting. I watched some older boys shoot up on the roof at first. They would skin pop me. People in our building would stash "works" [syringes and cookers] in the basement of the building. I would find them. That was how I got my first set of works. Before dope, it was really a nice neighborhood, nobody locked their doors. But with drugs, everything deteriorated, it became mean. (Quoted in Singer and Jia 1993: 231)

Characteristics of the youth who formed the first generation of Puerto Rican drug injectors suggest a pattern that Singer argues has typified many Puerto Rican addicts ever since. Most of these youth appear to suffer from a condition that Singer and his colleague Elizabeth Toledo have labeled *oppression illness*. They use this term to refer to the chronic traumatic effects of experiencing racism, classism (i.e., disdain and mistreatment of the poor and working class), and related oppression over long periods of time (especially during critical developmental periods of identity formation), combined with the negative emotional effects of intense self-disparagement associated with being the enduring target of social bigotry. Among Puerto Ricans suffering from oppression illness, Singer has described a pattern of feeling that they do not deserve to be respected while, nonetheless, intensely desiring respect (*respeto*) and dignity (*dignidad*), core values in Puerto Rican culture.

In addition to examination of the "demand" side of drug use (i.e., users) anthropologists have also looked at the supply side (i.e., dealers). This work began with Patricia Adler's (1993) study of a middle-class drug smuggling ring in a wealthy California neighborhood. Based on six years of fieldwork, Adler (1993: 144) noted, "Organized crime is a society that seeks to operate outside the control of the American people and their governments. It involves thousands of criminals, working within structures as complex as those of any large corporation, subject to laws more rigidly enforced than those of legitimate governments. Its actions are not impulsive but rather the result of intricate conspiracies, carried on over many years and aimed at gaining control over whole fields of activity in order to amass huge profits." Another extensive study in this regard is Enrique Arias's (2006) examination of drug trafficking, drug gangs, the police and political elites in Rio de Janeiro, Brazil. Unlike the dealers studied by Adler, drug traffickers in the shantytowns of Brazil are impoverished, poorly educated, adolescents of color. As individuals, they are disempowered, discriminated against, and tightly policed. Collectively, as drug gang members, however, they wield substantial power, sufficient to establish their own mini-states within the confines of a metropolitan city. In his research in Denver, Lee Hoffer (2006) focused on one small heroin distribution team that involved a partnership between two street drug addicts. They supported their addiction through the sale of small quantities of drugs to fellow users in their impoverished neighborhood. Using a different tack, Singer and Mirhej (2004) examined local systems of drug preparation and sales on the streets of Hartford, Connecticut, including the role of street gangs in this activity. Of concern in this study was the role of supply-side issues, including police control efforts, in creating drug-related health risks.

In addition to the major illicit drugs, in recent years drug users, from youth to experienced street drug addicts have turned increasingly to the use of diverted pharmaceutical drugs (Singer 2006a). In a study of nonprescription use of pharmaceutical drugs among youth, Quintero and Nichter (2012) found that youth obtain these drugs from leftover prescribed medications, peer networks, and parents or through burglary. Their appeal resides both in their ready availability and their established dosage, as well as the demand for self-medication in light of the growing pressures of unemployment distress, uncertain futures, and boredom in economically troubled times.

DRUG CAPITALISM

Although the production and worldwide flow of "legal" drugs such as tobacco, pharmaceuticals, and alcohol are included as part of the discussion of globalization, what of illicit drugs such as heroin, cocaine, and marijuana? Do contemporary processes of globalization—which generally are seen has being driven by corporate productive activities, restructuring of labor, communication technologies, and distribution of commodities—include illegal drugs? Are legal corporations one kind of production and marketing organization and illegal mafias and cartels another kind of production and marketing organization?

As David Courtwright (1991) notes, "Casks of rum, bundles of kola nuts, bricks of opium, and kilos of cocaine are so many commodities." All of these, as well as bales of marijuana, bottles of methamphetamine, sheets of LSD-laced paper, and jars of ecstasy pills, are consumable psychotropic commodities—that is to say, they are chemical substances that are commercially produced through a system of wage labor (although, like many farm products, some begin with the work of small farmers) and are commercially distributed (again through a system of wage labor) in a market economy, where they find their way into the hands and bodies of consumers. Having unique features (e.g., their legal status) does not mean they are not commodities any more than the fact that organizations engaged in the criminal production of illicit drugs are not corporations (if they are structured and generally act like corporations, even if they are not legally recognized). We argue that it is not the nature of its impact on the consumer that determines what is and what is not a commodity nor is it the legal status of the products it produces that defines a corporation (e.g., even legal corporations engage in a considerable amount of illegal and risky behavior, often on a repetitive basis). Consider the 2010 Deepwater Horizon Gulf of Mexico oil spill. This catastrophe, which was far from the first such spill in the Gulf, poured about five billion barrels of crude oil into the environment in the largest accidental release of oil into marine waters and "involved an oil rig built in South Korea that was operated by a Swiss firm under contract to a British company [BP] and was registered in the Marshall Islands, which held the primary responsibility for safety and other inspections" (Horowitz 2012: 21). This transnational decentralized corporate model is of note because illicit drug corporations increasingly are structured in the same way. This is not the only parallel between legal and illegal corporations, with many of the negative attributes attributed to illegal drug corporations being equally true of legal ones (Singer 2008).

This focus on commodities and their production raises a question: Why do commodities matter? One might say, aren't they just "things" we buy and use? Anthropologists Sidney Mintz (1985) and Eric Wolf (1982), however, both argue that the production and sale of things of value is far more than the mere economic exchange of inert objects because while society makes commodities, the opposite is true as well. As Alfred McCoy (undated) notes, "Since the rise of the modern world economy, commodities have—in a fundamental sense—shaped the politics, culture, and social structure of peoples around the globe." Thus, Mintz points out that the social adoption of an item like sweetened hot tea, a stimulant, as a mainstay of the diet of the British and later other working classes was a momentous historic event signaling the transformation of a whole society, including its economic configuration, its culturally constituted patterns of consumption, to say nothing of the daily routines of life and the cultural definitions of pleasure. The same is true of opium (the source of heroin), a commodity that from the eighteenth century on has strongly influenced relations and commerce between Asia, Europe, and North America (and now South America), becoming deeply embedded in the economies and cultures of all of these regions.

Many drugs have become truly global commodities; they originate in various places, pass through many others, and arrive for consumption in additional locations around the world. But not all parts of the world are equally affected by the flow of various drugs across national borders on their way from production, to refinement, to repackaging and shipment, and ultimately to the most lucrative terminal markets (i.e., wealthy countries), where high demand and risk inflate prices to consumers and profits to distributors. At the same time, global transformations of other sorts, such as international labor migration, have reshaped drug consumption patterns while workers are abroad and when (and if) they return home. Other global processes, such as transnational natural resource extraction, can undermine the physical environments and subsistence strategies of local populations having impact as a result on motivations for and patterns of drug consumption and involvement in drug production (as a new means of livelihood).

The commodification of drugs is driven by a dual drug industry involving both legal and illegal drug production and marketing (Singer 2008), with one segment being above ground producing and distributing casks of rum or cartons of cigarettes and the other being below ground producing and distributing bricks of opium or kilos of cocaine. Importantly, legal (above ground) and illegal (below ground) drug corporations are more closely linked and aligned than is commonly imagined. Furthermore, both can be analyzed as integral if somewhat different components of global drug capitalism and thus part of the wider capitalist economy. Whereas the above-ground sector of the dual drug industry tends to be wrapped in a cloak of social legitimacy, the underground sector generally suffers the stain of illegality, contrasting social positions that have significant consequences. For example, legal drug corporations can use the police to control their labor problems and the mass media to promote their psychoactive products. Illegal corporations have the same needs but must use other means to fulfill them (e.g., private armies, control of drug selling locations). Functionally, however, legal and illegal drug companies are but two sides of the same coin. They have common impacts on individuals and on society. For example, they both provide drugs to the poor and working classes and thereby help to maintain the existing pattern of pervasive social and health disparities among the socioeconomic strata.

CONCLUSION: THE TOMORROW
OF THE ANTHROPOLOGY OF ADDICTION

Although anthropology was in some ways a late arrival to the multi-disciplinary field of drug addiction research, it has gained purchase and substantial impact because of the strengths of ethnography; the power of the cultural model; the concern with emic understandings, lived experience, and subjectivities; the stress put on understanding pathways of bio-social interactions; the cross-societal breadth of its gaze; and the linkage of the microworld of experience and the macro-world of political economy and globalism. The future of the anthropology of drug use will be shaped by continued reexamination of the ethnographic approach in light of ongoing challenges, documenting the role of drug research as a valued arena of anthropological work, increasing ethnographic involvement in both examining and enhancing harm reduction, treatment and recovery, investigating user perception of drug risks and benefits, assessing the role of drug and alcohol use in work migrants and immigrant populations, assessment of discourses on drugs and security, ethnographically examining global drug distribution networks, and investigating societal response to the failure of the global war on drugs.

CHAPTER 9

AIDS and Infectious Diseases

HIV DISEASE: THIRTY YEARS AND COUNTING

At the time of this writing, the global HIV pandemic is now more than thirty years old. This disease is destined to take a greater toll on our species, proportionately and in terms of absolute numbers, than the bubonic plague, smallpox, and tuberculosis combined (Whelehan 2009). As a result, the pandemic has helped to shape the social, cultural, and health worlds of people living in all corners of the planet, whether they are always aware of it or not. Millions of people have grown up in a world in which AIDS has been present and known to them their entire lives. Yet since its discovery in 1981, there have been dramatic changes in our understanding of HIV as well as in our ability to treat the disease. One of the things that has been learned is that HIV is far older than thirty years. Also, we have come to understand that within the broader story of the devastating global impact of HIV, there are many differing local narratives that together comprise the complex mosaic of the global pandemic. In this chapter, we examine AIDS—or as it is increasingly called today, HIV disease—historically, socially, and biologically as a disease of a globalizing world and of local social settings. Also of critical importance to the chapter is the role anthropology has played in the pandemic globally and locally.

HIV Disease Today

Given the significant changes that have occurred in the world of HIV disease since this book was originally published in 1997, it seems appropriate to start at the front edge of the pandemic or where things are at more than thirty years since HIV disease was first discovered. In recent years, the HIV narrative has begun to shed its earlier catastrophic tone (replaced by the public health idiom of disease chronicity), major international health bodies like the World Health Organization and UNAIDS have suggested that the pandemic is losing momentum (as other daunting threats, like global warming, have moved increasingly into public focus), and even some established AIDS researchers have questioned the significant allotment of global HIV funding in light of the many other pressing health issues (e.g., lack of clean water, malnutrition, childhood diarrhea) faced by the developing world. Although it may be wishful thinking, and something that has been falsely assumed before in the pandemic, there is a celebratory sense among many people who work on HIV disease today that we are approaching the end of the pandemic as we have known it. For example, Anthony Fauci (2012), director of the U.S. National Institute of Allergy and Infectious Diseases at the National Institutes of Health, believes that the "scientific basis" exists to consider the possibility of a generation free of HIV disease. Around the world this disease has already killed more than 30 million people, 34.2 million people are living with HIV infection, 2.5 million people were first infected in 2011 (or almost 7,000 per day), in some populations rates of infection continue to grow, about one in five people who is infected does not know it, and the disease remains highly stigmatized. Thus, an AIDS-free generation would be no small accomplishment.

Yet even Fauci, who emphasizes the extraordinary accumulation of HIV knowledge since 1981, is cautious about overstating the elimination of HIV disease in the near future. Currently, HIV treatments, although an enormous advance (marked by ever more effect, ever more tolerable medicines, and the development of almost thirty approved antiretroviral drugs), must be continued for life, or the disease will rebound and the body will again be under attack from replicating the virus. These drugs suppress HIV, but the virus persists in reservoirs within the body. Curing the disease, however—that is, treating people and have them be virus-free afterward—remains a formidable scientific project for a number of reasons (Richman et al. 2009), including the virus' ability to "hide" in various sanctuary sites within the body, such the central nervous system, the lymph system, the intestinal system, and latently infected CD4 cells (in which HIV lies dormant—and out of reach of current HIV medications—until activated by various factors including infection with another disease; Lafeuillade 2011). Although there is some evidence that a drug called vorinostat that is used to treat some types of lymphoma may be able to dislodge hidden virus in patients receiving treatment for HIV, findings are still preliminary (Archin et al. 2012).

Additionally, there are four challenges that affect the effectiveness of HIV medicines. The first of these is the development of HIV resistance to existing drugs, as has occurred with medications used to treat other conditions such as tuberculosis. The second concerns the long-term toxicity of even new, low-toxicity HIV medications, resulting in the buildup of toxins in the body, which promotes heart disease, diabetes, liver disease, neurocognitive defects, frailty, and some forms of cancer. Third, there are the challenges of reaching certain populations with HIV medications and the societal will to do so (especially those that are poor and marginalized). Currently two-thirds of people living with HIV infection reside in poorer countries of the world, and significant disparities in HIV infection exist across groups defined by ethnicity, social class, and sexual orientation. Reaching the poor (in wealthy, middle-income, and poor countries), for example, requires a commitment of adequate funding, campaigns to overcome stigma, and conducive pro-health public policies—three things that have often been less than optimal since the beginning of the pandemic. Additionally, almost five million people aged 15 to 24 are living with HIV infection, and two-thirds of them are girls or young women, a group that in many contexts has especially constrained access to health and other social resources. Finally, there are the challenges of keeping people on medication for many decades, a psychosocial phenomenon called "pill burden" under changing economic circumstances, as people age, when they suffer multiple diseases each with their own treatment regimen, and when they are born with HIV disease and grow tired of always being a patient. Despite these issues, some HIV disease researchers now talk about the achievability of what they call a "functional cure," of the HIV pandemic as we know it (as contrasted with a full or sterilizing cure)—namely, a state, at the individual level of the infected patient, in which there is no disease progression, no virus transmission to others, and a life expectancy that is close to that of uninfected individuals. Other components of a functional cure would be the following: no new infants born with HIV, a sharp decrease in the global incidence (i.e., new cases) of HIV infection, and enrolling everyone who is infected in HIV treatment and assisting them to lead a relatively normal life and stay on medication.

Contributing to achieving a functional cure of HIV disease have been advances in prevention. Significant here are the administration of drugs to prevent in utero mother-to-child transmission of the virus; properly administered male circumcision (an approach first suggested by anthropologists; Bongaarts et al. 1989), which has been proven in clinical trials in Kenya and Uganda to reduce heterosexual men's risk of acquiring HIV by 50 to 60 percent (Bailey et al. 2007); antiretroviral-based preexposure prophylaxis (called PrEP) under controlled conditions (that is, administering HIV medications to uninfected individuals to protect them from becoming infected); use of microbicides applied on the genital mucosa during sex; and treatment as prevention (i.e., lowering risk of transmission of HIV to others through medication). These approaches too have their challenges. For example, medically administered circumcision or taking PrEP drugs can falsely convince people they are immune to HIV risk and are free to engage in highly risky behaviors without fear of infection. By way of analogy, in research in which anthropologists participated, it was shown that people who are administered oral HIV testing come to believe (incorrectly) that HIV can be readily transmitted orally (and hence, why bother with condoms; Clair et al. 2003, 2009). In other words, interventions can, unintentionally, send the wrong message resulting in increased not decreased risk. Additionally, PrEP drugs raise questions about participant adherence, the development of drug resistance, bodily tolerance, longer-term effects, drug interactions, real-life context factors that differ from clinical trial control contexts, and the impacts of other diseases a participant might have on PrEP effectiveness.

As this brief review of the state of the HIV-disease pandemic suggests, although we stand far closer than ever before to the functional elimination of the HIV disease pandemic (although have many years to go to achieve a full elimination of the disease), further progress continues not only to hinge on advances in biomedicine but also, as emphasized in this chapter, to involve the interface of health with political, economic, cultural, and social factors, arenas of special concern to medical anthropologists and the primary arenas of their contributions to responding to HIV. To emphasize this point, consider this example: there are a billion people in the world today, one out of every seven people on the planet, who do not get enough food to be healthy and lead an active life. Yet from a "treatment" standpoint we know exactly how to eliminate this grave threat to global health: provide an adequate diet. That we have not solved this problem suggests why biomedical solutions alone will not end the AIDS pandemic.

Beyond the now rapidly advancing biomedical developments in the field of HIV treatment (including recent use of bone marrow transplant as a means of clearing the body of the virus), there is the issue of *changes in the world* that also shape the face of the pandemic. Globalization (and, especially, corporate globalization), for example, has produced a rapid flow of information (and advertisement) around the world. One effect this is having on HIV is that ideas about modernity, based usually on Western images, are impacting the behavior of people everywhere, especially youth and young adults. The term *global youth culture* has been used to refer to the emergence of a complex (and locally varied) hybrid popular culture and identity found increasingly among youth and young adults (the 1.1 billion people between fifteen and twenty-four years of age) throughout the world as a result of the broad proliferation of electronic media including popular music and music videos, movies, television, the Internet, and other communication technologies. To cite one anecdotal (and overly homogenized) depiction of this phenomenon, a piece that appeared in *Marketing News* (2002) several years ago reported: "Last year I was in 17 countries, and it's pretty difficult to find anything that is different, other than language, among a teenager in Japan, a teenager in the U.K. and a teenager in China." One of the issues raised by global youth culture is the growing acceptance of HIV risk behaviors as part of living a modern lifestyle. For example, with reference to youth in Thailand, the Institute for Population and Social Research (2005: 1) reports

Young people in Thailand are struggling to navigate a rapidly changing environment, frequently experimenting as they go. This struggle is reflected in some alarming new trends, such as steadily increasing rates of new HIV infections among 15–24 year olds—in spite of declining rates among other age groups. . . . [A] "global youth culture" is exposing young people to goods and lifestyles that encourage risk-taking.

As a result of these changes, young people in Thailand (and elsewhere) are more likely than previous generations to have sex in dating relationships. While condoms may be available, drinking and drug use, also promoted in global youth culture, reduce the likelihood of their use.

Another example of changes in the world that impact the pandemic involves the emergence of "new populations" that are put at risk for HIV infection because of the nature of their social situation. A case in point is the sizeable group in China, the world's most populous country, known as the *floating population* (*liudong renkou*; B. Li 2007). This is a group of people, estimated to number 120 million workers (many of whom being rural-to-urban economic migrants), who are "floating" in the sense that they are not settled in permanent residences, may move from place to place seeking work and often have unstable work situations. This group has emerged in response to fast-paced development in China, including a significant demand for labor in construction, hotels, restaurants, and other industries. Another factor in the appearance of the floating population has to do with policy changes in China. Before the late 1980s, China's system of household registration, the *hukou*, constrained people living in rural areas from moving to other provinces or to urban areas. The need for labor to construct the new China, however, pushed for a lifting of travel restrictions.

For the most part, this group consists of young, poorly educated individuals who are in the most sexually active period of their lives but lack ready access to HIV prevention education and resources. Males comprise the majority of the floating population. Many are away from home most of the year, often live in single-sex dormitory housing structures, and work long hours under difficult conditions. Consequently, they offer a potential market for drug sellers and commercial sex workers (many of whom also are migrants from rural areas) and have motivation to seek out their escapes from the day-to-day burdens of their difficult lives. Being far from home and from traditional family behavioral controls, they are also less constrained by the conservative norms common in their hometowns and villages. There is considerable concern that the instability and vulnerability of this huge population may contribute to risky sexual practices or drug use that rapidly accelerates HIV disease in China (Anderson et al. 2003). Because of their mobility and involvement in risky practices, the floating population may serve as a bridge group for HIV to the general population and for spreading the virus from higher-prevalence to lower-prevalence areas of the country. The existence of floating populations is not unique to China (e.g., the term is also used in India), indicating the global significance of this sociodemographic shift.

As these two examples suggest, HIV disease today is different from when it emerged in the early 1908s, but not only because of medical advancements. Changes in social patterns, economic structures and relationships, and ideologies are of equal importance.

The Making of the Pandemic

After many years of debate about the origin of HIV infection as a human disease, the historic facts are now becoming clear. Current research suggests a history of at least a hundred years. Thus, an international team of scientists (Worobey et al. 2008) studying human tissue samples that had been preserved for nearly fifty years concluded that the disease moved into human populations between 1884 and 1924, at the same time that urbanization starting to take off in west central Africa. Urbanization of colonial Africa created the conditions that allowed the most pervasive strain of HIV, the HIV-1 group M, to spread rapidly among humans (e.g., dense city populations primarily composed of young, sexually active adults).

Previously, a viral ancestor of HIV had made the zoonotic jump from nonhuman primates to humans involving SIV (simian immunodeficiency virus) evolving into HIV. Notably, at least half, and perhaps far more of all known infectious agents are of nonhuman animal origin (e.g., tuberculosis, influenza, plague); in fact an assessment of more than 1,400 pathogens that afflict humans found that 61 percent spread to humans from animals (L. Taylor, Latham, and Woolhouse 2001). Over time, and as a result of contact, some pathogens acquired the ability to spread to, live in, and successfully reproduce in the bodies of a new host species: humans. In the case of HIV-1, the original host was chimpanzees, and the jump to humans probably occurred in the late nineteenth century. HIV-2 likely jumped to humans from sooty mangabey monkeys early in the twentieth century. More recently, a new type of HIV was discovered in Cameroon, and it appears to have evolved from SIV$_{gorilla}$.

One model of interspecies pathogen transmission is called the Hunter Theory. In this scenario, SIV$_{cpz}$ was transferred to humans as a result of chimps being killed and eaten (called *bush meat*) or their blood getting into cuts or wounds on the hunter. This practice is not uncommon worldwide, including hunting deer for meat in the United States. Normally, the hunter's body would have fought off SIV, but mutations in the virus allowed it to transition to the new human host and become HIV-1. Given the high mutation rate of the virus and growing human penetration of forested areas in Africa, this transition is not surprising.

An article published in *The Lancet* in 2004 (Wolfe et al. 2004), reveals how retroviral transfer from primates to hunters is still occurring today. In a sample of 1,099 individuals in Cameroon, they discovered ten (1 percent) were infected with SFV (simian foamy virus), an illness that, like SIV, was previously thought only to infect primates. But the role of social factors in the transfer of SIV (chimpanzee) to HIV (human) should not be overlooked. During the late nineteenth and early twentieth century, much of Africa was ruled by colonial forces. In areas such as French Equatorial Africa and the Belgian Congo, colonial rule was particularly harsh, and many Africans were forced into labor camps where sanitation was poor, food was scarce, and physical demands were extreme. These factors would have been sufficient to create poor health, so SIV could have infiltrated the labor force following exposure through consuming wild-caught bush meat and evolved into HIV.

The earliest known cases of HIV were found in plasma samples taken in 1959 and 1960 in the Democratic Republic of the Congo and subsequently stored. Analysis of genetic changes between these two samples and more recent samples of HIV suggest a history of HIV that dates to the late nineteenth century. This event may have coincided with the development of colonial cities like Kinshasa with high population density and radically increased opportunities for exposure over previous years. Present-day Kinshasa, in the Democratic Republic of the Congo, was once the hub of Belgium's colonial presence in Africa. The colony went through swift urban growth at the turn of the nineteenth century, as did the neighboring areas, during a period that matches the earliest spread of HIV among humans. Genetic diversity found in the virus by Worobey and coworkers (2008) suggests that a lot of people in the area were already infected by 1960, and from there it spread to the rest of the world, until 1981 when it came first to U.S. and then global public awareness.

Changes in human ecology (i.e., in our relationship to the environment, including changes we make in the environment, intentionally and unintentionally), like what happened in Kinshasa, results in changes in the microbes that populate our bodies and our infectious disease–related health. During much of our evolutionary history, hominid ancestors of modern humans foraged the African savanna as small, nomadic bands of foragers. Early hominid populations likely were too small and dispersed to support many of the acute communicable pathogens. Viruses, such as chickenpox and herpes simplex, however, may survive in isolated family units, suggesting that they could have been sustained in early dispersed and nomadic population.

The current distribution of parasite species common to human and nonhuman primates provides evidence for longstanding hominid-parasite relationships that predate the divergence of the hominid lineage. As humans have evolved, so too have their infectious diseases. Some diseases that once were rare have become common, others have disappeared completely, and new infectious agents have emerged over time. Each pathogen that has infected humans has produced its own effects. Human ancestors, for example, were covered with hair; why did (most of us) become hairless (say compared to a chimp)? Hairiness, of course, has its evolutionary benefits: warmth most notably, and unlike reptilians, ability to be active at night. One theory (first suggested in the 1800s) of our evolutionary move toward hairlessness is the advantages it conferred in dealing with ectoparasites (e.g., lice, ticks, flies, fleas) and the infectious diseases they transmit. Notably, research has shown an association between recent involvement in body waxing and a drop in ectoparasites (W. Armstrong 2006).

But, of course, all of our closest primate relatives still are furry; what about them? In fact, they are quite covered with ectoparasites but may control them by moving their resting places nightly, engaging in social grooming, and having long-term relationships with their pathogens be-cause of less mobility and slower-changing lifestyles than humans (who enter new territories and acquire new zoonotics). So the issue is not biting ectoparasites per se (which is an irritant but not decisive from an evolu-tionary perspective), but the many, potentially lethal, diseases they trans-mit as vectors (e.g., plague, spotted fever, typhus, Lyme disease) that may be of evolutionary importance because of the survival benefits of reducing opportunities for infection.

The Pandemic Begins

The beginning of the AIDS pandemic—not the point at which the virus began to spread in human populations but the point at which people began to recognize this was happening—is not in dispute. During 1980, fifty-five young men in the United States, primarily self-identified gay men, were diagnosed with various diseases that ultimately came to be linked to HIV infection. The health problems of these men were noticed because they sought medical care; their physicians, in turn, unable to halt the infection with standard remedies, sought approval to use a second-line antibiotic (pentamidine) from the Centers for Disease Control (CDC). The first report of an emergent health problem suggested by the diseases of these men appeared on June 5, 1981, in a widely read public health publication, the CDC's *Morbidity and Mortality Weekly Report* (MMWR). This article, which focused on five cases from Los Angeles, did not mention that the people who were coming down with an unusual form of pneumonia were gay men. On July 4, 1981, however, the same publication carried a second article titled "Kaposi's Sarcoma and Pneumocystis Pneumonia among Homosexual Men—New York and California." This linkage of a rare cancer with a rare pneumonia (caused by a harmless parasite for those with healthy immune systems) in a geographically dispersed population defined by sexual orientation was startling. The story was picked up immediately in both the *New York Times* and the *Los Angeles Times* and soon found its way into the mass media throughout the country and soon the world

But epidemiologists and other health researchers were puzzled by the epidemic that appeared to be breaking out around them. Although it was clear that the disease was linked to a breakdown in the body's natural defense system, the immune system, the cause of immunosuppression (i.e., a breakdown of the immune system) was unclear. Was it the result of environmental conditions, dietary practices, a promiscuous fast-lane gay lifestyle, or the inhalation of amyl or butyl nitrite poppers to enhance sexual or dance-floor arousal? No one was sure. There was less uncertainty, or so it seemed, about who was becoming ill. In December 1981, David Durack wrote an editorial for the *New England Journal of Medicine* proposing a multifactorial disease model that centered on the interaction between recurrent sexually transmitted disease and popper use as the cause of immunosuppression in gay men. Before long, the term *gay plague* had made its way into popular discourse. The new disease complex appeared to single out and attack only gay men, particularly those with a promiscuous lifestyle. Ultimately the term *gay-related immune deficiency* (GRID) was suggested to label the new syndrome descriptively. In short order, San Francisco, especially the heavily gay-populated Castro Street area, came to be thought of as "AIDS City, U.S.A." (Shilts 1987: 268) in the popular imagination.

In this way, gay lifestyle (or one variant of what itself is a quite varied set of behaviors) became an intensified object of mainstream social derision; not only was it seen by many as being immoral, but now it could be said to be life-threatening as well. Some people began to see the new disease complex as divine punishment for violating religious prohibitions against homosexuality. In time, the same language of blame and punishment would be applied to illicit drug users infected with HIV and Haitians as well. In this way—involving the social linkage of disease with denigrated behaviors or identities—AIDS came to be a heavily stigmatized disease.

The actual term *acquired immunodeficiency syndrome* (AIDS) was introduced in 1982, when the growing number of blood transfusion cases made it clear that GRID or other gay-specific terms were problematic. But the cause of acquired immunodeficiency was still not clear. A number of scientists on both sides of the Atlantic became committed to finding the common cause of AIDS among gay men, injection drug users (IDUs), blood-transfusion recipients, and, in Africa, large numbers of non-drug-using heterosexual women and men. Many were now sure that a distinct pathogen had to be involved because patients did not share a common lifestyle or set of environmental conditions.

Blood transfusion cases soon made it clear that the pathogen in question had to be found in the blood. Cases of sexual transmission suggested that other body fluids harbored the pathogen as well. Then, on April 23, 1984, Margaret Heckler, secretary of the Department of Health and Human Services, held a press conference to announce that what she referred to as the long honor roll of American medicine and science had recorded another miracle; the virus that caused the new disease had been discovered. Flushed with confidence and enthusiasm, she also added that a vaccine to stop the virus would be ready for testing in two years, and, by implication, ready for human inoculation a few years thereafter, an achievement that several decades years later has yet to be added to the "honor roll" of medicine and science. The Heckler announcement created an international debate as well. For several subsequent years, disagreement raged over whether HIV was first isolated in France at the Pasteur Institute laboratory of Luc Montagnier or in the United States at the National Cancer Institute laboratory of Robert Gallo. Both labs were working feverishly on discovering the pathogenic cause of AIDS. Heckler's press conference, in fact, was designed to cut off the French and patriotically claim American credit for the discovery of HIV as well as the profits to be gained by designing a blood test to detect the virus. Anthropologically, these events are of interest because they reveal the underlying political-economic nature of scientific work. No less than disease itself, the treatment of disease is far more than a clinical issue, it is at the same time a lucrative economic and a political one as well. Ultimately, Gallo and Montagnier agreed to share credit for the discovery, but tension continued for years. The April 11, 1983, issue of *Newsweek*, which carried a cover story labeling AIDS the "Public Health Threat of the Century," signified a new era in media coverage. Notes Shilts (1987: 267): "In the first three months of 1983, 169 stories about the epidemic had run in the nation's major newspapers and newsmagazines, four times the number of the last three months of 1982.

Moreover, from April through June, these major news organs published an astonishing 680 stories." The pandemic, as we have known it, had begun.

HIV disease was coming to be recognized as a major health problem, one that was not narrowly limited to any specific population subgroup. With this recognition, the level of public hysteria about HIV disease began to grow enormously. These might be thought of as the panic years in the HIV disease pandemic, a period when a growing list of well-known actors, sports stars, and other performers either died of AIDS or publicly shared their HIV status. A sense of mounting vulnerability developed in the general public, as did growing political pressure for massive government action to respond to the HIV crisis. Political activism around HIV disease was successful during this period in significantly increasing the level of government spending on research, prevention, and treatment.

Social Aspects of the Pandemic

Early in the epidemic, it was realized that HIV disease spreads "along the fault lines of . . . society and becomes a metaphor for understanding . . . society" (Bateson and Goldsby 1988: 2), and further, that it has exposed the "hidden vulnerabilities in the human condition" (Fineberg 1988: 128). In other words, while certainly a biological phenomenon, HIV disease cannot really be understood only in biological or clinical terms. The disease interacts with human societies and the social relationships that constitute them to create the global "HIV pandemic," that is, the unequal global distribution of the disease and the social response to it in particular groups and populations. By referring to HIV disease as a metaphor for society, Bateson and Goldsby draw attention to an issue that will be of central concern in this chapter—namely, the way in which the HIV disease crisis and the disturbing pattern of distribution of HIV infection expose the nature and consequences of social inequality within and between nations and groups in the contemporary world. Glaring disparities in the distribution of HIV disease have inspired a hunt for cofactors that facilitate the spread of HIV in groups with disproportionate rates of infection. For example, genital ulcerative diseases such as chancroid and syphilis, because they cause open wounds in the genital area that might allow the movement of body fluids and the pathogens they might contain (see Chapter 11), have been explored successfully as prompters of the person-to-person spread of HIV infection. However, notes Farmer (1999: 51–52):

To date, not a single one of these associations has been convincingly shown to explain disparities in distribution or outcome of HIV disease. The most well-demonstrated co-factors are social inequalities, which structure not only the contours of the AIDS pandemic but also the nature of outcomes once an individual is sick with complications of HIV infection.

Farmer's assertion is validated by existing studies of the relationship of AIDS to economic deprivation and poverty. These studies (conducted by different groups of researchers) consistently show that HIV infection occurs disproportionately and at a growing rate of disproportion among the poor and socially deprived. For example, Zierler (2000) and her coworkers in Boston found that neighborhood levels of economic deprivation and population density are strong predictors of incidence of AIDS in Massachusetts. Comparing the least and most economically deprived street blocks in the state, they found that poorest neighborhoods had an excess of 309 AIDS cases per 100,000 population. Similarly, the most densely populated blocks had an excess of 333 AIDS cases per 100,000 compared with the least densely populated blocks. The highest rates of AIDS were found among non-Hispanic African American men who lived in the most densely populated areas. The group with the second highest rate of HIV disease was composed of non-Hispanic black men and Hispanic men who lived in the most impoverished areas. The lowest rate of HIV disease in Massachusetts was among white women who lived in the wealthiest neighborhoods. In short, the greatest risk factors for HIV disease are being poor and being an oppressed ethnic minority; notably, these are not behavioral factors (of the sort that commonly are linked to HIV disease) but, instead, are reflections of the health effects of the reigning structures of social inequality.

In exploring the relationship between HIV disease and social structure, it is important to begin by emphasizing that the HIV crisis exploded rapidly. Soon after its discovery, HIV disease came to be recognized as a leading cause of death among men and women in the United States between the ages of twenty-five and forty-four. On a global scale, Jonathan Mann, director of the International AIDS Center of the Harvard AIDS Institute, and his coeditors of *AIDS in the World* reported:

In the first decade of response to AIDS, remarkable successes in some communities contrast dramatically with a sense of threatening collective global failure. The course of the pandemic within and through global society is not affected—in any serious manner—by the actions taken at the national or international level. . . . As we enter the second decade of AIDS, it is time to ask: Is the AIDS pandemic now out of control? (Mann et al. 1992: 1)

Certainly the sudden appearance of HIV disease in the early 1980s was a profoundly unexpected occurrence, "a startling discontinuity with the past" (Fee and Fox 1992: 1). Global public health efforts that date to the period before the beginning of the HIV disease pandemic, such as the successful smallpox eradication program, "reinforced the notion that mortality from infectious disease was a thing of the past" (McCombie 1990: 10).

Consequently, whatever the actual health needs of particular populations, the primary concerns of the biomedical health care system had been the so-called Western diseases, that is, chronic health problems, such as cancer and cerebrovascular problems, common in a developed society with an aging population. This surely has been the case in the United States, notes Brandt (1989: 367): "The United States has relatively little recent experience dealing with health crises. . . . We had come to believe that the problem of infectious, epidemic diseases had passed—a topic of concern only to the developing world and historians." However, with the appearance and spread of HIV disease and a growing number of other "emergent infectious diseases," like ebola, Lyme disease, or Brazilian purpuric fever, there has been a complete rethinking of disease risk globally.

As a result of HIV disease, in particular, but other diseases as well, the term *epidemic* was thrust back into the popular vocabulary. Many definitions of this term exist. Marks and Beatty (1976), in their history of the subject, adopt a broad approach and include both communicable and noncommunicable diseases that affect many people at one time. Epidemics (a word formed by joining *epi* or "in" with *demos* "the people") are conceptually linked to other words in the *demic* family of terms, including *endemics* (from *en* or "on"), which are nonexplosive, entrenched diseases of everyday life in particular communities, and *pandemics* (from *pan* or "all of"), which are epidemics on a widespread or global scale.

HIV disease in this sense is best described as a pandemic. It is found in every nation and every populated location on the planet. Further, it has spread to people of every age, ethnicity, class, gender, sexual orientation, political perspective, and religion. However, as noted in Chapter 1, another term useful in thinking about HIV disease is *syndemic*, in that HIV disease is best understood in light of its interactions with other diseases and its biocultural and political economic contexts. Unfortunately, to date no country or community that has been struck by HIV disease since the early 1980s has been successful in stopping the spread of the disease. Thus, although no longer seen—as it was in earlier years—as a "death sentence," HIV disease remains a global disease that significantly shapes the health of millions in various ways. Over the course of time, with the transmission of the virus to diverse new populations through a number of routes of contagion tied to a range of behaviors, the pandemic has become ever more complex and can be said to be composed "of thousands of smaller, complicated epidemics" in local settings and populations (J. Mann et al. 1992: 3). These local epidemics reveal that in each setting, somewhat different subgroups are put at highest risk, but almost always it is those who have the least power in society or are otherwise subject to social opprobrium and public disparagement who are the most likely to be infected.

Throughout its known history, HIV "has repeatedly demonstrated its ability to cross all borders: social, cultural, economic, political," but this often has not brought people closer together to appreciate their common plight and their shared needs as human beings (Mann et al. 1992: 3). Rather, the pandemic often has led to increased conflict and social contestation, usually on preexisting lines of tension. Indeed, since it first appeared, HIV disease has probably become the most political affliction visited on the human species in modern times. The disease caused by this "strange virus" (Leibowitch 1985) reminds us, in fact, just how political are all facets of health, illness, treatment, and health-related discourse. This is an important point. Public health is never merely a medical issue, it is always shaped and molded by structures of power and struggles over power locally, nationally, and internationally.

In sum, HIV disease has revealed itself as a disease of social relationship—not merely a social disease, but a disease of society as it is constituted as a markedly stratified and widely oppressive structure. This occurs locally within communities, nationally within the social systems of individual countries, and internationally within the global system of nations. As pointed out by the United Nations Research Institute for Development (2005), "From early on, national governments often denied the existence of HIV/AIDS, dismissed its potential harm or moved slowly to offer supplementary health services to people living with HIV/AIDS." Moreover the institute (2005) observes:

Of the many social, economic and political factors that drive and determine responses to the HIV/AIDS pandemic, structures of national and international political economy are among the most significant. Various decision makers and stakeholders assess what they expect to gain or lose by speaking out and taking substantive action on HIV/AIDS issues. These political considerations and decisions have remained largely hidden in analyses of the pandemic, but many have long-term implications for more fully shaping effective responses to HIV/AIDS.

Stigma

One of the most important and enduring aspects of the HIV disease pandemic has been stigmatization of sufferers or even assumed sufferers. The extent of the stigmatization of AIDS was evident in the findings of a nationally representative public opinion internet survey in which nearly one in five U.S. respondents (19 percent) agreed with the statement "People who got AIDS through sex or drug use have gotten what they deserve." The stigmatizing attitude was found more often among men, whites, individuals aged forty-four years of age and older, people without a high school diploma, and individuals who have annual incomes of less than $40,000. Additionally, those who were less knowledgeable about HIV were almost twice as likely to agree with the stigmatizing statement as those who were correctly informed. Thus, 25 percent of those who answered incorrectly that "it is likely for HIV to be transmitted from sharing a glass with someone who is HIV-infected" or "by being coughed or sneezed on by an HIV-infected individual" were in agreement with the stigmatizing statement, whereas only 14 percent of those who knew that HIV cannot be transmitted in these ways agreed with the stigmatizing statement (CDC 2000). The stigmatization of people living with HIV disease is not a unique American pattern but rather has parallels in many places around the world.

As a result of stigmatization, people living with HIV disease often come to experience what has been called "a damaged sense of self." Arliss (1997: 56) encountered an ethnographic example of this process during an interview with Jack, an AIDS nurse who himself is infected with HIV:

I felt unclean like a leper or something, and the sort of prevailing attitude that comes through from different people, particularly who should know better, who don't know better because they haven't the disease yet, and you feel unclean.

Jack's analogy to leprosy is telling. Leprosy historically has fallen into the category of chronic diseases that medical anthropologist Sue Estroff (1993: 257) calls "I am" diseases, meaning diseases that by the very way they are talked about ("He is a leper") are marked as "more mysterious and more stigmatized" and "where attributions of blame for the condition rest with the individual" sufferer. By contrast, "I have" diseases are not seen as embedded in the personhood of the sufferer, who is absolved of blame for his/her condition. For example, one says, "he has arthritis" not "he is arthritis," with the term *arthritic* being reserved for delimited body parts, not the whole person. Arthritis, in turn, is generally not stigmatized and sufferers are not blamed for causing their own sickness through immoral beliefs or deeds. While in public discourse HIV came to be talked of as an "I have" disease (reflecting, according to Estroff, the effort of organized HIV sufferers and their supporters to destigmatize the disease and to counter punitive efforts to blame people with the disease for their own suffering), in actual street conversation, the "I am" usage is common. Thus, in his ethnographic work with African American and Latino drug users, Singer found that infected individuals often say "I am HIV" rather than "I have HIV," suggesting the experienced stigmatization of infected individuals. Typical is a study participant referred to as Carlos who was interviewed by Singer (1998: 69) shortly after learning of his HIV status. "The questions just came into my head again and again; am I good, am I bad? Back and forth. I used drugs. I have problems. I ain't a kid who cares. And now she [his wife] is in jail [on a drug charge that Carlos avoided by leaping from his bedroom window]."

As Lindenbaum (1998: 51) points out, "The notion that AIDS punishes socially marginal people for deviant behavior echoes widely held nineteenth-century American views that the 'vicious poor' and lower orders rightly suffered most during the cholera epidemic of 1832 . . . The moral view that established or governing groups have better health by dint of their position in society . . . thus has a long history in Western thought and experience." Such views of disease, in fact, can be seen as part of the ideological support system that helps maintain the existing structure of society. In effect, the stigmatizing of HIV disease or other diseases reflects the effort to corral biology in the service of the politics of inequality. As noted, enforcement of HIV disease stigma has not gone unchallenged, nor did a moralist or religious interpretation of the disease as divine punishment. That the disease initially appeared to target gay men but largely avoid lesbian women who were not otherwise at other risk for the HIV infection also created a dilemma for the divine punishment argument. The rapid appearance of the disease among blood-transfusion patients, individuals who seemingly were not guilty of any known moral transgression, further undercut but has never fully eliminated the appeal of a punitive view of the disease. As Parker and Aggleton (2003: 13) emphasize, "negative social responses to the epidemic remain pervasive even in seriously affected communities."

Of special note is the response to HIV infection among individuals from groups that hold higher social status and are not otherwise marked by stigma. In a study of white, middle class women with HIV infection in San Diego, Stanley (1999) found that many woman adopted a spiritualized view of the disease seeing it as a higher calling (e.g., to become an HIV educator or community activist), as redemption (saving them from a life of sin), or even as a blessing (and personal rebirth). One interpretation of these findings is that people with adequate access to resources are able to minimize the experience of HIV stigma through "moral management strategies . . . [that] facilitate reconnection to an ideal, pre-HIV representation of self to which their self-esteem is intimately linked" (Stanley 1999: 119). Ironically, as a result, it appears that it is not only HIV that is unequally distributed in society but the social suffering that is a consequence of HIV stigma as well.

Research on stigma makes it clear that in the eyes of many people living with HIV disease, the social damages of stigmatization are equal to if not more painful than the medical consequences of the disease. One factor that has slowed our progress in understanding HIV stigma, according to anthropologist Gilbert Herdt, is the lack of a unified and cross-culturally applicable conception of "harm." Indeed, rectifying this shortcoming in our conceptual framework would be useful more generally in efforts to understand the role of inequality and oppression in health. To address this dilemma, Herdt (2001: 146), building on the classical study of stigma by Goffman (1963), offers the following definition:

Harm . . . constitutes the state of being vulnerable to scapegoating, shame, and silence, to being the object of accusation and unwarranted, displaced fear, anxiety, and contagion. Harm includes the loss of social status and community belongings . . . but even more, it suggests the loss of basic personhood, of existence itself.

To this definition might be added the loss of health and well-being as a consequence of blame and mistreatment, subordination, and denial of equal access to items, places, and statuses of value or basic need. The narrow focus on gay lifestyle during the early years of the pandemic overlooked a growing body of evidence that immunodeficiency diseases like Kaposi's sarcoma and especially pneumocystis carinii pneumonia also were showing up in increasing numbers among heterosexual drug injectors, their lovers, and their children, especially in New York and New Jersey. In December 1981, for example, when Arye Rubinstein, chief of Albert Einstein's medical college Division of Allergy and Immunology, submitted a paper to the annual conference of the American Academy of Pediatrics suggesting that the African American children he was treating in the Bronx, New York, were suffering from the same disease as immunodeficient gay men, he was rebuffed. Such thinking, he said,

was simply too farfetched for a scientific community that, when it thought about gay cancer and gay pneumonia at all, was quite happy to keep the problem just that: gay. The academy would not accept Rubinstein's abstract for presentation at the conference, and among immunologists, word quietly circulated that [Rubinstein] had gone a little batty. (Shilts 1987: 104)

The same pattern occurred historically among inner-city adult drug injectors, who began exhibiting immunodeficiency disorders in the early 1980s. Consistently, health officials "reported them as being homosexual, being strangely reluctant to shed the notion that this was a gay disease; all these junkies would somehow turn out to be gay in the end, they said" (Shilts 1987: 106).

By 1983, however, IDUs constituted the majority of immunodeficiency cases in the Northeast. Still, among epidemiologists focused on the gay-lifestyle explanation, "There was a reluctance to believe that intravenous drug users might be wrapped into this epidemic" (Shilts 1987: 83). Nonetheless, the first clinical description of immunosuppression and opportunistic infection among IDUs appeared in MMWR in December 1981, followed by a second report in June 1982 that indicated that 22 percent of new patients with Kaposi's sarcoma and pneumocystis carinii pneumonia were heterosexuals, the majority IDUs. Crimp (1988: 249), in fact, has suggested that "the AIDS problem did not affect gay men first, even in the United States. What is now called HIV disease was first seen in middle-class gay men in America, in part because of [their] access to medical care. Retrospectively, however, it appears that IDUs—whether gay or straight—were dying of AIDS in New York City throughout the 1970s and early 1980s, but a class-based and racist health care system failed to notice, and an epidemiology equally skewed by class and racial bias failed to begin to look until 1987." Put otherwise, IDUs, who live on the social and economic margins of society, were (and are) already so stigmatized that no one paid much attention to their deaths, and no one initially recognized that an infectious disease was spreading among them.

Indeed, as Parker and Aggleton (2003) point out, the sources of HIV disease stigmatization are multiple, including the sudden appearance of a deadly contagious disease, the association early on of this disease with individuals who already endured preexisting sexual stigma associated with sexually transmitted infections, homosexuality, prostitution, and promiscuity; linkage of the disease with condemnatory attitudes about "loose" women; prevailing stereotypes about ethnic-minority sexuality; and finger-pointing at the poor for being lazy, lacking in morals, and dangerous. All of these preexisting sources of stigmatization reflect socially constructed, but factually problematic, attitudes. In turn, they rationalize blatant discrimination across societal institutions including the criminal justice and legal systems, social welfare programs, education, religion, and health care. In this way, stigmatization and accompanying discrimination, by differentiating those considered normal from those considered deviant (or a burden, or a threat) form part of the often hidden structuring and control of society. In other words, stigmatization helps produce, legitimizes, and perpetuates social inequality; indeed, it is a nefarious force in the making and progression of disease, the production of individual and social suffering, and the creation of (unequal) society.

Notably, Castro and Farmer (2005: 53) report "that the introduction of quality HIV care can lead to a rapid reduction in stigma." Their point is that while stigma contributes to individuals avoiding HIV testing and adherence to treatment and is a significant source of social suffering, its existence is not a social excuse for not implementing quality care among stigmatized populations. Research, they note, from Haiti and the Dominican Republic, suggests, for example, that the implementation of effective HIV treatment for mothers has helped to diminish patient stigmatization.

LESSONS OF HIV

Science has produced more knowledge about HIV than any other known virus. Because of this disease, we now realize that "infectious diseases are not a vestige of our premodern past; instead, like disease in general, they are the price we pay for living in the organic world" (Morse 1992: 23). However, because of HIV, we also know that the price of living in an organic world is not paid equally by all of those who live in that world. Indeed, although the virus is a product of the organic world, the pandemic (i.e., who is likely to become infected and who is not, and what happens to people after they are infected) is a social creation. In other words, as William McNeill (1976) suggests in his book *Plagues and Peoples*, it is important to differentiate between microparasitism and macroparasitism and to examine interrelations between the two.

Microparasites are tiny organisms like HIV that find the resources for sustaining their vital processes in human tissues and in the process may cause sickness or even death. In the case of HIV, it appears that the virus needs host-cell proteins to be able to transcribe its RNA genome (i.e., its genetic code for making copies of itself), synthesize its glycoprotein outer coat that shields the genome, and assemble new infectious virons that can, in turn, seek out new host cells for continuing the process of replication. As it invades a host-cell, HIV harvests proteins that it finds there, including cyclophilin A, actin, and ubiquitin. Without these stolen proteins, HIV would not be able to reproduce itself or successfully avoid destruction by the body's immune system (e.g., it is thought that by covering itself in the type of proteins found on the surface of human cells, HIV virons may evade the immune system by masquerading as human blood cells).

Macroparasites, by contrast, are larger organisms that prey on humans, "chief among which have been other human beings" (McNeill 1976: 5). In the course of human history, macroparasitism has become ever more important in determining human health. In early times, the skill and formidability of human hunters outclassed rival predators. Humanity thus emerged at the top of the food chain, with little risk of being eaten by predatory animals. Later, when food production became a way of life for some human communities, a modulated macroparasitism became possible. A conqueror could seize food from those who produced it, and by consuming it himself become a parasite of a new sort on those who did the work. In especially fertile landscapes, it even proved possible to establish a comparatively stable pattern of this sort of macroparasitism among human beings.

The emergence of a class structure, as McNeill shows, institutionalized macroparasitism. Moreover, as the case of HIV suggests, microparasitism and macroparasitism interact, an interaction we have referred to as a syndemic. As a consequence of the effects of macroparasitism some human beings—those who have less power and resources in society—are put at greater risk for exposure to and infection by various microparasites like HIV. This interconnection explains why poorer, less powerful classes in society and nations in the global system suffer more from disease than their richer, more powerful counterparts.

During the mid- to late 1990s, the era of the "AIDS panic," particularly in the developed world, came to a close. Because of improved treatments, the death rate for HIV disease in wealthy nations began to drop rapidly. Newspapers started carrying stories about individuals who were at death's door only to be swept back to reasonable health and activity as a result of available medical treatments. People who were preparing to die suddenly found themselves going back to their old lives, to their previous jobs, and to their remaining social relationships. A report released in March 2001 noted that U.S. AIDS patients diagnosed in 1984 lived an average of eleven months after diagnosis, compared with almost four years for those diagnosed in 1995. For those diagnosed in 1997, 90 percent were still alive two years later. One effect of this dramatic change was that HIV came, for some, to seem like less of an important problem for society; just another chronic disease among many. HIV-negative men interviewed in a San Francisco study reported seeing it as more of an "inconvenience" than a killer, and HIV-positive men said that they were no longer spending as much time warning their friends to be careful about AIDS.

In response, in wealthy nations, by the late 1990s a kind of "AIDS fatigue" set in, with people no longer wanting to hear or think about the disease. This attitude seemed to be particularly strong among young gay men, some of whom began to see condom use as unnecessary or even oppressive. Avoiding condoms, a practice that came to be called barebacking, developed a set of vocal advocates. The consequence was a notable rise in risk behavior in this population with expectable consequences. By 2001, the CDC reported that the new infection rate for twenty-three- to twenty-nine-year-old white gay men in the United States had almost doubled since 1997, going from 2.5 percent per year to 4.4 percent. Research reported at the 2012 XIX International AIDS Conference found a 5.9 percent incidence rate (i.e., new infections) among African American men who have sex with men and are eighteen to thirty years of age. Furthermore, CDC data indicate that young black men who have sex with men and are aged thirteen to twenty-nine years had a 48 percent increase in new HIV infections from 2006 to 2009 (NIH News 2012).

Among people living with infection and their loved ones, activists, researchers, and others still strongly focused on the epidemic, the fear began to grow that HIV programs would begin to face significant cutbacks. The height of this fear was reached in the weeks after September 11, 2001, in the wake of the brutal terrorist attack on the World Trade Center in New York City and on the subsequent bioterriorist anthrax assault using the U.S. postal system. As a result, the U.S. government initiated a massive budget restructuring, pouring billions of dollars in a war against Afghanistan and in a radical beefing up of what came to be called homeland security. The subsequent war in Iraq, and intensely challenged federal effort to link the war to the fight against terrorism, became another military drain on federal dollars. The prevailing fear among those concerned about ' the ever-rising number of people living with HIV was that terrorism would become "the new AIDS" in terms of federal spending and public attention. Further dampening enthusiasm were reports of growing drug resistance, as the virus mutated and became immune to some of the best medicines available. Fortunately, although the worst case scenarios did not occur, HIV is now part of a more complex health and funding world, amid recognition that one more big push might, as noted earlier, push this disease onto the trash heap of human history.

ANTHROPOLOGY AND THE PANDEMIC

The emergence of an "anthropology of HIV disease" dates to the early to mid-1980s, a transitional period during which our basic understanding of this disease was still forming, its devastating potential had not yet been fully realized, and uncertainty about the contributions that anthropologists could make in this arena was widespread within the discipline. Still, a small number of anthropologists took up HIV/AIDS-related work during the 1980s, leading in the United States to the formation of the AIDS and Anthropology Research Group (AARG) in 1987. This association remains active more than twenty-five years since its formation, and it is still committed to elevating a disciplinary focus on HIV disease and to offering support to those working in this field. At the suggestion of Roy Rappaport, then president of the American Anthropological Association (AAA), at an AARG meeting in November 1987, the AIDS and Anthropology Task Force of the AAA was created in April 1988 with the purpose of encouraging anthropological work on HIV and AIDS. The task force was charged with building awareness of HIV disease among anthropologists at a time when many had not yet recognized the relevance of the pandemic to their own areas of work, and thus with expanding anthropological impact on responses to the pandemic. The task force operated until 1993 when its allotted time ended, but, in response to questions about whether its termination signaled that the AAA was turning away from promoting HIV disease awareness, the association established the Commission on AIDS Research and Education. The mission of this new body was to coordinate AAA educational and advocacy efforts regarding HIV and AIDS, recommend priorities for the AAA regarding HIV/AIDS-related policies and research agendas, and evaluate proposals by AAA members for HIV/AIDS-related initiatives.

By the time the commission ended its work, the anthropology of HIV disease was well established, but the initial efforts to gain a foothold in this arena had encountered various obstacles. In 1986, the first set of anthropological papers on HIV-related research and application appeared as a special issue of *Medical Anthropology Quarterly*. In a concluding essay to that set of papers (not all of which were by anthropologists), Douglas Feldman (1986: 38), among the earliest anthropologists to conduct research on the epidemic, observed: "It is surprising that only a dozen or so medical anthropologists have become involved in AIDS research." This delay in the involvement of any sizeable number of anthropologists reflected a hesitation within the discipline that occurred while researchers in other fields were beginning to carry out large HIV/AIDS-related research initiatives and publish extensively on the pandemic (Bolton and Orozco 1994). Uncertainty among anthropologists reflected the combined effects of a crisis of confidence that gripped the discipline in the wake of postmodernist critiques of theory and application, a lack of anthropological attention to the present, and a failure on the part of social and behavioral scientists in other disciplines to see the value of anthropological approaches to an infectious disease epidemic.

Since then, much has changed. HIV disease has become one of the most studied infectious diseases. The devastating magnitude of the pandemic came to be fully recognized—although debates emerge anew about the appropriate level of resource allocation, especially in developing countries with complex health and social problems. A large number of anthropologists have since conducted on-the-ground research, been active in HIV-prevention and intervention initiatives, or played other roles in addressing HIV epidemics in diverse landscapes. The sheer scale of the impact of the pandemic on people and places long studied by anthropologists, and recognition of the failure to fully incorporate observational methods, exploration of emic perspectives (e.g., the views of HIV-infected/affected people), and other common anthropological approaches (e.g., use of key informants and social networks in data collection, comparison of cultural ideals, and actual behaviors) within the prevailing nonanthropological research, contributed to this critical turn in anthropological work. Of equal importance have been the emergence of weariness with the postmodernist conundrum in anthropology (i.e., how to do anthropology if anthropologists cannot ever really fully know another way of life and meaning beside their own) and a subsequent embrace of "good enough" ethnographic standards that combine objective observation, reflexivity, and recognition of the responsibilities of conducting research within a global health crisis.

Today there is a strong sense that anthropologists have made some significant contributions to the theoretical and applied study of HIV disease. Central among these is the development of ethnographically informed accounts of everyday behavior in local contexts affected by HIV disease, which often are at odds with views developed from afar (or from "above") that are based only on quantitative survey data or on official health information sources (Lee and Susser 2008). One of the first contexts in which a move to include on-the-ground ethnographic research was in HIV prevention research among IDUs.

Between 1987 and 1988, forty-one projects in sixty-three U.S. sites were funded by the National Institute on Drug Use to conduct outreach-based research on HIV among IDUs. The approach used by these projects was formulated by social and behavioral scientists in drug abuse, who, when faced with the opportunity to obtain new sources of funding by focusing on HIV disease among IDUs, conceived research strategies that combined ethnography, HIV testing, catchment surveys, and intervention trial technologies into overarching research plans aimed at stemming the spread of disease in IDU populations throughout the United States. These investigators realized that to engage street-based IDUs in a research study and enable them to respond candidly to one-time, short-answer surveys, the questions had to reflect the researchers' informed understanding of the behavior patterns and contexts of interest. The researchers therefore designed a study model that investigators in various cities could emulate. Ethnography was to be a key component of the model, because the framers correctly surmised that the potentially varying patterns of injecting drug use in different cities would require researchers to obtain locally grounded specific information on how, when, where, and with whom IDUs injected themselves with drugs. Numerous anthropologists entered into HIV research through this initiative.

Two collections of articles and numerous other publications in peer journals resulted from this project. These various publications focused on issues such as the role of social networks on the relationship between HIV infection and drug use, the uses of ethnography in the study of men who have sex with men who use amphetamines (Gorman, Morgan, and Lambert 1995), ethnography in the study of women's drug use and risk (Sterk 1995), advanced ethnographic methods (Trotter 1995), use of research teams in studying emergent patterns of HIV risk and drug use (Ouellet, Weibel, and Jimenez 1995), multimethod studies that use ethnography (Bluthenthal and Watters 1995), and the use of ethnography in the evaluation of community intervention strategies (Singer et al. 1995). A consensus article on the reuse of potentially contaminated injection equipment also emerged from this process (Needle et al. 1998). This article relied heavily on ethnographic perspectives to trace how individual IDUs come to use contaminated paraphernalia, despite exposure to dire warnings of danger. Flowing from this work, Page's studies of HIV risk among IDUs in Miami were the first to utilize direct observation of self-injection behavior in settings where IDUs gathered to inject drugs (e.g., Page, Smith, and Kane 1990).

Similarly, Koester (1994) added to our understanding of why IDUs are unwilling to carry personal needles/syringes. He conducted the observations and in-depth interviews necessary to delineate personal histories of IDUs in which there was no room for error when one intended to inject drugs. Because most of his interviewees had extensive and often unresolved histories of petty crime, their possession of a needle/syringe could, if they were detained for any reason, lead to the invocation of some or all of the prior charges, leading to extensive jail time. Rather than risk what for an ordinary citizen would be a minor inconvenience, the IDUs interviewed and observed by Koester and his associates preferred to rely on whatever needles/syringes their associates might have available at the locale where injection took place. Koester's work also verified Page's observations of what have come to be called indirect sharing behaviors.

In addition to closely focused studies in local contexts, anthropologists working on HIV disease have looked at the impact of structural factors on local behaviors. For example, ethnographic research has confirmed that structural-adjustment policies imposed by international lending institutions, on the grounds that market-based economic practices would lead to higher standards of living and better health in lesser developed countries, has instead at times led to increases in HIV-related risk (Lurie, Hintzen, and Lowe 2004; Susser 2009). This was found to occur for several reasons, including (1) these policies undermined rural economies and increased the cost of food, leading to individuals' reduced nutritional status and weakened immunocompetence; (2) as a result of increased urban labor migration, the policies caused a separation of families and thereby contributed to the involvement of isolated urban workers and impoverished rural women as the respective customers and sellers of commercial sex; and (3) the policies supported cuts in HIV-prevention and health care budgets, which have further limited access to care in resource-poor settings. Structural factors that interact with local cultural constructions of appropriate sexual behavior, gender roles, and other factors have been found to underlie patterns of HIV-related risk (Rwabukwali 2008). In many parts of Africa, for example, a combination of economic and cultural factors "circumscribe the ability of women, married or single, to refuse sex with a steady partner, even if they suspect he may be [HIV-]infected, or to insist on condom protection" (Schoepf 2004: 131).

Another contribution of anthropological research involves investigation of "the interrelations between macro-level conditions [e.g. structural adjustment policies] . . . and the lived experience of individuals and social groups" (Schoepf 2004: 123), that is to say, interactions between social structure and individual agency. One product of such research is the increased awareness of an often wide gap between what people say they do and what they actually do. Asked about their own behavior, people will often report what they intend to do under optimal conditions. However, circumstances, including the force of structural factors (such as structural violence or the social construction of "risk environments"), do not always allow people to act in accord with their intentions. Rather, they select behaviors among those that are possible within structurally imposed constraints, some of which may be quite risky from the perspective of HIV infection. Exemplary is Schoepf's (1988) observation that one of the important consequences of the global economic crisis of the 1980s was the movement of women in central Africa toward commercial sex exchanges, with an attendant increase in exposure to HIV. This behavior change is best understood not as an individual-level event nor as the consequence of individual-level characteristics; instead, it reflects a widespread survival strategy of individuals with limited resources facing a common structural threat.

Anthropologists have helped influence the shift in the HIV/AIDS literature away from an emphasis on "risk groups" to "risk behaviors." While early epidemiological publications on HIV conceptualized the existence of groups of people who shared patterns of inherently "risky" behavior (e.g., men who have sex with men, IDUs), based on their own research, anthropologists have stressed that empirically bounded "risk groups" do not exist. Rather, it is various behaviors, such as unprotected sex, that put people at risk, not particular kinds of relationships, statuses, or identities. Thus, some individuals involved in sex work may or may not insist on condom use depending on their structurally determined ability to exercise agency (McGrath et al. 1993). Moreover, anthropologists have helped to clarify many realities of gender relations and the ways that specific patterns of male-female interaction, as well as other gender identities, play important roles in the construction of risk behaviors and in patterned ways of living with HIV infection (Ingstad 1990; Kornfield and Babalola 2008). Furthermore, insights about the nature of culture as a factor in human reproductive behavior have been used by anthropologists to help develop culturally attuned HIV-prevention and intervention models, including models that move beyond knowledge promotion to those that address structural, environmental, situational, and personal barriers to HIV-risk reduction.

For example, a number of anthropologists (Buchanan et al. 2004; Green et al. 2010) have been involved in the development and evaluation of syringe exchange programs as a harm reduction approach designed to assist injection drug users from becoming infected because they lack clean (sterile) syringes and reuse syringes used by others. Whelehan (2009), for example, worked with syringe exchange in San Francisco during the late 1980s. Although a series of studies have documented the value of syringe exchange in lowering HIV transmission among drug injectors, syringe exchange has long been a controversial issue in the United States. It was only with the election of Barrack Obama as president, in fact, that the United States finally stopped prohibiting the federal funding of this proven public health strategy. Full funding of syringe exchange at the level needed to radically reduce the frequency of new HIV infections, especially among newer and younger drug users, remains to be realized. In her discussion of syringe exchange, Whelehan reviews the role of syringes in the person-to-person spread of HIV, the ways existing laws and stigmatization contribute to syringe-related risk among injection drug users, the need for understanding drug use and related health risks within the wider frameworks of sociopolitical and economic relations, and why it is easier to modify drug-related risk than sexual risk for HIV infection.

Through their effort to find a useful place in HIV responses, as well as in other arenas of global health work, anthropologists have become strong advocates for multidisciplinary approaches. Whelehan (2009: 253), for example, notes: "The response to [HIV disease] . . . needs to be comprehensive, collaborative, and continuous. A holistic, integrated, and interdisciplinary approach is necessary to address the pandemic." Although not hesitant to point out the limitations encountered in constricted biomedical paradigms of disease, top-down prevention/intervention models, a narrow epidemiological focus on individual behaviors that ignores the social embeddedness of vulnerability, and nonparticipatory research and intervention strategies—traditionally independent anthropologists have learned the value of cross-disciplinary team efforts. Indeed, as Kleinman (2009: vi) indicates: "The new global era of central concern with AIDS, other emergent infectious diseases, disability rights, tobacco-related diseases, epidemic diabetes, trauma from political and social violence, substance abuse, suicide and dementia [has been] the time for medical anthropology." Central to the newfound importance of multidisciplinarity is an understanding that not only is the HIV pandemic a biosocial complex that involves multiple intersections among global political economy, local environments, cultural patterns, local social structures (including class, ethnic, and gender inequalities), war, human evolutionary biology, and viral pathogenesis, but also that the pandemic did not emerge in a disease vacuum. Rather, HIV disease always comes entwined with a wide range of other diseases and threats to health and well-being. Critical among these are malnutrition, malaria, sexually transmitted diseases, tuberculosis, and a group of afflictions associated with poverty that have come to be called "neglected tropical diseases." As a result, many countries face a daunting constellation of interacting and mutually exacerbating epidemics, epidemic-enhancing social conditions, and socially adverse disease syndemics (Singer 2009a).

A case in point involves the distribution of antiretroviral treatment to HIV patients in Mozambique. Between 2004 and 2010, there was a 1,500 percent increase in the number of people accessing free and publically accessible HIV treatment in the country, a sign of both the level of need and the effort by the international community to make HIV medications available in poor countries. However, as Kalofonos (2010) argues, hunger is the principal complaint voiced by those receiving antiretroviral treatment. The inability of HIV interventions to adequately address this pressing issue has created intense competition among infected individuals for scarce resources, undermining both social solidarity and the potential for further community-initiated action to address HIV challenges. This case, stands as a reminder that

even while they save lives, AIDS treatment programs can paradoxically have dehumanizing effects if the broader social structures that contribute to suffering and impoverishment remain hidden and intact. . . . By targeting a biological condition, political and economic concerns are sidelined, and local forms of solidarity are undermined as disease-related distinctions determine eligibility for scarce resources. (Kalofonos 2010: 364)

Voicing a somewhat similar theme, Jones (2011), based on fourteen months of field research in South Africa, argues that prevailing economic inequalities and structural barriers to resources among the poor have created dire situations in which people living with HIV disease often must choose between economic security and health security. In this case, infected individuals who are too sick to work rely on social assistance grants from the government as their only form of income. To qualify for these "disability grants patients must have a CD4 cell count of 200 or lower. Taking and carefully adhering to HIV medications, however, can improve a patient's CD4 count above the 200 cutoff point, resulting in an HIV patient losing his or her only means of livelihood. As Jones titles her article on these findings, from the perspective of the patient, "If I Take My Pills I'll Go Hungry."

Anthropologists often identify these kinds of contradictions because they are trained to pay keen attention to local patterns of culture and the intricacies of social organization in the course of research on HIV as well as on other health and social issues. Anthropologists, for example, have repeatedly seen that intervention programs that treat indigenous culture as either irrelevant or as an obstacle to be overcome fail to achieve planned changes. Speaking of Africa, for example, Gausset (2001:509) remarks: "The fight against AIDS in Africa is often presented as a fight against 'cultural barriers' that are seen as promoting the spread of HIV. This attitude is based on a long history of Western prejudices about sexuality in Africa which focus on its exotic aspects only (polygamy, adultery, wife exchange, circumcision, dry sex, levirate, sexual pollution, sexual cleansing, various beliefs and taboos, etc.)." Anthropologists are well aware that cultural beliefs and practices at times contradict HIV-intervention agendas, although often the problem is simply a failure by interventionists to learn about and fully appreciate the cultural logics that underlie behavior in target communities. Consequently, anthropologists commonly play an active role as "revealers" of culture by stressing its structure and meaningfulness and the fact that that culture should not be ignored by interventionists. Moreover, anthropologists have sought to demonstrate that including sincere attention to local culture and (more challengingly) its incorporation in some (locally appropriate) fashion into intervention design can contribute significantly to improving program appeal and efficacy. Generally, anthropologists stress that full community participation at all levels in a program is the most productive approach (Schensul, Weeks, and Singer, 1999). As Bennett (2007) comments:

An education in applied anthropology requires training in engaged scholarship, which mandates community participation from the beginning of a research project as opposed to the community's having a more passive role, simply receiving research results. The more students are involved in engaged scholarship, the more successful they will be as applied or practicing anthropologists.

Even in cases in which specific cultural practices appear to increase HIV risk, as Gausset (2001: 517) points out, "Prevention campaigns . . . [should] try to make cultural practices safer, rather than to eradicate them," for the sake of both ethics and efficacy. For example, based on research in Zambia, Emily Frank (2009) observes that getting tested for HIV infection is not a simple or straightforward health-seeking behavior, as might be assumed by interventionists who know the health benefits of learning one's HIV status. Rather, getting tested for HIV is often enmeshed in layers of cultural meaning and significance, which may be beyond the recognition of public health or biomedical providers seeking to address the HIV epidemic. On the basis of ethnographic research, Frank (2009) suggests that Zambians' fear of and resistance to HIV testing and treatment does not reflect a lack of desire for healthier lifestyles and improved well-being, but rather that the emotions, attitudes, and behaviors attached to testing express resistance to a system that prioritizes individual and scientific outcomes over locally valued goals, such as protecting community identity and ensuring community sustainability in a globalizing world. Frank argues that resistance to HIV testing and treatment is part of a communal effort to defend against an international system that hurtfully depicts Zambia as a nation characterized by economic failure and a devastating HIV epidemic. From the cultural logic that informs the Zambian perspective, HIV-intervention programs are not impartial players in a world of international social relations and economic development. Instead they may be experienced as one of the adverse ways in which international powers impact on the most personal domains of everyday life and identity. As this example suggests, ethnography, which has long served as the core methodology of anthropological research, has proven to be an adroit approach for allowing cultural outsiders to grasp and appreciate the inner logics that inform people's behavior and attitudes. Additionally, ethnography has contributed to our understanding that, in addition to reflecting webs of meaning, behavior is shaped by networks of power and the history of power relations as locally experienced.

In South Africa, Robert Thornton (2009) similarly identifies an overlap between known patterns of risk for sexual transmission of HIV and prevalent behavioral patterns in communities. Thornton examines underlying culturally meaningful reasons for maintaining multiple concurrent sexual partners, even though this is an identified HIV-risk pattern among public health experts and educators. He found that rather than being irrational or obstructionist, this behavior could be a realistic response to limitations in access to social and economic goods because it enables people to increase both the size and the diversity of their social networks. In a world in which social networks are critical in accessing needed resources, enhancing one's ties to others through any available means may be key to immediate survival, even though this may increase one's health risks in the long run. Notably, there are parallels here to the findings of Singer, Erickson, and colleagues (2006) on the reasons low-income, inner-city African American and Puerto Rican young adults in Hartford, Connecticut, engage in risky behaviors. There are multiple threats facing the people studied by Singer et al., and multiple arenas to experience social failure as ethnic minorities. Sexual and romantic relationships, may be one arena—one over which they feel they have some control—in which failure (e.g., being rejected) may be avoided by engaging in risk (e.g., having multiple sex partners).

Not only do anthropologists pay particular attention to culture, they also listen to people talk (or avoid talking) about particular issues as clues to underlying cultural dynamics. Kate Wood (2008), for example, studied local discourse about HIV in a South African township. She found that discussions about the disease and of affected individuals where generally coded and indirect. Rather than denial of the disease, which is a common assumption when it is found that people avoid talking about

HIV, she concluded that verbal silence and elision about a stigmatized disease reflect a felt need to maintain hope and a traditional injunction against naming dangerous diseases.

Ramin (2007) asserts that two competing schools of anthropological thought have contributed valuable and concrete knowledge to our understanding of the HIV disease pandemic. The first are labeled traditional anthropologists, people who see their role as adding cultural depth and social grounding to biomedical and public health knowledge through the detailed examination of local cultures in interaction with the pandemic. The second group of anthropologists is influenced by political economy and believes that it is the political and economic structure in which individuals act that most shapes their behavior. This second school "proposes structural violence, the notion that societal structures such as racism, sexism and inequality cause direct and indirect harm to individuals, as the principal perspective for understanding HIV/AIDS" (Ramin 2007: 128). In fact, the critical medical anthropology model that guides this book emphasizes the importance of marrying political economy and ethnographically informed studies of local cultures, or what is termed a *micro-macro model* of the pandemic.

The following "A Closer Look" provides another angle on studying sexual relationships from the standpoint of HIV risk.

"A Closer Look"

ETHNOGRAPHICALLY STUDYING PRIVATE SEXUAL ENCOUNTERS

Given the importance of sexual behavior in the transmission of AIDS, we need to have a clear understanding of what actually happens when two (or more) people have sex in diverse cultural settings. However, the privacy of sex in most cultures makes it difficult to collect this kind of observational data. One innovative response to this dilemma was undertaken by Ralph Bolton in his study of AIDS risk among gay men in Belgium. He reports:

I spent most of my time, at all hours of day and night . . . in settings where gay men in Brussels hang out: bars, saunas, restaurants, parks, tearooms [public bathrooms where sex occurs], streets, and privates homes. . . . My presentation of self was simple and straightforward: I was a gay man doing research as a medical anthropologist on AIDS and sex. . . . In my casual sexual encounters with men I picked up in gay cruising situations, my approach during sex was to allow my partner to take the lead in determining which sexual practices to engage in. Low-risk activities posed no problem, of course, but to discover which moderate and high-risk behaviors they practiced, I assented to the former (oral sex, for example) while declining the latter (unprotected sexual intercourse). (Bolton 1992: 133–135)

Through this strategy, Bolton was able to determine that high-risk sexual behavior was quite common and quite accepted in the privacy of the bedroom among gay men in Brussels. This finding was of importance because health officials in Belgium had come to the conclusion, based on several surveys, that gay men had significantly curtailed risky sexual behavior and that it was no longer necessary, therefore, to focus prevention efforts on the gay community.

Another way in which anthropological research on HIV has developed program and policy-relevant insights is revealed in the next "A Closer Look" at the "war stories" of drug users.

"A Closer Look"

THE STORIES PEOPLE TELL

In their attempt to identify effective ways of curbing the AIDS epidemic among drug users, public health researchers have been especially concerned with expanding understanding of (1) the precise nature of risk behaviors among drug-users (i.e., specific acts that increase the chance that a drug user will be infected with HIV and/or transmit the virus to others), (2) the social contexts that facilitate risk behavior, (3) the social structural factors that contribute to risk taking, and (4) the role of social networks and relationships in promoting or inhibiting risky acts. Anthropologists working in AIDS have attempted to advance our understanding of these issues by directly observing behavior, fully describing the immediate and broader social environments in which risk occurs, and exploring insider drug user perspectives about their lives and behaviors. The latter effort has produced a rich corpus of narrative data of various kinds, including stories told by drug users about their day-to-day activities and adventures, the challenges and suffering they face, and their relations with other people. War stories, as these narratives are known on the street, provide a window into the often hidden worlds of active illicit drug users. Storytelling has been recognized by anthropologists and others as central human social activity that functions to help people to work through, organize, and invest meaning in their experiences. Moreover, narratives situate people in "local moral worlds," constructing borders and pathways of valued and devalued conduct. Analysts of narratives have argued that they can be decomposed into a series of mini-events and intermediary states and that a vast number of different but similar events may be included under a single event label. In this light, in listening to numerous drug user war stories over ten years of HIV research, Singer and his colleagues (Singer et al. 2001) realized that they could be grouped into a number of distinct categories. Using etic event labels (i.e., designations developed by the researcher team), they constructed a typology of drug user stories by twice reading through interview transcripts and field notes from one of their studies and identifying distinct themes, messages, or plot elements. Examination of these themes suggested a typological organization of primary (namely, learning the ropes, adventurous experiences, miraculous gains, not like the old days, the power of drugs, and suffering and regret) as well as various secondary and tertiary categories. One subtype of adventurous story, for example, focused on the display of useful survival skills, as depicted in the following narrative told to research team members by Kyle, a middle-aged African American man:

I used to work in the hospital [in prison]. My job was in the hospital. I set up all the stuff for the doctor [e.g., syringes]. So, I was the guy selling the needles [to other inmates]. I had access to needles; they'd tell me to destroy them [after use with a patient, but] I'd put them [aside instead]. . . . You know . . . they sent you up on different floors, like guys with low crimes on the first floor. Bigger crimes on the second floor, bigger crimes on the third floor, highest crimes on the top floor. . . . So, I always went straight to the top floor. Those were the guys that had the C.O.s [correction officers] running the drugs [in] for them. So, I'd go over to them and . . . every morning those guys would say, "Look man, I need fresh needles every day." So, that's how I took care of myself [i.e. his drug addiction] in jail. "You need five set ups [syringes] every morning, you got them. Now grab me a couple of bags [of drugs]." And they'd give it to you man, no questions, no wait. When I got there [to the cells of customers], they'd slide that shit [drugs] under the door . . . I took care of the guys! It's something that you learn. (Singer et al. 2001: 595)

Stories like these invert the socially dominant image of street drug users as social failures and people lacking the intelligence or skills to succeed in regular society. Rather, narratives like this one portray efficacious individuals with notable abilities, people who make things happen and get things done even under trying circumstances. Whatever the veracity of such stories, they reveal, by the cultural elements they express, that contrary to the assumptions of "straight society," drug users embrace conventional action- and achievement-oriented cultural values. Although street drug-users commonly are seen as socially marginal individuals, their stories appear to give voice to noticeably mainstream concerns and ideas.

Also found among the adventurous narratives of drug users are stories that tell of close calls, narrow escapes, and heroic rescues. Commonly, these narratives emphasize the grave threats that drug users face each day on the street. Oftentimes, narrow escape narratives involve mistaken identities in which the wrong person or, alternately, a substitute (e.g., an accessible friend of the intended victim) is targeted for some form of retribution stemming from a violation of trust in the drug trade (e.g., receiving drugs to sell and not turning in the money).

Great escapes from the police are also common as seen in the following story told to the field team:

So, we was on the highway. I was smoking [rock cocaine] just looking around. He was just driving. He was like doing fifty on the highway at night. The next thing you know the narcs were pulling us over. I rolled down my window, I just shot the stem [cocaine pipe] right out the thing and the lighter out the window. My brother, I don't know what he did with the cooker or whatever. I think he slipped it under the seat or something. The needle, I don't know what he did with it. They took us out of the car. They searched us and everything. They made us drop our underwear, lift up our socks, everything. And they didn't find nothing!

The literature on narratives would certainly suggest that in formulating their tales, drug users, like all storytellers, merge their immediate experiences with culturally constituted imagination, objective fact with colorful fantasy, and the details of real events with rhetorical devices and culturally meaningful themes. In analyzing the narratives in their sample, Singer and his colleagues found that they appear to group around a number of contrastive experiential sets: high (psychotropic effects) versus low (drug withdrawal), kindness versus abuse, trust versus betrayal, success versus failure and regret, and excitement and surprise versus burdensome routines (things you have to put up with) and enduring suffering. Whatever the historic truthfulness of any particular narrative, the dynamic and oppositional tension of the narratives seems to very accurately reflect the actual experience of street drug use: drug users both love and hate being on drugs and all that focusing their lives on drugs entails. The intensity of this conflicted involvement enlivens their stories, just as their stories construct and encapsulate core cultural meanings in their lives. The research team identified three of these core cultural meanings that they believe have relevance for HIV prevention as well as drug treatment.

First, it is evident from the narratives that acts of generosity and caring are not expected, and hence, when they occur they are seen as a pleasant surprise. The stories underline the degree to which street drug users expect to be mistreated and abused in their social interactions, producing, as a result, a narrational celebration of unforeseen acts of kindness. One lesson of this realization is that in drug treatment or AIDS prevention work with drug users consistently treating participants in a caring fashion, based on a genuine appreciation of them as fellow human beings, would be warmly received. Although service providers who work with street drug users come to grow wary of their survival-oriented tendency to engage in manipulation or be undependable, their narratives reveal both a hunger for acts of patient kindness and a strong valuing of caring behavior.

Second, drug-user stories emphasize that they are quite wary of betrayal. Their personal narratives suggest that they expect others to fail them, although it is always, nonetheless, a painful experience. Avoiding actions that can be construed (rightly or wrongly) as betrayal, therefore, should be a critical program element in AIDS prevention.

Finally, the narratives emphasize the skills and abilities of drug users, attributes that fly in the face of their usual denigration as unproductive individuals who lack desirable qualities or useful talents. Reversing the usual course, by treating drug users as socially resourceful, knowledge-able, and goal-oriented individuals is a way of engaging drug users in AIDS prevention. At the same time, the narratives suggest the value of recognizing and appreciating demonstrated acts of generosity and caring by drug users, traits that similarly are denied by social stereotypes that portray them as aggressively self-focused and completely controlled by their drug dependencies.

CONCLUSION

Since about 2000, in particular, there have appeared an impressive number of compelling books by anthropologists immersed in ethno-graphic research on HIV disease in places big and small around the world. Generally, these books have attempted to unpack the complexities of the pandemic as a form of lived experience in local context, as a product of social relations within and between societies, and as an issue in human decision making and action. Often, an underlying topic is: why do these people in this place at this time act and think the way they do in the con-text of the HIV pandemic? Anthropologists with a special interest in HIV have pursued a wide range of topics and issues (characteristic of the dis-cipline), from patterns of male condom use and female condom accept-ability to the benefits (and unintended risk consequences) of circumcision; from the roles of ethnomedical practices and practitioners in HIV disease treatment to the consequences of the stigmatization of people living with HIV infection; and from the role of gender relations in the structuring of HIV vulnerability to the health and social impacts on children orphaned by the disease. They have also studied the daily experience and struggles of having AIDS and community response to the epidemic and people living with infection, and they have worked as advocates, intervention program administrators, program evaluators, and community outreach coordinators. This is only a short list of the many relevant concerns in-vestigated by anthropologists and types of work anthropologists working in the pandemic have done across the globe. Indeed, inventories like this are always incomplete, both because anthropologists have participated in HIV-related work in diverse countries, regions, and local contexts and also because HIV remains an ever-changing domain with a continuous array of emergent issues.

CHAPTER 10

Syndemics and the Biosocial Nature of Health

THINKING ABOUT THE NATURE OF DISEASE

What is disease? It is generally recognized that the traditional biomedical approach to disease, an approach that has dominated thinking about health since the late nineteenth century, was erected through an effort to diagnostically identify, closely study, and therapeutically treat individual cases of specific diseases. This approach is based on an understanding that each disease (e.g., cholera, diabetes) is a distinct entity that exists in nature separate from other diseases and independent of the biosocial contexts in which it is found. In the case of infectious disease, illness is understood as a consequence of a specific pathogenic agent, be it a bacteria, virus, parasite, or other microorganism or helminth (worm).

This approach, at the heart of biomedicine, proved useful historically in focusing medical attention on immediate causes and biological expressions of disease (seen as any harmful change that interferes with the normal form or function of the body or any of its parts or systems). It contributed as well to the emergence of diverse pharmaceutical, surgical, and other biomedical treatments for specific diseases, some of which have been enormously successful, especially for acute conditions, particularly those preventable with vaccines and hygienic practices or treatable with antibiotics. However, adopting this orientation to disease has meant that "our health and research paradigms have been shaped by reductionist ways of thinking in which one aims to isolate diseases, control the environment, and single out exposures" that cause individual disruptions, breakdowns, and infectious of the body (Maria González-Guarda et al. 2011: 114).

Consequently, in public health, "[t]raditionally, research protocols, prevention programs, policy interventions, and other aspects of . . . practice have focused on one disease at a time, leaving other health problems to be addressed by parallel enterprises" (Syndemics Prevention Network 2005). Moreover, as infectious disease physician John Bartlett (2007: S125) points out with specific reference two infectious diseases of considerable contemporary global importance, "experts in TB and experts in HIV infection live in different worlds. . . . This great divide applies to clinical care, research, and training; it is lessened by the overlap between the two diseases but not as much as it should be." The same point applies as well to other disease overlaps where the copresence of two or more diseases critically shapes the well-being of the patient or population experiencing a congress of diseases.

Even in the development of new medications, the emphasis has been on isolating one disease from another, as if that were how diseases exist in the world (which is not the case). Thus, an examination of randomized clinical control trials for new medications by Harriette Van Spall and coworkers (2007) found that 81 percent of the randomized trials published in the most prestigious medical journals excluded patients because of coexisting medical problems. In other words, clinical trials, the gold standard for testing new drugs or other treatment approaches before bringing them onto the market, avoid investigating the health effects of copresent diseases. In a 2005 study, Cynthia Boyd and colleagues (2005) analyzed influential, evidence-based clinical practice guidelines used to inform physicians on how to best treat nine of the most common chronic diseases in the United States, including osteoporosis, arthritis, type 2 diabetes, and high cholesterol. These researchers found that fewer than half the guidelines specifically addressed patients with more than one disease, and most were limited to patients with only one coexisting disease or a small number of closely related diseases, even though two-thirds of people over age sixty-five have multiple chronic diseases. These kinds of findings are of significance because they reveal the degree to which biomedicine traditionally has seen and acted on the world of disease as a place in which copresent diseases have no impact on each other or the well-being of the patient. The same is true within public health, which has been strongly influenced by biomedicine, each disease in a population is responded to as if it were encapsulated by itself rather than linked to and affected by other diseases. Consequently departments of public health at city, county, and state levels comprise disease-specific silos with their own budgets, staff, agenda, bureaucracy, and programs, with little communication between departments as if they were separated by protected borders.

Biomedical and public health consideration of the importance of a person having two or more diseases at the same time is relatively recent. The term *comorbidity* was introduced into the medical literature by Feinstein (1970) to denote the fact that diseases do not tend to appear in isolation but rather as two or more copresent conditions that befall a sufferer at the same time. The concept of comorbidity has proved to be useful in medicine as a means of allowing clinicians to develop a framework for treating patients with multiple diseases. It has been used in helping them to make critical decisions about which disease to treat first and whether treating one disease by itself will outweigh the negative effects of not treating other copresent conditions. Feinstein's approach reflects a conception of comorbid diseases as copresent but still independent entities. It fails, however, to draw attention to the importance of *comorbid disease interactions*.

INTRODUCING THE SYNDEMICS PERSPECTIVE

The syndemics perspective challenges the conception of the world of disease described in the previous section. Rather than focus on discrete, bounded disease units, it focuses instead on connections, interactions, flows, and underlying unities. The syndemics perspective, moreover, moves beyond conventional focus in epidemiology on groups at high risk or individuals who engage in risky behaviors to environments of risk and agents and social structures that promote risk and adverse disease interaction. Its concern is with *epidemiological synergism*, i.e., reciprocal relationships that propel a spiral of disease within a population.

One way of grasping the core idea of this alternative perspective (and body of theory) is to consider what nature writer Douglas Chadwick had said about the common lichen that grows on trees and rocks (assuming the air is not filled with lichen-killing pollution) giving them a splotchy brown and green coloration. Lichen, as Chadwick notes, and contrary to popular assumption, are not a single organism but rather an interacting group of species, a community composed of two quite different species. Thus lichen can be seen "as kind of a doorway between organisms [or individual species] and ecosystems" (Chadwick 2003: 106). "Look out one direction, and you see individual things; look the other way, you see processes, relationships—things together. This is the new level in understanding biology" (Chadwick 2003: 106). In the words of theoretical physicist, Fritjof Capra (1984: 57), Quantum theory . . . shows that we cannot decompose the world into independently existing smallest units. As we penetrate into matter, nature does not show us any isolated 'building blocks,' but rather appears as a complicated web of relations between the various parts of the whole."

Many other observers of the world of nature also have commented on the importance—indeed, the centrality—of interconnections in nature. The world renown Scottish-born American naturalist and conservationist leader John Muir (1911: 110) noted in his quaint style, "When we try to pick out anything by itself, we find it hitched to everything else in the Universe." More recently Clive Jones (National Science Foundation 1998), a terrestrial ecologist at the Cary Institute of Ecosystem Studies, observed with specific reference to the issue of health, "A remarkable amount of nature is interconnected, with unexpected players and interactions over time that have important implications for human health." This is the perspective on what nature is like informs the conception of syndemics, which incorporates both biological and social interactions, but also the interactions between biology and social forces, to understand immediate and ultimate causes and processes in disease. Notably, in this regard, Capra has likened the reductionistic approach that syndemics theory challenges to the experience of a housefly who lands on a television screen and only sees the little dots (pixels) and not the big picture (which is the reason for the specific configuration of the little dots). A fly with syndemic vision, by contrast, could fly through a crowded room and see not only all the individuals in the room but also all of the ways they are connected to each other (e.g., friends, coworkers, enemies), interact with each other (e.g., date, play tennis together on Tuesdays, intentionally ignore each other), and have impact on each other (e.g., cause happiness, make nervous, frustrate).

Defined as a set of enmeshed and mutually enhancing epidemic diseases and other health problems that, *working together* within the influencing context of noxious and unjust social and physical conditions, syndemics significantly and adversely affect the disease burdens of populations as well as the disease experience of individual sufferers (Singer 2009a), as illustrated in Figure 10.1.

It is important to be clear on the key differences between the concepts comorbidity and syndemic. As Mustanski, Garofalo, Herrick, and Donenberg (2007: 40) aptly point out, "[I]t is possible for two disorders to be comorbid, but not . . . syndemic (that is, the disorders are not epidemic in the studied population or their co-occurrence is not accompanied by additional adverse health consequences)." Thus, diseases have been found to interact in ways that do not produce additional negative outcomes. Moreover, it is possible for one disease to inhibit the negative effects of another disease, a relationship that is termed a *counter-syndemic*. In syndemics, by contrast, two or more diseases or other health conditions (e.g., trauma, malnutrition) interact in some fashion (biochemically, behaviorally, anatomically) to make one (unidirectional syndemics) or more than one of the involved diseases worse or more easily spread (bidirectional syndemics). Moreover, the term comorbidity does not require (and often does not involve) a consideration of social conditions that facilitate or are the ultimate causes of disease. For the syndemics perspective on health and disease, however, this consideration is fundamental.

Figure 10.1
The Syndemic Model

Syndemic Model

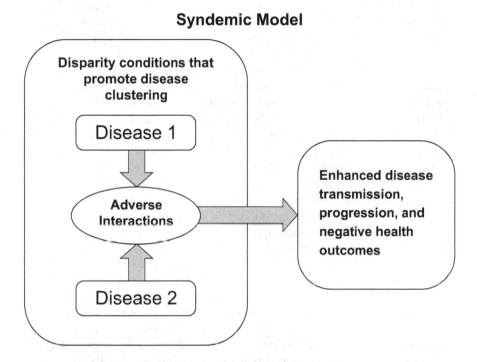

Introduction of the syndemics perspective has begun to have impact on the dominant biomedically influenced conception of disease. In no small part because of mounting syndemic awareness, biomedical boundaries between chronic and acute diseases are breaking down (Barrett 2010), concern has mounted about the heavy toll of interacting emergent diseases in marginalized populations (e.g., the H1N1/diabetes syndemic among indigenous peoples around the world), the effects of pathogen-pathogen interaction on disease virulence are being reexamined (Bulled and Singer 2011; Singer 2010b), the importance of animal populations and zoonotic diseases in human health have gained new prominence (Rock, Buntain, Hatfield, and Hallgrimsson 2009), and health promotion efforts are being redesigned to address adverse disease interfaces (e.g., the new South African strategic plan to target the HIV/TB syndemic for the period from 2012 to 2016; Ribera and Hausmann-Muela 2011). Moreover, add Reitmanova and Gustafson (2012: 404), "A syndemic approach unravels social and biological connections which shape the distribution of infections over space and time and is useful in de-racializing and de-medicalizing . . . epidemiologic models."

These developments reflect broader health changes that are underway, of which syndemics are an important component; namely, humankind is developing a global disease ecology that entails a convergence of disease patterns across diverse social environments. One role that syndemics play in this consequential epidemiological transition involves chronic/acute disease interactions, or what, for developing countries, has been called "the worst of both worlds" (Bradley 1993). As Berndard Choi et al. (2007: 832) emphasize, "Segregation of epidemiology into chronic and infectious diseases has led to a neglected area in public health—the interface between [these two disease conditions]. Indeed, this neglected area requires increased public health attention across a broad spectrum of activity, including research, surveillance, prevention[,] . . . control and health policy." Syndemics theory provides a framework for guiding such research (Singer 2009b).

Research since the dawn of the new century has shown that syndemics are having a significant impact on diverse populations currently and are likely to have continued consequential influence on the health profile of the twenty-first century. In no small part because of syndemics, contemporary health around the world looks rather different and in several ways worse than was expected before the turn of the twenty-first century. The reason is succinctly summarized by Littleton and Park (2009: 1679) in stressing that "syndemic relationships multiply risk," and greater risk tends to promote disease.

At the same time, it is now understood that many of the most damaging human epidemics across time and location, from the lethal influenza epidemic of 1918–1919 to the contemporary global AIDS pandemic, are the consequence not of single disease striking human populations but a congress of diseases acting in tandem under the influence of toxic social conditions (Kant 2003). As Mark Nichter (2008: 157) observed in his review of global health, the syndemic idea "is a useful conceptual framework for social science investigations into global health inequality that are sensitive to environments of risk and agents promoting risk, [and that take us beyond a narrow conception of] groups at risk and risky behaviors." In short, syndemics has opened up a new way of thinking and responding to health challenges faced by human communities through time and space.

Moreover, as a *biosocial approach to disease*, seeing the world through a syndemics lens does not narrowly reduce disease to biology but rather is focused on the ways in which biology and society interact to shape health (see Figure 10.2).

Indeed, the syndemics approach is concerned especially with three types of interaction:

- Micro-level of disease interaction: the specific pathways and mechanisms of contact and exchange between two or more comorbid health conditions clustered within a population that result in enhanced disease morbidity and morality

Figure 10.2

The Syndemics Biosocial Model of Disease

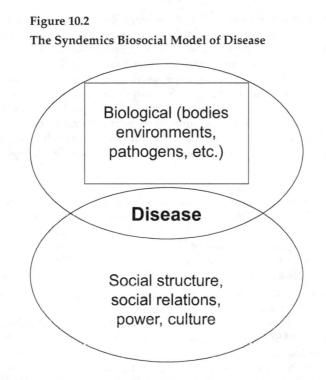

- Meso-level of disease interaction: the cultural beliefs and practices that comprise local knowledge about the diseases in question that shape on-the-ground behaviors in a syndemic with the effect of enhancing or diminishing disease interaction and disease course
- Macro-level of disease interaction: the social and environmental determinants of disease spread and clustering that enable synergistic micro-level disease exchange.

Each of these levels are now discussed in turn.

THE MICRO-LEVEL: PATHWAYS OF DISEASE INTERACTION

How do diseases interact? Multiple pathways of syndemic interaction among diseases have been identified, including the following:

- Changes in biochemistry or damage to organ systems caused by one disease promote the progression of another disease. An example of this pathway is seen with influenza. Viruses that cause this disease target and kill cells that comprise the ciliated epithelia that line the surface tissue of the respiratory tract. These cells have five- to ten-micrometer-long hairlike projections that beat in coordinated waves, sweeping mucus (which traps small particles such as bacteria), dirt, and other foreign matter out of the lungs and thus perform a critical immune function. Smokers, for example, are more prone to infection because tobacco smoke destroys these ciliated cells. Because influenza also kills these cells, it "can pave the way for other microbes to enter areas of the upper respiratory system damaged by the virus and spread into the lungs or occasionally other parts of the body" (Barnes 2005: 338). Similarly, suffers of cystic fibrosis undergo alterations of the respiratory tract, which appears to predispose their lungs to diverse bacterial infections, including from Burkholderia cepacia, a family of bacteria first identified as the cause of soft-rot on onions. Chronic pulmonary infection is one of the leading causes of death among people with cystic fibrosis (Lipuma 2005).

- One disease enhances the virulence of another disease. An example of this process is seen among individuals dually diagnosed with HSV (herpes simplex virus) and HIV. Studies show a significantly more rapid pathogenesis of AIDS in such individuals. This amplification appears to be caused by specific effects that the herpes virus has on the pace of HIV viral replication. These effects appear to be shaped by certain proteins found in HSV (e.g., ICP-0, ICP-4, and ICP-27) that boost HIV replication efficacy (Schacker 2001).

- One disease assists the physical transmission of another. In a literature review of 163 published studies on the interrelationships between HIV infection and other sexually transmitted diseases (STDs), Wasserheit (1992) identified 75 studies on the role of STDs in the facilitation of HIV transmission of which 15 analyses provided laboratory evidence of STDs (adjusted for sexual behavior) that affirmed that both ulcerative and nonulcerative STDs (i.e., those diseases that do and do not cause lesions on the genitals) increase the risk of HIV transmission by approximately three- to fivefold. This syndemic interaction, the author concludes, may help account for the explosive growth of HIV infection in some populations. Genital ulcers, for example, may increase susceptibility to HIV by disrupting mucosal integrity (breaking the body surface allows HIV entry) and by increasing the presence and activation of HIV susceptible cells found in the genital tract where they can be attacked by HIV upon exposure (Fleming and Wasserheit 1999).

- Coterminous body injection. Through several pathways, it is possible for two or more interacting diseases to be injected into the body at the same time. One of these, involving the injection of multiple tick-borne infectious diseases, is described in the "A Closer Look" later in the chapter. Another method involves infected syringes used by injection drug users who do not have access to sterile syringes. Studies show that in addition to HIV, syringes can be involved in the spread of a number of other diseases including hepatitis B, hepatitis C, parvovirus, leishmaniasis, and malaria. Using a syringe previously used by someone infected with two or more of these diseases can transmit them concurrently to the new syringe user. For example, between 25 and 30 percent of HIV infected individuals suffer from chronic hepatitis C virus infection. A study of injection drug users in China found that infection with HIV increased the probability of HCV infection by seventeen-fold (Xia et al. 2008). In the Vancouver Injection Drug User Study, C. Miller et al. (2004) found that among younger injectors (those under thirty years of age), sixteen percent were coinfected with HIV and HCV at baseline, and an additional 15 percent were coinfected at follow-up. Simultaneous coinfection through injection with dually infected syringes appears to help drive this potentially deadly syndemic.

- Gene mixing or assortment among pathogens. This pathway is created by the capacity of microorganisms to exchange genetic material, including both the movement of genes from one strain or subtype of a species to another strain and the movement across species (e.g., one bacterial species to another), or even across types of microorganisms (e.g., from a bacteria to a virus). Mixing across "species" is of particular importance in influenza. The 2009 H1N1 influenza pandemic was caused by a triple assortment of viruses involving genes from avian, human, and swine influenza viruses coming together to form a new viral pathogen. Similarly, both the H2N2 (which caused an influenza epidemic in 1957) and H3N2 (which caused an influenza epidemic in 1968) were generated through gene mixing events in mammalian hosts and involved genes coming together from multiple avian viruses and the zoonotic infection of humans. Mixing also can promote drug resistance in pathogens, as is currently happening with strains of tuberculosis that are now resistant to multiple frontline TB drugs.

- Emotional pathways. Not all pathways are biological; psychological factors can also drive syndemics. A case in point is a syndemic condition that has been called diabulemia. The first part of this term comes from diabetes. It is well established that type 1 diabetes and many cases of type 2 diabetes can be controlled through the routine injection of manufactured insulin. This usually requires diabetes sufferers to administer regular doses of insulin through self-injection with a plastic diabetes syringe. Studies of medical adherence in people with diabetes show that various psychosocial factors, including depression, certain personality attributes (e.g., poor internal locus of control), poor memory, inadequate health literacy, and conflicted family environments reduce the quality of self-care in diabetes sufferers. By contrast, in cases of diabetes, patients who also suffer from eating disorders like bulimia and anorexia nervosa may consciously select to limit insulin intake to achieve weight loss (as well as avoid the weight gain that can be associated with insulin use). Sufferers of these often brutal disorders, which involve abnormal body perception and intense sensitivity to being perceived as fat, engage in various techniques (depending on the particular disorder) such as obsessive dieting, intensive exercise, compulsive use of laxatives, and regular vomiting as strategies for experiencing a sense of control in their lives (Singer and Singer 2008). As Stuart Brink, a senior pediatric endocrinologist at the New England Diabetes and Endocrinology Center in Massachusetts observes, "You don't have to vomit. You don't have to purge. You don't have to use laxatives. . . . You just have to let your sugar stay high" (quoted in Mendelsohn 2008). The end result is a worsening of diabetes with potentially severe consequence from blindness to loss of feet to death.

- Iatrogenic pathways. Iatrogenesis refers to an inadvertent adverse effect or complication resulting from medical treatment. For example, McFarland (1995) carried out a study in a general medicine ward of a county hospital that involved recruiting all consenting patients in the study ward over an eleven-month period. Of the 382 patients enrolled in the study, 32.9 percent developed severe diarrhea while in the hospital; 57 percent of these cases were iatrogenic in origin as a result of antibiotic therapy for another disease. The most common cause of the diarrhea was an infection, often by the pathogenic agent *Clostridium difficile*. This pathogen is known to cause intense diarrhea (through the release of toxins), as well as other intestinal diseases, when competing normal (and needed) bacteria in the gut flora have been wiped out by antibiotics allowing the intestines to be overrun by *C. difficile.* McFarland (1995: 295) concluded that in the study sample "diarrhea was found to be common and associated with an additional burden of comorbidity."

THE MESO-LEVEL: THE ROLE OF CULTURAL KNOWLEDGE AND PRACTICE IN SYNDEMICS

Human communities the world over possess locally produced or borrowed and adapted knowledge about health and various healing practices. Are these ever a factor in the development or avoidance of a syndemic? A case in point is the great influenza pandemic of 1918–1919 (caused by the syndemic interaction of a viral strain of influenza with a bacterial lung infection), a calamity that killed 50 to 100 million people worldwide. During this pandemic, various local health strategies were tried to protect people or to cure their infection. In Utah, for example, people adopted a variety of home and doctor remedies. Alcohol, which was normally banned in the state because of Mormon influence, was sold to doctors who used it to treat patients. In the town of Panguitch, Margaret Callister, who was a young child when the pandemic hit the area, "remembered 'dead people were all around us, three or four to a family.' Following a typical folk practice, her mother put sacks of herbs around her neck and those of her siblings to prevent influenza" (Department of Health and Human Services, undated). In the small town of Meadow, Utah, local residents understood that "germs" caused the disease; however, they were unsure of just what germs were or how they were transmitted from one person to another. As a result, families locked themselves in their homes and sealed their keyholes and the cracks around their doors with cotton. When these strategies proved ineffective because individuals who had already been exposed fell ill, townspeople resorted to herbal remedies concocted by a local healer. These too did nothing to stem the tide of the pandemic.

As these folk practices were being tested at the lay level, Utah public health officials passed laws requiring citizens to wear masks. Throughout the state, wearing of masks became common practice. During this period in the town of Cedar City, Utah, a parade celebrating the end World War I featured a statue of Lady Liberty wearing a mask. As was the case many decades later with the H1N1 influenza pandemic, people were mistaken in thinking that masks would prevent the spread of the disease.

Various folk practices also were in vogue centuries earlier when the Black Plague (bubonic plague) swept in several waves through Europe between the sixth and seventeenth centuries. Generally attributed to the bacterium *Yersinia pestis*, the plague is believed by Cantor (2002) to have been caused by a syndemic uniting the effects of *Y. pestis* with those of anthrax and by DeWitte and Wood (2008) between the *Y. pestis* bacterium and malnutrition. Whatever the exact cause, one folk talisman used to ward off this highly virulent disease involved nailing a horseshoe above one's door, a practice that is still in use to bring good luck. In Scotland during in the fourteenth century, loaves of bread were hung on poles and left to become moldy, after which they would be burned. The rationale for this practice was the belief that the bread became moldy because it had collected the entities causing plague. More drastically, bloodletting through the cutting open of veins was in common practice as a plague treatment. Herbs were also used. Garlic, for example, was consumed heavily for various diseases, and people believed that it offered protection from the Black Plague. In fact, almost everyone who became infected with the plague died, so it is unlikely that any of these behaviors offered more than emotional relief.

Although the local knowledge that fueled such practices only played a role in the syndemics to the degree to which they blocked the adoption of other behaviors (e.g., killing the rats that spread *Y. pestis*) that might have been more efficacious or encouraged people to engage in risky behaviors because they thought they were protected, they probably were not a major factor in disease interaction. In other cases, meso-level cultural practices may play a more active role in syndemic development. For example, lead has been found in a number of traditional medicines used among some East Indians, Native Americans, Middle Easterners, West Asians, and Hispanics. An example is Hispanic use of ethnomedicines that contain substances known to users as *greta* or *azarcon* for upset stomach (*empacho*), constipation, diarrhea, vomiting, and irritability among teething babies. These substances are both fine orange powders that have a lead content that sometimes reaches 90 percent (Trotter 1985). The health-related consequences of lead exposure include the disruption of three biological processes: (1) molecular interactions, (2) intercell signaling, and (3) cell functioning, which can lead to nervous system damage, decreased IQ, decreased growth, sterility, hyperactivity, impaired hearing, and seizures. Lead damages all body systems, including the immune system, creating the possibility of a lead poisoning/infectious disease syndemic, an outcome already known from animal model studies and to a lesser degree from research with humans (Singer 2011a).

In short, the folk use of ethnomedicines to treat upset stomach could be a factor in a syndemic driven by the interaction of lead poisoning and various infectious diseases. This might be expected to be most likely in cases where the community using lead-bearing ethnomedicines also lives in poor inner-city areas in which the local housing stock has a high lead content because of having been painted in the past with now decomposing leaded paint, a not-uncommon situation across the United States. These statements remain somewhat tentative because there remain major gaps in our understanding of lead as a factor in human immunodeficiency disease.

Another example of how local cultural knowledge may facilitate a syndemic is illustrated by a study carried out by anthropologist Vinay Kamat (2009) on why large numbers of children infected with malaria in sub-Saharan Africa die because they do not get prompt (within twenty-four hours of onset) medical attention. Based on sixteen months of ethnographic research in a community (population = 5,550) near Dar es Salaam, Tanzania, with high malaria rates, Kamat found that most children with a fever were not brought to a medical facility until forty-eight hours after onset. Furthermore, he found that when a child developed a fever, most parents (usually mothers because fathers tend to stay out of it) adopt a "wait and see" policy, as there are many causes of fever in the area and most are self-limiting conditions. Upon interview, parents said their first reaction to childhood fever was to assume the symptoms were caused by "an ordinary illness" (*homa ya kawaida*) rather than a "life-threatening illness" (*homa kali*) or malaria (*homa ya malaria*), which was certainly a known disease in the community. Parents commonly spoke about childhood illness as routine, something that was part of everyday life for children in their world. Even past experience with malaria did not change this pattern, and mothers were surprised when their children were ultimately diagnosed with malaria. Even when their child became quite sick, some mothers did not recognize malaria but thought their child suffered from a condition they called *degedege* (which literally means "bird-bird"), a folk illness with symptoms that parallel malaria and thought by community members to be caused by a coastal spirit that takes the form of a bird that casts its shadow on vulnerable children and makes them sick. Many of the parents interviewed by Kamat believed that an injection, of the sort children might be given in the hospital, could cause a child with *degedege* to go into convulsions, leading to death. Also parents were concerned about the prohibitive costs of diagnoses that required multiple injections, in addition to the travel costs of having to return to the medical facility for multiple injections, an issue of no small concern to a poor family that must make judicious decisions about resource allocation. In that malaria is known to act together adversely with other threats to health (e.g., helminth infection, HIV), delays in its treatment could facilitate the progress of this disease and its interaction with other comorbid diseases.

At the same time, in another setting, ethnomedical treatment for malaria, may have helped to avoid malaria-driven syndemics. Quinine, derived from the bark of the cinchona tree, a reasonably effective antimalarial drug, was originally discovered by the Quechua Indians of Peru and Bolivia; Jesuit missionaries learned about the drug from indigenous people and began shipping it to Europe, where it long served as the primary preventive and treatment for global travelers in malarial areas.

THE MACRO-LEVEL: THE SOCIAL ORIGINS OF SYNDEMICS

According to the World Health Organization, there is a

growing body of evidence accumulated over the last 20 years which shows that people who live in disadvantaged social circumstances are more prone to illness, distress and disability and die sooner than those living in more advantaged circumstances . . . . Evidence from around the world points to an increase in the gaps in health status and health care by socioeconomic status, geographical location, gender, race, ethnicity and age group. (Currie et al. 2008: 2)

Adds Harvard epidemiologist Nancy Krieger (2005: 15):

Social inequality kills. It deprives individuals and communities of a healthy start in life, increases their burden of disability and disease, and brings early death. Poverty and discrimination, inadequate medical care, and violation of human rights all act as powerful social determinants of who lives and who dies, at what age, and with what degree of suffering.

One of the important ways this occurs is through the *multiplying effects of syndemics* in promoting disease clustering within a population, facilitating disease spread among members of a population and propelling disease progression to more advanced and damaging disease states in comorbid patients.

The causal relationship between social inequality and poor health has been documented in numerous studies. Such research shows that if you measure the inequality of any society and you correlate that with key epidemiological variables such as infant mortality, death from violence, or life expectancy, the correlation is highly significant. Kaplan and coworkers (1996), for example, examined health records and found strong correlations between income inequality and low birth weight of children, rates of homicide, exposure to violent crime, work disability, rates of stress-driven smoking, and imprisonment. These associations are confirmed by the various studies reported in *The Society and Population Health Reader* (Kawachi, Kennedy, and Wilkinson 1999, among many other references, e.g., Budrys 2011). Why is inequality so toxic? In part because it subjects people to chronic (daily) stress (e.g., from overcrowding, living in conditions marked by threat of physical violence, being subjected to the adverse psychosocial effects of continual exposure to deteriorated physical environments, suffering deprivation and relative deprivation) that wears down the effectiveness of the immune system to fight disease by overwhelming the body's ability to cope. Such conditions also have a negative impact on the circulatory system, cause hormonal imbalances, and contribute to depression. Another reason is malnutrition, a common consequence of inequality, which contributes to subpar functioning of the immune system. This is because the body needs specific macro- and micronutrients to build the various kinds of cells (e.g., CD4 cells) that comprise the immune system. Physical trauma, witnessing violence, and the threat of street violence also are higher in poor neighborhoods and constitute another factor in immune system dysfunction. Moreover, subordinated populations are more likely to be exposed to toxins in their immediate environment. Industrial dumping of hazardous waste from production, for example, is much more likely to occur in poor areas than in wealthier ones, and wealthier nations actually sell their hazardous waste and other discards to cash-starved nations willing to accept and dispose of toxic waste in exchange for needed cash. Some of the poorest people in the world, in fact, live near urban trash piles so that they can scavenge a meager living (by recycling found items) off of the trash of wealthier families. The breakdown of social support networks, which are vital to the health of a social species like humans, may also tend to occur under the kinds of stressed and unstable conditions common to poor and subordinate social groups. Without good support networks, people tend to be alone and vulnerable, emotional states that contribute to sickness. As this list of factors suggests, humans biologize their life experience: that is, whatever they experience and feel finds expression in the health state of their physical bodies. Additionally, poorer, more marginalized people tend to have less access to public health prevention measures and biomedical treatment of existing diseases. Because of poverty, for example, the poor may not get into treatment until a disease has progressed to an advanced stage. Even the cost of a bus ride to a clinic may become a barrier to health care access. Finally, poor and marginalized populations face discrimination in health care institutions, subjecting them to less and lower quality care than wealthier or more dominant groups in society. These factors have grown in recent decades because of pressure from development lender institutions like the World Bank to pressure governments not to subsidize health care or operate government health care.

In light of these multiple pressures on the health of subordinated groups, syndemics theory draws attention to the ways health and biology are significantly shaped by social inequality, the great disparities in the conditions in which different populations or segments of populations live, and the ways power is used to create and maintain the structure of social inequality for the benefit of the wealthiest and most elite groups in society and globally. A syndemics framework, in short, describes situations in which adverse social conditions, such as poverty and oppressive social relationships, stress a population, weaken its natural defenses, and expose it to a constellation of potentially adversely interacting diseases. Furthermore, syndemics theory focuses attention on why disease concentrations or time-space clusters of disease (i.e., at least two but possibly multiple comorbid diseases and other health conditions in a population sequentially or simultaneously), the various pathways and processes through which diseases interact biologically within individual bodies and socially within populations, as well as the ways this interaction increases disease burden beyond what would be expected from the sum of the involved diseases acting alone.

As this discussion suggests, ignoring social conditions as a factor in health status is the equivalent of ignoring clouds, topographical, and climatic patterns in the study of rain. Social conditions are *central to syndemics* for two reasons. First, as indicated, they have impacts on various body systems and can leave groups highly vulnerable to disease. Second, unhealthy social conditions (and the structural social relationships that facilitate unequal living and working conditions) promote the clustering of multiple diseases in subordinate populations while diminishing ability to resist disease.

THE ANTHROPOLOGICAL ORIGIN OF THE SYNDEMICS CONCEPT

The term *syndemic* is a portmanteau, a word that brings together two distinct concepts to convey a new meaning. The first constituent of this term is *synergy*, which is derived from the Greek word *synergo*, meaning two or more agents working together to create a greater effect than the sum of each working alone. The second component is *demic*, which comes from the Greek word *demos* or "people," as in epidemic, pandemic, and endemic.

The origin of the syndemics concept lies in medical anthropology during the early 1990s. Within medical anthropology, this era was shaped by a significant rise in work on the AIDS pandemic, as funding for anthropological research became available from the National Institutes of Health, the Centers for Disease Control and Prevention, private foundations, state governments, and other sources. Working with AIDS-impacted populations called attention to the consequence for health of being immunocompromised—namely, the serial onset of multiple diseases—raising the question: what happens in a human body suffering multiple threats to health?

The first syndemic described by anthropologists in the literature is a tripartite health condition called SAVA, a product of the complex interactions that researchers were beginning to realize occur among substance abuse, violence, and AIDS (Singer 1996a, Singer 2006b). From the syndemic perspective, AIDS, drug use, and violence in particular social contexts are so entwined and codeterminant that it became difficult to conceive of them as distinct or isolated sources of illness. In SAVA, all three disease/health-related components interact in mutually accelerating ways, as was evident in field observations of people engaged in risky behaviors like "street drug use," a term adopted in the health and research literature to refer to the drug-related behaviors of marginalized, inner-city drug users who are forced by poverty, discrimination, and addiction into a visible and public pattern of drug acquisition and consumption. Consequently, in addition to provoking questions about the nature of interactions among co-occurring diseases, it came to be realized that the actual expression of the SAVA syndemic is intimately shaped as well by social context factors such as the social treatment of poor drug users by the larger society, including institutions like the health care system, law enforcement, the courts, and other sections of society.

This set of initial insights about the importance of disease interactions, the development of the syndemics concept to label the intersections of disease, the incorporation of social factors as a central component of the syndemics model, and the initial research on SAVA was initially carried out by a small group of community-based medical anthropologists and other research-ers working on a set of AIDS studies led by Merrill Singer at the Hispanic Health Council (Singer 1996a; Singer and Clair 2003), a community-based health research and service organization in Hartford, Connecticut.

Subsequently, SAVA-related research by Brian Mustanski and cowork-ers (2007) with drug-involved urban young men who have sex with men found that various psychosocial health problems (e.g., binge drinking, sexual assault, psychological distress) additively increased risk for HIV among urban young men who have sex with men. Multivariate analyses by his team found that substance use and being the victim of violence showed the strongest relationship to sexual health and HIV risk. Overall, they found that each psychosocial health problem suffered by an indi-vidual increased the odds of an HIV positive status by 42 percent and also increased the odds of sexual health risk behaviors. On the basis of these findings, they argued that the more diseases suffered by an individual in a population facing HIV/AIDS, the greater the odds of becoming infected.

Similarly, Ron Stall and coworkers (2003) began investigating SAVA in populations of men who have sex with men using a household telephone survey of almost 3,000 men in New York City, Chicago, Los Angeles, and San Francisco. They found that the SAVA syndemic among men who have sex with men is rooted in childhood sexual abuse, which contributes to the development of depression in adulthood and subsequent entrance into abusive adult relationships, use of multiple drugs, and high levels of HIV risk and infection. Furthermore, being the victim of homophobic attacks contributes to serious health problems among adult gay men. These psychosocial factors interact and are mutually reinforcing. The work of Stall and coworkers helped to build broad interest in syndemics. Also critical to awareness about the syndemics approach was the formation of the Syndemics Prevention Network (and website) by the Centers for Disease Control and Prevention under the guidance of Bobby Millstein (2001).

The development of the syndemics concept and syndemic theory extended the work of health researchers who had previously recognized the fundamental importance of disease interaction in social context. Most notably, in an important series of papers on health in New York City, Deborah Wallace and Roderick Wallace (1998) called attention to what they termed the "synergism of plagues" produced by public policies designed to restrict municipal services in poor neighborhoods as a way of pushing people out, thereby freeing up the land they lived on for economic development (i.e., turning the land occupied by the poor into profits for the wealthy). The tragic outcome was a mass movement of people to new (but also poor) areas, resulting in overcrowding and an unraveling of supportive community relationships and support structures, as well as a set of linked and interacting epidemics of tuberculosis, measles, substance abuse, AIDS, low-weight births, and street violence.

TOWARD MULTIDISCIPLINARITY

Since the initial work on syndemics that we have reviewed here, syndemics has become an increasingly widely used multidisciplinary disease concept and associated body of disease theory. The web-based Syndemics Prevention Network developed at the CDC, the use of the syndemics perspective in various CDC publications (Millstein 2001), and attention-generating public presentations by various CDC-affiliated researchers, including the director of the CDC, disseminated the syndemics perspective broadly among researchers from various disciplines as well as among public health officials and providers. At the same time, epidemiologists like Ron Stall and coworkers (2003, 2007) and Freudenberg et al. (2006) published influential papers that helped spark further interest in syndemics across several disciplines. Additionally, various anthropologists not affiliated with the Hispanic Health Council and dispersed across several countries also began adopting a syndemics approach to health research, helping to create a global interest in this phenomenon (M. Marshall 2005, 2013; Herring 2008; Everett 2009; Himmelgreen et al. 2009; Littlefield and Park 2009; Rock et al. 2009; Sattenspiel and Herring 2010; Mendenhall 2012).

The resulting growth in the recognized utility of the syndemics approach is seen in its adoption across multiple health-related disciplines and the ever-increasing pace of syndemics publications within and beyond medical anthropology, including public health, biomedicine, psychology, nursing, dentistry, behavioral health, and veterinary medicine, among others (Stall et al. 2007; Kurtz 2008; Gonzáles-Guardia 2009; Gonzáles-Guarda et al. 2011; H. Klein 2011). Although still not universally used among reseachers studying the effects of interaction among comorbid conditions, the notion of syndemics has become broadly established in the world of global health.

Understanding the idea of syndemics is facilitated by a closer examination of a specific example, as seen in the following "A Closer Look."

"A Closer Look"

GRASPING THE SYNDEMIC INTERACTION: SCHISTOSOMIASIS AND HIV

Schistosoma are tiny blood-consuming worms (trematodes) that derive their name from the fact that they travel through human bodies in pairs, male and female, with the male living in a slit in the body of the female. An individual can become infected by schistosoma when the water-dwelling parasite, which is carried by a freshwater snail vector, penetrates the host's skin. This can happen, for example, when the individual is standing in water that is home to the snail, as when a woman washes her family's clothes or pots in a river, a common practice in lesser developed nations or regions without running water in poorer areas. In girls and women, this can occur through a urinary tract penetration by the parasite (see Figure 10.3). Schistosomiasis, the disease caused by schistosoma, also known as bilharzia, is not found in the United States, but more than two hundred million people are infected worldwide. Long-term infection with schistosomiasis reduces the capacity of sufferers to work and in some cases can lead to death; perhaps claiming as many as two hundred thousand lives per year in sub-Saharan Africa alone. In children, schistosomiasis can cause anemia, growth stunting, and a reduced ability to learn. In recent years, as ecotourists have sought new experiences by traveling "off of the beaten track" to less traditional tourist areas, they have also been infected with this disease. At times, infected tourists (who have never had previous immune system exposure) present with severe acute infection and may develop paralysis.

Figure 10.3
Life Cycle of Schistomes (Developed by Taina Litwak. From John I. Bruce, Schistosomiasis: VBC Tropical Disease Paper No. 2. United States Agency for International Development, Vector Biology Control Project. 1990. p 4. Available at http://pdf.usaid.gov/pdf_docs/PNABI935.pdf)

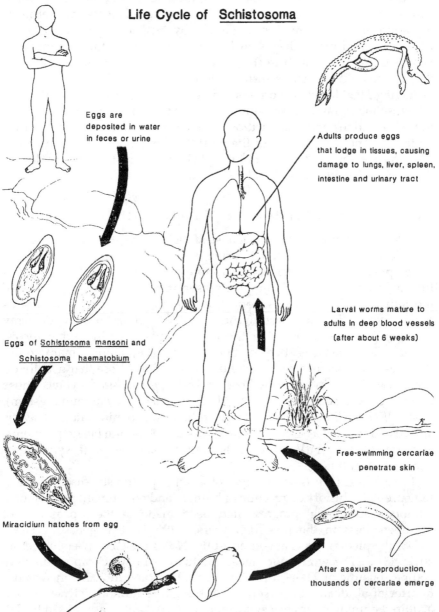

Life Cycle of <u>Schistosoma</u>

Eggs are deposited in water in feces or urine

Adults produce eggs that lodge in tissues, causing damage to lungs, liver, spleen, intestine and urinary tract

Eggs of <u>Schistosoma</u> <u>mansoni</u> and <u>Schistosoma</u> <u>haematobium</u>

Larval worms mature to adults in deep blood vessels (after about 6 weeks)

Free-swimming cercariae penetrate skin

Miracidium hatches from egg

After asexual reproduction, thousands of cercariae emerge

Penetrates soft tissues of snail

It is estimated by the World Health Organization (2012b) that ninety million women in Africa are infected with schistosomiasis and that in southern Africa, 75 percent of women infected with urinary schistosomiasis develop genital lesions. Importantly, these lesions provide HIV (upon exposure) with ready access to the body's deeper cell layers. Furthermore, the abundance of immune cells sought by HIV for reproduction (e.g., CD4+ cells and macrophages) at lesion sites increases rapid binding by HIV. Research in Zimbabwe (Kjetland et al. 2006), for example, showed that women with urinary schistosomiasis have a threefold increased risk of having HIV. In other words, syndemic interaction between HIV and schistosomiasis (as well as with other diseases, such as sexually transmitted infections and malnutrition) is a significant factor in why Africa, which has about 15 percent of the world's population, was estimated in 2007 to have almost 70 percent of people living with HIV worldwide and 75 percent of all global AIDS-related deaths.

HIV/AIDS: THE ULTIMATE SYNDEMOGENIC DISEASE

HIV/AIDS has a special status in *syndemology* (the study of syndemics) historically. Not only, as noted earlier, was its emergence critical to the development of the syndemic perspective during the early 1990s, but the full impact of HIV/AIDS, and the reason it became a leading cause of mortality worldwide, stems from its syndemic interaction with various other diseases. HIV has been found to work together with a wide array of other pathogens, including those that cause hepatitis, tuberculosis, malaria, leishmaniasis, herpes, and other STDs, among many other diseases. This includes both *opportunistic infections* (those that usually do not cause disease in a healthy host) and *nonopportunistic infections* (those that can cause disease even in individuals with a healthy immune system). Also, HIV/AIDS interacts adversely with various noninfectious diseases and disorders such as kidney disease, cancer, behavioral health problems, and malnutrition. HIV, in short, is highly *syndemogenic* (a syndemics-generating condition).

Tuberculosis (TB) is an example of a nonopportunistic disease with a long pre-AIDS history of infection of human (and nonhuman) populations. Although substantial progress had been made in the global control of tuberculosis in the pre-AIDS years, with the emergence of HIV/AIDS, the picture has changed abruptly. Notes the CDC (Getahun et al. 2012: 484), "The world now faces a situation in which approximately 160 persons die of TB each hour (1.45 million died in 2009), in which a quarter of all deaths in persons with human immunodeficiency virus/acquired immunodeficiency syndrome (HIV/AIDS) . . . are caused by TB, and in which the evolution of the bacteria has outpaced the evolution of its treatment to such an extent that some forms of TB are now untreatable." Overall, it is estimated that of the 7 billion people on Earth, 2.3 billion are infected with TB and 9 million new cases are added to this total each year. However, most of those who are infected do not have active TB (known as TB disease) but rather have TB in latent form because it is kept in check but the body's immune system. However, "HIV infection is the most powerful risk factor for progressing from TB infection to disease" (Pawlowski et al. 2012).

ECOSYNDEMICS

In keeping with its focus on connections, intersections, and crossing points, syndemics theory conceptualizes disease in terms of the encompassing biocultural/biosocial environment. Unlike traditional environmental models, however, nature is not conceived in syndemics theory as "natural," in the sense of being in any sense pristine or separate from and independent of human action; nor is it seen as an isolated reserve of nonhuman things and processes (Singer 2010a). Rather, there is a strong concern among those who embrace the syndemic perspective about the historic ways that the physical environment has been shaped and influenced by human action, intentional and otherwise, including the ways human impact on "natural" environments no less than on built environments are a reflection of inequalities within and across societies (Herring and Satenspiel 2007; Baer and Singer 2009). Moreover, syndemics theory is concerned with understanding how social conditions "get under the skin" (i.e., are biologized) and leave their imprint in the form of diseases and disabilities. These points are of keen importance in syndemics theory because (1) as noted syndemics commonly are found among subordinated groups—precisely because of their social status and their physical location or conditions of living; (2) the exercise of power in society shapes the human imprint on the physical environment and the social imprint on the human body (e.g., powerful transnational corporations such as BP have huge impacts on the environment); and (3) effective public health response to syndemics requires focus on underlying causal factors including environmental conditions such as air pollution or global warming (Singer et al. 2011). As Kreiger (2001) comments, thinking "critically and systematically about intimate and integral connections between our social and biological existence—and, especially in the case of social production of disease and ecosocial theory, to name explicitly who benefits from and is accountable for social inequalities in health."

To call attention to the important role of the environment in many syndemics, Singer (2009a) introduced the term *ecosyndemic*, which is defined as the ever-growing impact of global warming and other anthropogenic ecocrises (e.g., oil spills) on the spread of disease and on deleterious interactions among diseases. An example of an ecosyndemic is seen in the deleterious interactions that occur between malaria and filarial worm infection.

Every day in the "malaria belt" that runs through central Africa (and extends around the equator from South America, through the Middle East to Southeast Asia), thousands of people are bitten by the female mosquitoes that serve as vectors of the parasites that cause malaria. The one-celled organisms are so tiny that 50,000 could swim in a pool of water the size of the period at the end of this sentence. Although several dozen make the journey from vector to host with every bite, it only takes a single pathogen to cause malaria and potential death. For example, in the Northwestern Province of Zambia, a forested region sandwiched between the borders of Angola and the Democratic Republic of the Congo, for every 1,000 children under the age of five in Providence there are 1,353 cases of malaria annually, a statistic clarified by the fact that some children are infected more than once per year.

Once in a new human victim, the parasites migrate quickly to the host's liver and embed themselves in liver cells, where they feed and multiply. Within a week, each parasite has consumed a liver cell and replicated as many as forty thousand times. At this point, infected cells explode, and the parasites reenter the host's blood stream. This time their target is red blood cells, in which they continued to feed and replicate. By this point, the few parasites that first entered the host have grown to hundreds of thousands of invaders, each targeting a red blood cell, which it consumes. Before long, the host begins to show the outward symptoms of the destruction going on inside his or her body, including headaches, muscle pain, fever, soaking sweats, and seizures.

Today it is estimated that there are 300 to 500 million cases of malaria each year in Africa alone, resulting in between 1.5 to 2.7 million deaths, more than 90 percent occurring among children under five years of age. Malaria is the reason nearly 20 percent of Zambian babies do not live to see their fifth birthday. This pattern has been going on for so many centuries that humans living in the malaria zone (a temperature zone that is hospitable to mosquitos) have undergone genetic changes that diminish the impact of malaria for some individuals. However, things are changing as malaria appears to be on the move. It is estimated that as many as 100 million extra cases of malaria had occurred worldwide by the close of the twentieth century than would have occurred without the environment-changing effects of global warming. As a result, malaria is now showing up in places it was never seen before or not for many decades. Houston experienced a malaria outbreak in recent years, and cases have been diagnosed as far north as New Jersey, Queens, New York, and Michigan.

Additionally, as it spreads to new areas, malaria may come to interact with diseases that it was not, or not frequently, coterminous with in the past. The potential for such interaction is seen in people who simultaneously suffer malaria and filarial worm infection. Both of these threats to human health can be transmitted by the same mosquito vector. Helminth coinfection appears to affect how well the immune system responds to malaria. Using animal models, it has been shown that coinfected individuals develop more severe disease, assessed both in terms of level of anemia and loss of body mass, compared to individuals infected with malaria alone (Graham et al. 2005). Human research in Georgetown, Guyana, in South America, found that of almost eight hundred people tested for filariasis over the course of a year, 13 percent were positive for worm infection; 3 percent of those with helminth infections were coinfected with malaria (Chadee, Rawlins, & Tiwari, 2003). Similarly, of more than five hundred people tested for malaria, four percent were positive for the disease, of which 3 percent were coinfected with filarial worms. In a hospital study of pregnant and postpartum Nigerian women, Egwunyenga and coworkers (2001) found that mothers infected with malaria but free of intestinal helminths delivered babies of a higher birth weight on average than did mothers coinfected with malaria and worms. This difference was enhanced in first-time mothers. Although coinfection infection in the samples reported here was low, occasions for interaction between these two diseases could rise significantly as global warming enables mosquitoes to carry these two pathogens to new areas.

Ecosyndemics can also involve populations that move, including *climate refugees* who are forced to flee their traditional lands because climate factors (e.g., prolonged drought, rising oceans, extreme weather) make immediate or even long-term life there impossible. Refugees not only encounter new diseases in new environments, but they tend to be highly stressed, undernourished, and vulnerable populations, factors that facilitate syndemic disease interactions. From a syndemic perspective, what is critical is not that diseases or people move (movements of both have happened many times throughout human history), but rather where and why they move, and what happens to them in their new environments. Critical questions in infectious ecosyndemics include the following:

- What are the specific sources responsible for adverse environmental change?
- What are the environmental factors that result in diseases or people going to new places, and to what degree do anthropomorphic factors play a role in this change?
- To what degree will diseases "on the move" cluster with other diseases in new host populations?

- What diseases do people "on the move" take with them?
- Which other diseases will moving populations encounter in the new environment?
- How will moving diseases or the diseases moving people bring with them interact with newly encountered diseases in the new environment?
- What consequence will these interactions have for human health?

Climate change and other forms of environmental degradation and ecocrises can also cause ecosyndemics involving noninfectious diseases. For example, extreme weather caused by global warming can lead to malnutrition because of crop and herd loss and to the pollution of the only available water sources. As a result of drinking water that is polluted by pathogens or toxins, malnourished children may suffer from reduced appetite and diminished intestinal absorption of nutrients. Also, their bodies may suffer from increased catabolism (the breakdown of body tissues). Mathematical models have calculated that a quarter to a third of cases of retarded growth in children is due to intestinal infections, and drinking contaminated water is a primary source of such infection. Diarrhea, in turn, is known to prevent children from achieving normal growth, "while malnutrition increases the frequency and the duration of diarrheic events, thereby creating a vicious [syndemic] circle" (Action Hunger 2007: 3).

Finally, as, suggested earlier, a critical issue within ecosyndemic research and related public health concern are the climate trends that have been building for more than one hundred years. The many environmental changes being introduced by global warming are subjects of considerable concern from the standpoint of syndemics. Indeed, it is precisely because global climate change has impacts on so many health and health-related issues—including nutrition, stress, air quality, water availability and pollution, allergies, flooding, wildfires, loss of tundra, vector-borne diseases, creation of refugee populations, heat stroke and related conditions, mold exposure, war—that it is not inappropriate to talk about the diseases and syndemics of global warming (Baer and Singer 2009). As we move deeper into the twenty-first century, the syndemics of global warming will likely become a primary global health issue, if not the single most important global health issue facing humankind.

One type of ecosyndemic is seen in the following "A Closer Look."

"A Closer Look"

TICK-BORNE SYNDEMICS

Ticks are small arachnids (a term derived from the Greek word for spider and referring to eight-legged organisms). In humans and other mammalian, bird and reptile species, they are *ectoparasites* (i.e., they are parasitic on the outside of the body). Ticks feed on blood, a behavior known as *hematophagy*. They gain access to the blood of other species by hanging onto them while cutting a hole in the host's skin into which they insert their hypostome, which is a calcified harpoon-like structure near the tick's mouth, and suck out blood. While feeding, if infected, they serve as vectors for the spread of a number of infectious diseases, including Lyme disease, babesiosis, anaplasmosis, Colorado tick fever, Rocky Mountain spotted fever, African tick bite fever, tick-borne relapsing fever, ehrlichiosis, and tick-borne meningoencephalitis. Importantly, ticks can be infected simultaneously with more than one type of disease-causing pathogen. As a result, tick bites can be the source of coinfections, including coinfections that interact with adverse outcomes—that is, syndemics.

ANTHROPOLOGISTS WORKING ON SYNDEMICS

In addition to the ongoing contributions of Singer and colleagues, a growing number of anthropologists have begun studying syndemics. To convey a sense of this work, in this section, we review the studies of four anthropologists (two of whom work as a team) investigating syndemics at several locations around the world.

Ann Herring, a biological anthropologist at McMaster University, focuses her research on health, which she calls "the fundamental human condition" (Waldram, Herring, and Young 2006: 3), especially on the anthropology of infectious disease. This involves studying the evolution of pathogens and the biosocial processes that promote epidemics and facilitate their spread. Also of concern are the causes of epidemics and the way populations and communities—in the past and at present—are transformed by epidemics. In their work on syndemics, Herring and her colleagues have investigated the interacting epidemics and deteriorating life conditions historically among northern aboriginal communities in Canada, a population "[l]ong considered to be the most disadvantaged group in an otherwise affluent society." In particular, Herring has argued that epidemics suffered by aboriginal communities in Canada in the early twentieth century were not simply a consequence of exposure to new, imported pathogens but rather a syndemic involving complex social and biological processes (Herring and Sattenspiel 2007). These processes include ecological changes that are the result of the importation of new plant and animal species (including pathogenic species); imposition of social, political, economic, and religious structures and policies by government officials, missionaries, and traders; an increasing number of nonaboriginal settlers farming aboriginal lands; growing marginalization of aboriginal people relative to Canada's centers of economic and political power and mainstream cultural life; assimilationist government policies; and resulting social fragmentation of aboriginal communities. Three other factors also were of importance. First was the growth in the frequency of diseases such as measles that are dependent on population density and the improvement of Canada's transportation systems that allowed a wider spectrum of diseases to travel from urban centers to more remote areas (in the bodies of individuals or on or in the flow of vehicles and commodities traveling the new roads). As a result, northern aboriginal communities came, over time, to be increasingly connected to global disease networks. Second were the effects of centuries of hunting and trapping of fur animals for export, leading to a depletion of animal resources in the Canadian north, a consequent closing of fur-trading hubs by transnational businesses such as the Hudson Bay Company, and the erosion of the historic economies of most northern aboriginal communities. Third were government policies that led to the crowding of aboriginal peoples into reserve housing, the growing concentration of children in government-funded residential schools, and the change from a more mobile to sedentary life. A direct effect of these changes was aboriginal impoverishment and increasing vulnerability to malnutrition and to diseases imported from other places.

One of the critical health issues that emerged as a consequence of the multiple changes described here was tuberculosis, which became a leading cause of death among aboriginal peoples, especially children, in the early twentieth century. Moreover, tuberculosis played a significant part in the syndemic conditions that developed in this population. Exemplary of this development and of Herring's work on syndemics are the circumstances at York Factory, a Cree community located on the western edge of Hudson Bay in northeastern Canada. Specifically, Herring and Sattenspiel (2007) illustrate how syndemic processes operated through endemic TB and two acute respiratory epidemics in the spring of 1927.

By this point in time, tuberculosis was endemic among the people of York Factory. Under these conditions, they were suddenly overwhelmed by a severe epidemic of influenza. The death rate associated with this outbreak was highest among adults twenty-one to sixty-five years of age, who comprised 87 percent of the deaths (which occurred at the rate of 120 deaths per 1000 population). By mid-February, influenza had devastated everyday community life. Not only was everyone sick or dying, but the sudden death of so many adults of productive age at a vital point in the annual fur harvest (a critical survival activity) led to the fur trade that year becoming a notable disaster.

The following autumn, a virulent epidemic of highly contagious whooping cough swept through York Factory. The worst effects were suffered by children under age six in particular. In this age group, the toll was severe (237 deaths per 1000 population). While children were dying from whooping cough, adults were suffering from what was described at the time as "very bad colds." These two outbreaks occurred during another crucial time in the annual subsistence cycle when families were preparing for the fall fishery.

In short, in 1927, the people of York Factory suffered three significant respiratory diseases, one endemic (tuberculosis), and two epidemics (influenza and whooping cough), which, acting together and sequentially, amplified each other's effects on the lungs of community members. It is well known that active tuberculosis can exacerbate influenza infection (Noymer and Garenne 2000). Influenza, in turn, enhances bacterial lung disease, impairs normal recovery processes, and damages the immune system. It can also trigger latent tuberculosis into an active state of infection. Whooping cough, in turn, destroys the respiratory lining (by killing ciliated cells), making it necessary to cough to remove mucous. This can exacerbate tuberculosis. Additionally, adults already suffering with tuberculosis at York Factory may have been more likely to experience whooping cough (i.e., the "bad colds") than is normal among adults. The impact of this respiratory syndemic made it far more difficult for the people of York Factory to make a living off the land under what were already difficult circumstances of increased competition and resource depletion. By the 1950s, York Factory was abandoned as surviving residents moved away hoping to find a better—and healthier—living elsewhere.

David A. Himmelgreen and Nancy Romero-Daza are faculty members in the Department of Anthropology, University of South Florida. These researchers, the first a biological anthropologist, the second a medical anthropologist, have carried out syndemics studies together in both Lesotho in Southern Africa and in Costa Rica in Central America. Based on their research, they have drawn the conclusion that nowhere "is the example of a syndemic more evident than in sub-Saharan Africa (SSA), where multiple epidemics conflate and seriously compromise the survival of individuals and communities" (Himmelgreen et al. 2009: 402). In the case of food insecurity and HIV disease, "food insecurity is a risk factor for both HIV transmission and worse HIV clinical outcomes" and, at the same time, "HIV increases the risk and severity of food insecurity for HIV-infected individuals and the members of their households" (Himmelgreen et al. 2009: 404). This interaction of two major threats to health occurs under social conditions characterized by widespread poverty, gender inequality, inadequate health care, lack of education, and a set of cultural attitudes toward sexuality and reproduction (e.g., the inappropriateness of sex as a topic for discussion among parents with their children).

The Kingdom of Lesotho is a small land-locked mountainous nation (about the size of the state of Maryland) positioned entirely within the boundaries of South Africa. The country's inhabitants have a life expectancy of only forty-five years, an estimated twenty-one years below what it would have been without the AIDS epidemic. The scale of the epidemic in Lesotho is staggering. The country has the third highest prevalence of adult HIV disease in the world, with 23.3 percent of people between the ages of fifteen and forty-nine years being infected. Only the countries of Botswana (24.1 percent) and Swaziland (33.4 percent) have high rates of infection (UNAIDS 2010).

Poverty in Lesotho reflects the country's colonial legacy. Much of the most fertile land in traditional Lesotho was taken by Afrikaners (people of Dutch heritage who settled in southern Africa during the seventeenth century) and became part of South Africa. A lack of adequate farmable land in mountainous Lesotho forced many men of the country into labor migration and work in the mines of South Africa. Despite remittances from miners, Lesotho is one of the poorest nations in the world. The vast majority (85 percent) of its 2.3 million inhabitants live in rural areas and over half are impoverished. Moreover, food insecurity is widespread. Note Himmelgreen et al. (2009: 407):

The ability of Lesotho households and communities to cope with food insecurity is severely limited in the face of HIV and AIDS, which disproportionately affects young adults, the most productive segment of the population. As adults become ill or die, vital skills and activities needed for production are lost. Through time, material and social assets become exhausted and it becomes much more difficult to recover from stresses and shocks in the environment.

As seen as well in the Aboriginal case from Canada, the syndemic in Lesotho involves entwined social and biological factors, resulting in a significant health cost for the affected population.

Central to the concerns of Himmelgreen and Romero-Daza is the identification and implementation of strategies to overcome the food insecurity/HIV syndemic in Lesotho. As applied anthropologists—individuals who seek to use the findings, methods, and on-the-ground insights of anthropology to address real-world human needs—they believe that for interventions to be effective they must be multidimensional rather than traditional single-issue initiatives. Moreover, interventions must go beyond changing individual behaviors to addressing larger structural issues, such as facilitating access to food, land, and employment. Few existing interventions deal simultaneously with poverty, food insecurity, gender inequality, and HIV/AIDS. One approach they propose involves testing integrated models of sustainable agricultural and poultry production; community nutrition education; social, physical, and human capacity development; and evidence-supported HIV/AIDS prevention strategies in the Lesotho context. Special emphasis in such programs, they stress, must provide women with viable economic alternatives to reduce their vulnerability to the dull burdens of poverty and HIV infection. A potential scenario would involve the following three components: (1) a food enhancement program designed to increase household production of reliable sources of nutritional food items (e.g., items like green-leaf vegetables, legumes, and poultry) using established sustainable agriculture and animal raising strategies; (2) an HIV/AIDS education initiative that begins with the assessment of using HIV knowledge and cultural understandings and addresses gaps in knowledge and access to prevention resources, including safe infant feeding practices; and (3) a linked nutrition education effort organized around the importance of adequate nutrition in the context of HIV and the specific nutrient needs of people living with HIV disease. International donor-support is critically needed in Lesotho for integrated multidimensional programs in light of the country's difficult economic condition.

Mac Marshall is emeritus professor of anthropology at the University of Iowa. His research focuses on the people of the islands of Oceania. He has done ethnographic research on many Pacific islands, including Truk (Micronesia), Papua New Guinea, Namoluk Atoll in the Eastern Caroline Islands (Micronesia), and in the diasporic communities of Chuukese in Hawai'i and the United States. His work on syndemics began with a study of smoking on Namoluk Atoll, a tiny island with a population under eight hundred people that he has returned to repeatedly for research over thirty years. A topic of interest to Marshall on the atoll is the issue of smoking. He found that a higher percentage of males (47 percent) than females (6 percent) were current smokers (Marshall 2005). High rates of smoking reflect the fact that "Micronesian smokers [particularly males] are hooked on cigarettes, and they expend a considerable portion of their limited cash resources on their addiction" (Marshall 2005: 369). This addiction traces to the colonial era when vessels from various European countries brought tobacco to trade for island resources. Although it is possible to grow tobacco on Namoluk, since the late 1940s, they have smoked industrially manufactured cigarettes that come either directly from the United States or from U.S.-owned subsidiaries in the Philippines. The cigarettes brought to this tiny atoll in the Caroline Islands produce profit for three tobacco companies based in North Carolina (and hence the title of Marshall's article "Carolina in the Carolines"): Philip Morris, RJR Nabisco, and Brown and Williamson/British American Tobacco.

In his research Marshall found that tobacco incorporates a number of cultural meanings:

it is a comestible, it is something that provides strength and vigor (although people are now well aware that it can contribute to ill health . . .) and it is something to be shared with others as a way to demonstrate generosity and to cement ties of kinship and friendship. (Marshall 2005: 374–375)

And it is a primary factor in illness and death on the atoll, including ever more frequently from chronic diseases like cardiovascular disease, cancer, cerebrovascular disease (stroke), and acute and chronic respiratory ailments such as pneumonia, influenza, bronchitis, emphysema, and asthma. Adding to the health risks of the island is its imported diet of frozen meat, including high-fat items such as turkey tails, high carbohydrate polished rice, salty and sugary items, and beer. Along with tobacco, the diet of atoll residents plays a role in "a new chronic disease syndemic that now afflicts Micronesian" (Marshall 2005: 375). This syndemic of consumption reflects Namoluk's position in the global transnational corporation-driven flow of food commodities worldwide, a flow that has the reputation of modernity but delivers mortality.

CONCLUDING REMARKS:
THE TOMORROW OF SYNDEMICS

Over the past forty years, medical anthropology has come of age, developing into a primary arena of work among biological and cultural anthropologists focused on addressing real-world problems and challenges. Although this transition was initially driven primarily by factors such as the value of the cultural model, the power of the ethnographic method, and a focus on attending to the experiential aspect of health and the emic point of view, in recent years, medical anthropologists have moved from providing supplemental insights on global health to contributing to general interdisciplinary health theory. Syndemics theory represents an explicit case of anthropological work helping to reshape contemporary ideas and applied responses in global and public health (Singer 2009a).

Viewed from the vantage of the syndemics perspective, the global threats to health of the twenty-first century are not isolated infectious diseases (including new diseases that will emerge over time, as HIV/AIDS did during the twentieth century) or even the growth in chronic diseases expected of an aging population, but an ever more complex array of syndemically interacting diseases, infectious and chronic (including chronic infectious diseases such as HIV/AIDS). Moreover, there is little reason to doubt that human inequality will continue to be a primary determinant of how this new era of disease and syndemics is differential experienced and differential produced through human action and relationship. Consequently, to avert worst-case scenarios, syndemics must become central to efforts to build a healthier future.

PART IV

Medical Systems in a Social Context

CHAPTER 11

Medical Systems in Indigenous and Precapitalist and Early Capitalist State Societies

The conceptions of human existence held by people cross-culturally reflect their relationship to the forces of production. Traditional foragers tend to view themselves in a friendly and cooperative relationship with their society and their habitat. The Mbuti pygmies (also known as the Bambuti) of the Ituri Forest in the Democratic Republic of the Congo view the forest as their mother and father and the source of all goodness in life. Horticulturists tend to view nature in more precarious terms. The Bantu villagers, neighbors of the Mbuti, who are relative newcomers to the Ituri Forest, view it as a place that has to be transformed and overcome to survive. They believe that the forest is filled with malevolent spirits and dangerous animals—a view that probably is reinforced by the Mbuti as a means of keeping the Bantu villagers from encroaching even farther upon their ancient home. Foragers believe that most misfortunes are self-inflicted by careless behavior in their otherwise harmonious relationship with nature but also attribute unexplainable accidents and severe diseases to external forces, particularly supernatural ones. Conversely, horticulturists, who live in larger and more densely populated settlements, believe that misfortune, often in the form of witchcraft or sorcery, emanates from strained relationships with people in their own or neighboring communities. Urban dwellers in agrarian state societies often express their alienation from the natural habitat and their political powerlessness by perceiving misfortune as emanating from the whim of the gods, the constellation of the stars, or fate.

Disease or physical injury is one of the misfortunes that may befall people in any society. Humans universally have developed theories of disease etiology and health care systems that reflect their living conditions and resources. As Young (1976: 19) observes, "while serious sickness is an event that challenges meaning in this world, medical beliefs and practices organize the event into an episode that gives it form and meaning." The medical systems devised by various peoples in all societies include healing techniques that may be employed either by ordinary persons or by healers of one sort or another. These healing techniques include a pharmacopoeia as well as at least rudimentary medical techniques. Ari Kiev (1966) has argued that the configuration of healers found in various societies varies according to their economic basis. Whereas shamans tend to prevail in foraging societies, such as the Inuit, Shoshone, Australian Murngin, and Andaman Islanders, horticultural societies manifest the beginnings of a medical division of labor with the appearance of diviners, herbalists, midwives, and medical guild members.

Anthropologists have often used the term *ethnomedicine* to refer to the multiplicity of medical systems associated with indigenous societies as well as peasant communities and ethnic minorities in complex or state societies. Charles Hughes (1978: 151) defines ethnomedicine as "those beliefs and practices relating to disease which are the products of indigenous cultural development and are not explicitly derived from the conceptual system of modern medicine." Yet there is something implicitly ethnocentric about making a sharp distinction between indigenous medical systems and "modern medicine." Indeed, Hahn (1983) argues that biomedicine emerged as a form of Euro-American ethnomedicine that diffused to many other parts of the world. In the ethnomedical systems of the "little peoples"—indigenous peoples, peasants, working-class people, and ethnic minorities—whom anthropologists typically study, biomedicine constitutes an ethnomedical system of a special sort—one that has undergone a process of professionalization and etiological specificity that makes it acceptable to ruling elites around the world in that it downplays the social origins of disease. Whether we are referring to the indigenous medical system of a foraging society or to biomedicine as it is practiced in a particular national setting, each can be viewed, as Grossinger (1990: 75) so aptly observes, as "an elegant and comprehensive response to social and ecological resources and a patchwork of desperate solutions to an ongoing crisis of health and survival." As Erickson (2008: 99) emphasizes, "The comparative study of ethnomedicines provides a foundation for understanding the range of ethnomedical theory and practices that can help us to understand why healing can and does occur within all ethnomedical systems." Conversely, each ethnomedical system has its limitations, even biomedicine, the practitioners of which regard it as vastly superior to local and regional medical systems, although not all observers share this view.

In contrast to earlier conceptions of ethnomedicine, which tended to delimit it to indigenous, folk, or traditional medical systems, Quinlan (2011: 381) defines it as the "area of anthropology that studies different societies' notions of health and illness, including how people think and how people act about well being and healing." From this perspective, ethnomedicine consists of various subsets. *Ethnophysiology* and *ethnoanatomy* focus on cultural conceptions of body structure and function as well as internal organs. *Ethnopsychiatry* or cultural psychiatry examines cultural conceptions of mental illness and appropriate ways to treat it and essentially "forms a bridge between and fits equally within the purview of both medical anthropology and psychological anthropology" (Quinlan 2011: 387). Finally, *ethnopharmacology* "examines drugs or medicines used within a particular culture" and relies not only on medical anthropological research but also draws insights from ethnobotany and biochemistry (Quinlan 2011: 393).

ETHNOMEDICINE AS A RESPONSE TO DISEASE IN INDIGENOUS SOCIETIES

Ultimately, professionalized medical systems have their roots in the ethnomedical systems of indigenous societies, which intricately combine empirical and magicoreligious beliefs and practices. Grossinger makes a distinction between "practical medicine" and "spiritual medicine," noting that the tension between traditional healing and biomedicine "begins in the occupational distinction between faith healers and surgeons, and shamans, medicine men, and voodoo chiefs, on the one hand, and herbalists, wound dressers, and midwives on the other" (Grossinger 1990: 76). He delineates three forms of pragmatic medicines: (1) pharmaceutical medicine, which consists primarily of a wide variety of herbal remedies; (2) mechanical medicine, which consists of surgical techniques as well as techniques that simulate physiological processes such as bathing, sweat-bathing, shampooing, massage, cupping, emetics, burning, incision, and bloodletting; and (3) psychophysiological healing, which relies on a wide variety of magical and psychotherapeutic techniques such as the classic "sucking cure" (Grossinger 1990: 76–95), in which a shaman orally extracts intrusive objects from a patient body. The distinction between psychophysiological healing and spiritual medicine is blurred. For the most part, however, spiritual medicine emphasizes the spiritual origin of disease and views it as the "primary weapon of the spiritual world" (Grossinger 1990: 99).

INDIGENOUS THEORIES OF DISEASE ETIOLOGY

All medical systems seek to answer ultimate questions, such as, "Why did I get sick—why did it happen to me?" or "What meaning does disease have in the larger scheme of things?" Indigenous peoples often do not make a sharp distinction between disease per se and other kinds of misfortune. All undesirable events may be lumped together, both in a theory about why they occur and in practices directed at alleviating or preventing them. Indigenous peoples rely heavily, but not exclusively, on supernaturalistic explanations of disease. This prompted Ackerknecht (1971) to view "primitive medicine" as "magic medicine." Nevertheless, indigenous medical systems contain a strong dose of naturalism in terms of both disease etiology and treatment. The Azande of southern Sudan, for example, do not resort to oracles as a means of detecting the source of witchcraft except when naturalistic explanations have failed to explain why people experience a misfortune. Indigenous societies generally do not compartmentalize their cognitive systems in the manner that Western societies do. Ultimately, indigenous disease theories generally have major relevance to the moral order of a society. Disease compels people to reflect on certain aspects of the social order.

Forrest E. Clements (1932) proposed the first cross-cultural classification of emic theories of disease etiology. These are sorcery, breach of taboo, intrusion of a foreign object, intrusion of a spirit, and soul loss. Many societies emphasize one or a combination of causes. The San, a foraging society that resides in the Kalahari Desert of Namibia, believe that disease is caused by a specific intruding substance, sometimes placed in the body by spirits or a witch but often not (Katz 1982). The spirits involved are sometimes specific ancestors who desire the company of their loved ones or maybe the great god or a lesser god. The Inuit generally attribute disease to soul loss or breach of a taboo. Soul loss also serves as an explanation of disease among many groups in western North America.

Among the Murngin, an Australian aboriginal people located in northeastern Arnhem Land, various forms of witchcraft are considered to be the causes of many serious diseases and of almost all, if not all, deaths (J. Reid 1983: 44). The Jivaro Indians of the Amazon Basin also believe that witchcraft is the cause of the vast majority of diseases and nonviolent deaths. Many African societies tend to attribute disease to the malevolence of sorcerers or witches. Although disease etiology is important among the Gnau, a horticultural society of the Sepik River region of New Guinea, Gilbert Lewis (1986), a physician-anthropologist, notes that they often merely accept disease as a fact of life, without attempting to explain or treat it. The Gnau explain wounds, burns, and the like in obvious naturalistic terms but generally ascribe most diseases to offended spirits.

Clements concluded that the attribution of disease to soul loss or a magical intrusion of a foreign object had only a single point of origin, from which it spread over the rest of the globe. He argued that attributing disease to violation of a taboo had probably started independently in three different places: Mesoamerica, the Arctic, and southern Asia. More recently, Murdock (1980) argued that regional variations suggest an important influence of diffusion of ancient ideas, noting the failure of some explanations to appear in places isolated from the societies that already share them. He observes that attribution of disease to the action of spirits is almost universal, appearing in all but 2 of a world sample of 139 societies. Murdock examined the relation between the importance of spirit explanation and several variables of general societal characteristics.

G. M. Foster and Anderson (1978) make a distinction between *personalistic* and *naturalistic* theories of disease. In a personalistic system, disease emanates from some sort of sensate agent, such as a deity, a malevolent spirit, an offended ancestral spirit, or a sorcerer. Naturalistic theories posit disease in terms of an imbalance among various impersonal systemic forces, such as body humors in ancient Greek medicine or the principles of yin and yang in traditional Chinese medicine. In Greek medicine as delineated by Aristotle, the universe consists of four elements: fire, air, water, and earth. People represent a microcosm of the universe and are composed of four humors with four corresponding personality types: blood is associated with high-spiritedness, yellow bile with bad temper, black bile with melancholia, and phlegm with sluggishness. Disease results from an imbalance of the humors. The physician attempts to restore health by correcting this imbalance.

In Chinese medicine, *yang* is associated with heaven, sun, fire, heat, dryness, light, the male principle, the exterior, the right side, life, high, noble, good, beauty, virtue, order, joy, and wealth. *Yin* is associated with the earth, moon, water, cold, dampness, darkness, the female principle, the interior, the left side, death, low, evil, ugliness, vice, confusion, and poverty. A proper balance of yang and yin results in health. Excessive yang, associated with heat, produces fever; and excessive yin, associated with cold, produces chills.

Although Foster and Anderson do not see the two types of etiological systems as mutually exclusive, they argue that personalistic explanations predominate among indigenous peoples as well as in certain state societies such as West African ones and the Aztecs, Mayans, and Incas. Conversely, naturalistic theories historically have been associated with certain great traditional medical systems, such as traditional Chinese medicine and Ayurveda and Unani in South Asia.

Morley provides a more elaborate typology of indigenous "etiological categories" of disease in the form of a four-cell matrix, illustrated in Figure 11.1.

Figure 11.1
Etiological Categories (Morley (1978:3)

Supernatural Causes	Nonsupernatural Causes
Ultimate Causes	Immediate Causes

Supernatural causes ascribe disease etiology to superhuman forces, such as evil spirits, ancestral spirits, witches, sorcerers, or the evil eye. Nonsupernatural disease categories are "those based wholly on observed cause-and-effect relationships regardless of the accuracy of the observations made" (Morley 1978: 2), such as profuse bleeding. Immediate causes follow from nonsupernatural sources and account for sickness in terms of perceived pathogenic agents. Ultimate causes posit the underlying sources of misfortune as it affects a specific individual. Based upon comparative data from 186 societies listed in the Human Relations Area Files, George P. Murdock (1980) delineated an elaborate typology of "theories of illness," which is summarized in Figure 11.2.

Although many of the categories in Murdock's scheme are self-explanatory, others are not. Theories of mystical causation posit illness to "some putative impersonal causal relationship" (Murdock 1980: 17). Theories of animistic causation posit illness to "some personalized supernatural entity—a soul, ghost, spirit, or god" (19). Theories of magical causation posit illness to the "covert action of an envious, affronted, or malicious human being who employs magical means to injure his victims" (21).

Murdock's scheme of illness or disease etiology has the advantage of illustrating the wide repertoire of explanations that peoples around the globe have devised to explain their maladies and ailments. Conversely, it is much more cumbersome than both Foster and Anderson's scheme and Morley's scheme. At any rate, Murdock's sample draws primarily from indigenous societies but also from some archaic state societies such as the Egyptians, the Babylonians, the Romans, the Japanese, the Aztecs, and the Incas. Many societies rely on multiple causes of illness or disease. Murdock also reports on the relative frequency of theories of disease etiology in various culture areas. Africa ranks high in theories of mystical retribution. North America "outranks all other regions in theories of sorcery, which occur in all of its societies without exception and are reported as important in 83 percent of them" (Murdock 1980: 49). Conversely, South America "ranks high in theories of spirit aggression, which are recorded as present in 100 percent of its societies and as important in 91 percent of them" (52).

Figure 11.2
Theories of Illness (Murdock (1980))

A. Theories of Natural Causation

    1. Infection

    2. Stress

    3. Organic deterioration

    4. Accident

    5. Overt human aggression

B. Theories of Supernatural Causation

    1. Theories of mystical causation

        a. fate

        b. ominous sensations

        c. contagion

        d. mystical retribution

    2. Theories of animistic causation

        a. soul loss

        b. spirit aggression

    3. Theories of magical causation

        a. sorcery

        b. witchcraft

Horacio Fabrega (1997), a biocultural anthropologist, has posited a rather elaborate evolutionary discussion of medical systems in various types of societies. He employs the acronym SH for referring to a hypothesized biological adaptation for sickness and healing. Fabrega maintains that chimpanzees exhibit some basic behaviors, such as the use of leaves to wipe themselves and the use of leaf napkins to dab at bleeding wounds, associated with the SH but also observes that they exhibit some non-SH responses, such as aversion to and exploitation of sick group members. He suggests that many of the SH characteristics of chimpanzees existed in early hominid societies and that SH became more refined during the Neanderthal stage, as is implied by the presence of healed fractures in some Neanderthal remains. Asserting that "SH constitutes the foundational material for the elaboration of medicine as a social institution," Fabrega (1997: 70) posits that the provider of SH in early foraging societies tended to be a relatively insightful individual who possessed an elaborate knowledge of the social organization and culture of his or her society. He introduces the notion of *meme*: a unit of cultural information that is stored in the brains of individuals and passed on to others through enculturation. With regard to sickness and healing, medical memes serve as mechanisms for orienting to, thinking about, and responding to disease and injury. Unfortunately, although the concept of medical meme may be a useful analytical device, Fabrega provides no concrete evidence that it has any physical reality, and thus this idea remains within the realm of creative speculation.

At any rate, he characterizes SH in foraging societies as family and small-group oriented, based on "nonsystematized knowledge" and focused on immediate restoration of well-being or accommodation to death through ritual activities and social practices. SH in village-level societies is characterized by the presence of specialized healers, elaborate healing ceremonies attended by community members, and an expansion of the sick role—that is, exemption from expected work and social obligations, for example, in growing attention to psychosocial needs and sick individuals. According to Fabrega, chiefdom, prestate, and early state societies exhibit the beginnings of the "institution" or "system" of medicine that includes (1) an elaborate corpus of medical knowledge that continues to embrace aspects of cosmology, religion, and morality and (2) the beginnings of medical pluralism, manifested by the presence of a wide variety of healers, including general practitioners, priests, diviners, herbalists, bonesetters, and midwives who undergo systematic training or apprenticeships.

Despite the existence of these various schemes for typologizing the disease causation theories of indigenous ethnomedical systems, as Erickson (2008: 55) points out, "Ethnomedical systems do not tend to maintain rigid a single cause model of illness." Instead, within the same system, different kinds of illness may be seen as being caused by different forces, and any individual case of illness may be diagnosed by indigenous healers as having several interacting causes.

Indigenous Healing Methods

In facing any kind of crisis, humans characteristically feel compelled to take some kind of action, if for no other reason than to alleviate their anxiety and sense of powerlessness. Healing is the response that humans characteristically adopt in coping with disease. Hahn (1995: 7) defines healing as "not only the remedy or cure of sickness—that is the restoration of a prior healthy state—but also rehabilitation—the compensation for loss of health—the palliation—the mitigation of suffering in the sick." In reality, most ailments are self-limiting and eventually end with recovery. In their effort to exert control over disease, however, human societies have developed a wide array of therapeutic techniques. Therapies are not only a means of curing disease but also, equally important, a means by which specific diseases are culturally defined. Although indigenous medical systems rely heavily on various forms of symbolic healing, they also exhibit a storehouse of empirical knowledge. Laughlin (1963) argues that the acquisition of anatomical knowledge started at an early stage in human history and was based on the crucial significance of the meat-eating diet, relating practices of hunting and the processing of animals.

Even Ackerknecht (1971), who we noted earlier viewed indigenous medicine as "magical medicine," recognized the existence of a wide array of "primitive surgical procedures," including wound treatment, the setting of fractures, bleeding, incision, amputation, cesarean section, and trephination. The Masai, cattle pastoralists in East Africa, were master surgeons who operated on both humans and animals. The indigenous populations of the Aleutian Islands and Kodiak Island off the coast of Alaska developed a sophisticated anatomical knowledge and surgical competence (Laughlin 1963: 130). Various Native American groups, including the Carrier Indians of the Pacific Northwest, the Mescalero Apaches of New Mexico, the Teton Dakota of the Plains, and the Winnebago of the Great Lakes region, sutured wounds with sinews. Wounds were sutured with thorns by the Masai and with the heads of termites by various indigenous peoples of New Mexico, the Azande of West Africa, and the Melanesians, as well as among many other societies around the world. Other empirical techniques associated with indigenous medicine include massage, sweat baths, mineral baths, and heat applications. *Trephination* or *trepanning* refers to a surgical procedure in which a hole is drilled or scrapped out of the skull to remove a tumor or swellings from accumulated blood. The earlier archeological record of trephination comes for a 7,000-old burial at Ensisheim in the Alsace region of France (Womack 2010: 177–178). The Incas of the Andean region practiced trephination, possibly to release a malevolent spirit.

All human societies have a pharmacopoeia consisting of a wide variety of materials, including plants, animals (including fish, insects, and reptiles), rocks and minerals, waters (salt and fresh, surface and subterranean), earths and sands, and fossils, as well as manufactured items. An estimated 25 to 50 percent of the pharmacopoeia of indigenous peoples has been demonstrated to be empirically effective by biomedical criteria. Various biomedical drugs, including quinine and digitalis, were originally derived from indigenous peoples. The older people of northeastern Arnhem Land in Australia reportedly know how to locate and prepare at least a hundred herbal medicines (J. Reid 1983: 92). Indigenous pharmacy blends together herbal medicine and spiritual medicine. As Grossinger (1990: 105) relates, "A doctor gains full control over pharmacy by making allies of the spirits who control the plants, animals, stones, and springs from which he makes his tonics."

Brian Morris (2011: 245) asserts that "medical herbalism is the most widespread and most ancient form of medicine" and discusses the role of both plant and animal medicinal substances in Malawi. Virtually every adult in Malawi, regardless of ethnicity, is "essentially a practicing herbalist, and knows a wide variety of herbs to treat common ailments," as well as personal problems (Morris 2011: 249). Indeed, herbalists often sell their products in markets and dispense plant medicines for problems ranging from venereal diseases, stomach ailments, rheumatism, children's diseases, menstrual and reproductive disorders, and the need for good fortune in economic and social affairs. Although practitioners may belong to herbalist associations, they tend to practice on an individual basis. Fruits are used as medicines and are offered to the spirits at village ancestral shrines and shrines directed at rain deities. Morris (2011: 145) goes so far as to argue that there "has been the tendency among anthropologists to emphasize the religious and symbolic aspects of ethno medical systems—almost to equate ethno medicine with spirit healing—and so bypass herbalism and the naturalistic and empirical components of medical therapy."

Recent research among five eastern Tibetan villages reveals the presence of considerable variation among ordinary people about medicinal plants (Byg, Salick, and Law 2010). Ten people from each village, an equal number of men and women, were shown twenty-three pictures of plants, all of which are used in traditional Tibetan medicine. Overall, the number of plants recognized was ten with a range from five to fifteen, and the number of plants recognized as medicinal was five with a range of three to seven. Residents of villages at higher elevations knew more medicinal plants than people living in lower villages. Men recognized both more plants in general as well as medicinal plants than women. The most common uses of medicinal plants were in the treatment of high blood pressure, general ailments, broken bones, alcoholism, rheumatism, coughs, fevers, eye disease, visual problems, headache, and women's diseases. Due to commercial pressures, some medicinal plants are being overharvested in Tibet, thus posing a threat to their availability for local use in the future.

As noted earlier, ritual or symbolic healing constitutes an important therapeutic technique in indigenous societies. Conversely, biomedicine and professionalized heterodox medical systems in modern state societies also rely on the manipulation of a "field of symbols" (Moerman 1979: 60). Dow proposes the possible existence of a universal structure of symbolic healing that consists of the following patterns:

The experiences of healers and healed are generalized with culture-specific symbols. A suffering patient comes to a healer who persuades the patient that the problem can be defined in terms of myth. The healer attaches the patient's emotions to transactional symbols particularlized from the general myth. The healer manipulates the transactional symbols to help the patient transact his or her own emotions. (Dow 1986: 56)

In other words, symbolic healing occurs when both healer and patient accept the former's ability to define the latter's relationship to the mythic structure of their sociocultural system. As this observation implies, healing by its very nature often entails an element of faith in both healer and patient. Healing rituals, however, have a broader field of concern in that they are designed to mend wounds in the body politic within which the patient is symbolically embedded.

One of the best examples of symbolic healing is the sing practiced among traditional Navajo residing in northeastern Arizona and north-western New Mexico. Conceptions of disease and therapy are central elements in their elaborate cosmology. Indeed, in large part Navajo religion consists of a set of some thirty-six healing ceremonies (often referred to as sings or chants), each lasting from one to nine nights and the intervening days. The Navajo attribute disease to various causes, including sorcery, intruding spirits, and inappropriate actions on the part of the afflicted person. In the singer's *hogan* (Navajo dwelling), he creates a mythic sand painting and then destroys it with his feet as a symbolic enactment of the restoration of harmony in both the patient and his or her social network. A Navajo sing blends together many elements—ritualistic items such as the medicine bundle, prayer sticks, precious stones, tobacco, water collected from sacred places, a tiny piece of cotton string, sand paintings, and songs and prayers. Sand paintings exemplify the centrality of symbols to Navajo healing in that they must carefully follow traditional patterns that

recall significant episodes of mythical drama. . . . The patient in his or her plight is identified with the cultural hero who constructed a similar disease or plight in the same way the patient did. . . . From the myth the patient learns that his or her plight and illness is not new, and that both its cause and treatment are known. To be cured, all the patient has to do is to repeat what has been done before. It has to be done sincerely, however, and this sincerity is expressed in concentration and dedication. The sandpainting depicts the desired order of things, and places the patient in this beautiful and ordered world. The patient thus becomes completely identified with the powerful and curing agents of the universe. (Witherspoon 1977: 167–168)

Ultimately, healing is directed toward restoring harmony in the patient's life and in the members of his or her social network present at the chant.

Faraway on the island of Madagascar in the Indian Ocean, spirits (*tromba*), sometimes from other cultural groups, may possess a "spirit-host" (Mack 2011). "Spirit speech," when accompanied by music, the burning of perfumes and incenses, the use of herbs, and other practices, is regarded as empowering, cathartic, and curative.

THE SHAMAN AS THE PROTOTYPICAL INDIGENOUS HEALER

What anthropologists generally refer to as the shaman constitutes the prototypical healer in indigenous societies. Shamanism has been the focus of an extensive corpus of anthropological literature and continues to be a topic of considerable interest, not only among anthropologists (see Hoppal and Howard 1993; Seaman and Day 1994; Jakobsen 1999; Kehoe 2000; Winkelman 2000) but also among certain historians, such as Mircea Eliade (1964), and writers who hope that shamanic traditions can provide spiritual guidance in our own troubled times. Bowie (2000: 192–196) delineates four basic approaches to the study of shamanism: (1) as a widespread form of indigenous ecstatic or trancelike behavior, (2) as a primordial or early form of religion dating back at least to the Upper Paleolithic, (3) as primarily a northern-Arctic phenomenon, and (4) as a revitalized form of religion referred to as neo-shamanism. With respect to the fourth approach, the writings of anthropologists such as Carlos Castaneda, Michael Harner, and Holger Kaiweit as well as numerous proponents of New Age philosophy, as is shown in greater detail in the next chapter, have transformed the shaman into a primordial and existential "culture hero." Within anthropology, shamanism has been for some time a topic of interest to those interested in either religion or healing or in the interface of these areas.

Ripinsky-Naxon (1993: 67) defines shamanism as a "specialized body of acquired techniques, leading to altered states of consciousness or facilitated ecstatic transformations, with the purposes of attaining mystical or spiritual experiences." Although shamans carry out a number of roles, such as culture hero, entertainer, judge, and repository of cultural values, healing appears to be their primary activity in those societies where they exist. As Harner (1980: 175) observes, shamanism "represents the most widespread and ancient methodological system of mind-body healing known to humanity." Although the category of shamanism is being reconstituted and rejuvenated by both academic and popular writers as well as holistic health and/or New Age practitioners, it is being deconstructed within anthropology (Atkinson 1992).

The term *shaman* is derived from the Tungusic-Mongol word *saman* ("to know"). It has become an etic category for a part-time magicoreligious practitioner who serves as intermediary between his or her sociocultural system and the Cosmic Environment. Mircea Eliade (1964), a renowned historian of religions, defines a *shaman* as one who has mastery over the "techniques of ecstasy" or the ability to attain or engage in magical flight to the heavens or to the underworld. In her working definition of shamanism, Townsend (1999: 431–432) delineates five "essential criteria" and four "related criteria." The former include direct communication with the supernatural realm, his or her ability to control the spirits, an altered state of consciousness, an emphasis on solving problems in this life, and soul flight. The latter include the functioning of the shaman as a medium for the voices of the spirits, and/or the ability of the shaman to call upon his or her spirits to be present at the séance without actually possessing him; the ability of the shaman to remember at least some aspects of his trance; and the ability of the shaman to cure physical, psychological, or emotional disorders.

With respect to the issue of communication with the spirit world, Rogers (1982: 6–7) delineates two types of shamans: (1) the inspirational or ecstatic shaman who engages in a theatrical battle with the spirits to heal the patient and (2) the seer who relays messages from the spirits to the people but in a less intense manner. Whereas the former is sometimes associated with "Arctic shamanism," the latter is associated with the "general shamanism" characteristic of many New World societies. Much ink has been spilled in the past attempting to identify true shamanism in terms of the level of the shaman's consciousness of his or her activities and other criteria, but more recent work on shamanism has attempted to understand it as a complex, diverse, and widespread phenomenon.

Much of the literature on shamanism has also focused on the social and psychological attributes of shamans. Whereas priests as full-time religious practitioners in chiefdoms or state societies generally are males, shamans may be males or females, although this pattern varies considerably from society to society. Whereas male shamans predominated in lowland South American societies, the Yakuts in the Kolmyck district of Siberia had a higher regard for their female shamans than for their male shamans (Rogers 1982: 27). In fact, Yakut male shamans adopted women's clothing and hairstyles. Sámi (referred to in the past as Lapp) shamans were generally men, often having female assistants, but some were women (Sexton and Stabbursvik 2010: 577). Conversely, shamans among neighboring agricultural communities were primarily women (Blain and Wallis 2000). Much of the literature on shamans indicates that many of them assume various unconventional lifestyles, such as homosexuality, bisexuality, or transvestism. Conversely, although transvestism apparently was common among shamans in various Siberian and North American cultures, it reportedly has been uncommon in South American indigenous cultures but did occur among the Mapache of Patagonia during the nineteenth century (Langdon 1992). Shamans in many societies are social recluses who choose not to enter into lasting social relationships with others. As Gaines (1987: 66) observes, shamans are not peripheral or marginal as a social category but rather as individuals.

Anthropologists and other scholars have characterized the psychodynamic makeup of shamans in the following three ways: (1) as pathological personalities, (2) as highly introspective and self-actualized individuals with unique insights about the psychosocial nature of their respective societies, and (3) as individuals who experienced an existential crisis but became healed in the process of becoming a shaman.

Various anthropologists, particularly in the past, have argued that shamans exhibit universally psychotic traits, such as hysteria, trance, and transvestism (Devereux 1956, 1957; Ackerknecht 1971). The Russian eth-nographer Waldemar Bogaras characterized Chuckee shamans as on the "whole extremely excitable, almost hysterical, and not a few were half-crazy" (quoted in I. M. Lewis 1989: 161). Weston LaBarre (1972: 265), who made a case for the shamanic origins of religion as a by-product of the use of hallucinogenic drugs, maintained "'God' is often clinically para-noiac because the shaman's 'supernatural helper' is the projection of the shaman himself." More recently, Ohnuki-Tierney (1980) has asserted that Ainu shamanism is often associated with *imu*, a culture-bound syndrome. Aside from the matter of the actual mental status of the shaman, shaman-ist healing séances often impose considerable strain on the practitioner. A California Indian shaman reported, "The doctor business is very hard on you. You're like crazy, you are knocked out and you aren't in your right mind" (quoted in Rogers 1982: 12).

In contrast to negative portrayals of shamans, anthropologists in more recent times have presented shamanic behavior as a category of universal psychobiological capacities. Shamans are often portrayed as insightful, creative, and stable personalities who, although freely drawing on in-digenous traditions, transcend the limitations of their culture by creating their own responses to new situations. In essence, shamans are viewed as having a capacity to interpret the events of daily life more adequately than the other members of the culture. Kalweit (1992: 222–224) charac-terizes the shaman as a "spiritual iconoclast" who learns about human-ity through solitude and as a "holy fool" who is holy because he or she has been healed. Murphy's portrayal of the mental status of Inuit sha-mans on St. Lawrence Island, Alaska, in the Bering Strait bear out this characterization:

The well known shamans were, if anything, exceptionally healthy. . . . As for the shamans who had suffered from psychiatric instability of one kind or another, it has been suggested that shamanizing is itself an avenue for "being healed from disease." Whatever the psychiatric characteristics that may impel a person to choose this role, once he fulfills it, he has a well-defined and unambiguous re-lationship to the rest of society, which in all probability allows him to function without the degree of impairment that might follow if there were no such niche into which he could fit. (J. Murphy 1964: 76)

In his study of Henry Rupert, Handelbaum (1977) reports that this Washo shaman exhibited a process of lifelong psychological growth. In his comparison of sixteen shamanistic healers and nonhealers among the !Kung of the Kalahari Desert, Richard Katz (1982) found that the former tended to exhibit a more expressive, passionate, and fluid conception of their bodies as well as a richer fantasy life than the latter. Winkelman adopts a neurophenomenological approach to shamanism and asserts shamanistic healing activates

normally unconscious or preconscious primary information-processing functions and outputs to be integrated into the operations of the frontal cortex. This integrates implicit understandings, socioemotional dynamics, repressed memories, unresolved conflicts, intuitions, and nonverbal—visual, mimetic [imitative], and representational—knowledge into self-conscious awareness. (Winkelman 2000: xiii)

Although there is evidence of heightened cognitive and psychic functioning among shamans, this second approach often tends to romanticize shamanism by overlooking the variability among shamans both within a specific culture and cross culturally. Apparently some shamans exhibited exploitative and sadistic tendencies in that they acted as bullies and terrorized their communities to the point that they were killed (Kiev 1966: 110).

A fair number of anthropologists have characterized the role of shaman as a culturally constituted defense mechanism. Whereas Kiev (1966) views some shamans as assuming a mature and integrated "normal" disposition, he maintains that other shamans use their calling as a method for working out their psychological problems. In a similar vein, Spiro (1967) argues that shamanism provides an opportunity for certain members of a community to satisfy sexual, dependency, prestige, and Dionysian needs. The shaman has been depicted as a "wounded surgeon" (I. M. Lewis 1989) or a "'holy fool' who is holy because he [or she] has been healed" (Kalweit 1992: 222). Walsh (1997: 117) asserts that the "shaman may not only recover from the initiation crisis but may emerge strengthened and enabled to help others."

Unlike the schizophrenic, the shaman is not alienated from society and performs a valued social role. Unfortunately, studies that emphasize the therapeutic benefits of shamanism for the practitioner often downplay shamanic practices of manipulation, deception, and, in some instances, destruction. In reality, indigenous people often exhibit an ambivalent view of shamans—on the one hand, holding them in high esteem and being in awe of their abilities and, on the other, fearing and resenting them. The Netsilik Inuit believe that if one can control the universe or its objects for good purposes, one can also use that power for evil designs (Balikci 1963). Hippler (1976: 112) makes an interesting point by asserting that shamanism "could provide a life-style for the insightful observer of his own community who could act easily within its cultural limits and still, on the other hand, provide a necessary identity to the individual who is almost schizophrenic."

Certain scholars have associated shamanism with foraging societies or specific cultural areas, such as Siberia and North America (Walsh 1990: 15–17). Other research, however, has tended to view shamanism as a "globalizing" and "dynamic cultural-social complex in various societies over time and space" (Langdon 1992: 4). Despite the voluminous literature on shamanism, most of the research on this topic has tended to be particularistic. From a critical medical anthropology perspective, shamanism as a form of indigenous healing appears to take different forms depending upon the economic base of the society. Unfortunately, this issue still has not received much systematic attention. Critical medical anthropologists still need to develop an analysis of health beliefs and practices in precapitalist social formations that parallels the general sociocultural analyses that various critical anthropologists have made of such societies. Bearing these thoughts in mind, we present a modest effort to provide a broad perspective on shamanism by examining it in the following contexts: (1) foraging societies, (2) horticultural societies, and (3) indigenous cultures that have come into intense contact with or have been absorbed by state societies.

The role of shaman or healer tends to be a relatively open one in foraging societies, as we will see in the following "A Closer Look."

"A Closer Look"

"BOILING ENERGY" AMONG THE !KUNG

Richard Katz (1982), a comparative psychologist, has conducted the most extensive study of shamanistic healing in a contemporary foraging society. His study of indigenous healing among the !Kung of the Kalahari Desert in southwest Africa is particularly valuable because it gives us a partial glimpse of what shamanism may have been like under more pristine conditions and also of how the outside world has impacted upon shamanism. Although some fifty thousand San live in Botswana, Namibia, and southern Angola, only about three thousand continue to live primarily as foragers. The !Kung, a subgroup of the San, are a highly egalitarian people whose women contribute from 60 to 80 percent of the caloric intake, participate actively in decision making, and have been known to engage in hunting.

Katz studied shamanism among the !Kung of the Dobe area of Botswana, an area that embraces nine permanent waterholes. Shamanistic healing constitutes a highly important ritual of solidarity and intensification in !Kung culture. The all-night Giraffe dance, which appears to be an ancient part of !Kung culture and is depicted on rock paintings in South Africa, occurs about four times a month and serves as the central event in the !Kung healing tradition. Several men, who are sometimes joined by women, dance around a fire and a group of singers. The ecstatic dancing stimulates the "boiling" of spiritual energy, or *num*, in the dancers, who begin to *kia* or trance. The healers may ingest plant substances that contain *num*. The fire that illuminates the dance also serves to induce trance in the healers, who may begin to shake violently and experience convulsions, pain, and anguish. The intensity of *kia* has been so great in some cases that it has caused a heart attack in the healer. While in a state of *kia*, healers treat people at the dance by struggling with their ancestral spirits for the body of a sick person. The most powerful healers sometimes travel to the great god's home in the sky. The !Kung believe that the gods originally gave them *num*, which resides in the pit of the stomach and the base of the spine. It boils fiercely within a person when activated and rises up the spine to a spot around the base of the skull, at which point *kia* results.

The !Kung believe that specific diseases are manifestations of some imbalance between an individual and his or her environment. Disease occurs when the gods and ancestral spirits try to take the sick person to their realm. The spirits have various ways of creating mishaps and even death, such as permitting a lion to maul a person. The !Kung believe that the dance may function as a preventive health measure, which keeps an incipient illness from being manifested, or may cure an illness, especially a severe one. Katz (1982: 53) maintains that the !Kung healing dance functions to "reestablish balance in the individual-cultural environmental gestalt." A healing dance may also be performed to celebrate the killing of a large game animal, the return of absent family members, or visits from close relatives or honored guests, such as anthropologists. Other !Kung healing techniques include herbal medicines and massage. Some fifteen medicinal plants are used by healers and nonhealers alike in treating minor ailments and for spiritual protection. They are mixed with charcoal and applied to the skin to alleviate aches and pains, to treat abrasions, cuts, and infections, and even to bring luck in hunting.

Most !Kung males and about a third of adult women seek to become healers at one time or another. More than half of the adult males but only 10 percent of females succeed in doing so. Women tend to experience *kia* at the Drum dance, at which they only may sing and dance but do not experience *num*, to the accompaniment of a male drummer. Women assert that *num* endangers the human fetus and therefore often postpone seeking it until after menopause. Most young women expect to learn *kia* for its own sake regardless of whether they will eventually learn to heal. Whereas the healing of the Giraffe is available to all, the healing in the Drum extends only to the dancers and singers but not to the spectators. Although the !Kung are often portrayed as one of the most sexually egalitarian societies in the ethnographic record, the differential access to shamanistic healing between men and women in this society provides some clues as to how healing over time became increasingly a predominantly male preserve. Conversely, Katz (1982: 174) suggests that the Drum may constitute a response to the "greater role differentiation between the sexes and the loss of status for women which accompanies sedentism" in !Kung society as it has come into contact with the outside world.

In contrast to foraging societies, healing appears to be a somewhat more privileged role in horticultural societies. In his generalizations about shamans among the peoples of the tropical rain forests of South America, most of whom are horticulturalists, Metraux observes (see Sharon 1978: 132) that male shamans may play a predominant role, with women shamans, if they exist, exhibiting a modest role in comparison. Among the Culina Indians of western Brazil, only men become shamans (Pollack 1992: 25). Approximately one out of every four Jivaro males becomes a shaman, but no women apparently do (Harner 1968).

OTHER HEALERS IN INDIGENOUS SOCIETIES

In addition to the shaman per se, many indigenous societies have other types of healers. Based on his cross-cultural analysis of magicoreligious practitioners, Winkelman (1992, 2000) proposes an evolutionary typology of "shamanistic healers" consisting of two main categories: the "healer complex" and the "medium." The healer complex consists of three subtypes: (1) the shaman, (2) the shaman/healer, and (3) the healer. The shaman represents the original institutionalization of trancelike behavior or altered states of consciousness (ASC) and is primarily associated with societies that rely on hunting, gathering, and fishing modes of subsistence. Of the societies surveyed, this subtype appears in two Eurasian pastoral societies as well—namely, the Chuckee and the Samoyed. Shaman/healer refers to a "group of cases which varied between the Shaman group and the Healer group under different measurement procedures" (Winkelman 1992: 26). This subtype is found primarily in horticultural societies and also occasionally in pastoral societies. Shamans and shaman/healers are predominantly male, but females sometimes occupy this position. The healer "shares some similarities with the Shaman role, but lacks major ASC, and occurs predominantly in societies with political integration beyond the local community." Mediums are predominantly female and are low in social status. Winkelman's distinction between the relatively high status of the shaman, shaman/healer, and healer and the relatively low status of the medium roughly parallels I. M. Lewis's (1989) distinction between "central morality cults" presided over by shamans or priests and "peripheral cults" consisting of mediums and other devotees undergoing possession. Whereas the former play a significant role in upholding the morality of society, the latter tend to involve people who are subject to strong patterns of discrimination, such as women in societies at various sociopolitical levels and ethnic minorities and commoners in rank or stratified societies. In peripheral cults, the sick person being possessed by a spirit receives the attention of a social superior and has an opportunity to ventilate her or his frustrations without directly threatening the established system of social relations.

The healing role appears to undergo a process that Max Weber termed "routinization of charisma" in its evolution from the shaman to the healer. As Winkelman (1992: 65) observes, "While the Shamans are selected for their roles on the basis of ASC experiences labeled as illness, visions, spirit requests, and vision quests, the Healers are selected on the basis of voluntary self-selection, and generally without major ASC experiences." This trajectory appears to parallel the evolution of religious leadership from that of the shaman into that of the priest. Whereas the shaman functions primarily as a medicoreligious practitioner, religion and medicine become increasingly differentiated in chiefdoms and state societies, with the former constituting the domain of the priest and the latter the domain of the healer or physician. Furthermore, shamans and healers "differ with respect to political power, with the Shamans having informal and charismatic political power and the Healers exercising political/legislative power, judicial power, and higher socioeconomic status" (Winkelman 1992: 65).

Wood (1979: 321–326) identified three types of "nonshamanic traditional curers": spiritualists, diviners, and herbalists. Like the shaman, the spiritualist possesses the ability to communicate with the spirits and to relay messages to the living. Conversely, the spiritualist lacks an ecstatic experience, whereas the shaman purportedly undergoes a dramatic visitation to the supernatural realm and struggles with his or her spirit guides. In reality, as we saw earlier, the distinction between the shaman and the spiritualist or seer is a fine line. Among the Temiar, a horticultural society in the Malay Peninsula, most spiritualists or mediums are males who call upon various spirit guides and sing in their communal healing ceremonies. The wife of the medium serves as the cornerstone of the chorus during healing performances and serves as a "particularly astute foil to the medium's wit during performances" (Roseman 1991: 76). Temiar mediums also heal patients on an individual basis and may call for a spirit séance.

In traditional Samoa, a horticultural chiefdom society, both men and women can function as *fojo*, or an indigenous doctor who often may also hold some other type of prestigious role, such as chief, the wife of a chief, a pastor, a deacon, or a teacher (Macpherson and Macpherson 1990: 102). *Fojo* can treat a wide array of illnesses and often have knowledge of medicinal plants. Samoans loosely differentiate "between different classes of *fojo* according to whether they deal primarily with illnesses with natural or supernatural origins" (Macpherson and Macpherson 1990: 118). In literal translation, *fojo* means "to apply massage," suggesting the importance of this practice in traditional Samoan healing.

Compared with the shaman and spiritualist, who communicate directly with the supernatural realm, the "diviner interprets symptoms, prognosticates, and prescribes courses of action through mechanical, magical manipulations" (Wood 1979: 323). Whereas in traditional Navajo culture the shaman or singer conducts a healing ceremony, various specialists diagnose disease through a combination of divination and visualization:

There are three ways of determining an illness: gazing at sun, moon, or star, listening, and trembling. Listening is nearly, if not quite, extinct; "motion-in-hand" indicates trembling induced by proper ritualistic circumstances. The diviner is seized with shaking, beginning usually with gentle tremors of arms or legs and gradually spreading until the whole body shakes violently. While in a trembling state, the seer loses himself. Guided by his power, he sees a symbol of the ceremony purporting to cure the person for whom he is divining. Gazing may be accompanied by trembling; usually the diviner sees the chant symbol as an after-image of the heavenly body on which he is concentrating. (Reichard 1950: 99–100)

According to Wood (1979: 325), the herbalist is "probably the most pragmatic of the traditional healers" in that "he or she frequently relies on the knowledge gained during a lengthy training from an experienced practitioner." Among the Subanum on Mindinao Island in the Philippines, virtually every adult functions as his or her own herbalist.

The shaman and other indigenous healers described in this chapter persist in both archaic and modern state societies. In these settings, however, they tend to serve primarily members of the lowest strata of society.

"A Closer Look"

FOLK MEDICAL SYSTEMS IN AUSTRALIA

Given that Australia has evolved particularly since World War II and after the dismantling of the "White Australia" policy in the early 1970s into a multiethnic or multicultural society, undoubtedly numerous folk medical systems exist there. Of these, Aboriginal medicine has received the greatest attention, particularly on the part of social anthropologists (Berndt 1964). John Cawte (1974) reported that some three decades ago, many Aboriginal doctors remained in remote Australia. He interviewed eight Walbiri healers at Yuendumu about their illness beliefs and curing techniques (Cawte 1974: 41). Somewhat later, Janice Reid (1983) conducted research on the medical system of the Yolngu people in northeast Arnhem Land in the Northern Territory. She reported that the Aboriginal doctor and the indigenous concepts of sickness and curing were still an integral part of social life in many remote Aboriginal communities. Indeed, the Northern Territory's Department of Health employs Aboriginal healers and has a program to collect and identify indigenous herbal medicinal plants. Reid located and interviewed four Aboriginal Yolgnu healers or *marrnggitj* in the Yirrkala environs, two of them men, one of them a young boy, and one of them a woman. Some individuals become a *marrnggitj* in the wake of a frightening supernatural experience in which a spirit confers healing powers on him or her. Ultimately, of course, the traditional healer must have the ability to counteract sorcery or the work of a *raglak* to consistently attract patients.

While indigenous Australians have been on the continent for an estimated forty to sixty thousand years, immigrants to Australia have imported their respective folk medical systems. The Chinese brought their traditional medical system to Australia beginning in the late nineteenth century when they immigrated to work in the gold fields of Victoria. Chinese medicine practitioners served patients in goldmine towns such as Ballarat and Bendigo as well as Melbourne's Chinatown (Bentley 2005: 41). Chinese medicine practitioners served not only fellow Chinese but also European Australians. Manderson and Matthews (1981, 1985) report that traditional medical beliefs and practices persist among Vietnamese immigrants because they provide cultural continuity in difficult situations. Big Lueng (2008) has also examined Chinese folk medicine in a similar light among Chinese immigrants from various countries. With respect to another Asian immigrant group, Han (2000) observes that the Korean community in Australia did not even have herbal doctors or acupuncturists until 1980. Undocumented Korean migrants, however, sought herbal medicine and acupuncture in Chinatown when in acute pain. Unfortunately, virtually no scholarly research has been conducted on either Anglo-Celtic Australian folk medicine or the folk medical systems of the many ethnic groups, such as the Italians, the Greeks, the Macedonians, Turks, the Lebanese, the Indians, the Sudanese, and the Eritreans, now residing in Australia. This is quite in contrast to the United States, where numerous studies have been conducted on various folk medical systems, such as southern Appalachian herbal medicine, African American folk medicine, *curanderismo* among Mexican Americans, *espiritismo* among Puerto Ricans, *santeria* among Cuban Americans, *vodun* among Haitian Americans, and Hmong folk medicine.

MEDICAL PLURALISM IN PRECAPITALIST STATES: MEDICINE FOR THE ELITES AND MEDICINE FOR THE MASSES

In contrast to the indigenous societies, where healing tends to be relatively accessible, elite practitioners in state societies attempt to monopolize this role for themselves. Nevertheless, counterparts of indigenous healers persist in state societies. Indeed, a hierarchy of healers that reflects social relations in the larger society was a characteristic feature of precapitalist state societies. According to Fabrega (1997), the sickness and healing system in early civilizations and empires is characterized by an complex pattern of medical pluralism consisting of two tiers: (1) an official, scholarly academic medical system oriented to the care of the elites and (2) a wide array of less prestigious physicians and folk healers who treat subordinate segments of society. The state plays an increasing role in medical care by hiring practitioners for elites and providing free or nominal care for the poor, especially during famines and epidemics. The literate or "great" medical tradition includes the formation of a medical profession, the beginnings of clinical medicine, and the increasing commercialization of the healing endeavor.

In archaic state societies, priests often functioned as physicians or healers of one sort or another. Ancient Sumerian civilization possessed three categories of cuneiform texts that included medical information: (1) therapeutic or medical texts per se, (2) omen collections or "symptom" texts, and (3) miscellaneous texts that included information on ailments and medical practices (Magner 1992: 18). Sumerian physicians reportedly diagnosed symptoms by taking health histories rather than performing direct physical examinations. Conversely, the "conjurer," "diviner," or "priest-healer" conducted a direct physical examination and viewed the patient's symptoms and life circumstances as omens that diagnosed disease (Magner 1992: 19). Sumerian prescriptions included some 250 vegetable and some 120 mineral drugs as well as alcoholic beverages, fats and oils, animal parts and products, honey, wax, and various kinds of milk.

In ancient Egypt, priests of the goddess Sekhmet treated a wide array of diseases, except for eye disorders, which were treated by the priests of Douaou (Ghalioungui 1963: 31). Certain Egyptian temples developed a reputation as healing centers. In the fifth century B.C., Herodotus, the famous Greek traveler, maintained that Egypt had the healthiest population in the world next to the Libyans, because of the state's commitment to health services. Egypt had a medical hierarchy consisting of three categories of practitioners: (1) the priest-physician or *wabw,* (2) the "lay physician" or *swnw,* and (3) the magician. Like the priest-physician, the ordinary physician followed the teachings of various sacred books. Lay physicians apparently functioned as state employees with medical appointments in various areas, including public works, residential areas, the military, burial grounds, religious sites, and royal palaces (Ghalioungui 1963: 106–113). Lay-physicians themselves were organized into a hierarchy consisting of the chief physician of the south and the north, chief physicians, physician inspectors, and physicians per se. The royal palace also had a medical hierarchy consisting of the Chief Physician of the King, the Chief of the Physicians of the Palace, and Court Physicians.

Some of the more influential physicians meddled in state politics. The financial remuneration received by physicians varied widely. In contrast to the palace physicians or physicians with rich clients, many physicians were little more than manual workers who basically earned the bare necessities of life. A few physicians in Egypt were female, and a woman physician known as Pesehet bore the title of "Lady Director of Lady Physicians" (Magner 1992: 28). Although Herodotus contended that among the Egyptians, "Every physician treats one disease, not many" (quoted in Ghalioungui 1963: 149), apparently some physicians specialized as surgeons and veterinarians (quoted in Ghalioungui 1963: 149). In some instances, physicians were assisted by aides, pharmacists, nurses, masseurs, physiotherapists, and bandagists (Nunn 1996: 132). In contrast to Mesopotamian medicine, Egyptian prescriptions were relatively precise. The Ebers papyrus lists about seven hundred drugs, which were made into more than eight hundred formulas (Magner 1992: 31).

Medical pluralism in China can be traced back to the Shang dynasty, which emerged between approximately the eighteenth and sixteenth centuries B.C. along the middle course of the Yellow River and continued into the eleventh century B.C. Unshuld (1985: 25–27) identifies two forms of therapy during this period—*wu* therapy and ancestor therapy. The *wu* petitioned the divine ancestor Ti for good winds and rain for crops and attempted to ward off evil winds, which may have also been viewed as the source of sickness. Under ancestor therapy, the emperor functioned as the physician of his subjects during epidemics and other catastrophes but was assisted in this task by various diviners.

Beginning with the Chou dynasty (1050–256 B.C.), the Chinese system of medical pluralism consisted of two broad categories of healers: state-employed physicians and folk healers. Physicians consisted of two types: court physicians and practitioners of public and street medicine. The rank and salary for government physicians were based on their success rate. The imperial medical corps during the Chou dynasty included food physicians, physicians for simple diseases, ulcer physicians, physicians for animals, and chief-of-physicians (Magner 1992: 52). Although most physicians trained as apprentices, the Chinese state established medical schools in virtually every province of the empire. The Imperial College of Medicine consisted of about thirty physicians attached to the imperial palaces. Ancient China had a stratum of physician-scholars who had access to the Imperial Library's collection of some twelve thousand works, lectured to their junior colleagues on these classic texts, and provided medical care to the elite class. Although physicians with scholarly training or aspirations tried to separate their practices from magicoreligious procedures, they sometimes compromised by resorting to the latter (Magner 1992: 53). Folk healers included surgeons, apothecaries, the *wu*, and other magicore-ligious practitioners, and fortunetellers.

During the Period of Warring States (481–221 B.C.), Confucianism and Taoism came to influence Chinese medical thought. Confucianism was associated with the "medicine of systematic correspondence," a syncretic system that incorporated the concepts of chi, ying and yang, and the Five Phases with homeopathic magic (Unshuld 1985: 52–67). This medical system "dominated Chinese medical literature and the approaches of educated practitioners and self-healing private citizens as well, at least among the upper strata" for most of Chinese history until the modern era (Unshuld 1985: 223). Taoism drew on demonic medicine and pragmatic materia medica and introduced macrobiotics. Somewhat later, Buddhist monks offered medical treatment to the Chinese people as part of their missionary efforts and as a fulfillment of their ethical obligation to assist human beings (Unshuld 1985: 139).

Medical pluralism in the Greco-Roman world expressed itself in part in the form of various medical sects. These included the rationalists or dogmatists who maintained that physicians should rely on reason to discern the roots of health, disease, and human physiology; the empiricists who argued that theory is ultimately useless in medical practice; and the methodists who asserted that medical care could be achieved by adhering to a few simple rules that could be mastered in half a year (Siraisi 1990: 4; Gourevitch 1998: 104–117). Galen, who was born in A.D. 129 in Pergamum in Asia Minor, attempted to rise above the medical sectarianism of the time by asserting that an imbalance of four bodily humors—hot, cold, dry, and moist—resulted in disease (Strohmaier 1998: 139–142).

Medical pluralism was well in place in the agrarian tributary regimes of the Arab world during the period A.D. 660–950 (Gran 1979). Islamic culture combined the Galenic theory of disease and prophetic medicine, which drew on Mohammed's views of health and disease (Strohmaier 1998: 146–153). Conversely, like earlier Christian mystics, Muslim mystics also distrusted physicians and looked to God or Allah as the source of cures. Islamic culture began to establish hospitals and hospices in the early eighth century. These hospitals appear to have drawn their inspiration from the assistance offered to the poor and sick at Christian monasteries and other establishments. The services of these hospitals were initially subsidized by philanthropy and later by public funds and reportedly were free regardless of age, gender, or social status (Reynolds and Tanner 1995: 249). The Adubi hospital in Baghdad, built in A.D. 981, had twenty-four physicians. The largest hospital in the Islamic world, with a capacity of eight thousand beds, was established in Cairo in A.D. 1286 (Magner 1992: 138).

These hospitals provided their patients with a systematic treatment based upon Greek notions of humoral medicine that included exercises, baths, dietary regimens, and a comprehensive materia medica. Islamic medicine also relied upon manipulation, bone setting, cauterizing, venesection, and minor eye surgery, but devalued major surgery because of the religious prohibition on human dissection. The Al-Faustat hospital, built in A.D. 872, organized its wards on the basis of gender, illness, and the surgical procedure to be conducted. Furthermore, as in contemporary biomedical hospitals, "patients were required to wear special clothes provided by the hospital authorities while their clothes and valuables were kept in a safe place until their discharge" (Reynolds and Tanner 1995: 250). Whereas Islamic or Yunani medicine was sponsored by the courts, mystical medicine served urbanites in the larger towns, and the healing system associated with the Zanj movement catered to slaves, peasants, and some artisans.

Mary Lindemann (2010) has written a fascinating account of medicine in what she terms "early modern Europe," or from our perspective, the early capitalist era (1500–1900), in which she acknowledges a diversity of medical practitioners. Women played a particularly important role in health care within the domestic setting where they administer an array of herbs and common remedies (Lindemann 2010: 121–124). Midwives delivered the vast majority of infants in Europe and in larger cities they found "enough regular employment to earn their living solely by delivering babies" (Lindemann 2010: 124). In contrast to physicians who often received their education in universities, apothecaries and surgeons or barber-surgeons receiving training as apprentices within the guild system (Lindemann 2010: 128–138). Not all physicians, particularly in England, were trained in universities. According to Lindemann,

Increasingly, in England, or rather in London, by the middle of the eighteenth century, private or commercial teaching and medical education outside universities had come to dominate medical training. Students frequented a number of private schools or "walked the wards" of the city's hospitals with attending physicians and surgeons. (Lindemann 2010: 148)

Regular physicians for the most part were middle class, and tended to come from families where heads of household were clerics, lawyers, merchants, as well as physicians. Although poor individuals occasionally studied regular medicine, this generally was not the case "because medicine was one of the more expensive degrees and there were fewer bursaries for them" (Lindemann 2010: 151).

At the lower end of the pluralistic medical system were a wide assortment of "irregular" practitioners, including the "cunning folk," "executioners," and "root-wives." Cunning folk relied on magical cures as well as medicinal plants and salves, lotions, and elixirs and in some instances functioned as bonesetters. Bonesetters often learned their trade from a relative or friend and some "viewed their abilities as a God-given gift rather than an acquired skill" (Lindemann 2010: 259). Although execution-ers tended to be viewed as dubious and even polluted characters due the morbid task they carried out, they also often possessed a knack for treat-ing burns, cuts, and dislocations and sometimes even sold bodily parts that were believed to have curative powers (Lindemann 2010: 259–260). Finally, medicine peddlers roamed the countryside to hawk their tinc-tures, lotions, pills, and powders alongside household items and some medicine peddlers created mail-order businesses. Occulists and dentists, however, provided their services on the road.

Although people, particularly biomedical practitioners, in modern so-cieties tend to view medical systems in past and present-day indigenous societies and precapitalist state societies as having been filled with "super-stitions" and faulty medical practices, from an evolutionary perspective, as Horacio Fabrega (1997) has systematically illustrated, they served as the antecedents of biomedicine as well as various other contemporary medi-cal systems, such as Ayurveda and Chinese medicine. Family-level forag-ing societies, such as Australian Aborigines and the Inuit of the Canadian Arctic, tend to have shamanic healers who often employ naturalistic and supernaturalistic techniques. Village-level societies, such as the Ainu of northern Japan and the Yanomamo of the Amazon Basin, are characterized by the appearance of specialized healers and elaborate healing ceremo-nies attended by community members. Similarly, pastoral societies, such as the Tuareg of the Saharan and Sahelian areas of West and North Africa, have a wide array of healers to which they can turn, including herbalists, bonesetters, religious healers, diviners, and exorcists. Chiefdom societies, such as those of Polynesia, and sedentary foraging societies of the Pacific Northwest Coast, and early state societies exhibit an elaborate corpus of medical knowledge and the beginnings of medical pluralism manifested by a wide variety of healers. These trends become even more pronounced in later precapitalist state societies.

CHAPTER 12

Biomedical Hegemony in the Context of Medical Pluralism

The emergence of capitalism in sixteenth-century Europe contributed to the development of a global world economy by the twentieth century. Biomedicine as an outgrowth of this development provided an ideological rationale by downplaying the roles that political, economic, and social conditions played in the production of disease while at the same time helping to restore sick or injured workers to production. The emerging alliance around the turn of the century between the American Medical Association, which consisted primarily of elite practitioners and medical researchers based in prestigious universities, and the industrial capitalist class ultimately permitted biomedicine to establish political, economic, and ideological dominance over rival medical systems in the United States and ultimately globally. Navarro asserts that the capitalist class came to support a version of medicine in which:

disease was not an outcome of specific power relations but rather a biological individual phenomenon where the cause of disease was the immediately observable factor, the bacteria. In this redefinition, clinical medicine became the branch of scientific medicine to study the biological individual phenomena and social medicine became the other branch of medicine which would study the distribution of disease as the aggregate of individual phenomena. Both branches shared the vision of disease as an alteration, a pathological change in the human body (perceived as a machine), caused by an outside agent (unicausality) or several agents (multicausality). (Navarro 1986: 166)

Biomedicine also achieved preeminence over alternative medical systems such as homeopathy in European societies and eventually throughout the globe. The argument on the part of homeopaths, for example, that disease could be best treated by administering small dosages of drugs that produced symptoms in a healthy person and by altering environmental conditions was incompatible with the reductionist, high-dosage drug treatment of biomedicine.

THE EMERGENCE OF BIOMEDICINE AS A GLOBAL MEDICAL SYSTEM

Historically biomedicine has played a central role in capitalist imperialism in efforts to maintain control of exploited populations. As Arnold (1993: 1396) asserts, "Western medicine was present from the outset and implicated in all the subsequent phases of colonialism: from exploration and conquest, to state formation and the exploitation of human and natural resources." Beginning in the 1880s, the major colonial powers embarked on a project of political control over much of the world. The British Empire alone at its peak in the 1930s encompassed approximately one-fourth of the world's land area. A tiny European colonial elite dominated the native population with a combination of military might and administrative control. In contrast to the tributary nature of earlier states, the modern colonial state aimed to contribute to the development of productive resources and expanding markets.

Disease as a major obstacle to European expansion in Africa, Asia, and the Americas prompted the attachment of medical personnel to merchant marines and the creation of rudimentary hospital facilities at overseas trading posts. Both British and German colonies in Africa initially were served by a handful of physicians who were directly employed by trading companies and provided medical treatment to the colonizers. Medical missionaries also functioned as early purveyors of health care in the colonies. Christian missionaries, for example, first introduced allopathic medicine into the territory of what today is called Tanzania in the second half of the nineteenth century (Turshen 1984: 140).

Colonial states eventually, however, assumed responsibility for health care. Joseph Chamberlain, the British Secretary of State for Colonies, promoted the establishment of the London and Liverpool schools of medicine in 1899, noting that "the study of tropical disease is a means of promoting Imperial policies" (quoted in Doyal with Pennell 1979: 240). Schools of tropical medicine were also established in Amsterdam, Paris, and Brussels (Banerji 1984: 258). Germany established colonial medical services in Tanzania initially to serve the army garrison stationed there, in part to counter indigenous resistance during the 1880s and 1890s, and later to provide health care for European settlers.

After World War I, Britain assumed control of colonial medical care in Tanzania. Four types of medical care were created in Tanzania during the period 1919–1961: (1) government services organized on the basis of a three-tiered structure of central, provincial, and district administration; (2) voluntary services, most of them missions; (3) employer-based (sisal plantations, mines, and factory) services; and (4) private practices that tended to be concentrated in urban areas and catered primarily to Europeans and a few privileged Africans. Although the colonial state implemented preventive measures in the form of public health programs, by and large colonial medicine tended to be highly curative in its orientation. In Tanzania, as Turshen observes:

Up to 72 percent of the health budget was spent on expensive curative facilities, as late as 1961. This is in part the origin of the "demand for curative medicine" identified by European physicians. But there were also factors connected with the wage-earning population that helped to determine the type of health service offered. The government adapted colonial medical services to the needs of private enterprise for a productive labor force. . . . Men with chronic diseases were likely to be dropped from the labor force or, if discovered on recruitment, not hired. This was especially true of tuberculosis, for which recruits were x-rayed routinely. (Turshen 1984: 149)

Secular biomedicine did not reach rural African communities in any form in many places until the 1930s, and sometimes even as late as the 1950s and 1960s (Vaughn 1991: 57). The system of indirect rule, in which native leaders were used to carry out colonial policies at the local level, provided the administrative framework for implementing colonial medicine. As Comaroff (1993: 324) observes, "medicine both informed and was informed by imperialism in Africa and elsewhere. It gave validity of science to the humanitarian claims of colonialism, while finding confirmation for its own authority in the living laboratories enclosed by expanding imperial frontiers." Biomedicine also ascribed the poverty of African peoples to the diseases that they contracted as a result of appropriation of their lands and the exploitation of their labor power. When Tanzania gained independence in 1961, its medical services lacked native trained personnel because of the racist educational policies of the colonial government (Turshen 1984: 161).

Despite the fact that Chinese medicine is probably the world's oldest body of medical knowledge and tradition, dating back some four thousand years, Western medicine gained a strong foothold in China with the assistance of European and U.S. colonial powers in the nineteenth and early twentieth centuries. Medical missionaries began to establish allopathic hospitals and clinics in China as early as 1835 (Leslie 1974: 84). The European and North American missionary societies and churches that financed the establishment of hospitals did so more for evangelical reasons than because they aimed to provide "exemplary models of Western healing to China" (Unshuld 1985: 240). John Kenneth MacKenzie, a Scottish physician, established the first allopathic school in China in Tianjin in 1881, and foreign governments followed suit over the course of the next thirty years by establishing several other medical schools (Sidel and Sidel 1982: 23).

Rockefeller philanthropists sponsored medical and public health projects as an alternative means to missionaries and armies for opening up new markets in China. The Rockefeller Foundation took over the Peking Union Medical College from the missionary society that had established it. According to E. R. Brown (1979), Rockefeller campaigns against hookworm in not only China but also the Philippines, Latin America, the West Indies, Ceylon, Malaysia, Egypt, and other countries were "blatantly intended, first, to raise the productivity of the workers in underdeveloped countries, second, to reduce the cultural autonomy of these agrarian peoples and make them amenable to being formed into an industrial workforce, and third, to assuage hostility to the United States and undermine goals of national economic and political independence" (Brown 1979: 259). As elsewhere, biomedicine in prerevolutionary China tended to be urban-based and curative in its orientation.

The introduction of Western medicine, or what evolved into biomedicine, met with strong resistance in most underdeveloped countries as was made evident by the continued demand for traditional medical care. Christian missionaries in Africa opposed indigenous medicine on the grounds that traditional practitioners were allegedly witch doctors. Western physicians also denied that traditional medicine might have any benefits because "such an admission would run counter to the belief that Victorian civilization was the acme of human achievement" (Turshen 1984: 145). Colonial governments often feared indigenous medical systems because their communal orientation held the potential for local populations to organize opposition movements.

DOMINATIVE MEDICAL SYSTEMS AS REFLECTIONS OF SOCIAL RELATIONS IN THE LARGER SOCIETY

Medical pluralism in the modern world is characterized by a pattern in which biomedicine exerts dominance over alternative medical systems, whether they are professionalized or not. The existence of dominative medical systems in complex societies, however, predates capitalism. As Charles Leslie (1974), an anthropologist who has conducted extensive research on South Asian medical systems, observes:

All the civilizations with great tradition medical systems developed a range of practitioners from learned professional physicians to individuals who had limited or no formal training and who practiced a simplified version of the great tradition medicine. Other healers coexisted with these practitioners, their arts falling into special categories such as bone setters, surgeons, midwives, and shamans. However, the complex and redundant relationships between learned and humble practitioners, and between those who were generalists or specialists, full- or part-time, vocational or avocational, naturalist or supernaturalist curers, is clarified by professionalization in the great tradition that defined the relative statuses of legitimate practitioners and distinguished them from quacks. (Leslie 1974: 74)

With European expansion, allopathic medicine or what eventually became biomedicine came to supersede in prestige and influence even professionalized traditional medical systems. Third World societies are characterized by a broad spectrum of humoral and ritual curing systems. Some of these, such as Ayurveda and Unani in India and traditional Chinese medicine, are associated with literate traditions and have schools, professional associations, and hospitals. Although the upper and middle classes resort to traditional medicine as a backup for the shortcomings of biomedicine and for divination, advice, and luck, it constitutes the principal form of health care available to the masses. As Frankenberg (1980: 198) observes, "The societies in which medical pluralism flourishes are invariably class divided."

India, the most populated country second only to China, is an outstanding example of a complex society exhibiting a dominative system. Leslie (1977) delineates five levels in the Indian dominative medical system: (1) biomedicine, which relies upon physicians with MD and PhD degrees from prestigious institutions; (2) "indigenous medical systems," which have within their ranks practitioners who have obtained degrees from Ayurvedic, Unani, and Siddha medical colleges; (3) homeopathy, whose physicians have completed correspondence courses; (4) religious scholars or learned priests with unusual healing abilities; and (5) local folk healers, bonesetters, and midwives. Although approximately 150,000 physicians practiced biomedicine in India in the early 1970s, they were outnumbered by an estimated 400,000 practitioners of the three principal traditional medical systems, namely, "Ayurveda, which is based upon Sanskrit texts; Unani, or Greek medicine, based upon Arabic and Persian texts; and Siddha, a tradition of humoral medicine in South India" (Leslie 1977: 513). In 1972, of some 257,000 state-registered practitioners of traditional medicine, about 93,000 had at least four years of formal training. At the same time, in addition to ninety-five biomedical colleges, India had ninety-nine Ayurvedic colleges, fifteen Yunani ones, and a college of Siddha medicine. Many of the traditional medical schools were small and poorly equipped, but twenty-six of them were affiliated with universities, and ten offered postgraduate programs. Modern Ayurvedic medicine is drastically different from the system delineated in its classic texts. Indeed, it has a long tradition of syncretism, which has drawn heavily upon the Galenic (Unani) concepts of Islamic medicine. Both professionalized Ayurvedic and Unani medicine have incorporated aspects of biomedicine. Many Ayurvedic colleges have been converted into biomedical ones, whereas others are trying to return to a more pristine tradition (C. Taylor 1976: 290). Although homeopathy entered India as a European import, the opposition to it by the British-dominated biomedical profession spared it association with colonialism (Leslie 1977: 513). Homeopathic practices have become a standard part of Ayurvedic medicine.

During the late nineteenth century, nobles, philanthropists, and caste and religious associations supported the establishment of Ayurvedic colleges and health facilities throughout India. After independence, the Indian ruling elite promised to take active steps to make the benefits of health services available to the masses, particularly to peasants and workers. For this purpose, they also promised a revival and strengthening of certain traditional medical systems, including Ayurveda (Banerji 1984). As Frankenberg (1981: 124) asserts, however, such elite support for traditional medicine is really only a "surface phenomenon" in that members of the ruling class actively rely primarily on biomedicine for treatment of their own ailments, and most government funds for health education and services are allocated to biomedicine. It appears that the populist, anti-imperialist rhetoric characteristic of elite support for traditional medicine was primarily intended to deflect popular unrest about oppressive social conditions rather than to try to eradicate the conditions contributing to widespread disease in India and other underdeveloped countries. At any rate, as part of an effort to legitimize the professionalized traditional medical systems, in 1970 the Indian government did establish the Central Council of Indian Medicine as a branch of the Ministry of Health for the purposes of registering indigenous physicians, regulating education and practice, and fostering research (Leslie 1974: 101). Leslie succinctly summarizes the contradictory role that traditional medical systems play in South Asia and elsewhere:

[Traditional] physicians . . . are sometimes painfully aware that cosmopolitan medicine [or biomedicine] dominates the Indian medical system, yet a substantial market exists for commercial Ayurvedic products and for consultations with practitioners. The structural reasons that medical pluralism is a prominent feature of health care throughout the world are that biomedicine, like Ayurveda and every other therapeutic system, fails to help many patients. Every system generates discontent with its limitations and a search for alternative therapies (Leslie 1992: 205).

In the early 1970s, Margaret Lock (1980) conducted ethnographic research on medical pluralism in Kyoto, Japan. In addition to biomedicine, modern Japan has a wide variety of East Asian medical systems and has undergone a revival of these systems, in much the same way that various Western societies have. The most popular of these is *kanpo* ("the Chinese method"), which was imported from China in the sixth century. In addition to prescribing herbs, *kanpo* doctors administer acupuncture, manipulative therapy, and moxibustion. Modern-day *kanpo* doctors are biomedical physicians who draw from a traditional medical system. Emiko Ohnuki-Tierney (1984) also examined Japanese medical pluralism. In addition to biomedicine and *kanpo*, she noted the existence of an array of religious healing systems in Japan. These include shamanism which still in practiced in remote mountainous areas; the traditional religions of Shintoism, Confucianism, Buddhism, and Taoism; and new religions that appeared in the wake of World War II and often subsumed shamanistic elements. Shinto and Taoist deities and Buddhas are worshipped in special shrines and temples and look after general health, prosperity, and even traffic safety, much as in the same way that Western Catholics regard St. Christopher the patron saint of travelers. These supernatural personages may be appealed to for specific diseases, such as eye, throat, dental, and musculoskeletal complications, and to ensure safe pregnancy and birthing, physical growth, and a successful marriage.

The Dutch introduced Western regular medicine or the forerunner of present-day biomedicine, during the late eighteenth century, and a German variant was introduced during the Meiji period beginning in 1868. In Japan, biomedical physicians often have offices in their homes with their wives often assisting as pharmacists or receptionists. They tend to work long hours and operate on a first-come, first-serve basis as opposed to an appointment system. Biomedical physicians who work in large clinics and hospitals generally claim more than one specialty, with academic physicians enjoying the highest prestige. Japanese hospitals expect family members to be involved in patient care, with at least one family member staying with the patient and attending to his or her personal needs, receiving visitors, and even providing meals.

Whereas some anthropologists such as Leslie, Lock, and Ohnuki-Tierney have examined medical pluralism at the societal level, Paul Brodwin (1996) examines medical pluralism in the Haitian village of Jeanty (pseudonym). In addition to access to biomedicine or "metropolitan medicine," the villagers turn to various other practitioners and healing systems in their search for better health. These include herbalists, bonesetters, midwives, the cult of Roman Catholic saints, Voodoo priests, and Pentecostal ministers. Morality and medicine are intricately intertwined in rural Haiti and poses questions of innocence or guilt. Brodwin asserts:

People must constantly choose which gods to worship, and which forms of healing power and moral legitimation to accept, and they know the practical consequences of embracing one over the other. People know that distaining the *lwa* [Voodoo gods] allies them with the centralized Catholic Church: a traditional source of legitimation and advance. They know that fundamentalist conversion leads away from local allegiances and would propel them into a transnational space, politically centered in North America. (Brodwin 1996: 199)

In another study of medical pluralism in Haiti, Singer, Davison, and Geddes (1988) examined the efforts of Haitian women to receive biomedical treatment for folk illness. Knowing Western-trained physicians scoff at folk health beliefs, the women present their symptoms in terms that are meaningful to physicians while still retaining their own beliefs about the sources of their ailment.

Despite the existence of biomedical practitioners in various African countries, indigenous medicine continues to thrive, in part because of "brain drain" of health workers to developed countries. Kenya, for example, has experienced the exodus of biomedical physicians, nurses, and other health workers from Europe, the United States, and even South Africa and Namibia over the past few decades (Konadu 2007: 10). In 2003 alone, 240 physicians and some one thousand nurses departed Kenya, a tragedy in that the country spent about $50,000 training each physician and about $25,000 each nurse. This "brain drain" phenomenon involving health workers is yet one more example of the unequal change pattern between the core on the one hand, and the semiperiphery and periphery on the other, of the capitalist world system. Many indigenous healers in Ghana and other African countries belong to various traditional practitioner associations (Konadu 2007: 57). In some instances, biomedical practitioners and indigenous healers borrow from each others' therapeutic techniques. Traditional and Modern Health Practitioners Together against AIDS based in Uganda constitutes an example of this type of medical syncretism.

Anthropologists have tended to examine medical systems that invariably are directly or indirectly dominated by biomedicine. The U.S. dominative medical system consists of several levels that tend to reflect class, racial/ethnic, and gender relations in the larger society (Baer 1989, 2001b, 2004b). In rank order of prestige, these include (1) biomedicine; (2) osteopathic medicine as a parallel medical system focusing on primary care; (3) professionalized heterodox medical systems (i.e., chiropractic, naturopathy, and acupuncture); (4) partially professionalized or lay heterodox medical systems (e.g., homeopathy, rolfing, and reflexology); (5) Anglo-American religious healing systems (e.g., Spiritualism, Christian Science, Seventh Day Adventism, and evangelical faith healing); and (6) ethnomedical systems (e.g., Southern Appalachian herbal medicine; African American ethnomedicines, Hispanic ethnomedicines such as curanderismo, espiritismo, Santeria, and Native American healing systems. As a result of financial backing of initially corporate-sponsored foundations and later the federal government for its research activities and educational institutions, biomedicine asserted scientific superiority and clearly established hegemony over alternative medical systems. Although American biomedical physicians continue to exert a great deal of control over their work, some scholars have argued that they have been undergoing a process of "deprofessionalization" or even "proletarianization."

Haug (1975: 197) argues that three forces may be contributing to this process: the computerization of diagnosis and prognosis; the emergence of new health occupations, such as physicians' assistants and nurse practitioners, which have assumed many of the task carried out by the physician in the past; and a growing public awareness of health matters and an associated distrust of biomedicine's limited ability to address a wide variety of diseases, particularly chronic ones. McKinlay and Arches (1985) argue that as a result of the bureaucratization that is being forced on biomedical practice by the logic of capitalist expansion, physicians are being "proletarianized" or becoming glorified workers, largely because of their still relatively high incomes. Before World War II, solo practitioners dominated American biomedicine, and the American Medical Association served their entrepreneurial interests well. Berliner (1982) asserts that between 1900 and 1970 biomedicine functioned as an "industrial mode of production" carried out by competing practitioners who produced a commodity purchased by patients.

In the past several decades, the political clout of the AMA has been diffused by various organizations of specialists. The house of biomedicine has been split into two establishments: the AMA and the hospital doctors—those physicians who are employees in high-prestige teaching hospitals, university hospitals, government hospitals, research centers, and health corporations. In other words, an increasing number of physicians are becoming salaried employees of massive medical empires under private or state control, a development that has contributed to the emergence of a "monopoly mode of production" in biomedicine (Berliner 1982: 172). American biomedicine has evolved into a big business in which health care has become increasingly concentrated in large health care corporations and medical centers. Some scholars see biomedicine as embedded within a "medical-industrial complex" (Wohl 1984). The penetration of capital into health care has become a highly contradictory process. As Krause succinctly observes:

Capitalism itself is divided . . . between the few sectors that make money as costs rise—medical technology, drugs, hospital supply—and the majority, which suffer increases in health coverage costs. The state acts with the majority of capitalist sectors and is gradually restricting for-profit medicine. Doctors thriving as owners of for-profit settings are already beginning to lose their advantage as regulation tightens (Krause 1996: 8).

Despite the tendency toward growing monopolization and concentration in biomedicine, other medical subsystems persist and even thrive, although often under precarious conditions. Indeed, biomedicine's dominance over rival medical systems has never been absolute. The state, which primarily serves the interests of the corporate class, must periodically make concessions to subordinate social groups in the interests of maintaining social order and the capitalist mode of production. As a result, certain heterodox practitioners, with the backing of clients and particularly influential patrons, were able to obtain legitimation in the form of full practice rights (e.g., osteopathic physicians, who may prescribe drugs and perform the same medical procedures as biomedical physicians) or limited rights (e.g., chiropractors, naturopaths, and acupuncturists). Lower social classes, racial and ethnic minorities, and women have often utilized alternative medicine as a forum for challenging not only biomedical dominance but also, to a degree, the hegemony of the corporate class in the United States as well as other advanced capitalist societies, such as Australia (Baer 2009b).

Regardless of the society, biomedicine attempts to control the production of health care specialists, define their knowledge base, dominate the medical division of labor, eliminate or narrowly restrict the practices of alternative practitioners, and deny laypeople and alternative healers access to medical technology. Despite the hegemonic influence of biomedicine, alternative medical systems of various sorts continue to function and even thrive not only in the countryside but also in the cities of the world, including those in the United States and Australia. Ultimately, the ability of biomedicine to achieve dominance over competing medical systems is dependent upon support from "strategic elites" (or certain businesspeople, politicians, and high-level government bureaucrats; Freidson 1970). In the case of Australia, regular medicine came to dominate rival medical systems during the late nineteenth and early twentieth centuries. It formed associations that challenged competition, lobbied the state to ban or at least restrict heterodox practitioners, built alliances with conservative forces in government, and monopolized state funding for education and research on health-related issues. The cost of regular medical education tended to serve as an important factor in the transformation of regular medicine into a high-status occupation. According to Willis,

Entry to [regular] medicine . . . required substantial family backing involving the purchase of both a private school and university education. Once qualified there were further costs which heightened this class restrictiveness, such as the cost of setting up a practice. As a result, three quarters of native born doctors who commenced practice during the 1880s were sons of professional men. (Willis 1989: 60)

However, biomedicine is unable to establish complete hegemony in part because elites permit other forms of therapy to exist but also because patients seek—for a variety of reasons—the services of alternative healers. Because of the bureaucratic dimensions of biomedicine and the iatrogenic situations or mishaps occurring in the course of biomedical treatment, alternative medicine under the umbrella of the holistic health movement made a strong comeback even in North America, Western Europe, and Australasia. This eclectic movement incorporated elements from Eastern medical systems, the human potential movement, and New Ageism as well as earlier Western heterodox medical systems.

"A Closer Look"

TWO NATURAL MEDICINE COLLEGES IN AUSTRALIA: THE SOUTHERN SCHOOL OF NATURAL THERAPIES AND THE ENDEAVOUR COLLEGE OF NATURAL HEALTH

In his position as an academic at the University of Melbourne since January 2006, Hans Baer has been well positioned to conduct research on Australian complementary medicine in that his office has been located close to the Southern School of Natural Therapies, situated about 2 kilometers or 1.2 miles to the east and the Melbourne branch of the Endeavour College of Natural Medicine. The Southern School of Natural Therapies started out as the Victorian School of the National Association of Naturopaths, Osteopaths and Chiropractors (established 1962) and later became the Southern School of Natural Therapies (SSNT) before eventually offering training programs in Chinese medicine and myotherapy, an alternative therapeutic system focused on muscle work which emerged in the Australian state of Victoria (Jacka 1998:2). It constitutes the longest single existing complementary medicine school in Australia and many of its graduates have gone to teach in other complementary medicine programs in the country, including Sue Evans, a herbalist/naturopath who teaches at the Southern Cross University in Lismore, New South Wales, and Stephen Myers who went to obtain a PhD in pharmacology and a biomedical degree and has become a pivotal figure in integrative medicine. SSNT operates a clinic staffed by fourth year students in which a wide array of natural therapies are utilized, including iridology, herbal medicine, homeopathy, flower essences, dietary advice, nutritional therapy, relaxation massage, acupuncture, moxibustion, and cupping.

The Endeavour College of Natural Health is the successor body of the Australian College of Natural Medicine (ACNM) and an excellent illustration of the strong profit-making orientation characteristic of much of Australian complementary medicine education. It emerged out of what had been the Brisbane branch of Acupuncture Colleges (Australia; Sherwood 2004: 224). Endeavour College today has campuses in Brisbane, the Gold Coast of the state of Queensland, Melbourne, Sydney, Adelaide, and Perth. The Melbourne branch is situated in the CBD of Melbourne, called City, and about two kilometers south of the University of Melbourne campus. The Melbourne branch campus houses a student clinic, a bookshop, and a small library. Since 1998, Endeavour College has offered bachelor's degrees in naturopathy, acupuncture, homeopathy, and offered advanced diplomas, diplomas, and certificates in numerous other complementary therapies. Peter Sherwood, the founder of what had been ACNM, claimed that it had been "probably the largest natural medicine college in the world" with its more than four thousand students.

As early as the late 1970s, an increasing number of biomedical and os-teopathic physicians in the United States as well as biomedical physicians in other countries, including the United Kingdom and Australia, along with nurses, began to recognize the limitations of the conventional ap-proach to disease and illness and that they were losing many of their more affluent patients to Complementary and Alternative Medicine (CAM) practitioners (Baer 2004a, 2009b). A group of MDs and osteopathic phy-sicians (DOs) established the American Holistic Medical Association in 1978. Nurses, in particular, given their person-orientation, expressed in-terest in holistic health, forming the American Holistic Nurses' Associa-tion in 1981. The Australian College of Holistic Nurses represents nurses committed to 'holistic nursing' and holds annual conference (Baer 2009b: 116). It supports the use of a wide array of complementary therapies in institutional, community, and private health care settings. Many nursing schools in Australia teach their students various natural therapies, such as aromatherapy, massage, and Therapeutic Touch (Jacka 1998:161). The School of Nursing at La Trobe University in Melbourne operated a joint nursing-naturopathy training program in collaboration with the Southern School of Natural Therapies (Baer 2009b: 117).

Ironically, holistic health as a popular movement has by and large been tamed, evolving into a professionalized entity referred to as *complementary and alternative medicine* or even *integrative medicine*. The shift from a dis-cussion of holistic health, or simply alternative medicine, to CAM since the late 1990s is perhaps most apparent in the titles of various books and periodicals. Since this time, numerous biomedical physicians and nurses have written overviews of CAM (Synder and Lindquist 2006; Micozzi 2007). Wolpe (2002: 165) argues that CAM is "what sociologists refer to as a residual category" in that it is "defined not by its internal coherence but by its exclusion from other categories of medicine." In some circles, the term *integrative medicine* has come to supplant *complementary and alternative medicine* and is often treated as a blending together of the best of biomedicine and CAM. Although alternative practitioners or complementary practitioners and laypeople have tended to speak of holistic health, CAM and integrative medicine are in large biomedical constructions. CAM, often within the larger rubric of integrative medicine, has become part and parcel of biomedical and nursing education, workshops, journals, clinics, and hospitals in many settings around the world. Training in CAM has become increasingly available in U.S., UK, and European biomedical and nursing schools.

Various medical social scientists have warned that holistic health or CAM faces the danger of being co-opted by biomedicine (Wolpe 2002; Baer 2004b, 2009b). Indeed, Rakel and Weil (2003: 7), both biomedical physicians and staunch proponents of integrative medicine, observe that biomedicine often views CAM as "tools that are simply added to the current model, one that attempts to understand healing by studying the tools in the tool box." The Office of Alternative Medicine (established in 1992) and its successor body, the National Center for Complementary and Alternative Medicine (NCCAM) have always been directed by biomedical physicians. While biomedicine has not gone nearly as far in its efforts to co-opt CAM in Australia as in the United States, biomedicine continues to exert dominance over what is generally simply termed *complementary medicine* down under. Indeed, Australian biomedical physicians are increasingly redefining complementary therapies as modalities under biomedicine or closely related to biomedicine. For example, some general practitioners have come to term chiropractic and osteopathy as physical medicine or manual medicine (Eastwood 1997: 14). Dietetics and nutritional advice as treatment modalities have been incorporated by biomedical physicians under the designation of nutritional and environmental medicine. According to Eastwood (1997: 14), "Acupuncture, in the context of general practice, has been redefined as medical acupuncture."

In addition to CAM training at biomedical and nursing schools, many biomedical physicians, nurses, and allied health professionals are receiving training in CAM at an array of conferences and workshops. Conventional physicians and other health professionals, both biomedical and CAM, acquaint themselves with CAM or integrative medicine by consulting journals such as *Alternative Medicine*, the *Journal of Alternative and Complementary Medicine*, *Advances in Mind-Body Medicine*, *Alternative and Complementary Therapies*, *Alternative Healthcare Management*, and *Focus on Alternative and Complementary Therapies: An Evidence-Based Approach*. A growing number of biomedical schools and university hospitals have created centers of integrative medicine or CAM where they treat patients. Most of the growing number of integrative medical centers, whether affiliated with biomedical schools or independent of them, tend to be directed by one or more conventional physicians and arrayed by an array of CAM practitioners, often on a part-time basis.

Complementary and alternative medical systems or heterodox medical systems often exhibit counterhegemonic elements that resist, often in subtle forms, the elitist, hierarchical, and bureaucratic patterns of biomedicine. In contrast to biomedicine, which is dominated ultimately by the corporate class or state elites, folk-healing systems are more generally the domain of common folk. In Ghana, for example, there reportedly is one indigenous healer for every four hundred people as opposed to one biomedical physician for every 22,000 people (Konadu 2007: 10). More than 80 percent of people in sub-Saharan Africa rely on medicinal plants to deal with their sicknesses; however, this indigenous carrying capacity for health care is being undermined by the expropriation of medical plants by developed societies (Konadu 2007: 4). Langwick reports that

[n]eoliberal restructuring and the insistence of international financial organizations that the poorest of countries produce their way out of poverty—traditional medicine has emerged as a new way into the global economy. Tanzanian officials are joining other African countries in a chorus that welcomes the commercialization of traditional medicine as a prospective path into the global market of herbal medicine, which the World Health Organization [in 2002 estimated] to stand at USD 60 billion and growing. (Langwick 2011: 10)

Unfortunately, according to Elling (1981b: 97), "Traditional medicine has been used to obfuscate and confuse native peoples and working classes." Ethnomedical practitioners in the modern world have shown an increasing interest in acquiring new skills and use certain biomedical-like treatments or technologies in their own work, a process in which they often inadvertently adopt the reductionist perspective of biomedicine. Many Third Word peoples receive regular treatment from injection doctors and advice from pharmacists who indiscriminately sell antibiotics and other drugs over the counter. Many Ecuadorians now purchase natural medicines, which often are advertised on radio programs and commercially prepared in advanced capitalist countries, rather than utilizing indigenous herbal remedies (Miles 1998). In essence, biomedicine, commercialized alternative remedies, and traditional medicine, despite antagonistic relations between them, exhibit a great deal of overlap and even fusion. Furthermore, both CAM systems, such as chiropractic and naturopathy in developed countries, and traditional healers' organizations in developing countries engage in internal turf battles, yet exemplifying Virchow's assertion that "politics is medicine on a grand scale." In his examination of "traditional medicine" in Tanzania, Langwick (2011: 83) reports the following:

The new forms of difference and diversity spurred by the institutionalization of traditional medicine are fraught with struggles for control. For instance, the organization of traditional healers consolidates control among its representatives. Authority is generated along bureaucratic lines rather than through practices of healing and initiation. Some healers have begun to shape the criteria for including and excluding others.

The growing interest of corporate and governmental elites in alternative medicine is related to the cost of high-technology biomedicine. Even in regions such as Hong Kong, where explicit financial and/or legal support for traditional medicine is absent, governments often prefer to support traditional medicine because they recognize that it takes some of the strain off Western doctors in dealing with self-limiting diseases or diseases that tend to run their natural course without treatment (Topley 1976). Moreover, in the urban setting, traditional medicine minimizes the trauma of acculturation associated with the familiar cycle of capital penetration, import-substituting industrialization, and rural to urban migration of the peasant population. Singer and Borrero (1984) found that *espiritismo* often helps its Puerto Rican clients deal with social adjustments associated with migration to the United States and to deal with related conditions such as alcoholism. In essence, traditional medicine is assigned to address many of the stresses associated with capitalist development that are not easily garnered into the diagnostic categories and treatment approaches of biomedicine.

Although CAM systems have expanded their popularity and influence in particularly developed but also developing societies, they continue to remain relatively weak. According to Saks (1994:100), "while access to the alternatives to medicine [biomedicine] may be expanded, the traditional monopolistic power base of the orthodox profession still seems highly likely to dilute the scope of what is available, even at a time when the profession is coming under ever greater challenge in an increasingly market-based society." Even when biomedical physicians express an interest in CAM, often under the rubric of *integrative medicine,* they continue to view CAM practitioners who work in their clinics as their inferiors or subordinates. Ellen J. Salkend (2005) found this to be the case in her study of the Holistic Medicine Institute (pseudonym), a Midwestern suburban clinic in the United States operated by four biomedical physicians who hired several CAM practitioners on a part-time basis who were expected to carry out various labor-intensive therapies.

Various anthropologists have criticized a strong tendency in the study of medical pluralism to discuss the relationship among allegedly discrete medical subsystems because it deemphasizes the phenomenon of medical syncretism or medical hybridization in which health practitioners and patients often blend together beliefs and practices from different medical traditions (Poole and Gessler 2005: 38-51; Lewis 2007). In reality, patients often do not clearly subscribe to one set of medical beliefs or another. Immigrant groups, for example, often tend to engage in "mixed therapy regimens" in which they move back and forth between biomedicine and folk medicine. Medical syncretism is illustrated in modern Ayurvedic medicine, which is drastically different from the system delineated in its classic texts. Both professionalized Ayurvedic and Unani medicine have incorporated aspects of biomedicine, and homeopathic practices have become a standard part of Ayurvedic medicine (Leslie 1992: 196). Ferzacca (2001: 210) views medical pluralism in Yogyakarta, an educational center in Central Java, as a "social practice that produces hybrid forms of medicine" utilized by people who lead "hybrid lives." In his discussion of Ayurvedic acupuncture in modern India, Alster (2005: 42) asserts that in reality "all forms of medicine are theorized as transcultural systems."

SHAMANISM AND OTHER INDIGENOUS HEALERS' ENCOUNTERS WITH THE WORLD SYSTEM

Whereas the shaman tends to be an integral part of indigenous societies as both a magicoreligious practitioner and a healer, the occupant of this role generally poses a threat to the priest and the physician in state societies, including capitalist ones. The shaman is a representative of an earlier, more egalitarian, and more democratic social order, and the latter two figures tend to function as hegemonic agents of state religion and medicine, respectively. Biomedical practitioners often accuse indigenous healers of perpetuating superstitious behavior and engaging in sorcery. Based on his examination of medical pluralism in Bolivia, Bastien describes a scenario that resembles the encounter of Western medicine or biomedicine in many other parts of the world:

After the Spanish conquest of Central and South America, ethnomedical practitioners were forbidden to function as such because their curing techniques were considered heretical. Around the middle of this century, doctors and pharmacists in Bolivia pressured the Bolivian legislature to outlaw ethnomedical practices by requiring licenses. Although a few noted middle-class herbalists obtained licenses, others were unable to and were jailed. (Bastien 1992: 19)

In a similar vein, Janzen (1978: 51) reports that colonial authorities as late as 1956 rounded up village healers in the Kibunzi and Mbanza

Mwembe region of Zaire when relatives removed a patient to receive indigenous medical care.

With the encroachment of the frontier in the United States, shamanism underwent a rapid decline among the Washo Indians of the Intermountain West. Siskin (1984: 171–72) reports that only ten Washo shamans remained in 1939, and in 1956 there was only one, Henry Rupert, who died in 1973. Rupert, who spent much of his life in white society as a printer, hypnotist, farmer, and entrepreneur, incorporated Hindu and Hawaiian personages into his pantheon of spirit guides and was the first Washo to eschew a belief in sorcery. In contrast to Rupert, John Frank, a Washo healer in his nineties in the early 1980s, was never in Siskin's (1984: 201) view a "full-fledged shaman," in large part because he was an elderly man when he began to doctor in 1974 after having watched Rupert cure over the years.

Although shamans and other indigenous healers historically have been suppressed in state societies, they have often adopted entrepreneurial characteristics with exposure to a capitalist market economy. Although Siskin (1984: 68) provides no direct evidence to this effect, this may have been what occurred among the Washo when he reports that shamans "knew no lack in a tribe which suffered not infrequent shortage of food and in which paucity of material goods is characteristic." During the contact period, shamans exploited Washo fear of sorcery to the limit. According to Siskin (1984: 180), peyotism, a syncretic, introversionist religion that views peyote as the transformative sacrament of Native American peoples, offered the Washo an escape from their "long-standing antipathy and simmering resentment against shamans."

The matter of fees has also become a controversial issue among the !Kung. As several !Kung shamanistic healers began to receive goods or cash for treating members of other ethnic groups, they came to expect the same from their own people (Katz 1982). Kaw Dwa, a healer who has a reputation of having strong *num*, reportedly gives special attention to patients who pay for his services at "professionalized" dances. Elsewhere in Africa, Anthony Thomas (1975: 271) observes that in Kenya "traditional and illegal practitioners are doing very well financially. Healing for profit is much more lucrative than growing crops and raising livestock." Eduardo Calderon Palomino, a healer representing the north coastal Peruvian tradition of *curanderismo* and the subject of publications and films by anthropologist Douglas Sharon, has become a renowned figure by conducting performances for foreign tourists in his community as well as participating in New Age workshops abroad (Joralemon 1990). As a result of these activities, Calderon has been able to build a restaurant and a tourist hostel across from his home and to better provide for his large family. Lest anthropologists judge this eclectic, postmodern shaman too harshly, Joralemon argues that

it would be hypocritical for anthropology to scorn others for profiting from traditions in other cultures. Our livelihood too is earned on the basis of a Western fascination with other cultures. We, like the tour operator, are in the business of exploiting our informants for profit; the principal difference is that we legitimize our activities by reference to the pursuit of scientific knowledge and produce publications in place of travel opportunities. (Joralemon 1990: 105)

Despite the existence of numerous instances of pecuniary activities on their part, indigenous healers also exhibit counterhegemonic tendencies within the context of the capitalist world system. Michael Taussig (1987) maintains that shamans mediate divisions of caste and class relations in modern societies. In his highly acclaimed *Shamanism, Colonialism, and the Wild Man*, he presents a detailed portrayal of shamanic responses to colonial and neocolonial domination in multiethnic Colombia. Shamanism survives because it recreates the egalitarian and democratic ethos of indigenous society by allowing patients to live in the shaman's home. According to Taussig:

Unlike the situation of a priest or a university-trained modern physician, for example, whose mystique is facilitated by his functionally specific role defining his very being, together with the separation of his workplace from his living quarters, the situation in the shaman's house is one where patients and healer acquire a rather intimate knowledge of each other's foibles, toilet habits, marital relations, and so forth. (Taussig 1987: 344)

As opposed to the biomedical physician, who often is viewed as a demigod, the shaman is a mere mortal who possesses a certain gift or skill, namely, that of healing.

Ayahuasca shamanism refers to a healing system involving the use of ayahuasca, a plant with hallucinogenic properties, which has developed in urban contexts in west Amazonia over the past three hundred years. Gow (1994: 91) maintains that it

evolved as a response to the specific colonial history of western Amazonia and is absent precisely from those few indigenous peoples who were buffered from the processes of colonial transformation caused by the spread of the rubber industry in the region.

Town shamans, who are *mestizos*, insist that they have obtained their knowledge from the forest Indians. Conversely, the forest Indians look downriver for the source of shamanic power, to the cities of Pucallpa and Iquitos and to the ayahuasca shamans of the lower Ucayali and Amazon rivers. In contrast to their view that the *ayahuasca* shamans possess the curing power of the forest spirits, they look at their own shamans as relatively impotent. On the surface, *ayahuasca* shamanism appears to function as a hegemonic force in that the forest Indians have adopted a prototypical colonial mentality. Conversely, the counterhegemonic component of shamanism lies in the belief that the forest spirits afflict people with disease as a punishment for environmental damage caused to their domain. Curing entails a mediation of this imbalance through use of *ayahuasca,* a vine that as both cultigen and wild plant symbolizes the transition from domesticated space to full forest. In essence, as Gow (1994: 104) observes, the "historical sorcery of ayahuasca shamanism is centered on that spatial category that connects the forest and the city: the river."

Shona spirit mediumship constitutes yet another example of how shamanism serves to mediate social tensions in colonial and postcolonial societies. Spirit mediums played an instrumental role in assisting guerrillas belonging to the Zimbabwe African National Liberation Army (ZANLA) to liberate the Shona people from the oppressive rule of the white-dominated Rhodesian colonialist state (Lan 1985). Guerillas lived with a number of spirit mediums in the Zambezi Valley and regularly received advice from their ancestors that was mediated by the mediums who favored the return of appropriated lands to the peasantry. After the revolution, many mediums encouraged women to participate in local politics. Unfortunately, various mediums feel that they were not properly rewarded for their support of the revolution after independence. According to Lan (1985: 221), the Traditional Medical Practitioners Act implemented by the Zimbabwean state "entrenches in law precisely that control over the mediums that political authorities of the past, whether chiefs or district commissioners, attempted to enforce in order to discredit mediums who opposed them."

In the case of another postrevolutionary society, the Soviet Union beginning in the 1930s waged a campaign against shamans among the North Khanty villagers of Siberia, labeling them "deceivers" and *kulaks* (rich peasants; Balzer 1991). Some shamans went underground or turned to drinking, and others rebelled against the repressive tactics of the Soviet state. Whereas in the past Khanty shamanic séances tended to be community events at which the patient received moral support from a large number of people, during the Soviet period they evolved into sessions which generally were conducted in secret or with only a few family members present (Balzer 1987: 1091). In 1990, Vladimir Alekssevich Kondakov, who identifies himself as a Sakha shaman (*oiuun*), established the Association of Folk Medicine as part of a revival of shamanism in Siberia (Balzer 1993).

Missionaries also made concerted efforts to expunge shamanism about the Inuit or related groups in the Arctic regions of Canada, Greenland, and Alaska. While contemporary Inuit no longer practice shamanism, many Inuit claim to feel the past shamans in their daily lives. In a book titled *Interviewing Inuit Elders: Cosmology and Shamanism*, various students at Nunavut Arctic College "reported that they experienced fear and anxiety in the course of learning about Inuit shamanism" and other aspects of Inuit religion (P. R. Stern 2010: 110). Indeed, in contrast to their parents and grandparents, many young Inuit are interested in learning about the shamanistic practices of their culture.

Taman shamanism or *balienism* in Borneo represents an example of what Winkelman termed the shaman/healer in the context of the capitalist world system (Bernstein 1997). *Baliens* tend to be women who have recovered from some sort of chronic emotional problem. They belong to healing societies but do not generally associate with one another on an informal basis. Some *baliens* do not actively engage in healing or attend other ritualistic events. Shamanism has also become closely associated with women in other state societies, such as eastern Asia, where, as Vitebsky (1995a: 118) observes, "it has been subordinated to a Buddhist or Confucian High Culture which is more male-centered."

As noted earlier, many New Agers in advanced capitalist countries, particularly the United States, are proponents of neo-shamanism, a movement that idealizes the shamanistic practices of Native American and other indigenous peoples around the world. Vitebsky graphically describes the juxtaposition of traditional shamanism and neo-shamanism:

In the jungles and the tundra, shamanism is dying. An intensely local kind of knowledge is being abandoned in favour of various kinds of knowledge which are cosmopolitan and distant-led. Meanwhile, something called shamanism thrives in western magazines, sweat lodges and weekend workshops. The New Age movement, which includes this strand of neo-shamanism, is in part a rebellion against the principle of distant-led knowledge. (Vitebsky 1995b: 182)

Anthropologist Michael Harner, a former professor at the New School for Social Research, has become a New Age guru as a result of his popular book *The Way of the Shaman* (1990) and his creation of the Foundation for Shamanic Studies. He became intimately acquainted with shamanism among the Jivaro and Conibo Indians of South America and has developed a synthesis of universal shamanic practices, called "core shamanism," which he teaches in workshops. On its website, the Dance of the Deer Foundation (established in 1979), based in the Santa Cruz Mountains of California, advertises its commitment to maintaining the shamanic traditions of the Huichol Indians of northern Mexico through seminars, pilgrimages, and study groups in the United States, Mexico, Europe, and other parts of the world. Some Native Americans, however, regard New Age dabbling into shamanism as an illegitimate and imperialist appropriation of their cultures. In early 1994, the National Congress of American Indians declared war on "non-Indian 'wannabes,' hucksters, cultists, commercial profiteers and self-styled shamans" (quoted in Glass-Coffin 1994: A48) for exploiting, distorting, and abusing American Indian religious traditions.

In contrast to the traditional shaman who is oriented to serving the group, New Age neo-shamans focus on serving the individualistic endeavors of their clients to "journey" to higher states of spiritual consciousness. Kehoe (2000: 33) asserts that neo-shamanism "offers a haven for educated, middle-class Westerners uncomfortable with conventional institutionalized congregations and unwilling to limit themselves to strictly materialistic pursuits." She also argues that neo-shamanistic workshops offer their clients "gregariousness, relief from anxiety, and myths to daydream with" (Kehoe 2000: 34). In his observations of neo-shamanistic workshops in Denmark and England, Jakobsen (1999: 167–203) found that many of the participants were physicians, nurses, social workers, psychologists, counselors, and teachers. Despite its lament that the modern world has lost a sense of community, neo-shamanism has become part and parcel of the capitalist marketplace in which a wide array of religious and healing systems offer people salvation either in the next life or in this life. For the most part, neo-shamans serve clients in group or private settings but not as members of specific congregations per se. Moreover, in keeping with capitalist market dictates, neo-shamanism is sold as a set of consumer items (e.g., tapes, CDs) through mass advertising at a profit.

Robert J. Wallis (2003), an archaeologist with a personal involvement in neo-shamanism, has written an exhaustive examination of the cross-fertilization between shamanism and neo-shamanism. Although he admits that some neo-shamans have essentially engaged in colonial acts by expropriating indigenous shamanistic practices, Wallis (2003: xiv) asserts that he is engaging in a form of *autoarcheology*, which he characterizes as being driven by postmodernism, postcolonialism, and queer theory theoretically and multisited ethnography methodologically. Wallis provides a tour de force of neo-shamanism in California, the U.S. Southwest, and Britain, particularly its Celtic and Nordic variants. He asserts that anthropologists and other academic scholars have tended to neglect neo-shamans who he asserts have written more extensively on shamanism, in large part due to their desire to learn from it. Ironically, neo-shamans have drawn upon the work of various anthropologists, such as Michael Harner and Douglas Sharon but in particular Carlos Castaneda, who obtained his PhD in anthropology at the University of California–Los

Angeles and whose accounts of a supposedly Yaqui shaman by the
name of Don Juan became standard fare in the countercultural movement around the world during the 1970s and 1980s. Conversely, some
neo-shamans adopt a mainstream and conservative stance by teaching "business executives how to contact 'spirit guides' which can help
them make more money," thus demonstrating that neo-shamanism may
"embody a number of socio-political locations" (Wallis 2003: 30). Indigenous healers have criticized neo-shamanism as but another form of
Western imperialism.

THE "THERAPEUTIC ALLIANCE"
IN THIRD WORLD COUNTRIES

Despite numerous instances of state hostility to indigenous or traditional healers, many Third World countries have been turning to an increasing reliance on them as a cheap alternative to capital-intensive, high
technology biomedicine. Indeed, despite the emergence of biomedicine
as a global medical system, indigenous healers reportedly continue to
function as the major health care providers for about 90 percent of the
world's rural population (Bastien 1992: 96). Joseph W. Bastien, an anthropologist who has done extensive ethnographic work in Bolivia, presents
a relatively favorable report of the efforts to integrate biomedicine and
traditional medicine in that country. He asserts that a "dialogue between
doctors and shamans would provide doctors with an open-mindedness
important to exploring the multifariousness of healing, and it would provide shamans with scientific knowledge in order to be a bit more earthly"
(Bastien 1992: 101). In a similar vein, Sharon (1978) maintains that the only
realistic solution to health problems in northern Peru rests upon a para-
medical program that entails "reciprocity between traditional and modern
medicine."

In contrast, Phillip Singer, a critical medical anthropologist, views the
"therapeutic alliance" between biomedical and traditional practitioners
as a manifestation of a "new colonialism." He contends that under this
arrangement, traditional healing functions as a "mediation or 'broker-
age' process between the individual and the dominant values, institutions, powers, agencies, etc., that exist and with which he has to cope"
(P. Singer 1977: 19–20). Singer also maintains that medical anthropologists who collaborate with biomedical practitioners, particularly psychiatrists, within the context of the "therapeutic alliance" contribute to
the status quo by offering symptom relief for patients. He views "good
health" as "largely a function of the social and economic conditions that
make possible the conditions for good health, i.e., nutrition, housing,

water, sewage, etc." (P. Singer 1977: 14). In a similar vein, Velimirovic emphasizes the need for structural changes that complement the utilization of indigenous healers:

There is no need to either copy a Western model or to settle for low-quality care in coping with the health problems of the developing world. Indigenous healers might perhaps be incorporated into a modern health care system in some places, but they are not the only answer to lack of coverage. What is needed is the imagination and the will to institute basic, low-cost health measures appropriate for a particular country's culture and level of socioeconomic development. For these measures to succeed, transformation of the social structure may be a precondition. (Velimirovic 1990: 59)

In essence, an emancipatory "therapeutic alliance" ultimately requires an egalitarian relationship between representatives of various medical systems, one that transcends the hierarchical structure of existing dominative medical systems associated with the capitalist world system. Despite the persistence of a hierarchical relationship in the therapeutic alliance in developing societies, numerous instances of the syncretism of biomedicine and traditional or indigenous medicine have been occurring in many developing countries. For example, the Institute of Traditional Medicine in the Muhimbili University Center for Health Services is providing training to biomedical physicians and nurses in traditional medical practices (Langwick 2011: 17–18). Furthermore, Langwick reports that traditional healers in Tanzania resist efforts on the part of biomedicine to subordinate or even co-opt them with the framework of the therapeutic alliance:

[H]ealers on the Makonde Plateau are constantly reconfiguring the boundaries that mark the inside and outside of biomedicine as they strive to address the complaints, debilities, worries, and pain of those that come to them. Through their everyday encounters, healers suggest forms of integration, coordination, and engagement with biomedicine that disrupt the hierarchies of medical institutionalization, challenge the privileged position of science to articulate matter, and reject divisions between the physical and the social. (Langwick 2011: 233–234)

Simply stated, although asymmetry persists in the therapeutic alliance, traditional healers are not passive actors within it.

THE HOSPITAL AS THE PRIMARY LOCUS OF BIOMEDICINE

The modern hospital has become the primary locus for the practice of biomedicine as well as certain alternative medical systems, such as homeopathy in Britain, Ayurvedic medicine in India, and herbal medicine and acupuncture in China. Michel Foucault (1975) views the hospital as a significant site of what he terms the "clinical gaze." He describes how the Hospital Generale, which was constructed in Paris in 1656, served as an institution where the poor, sex workers, vagabonds, and the mentally disturbed were institutionalized and subjected to various medical experiments and surveillance. In the United States at the turn of the century, hospital construction became a favored form of philanthropy on the part of very rich donors such as Johns Hopkins, Cornelius Vanderbilt, Eli Whitney, and John D. Rockefeller. By contrast, the state in many European countries funded the erection and operation of hospitals.

The basic structure of the contemporary hospital had taken shape by the 1920s (Raffel 1994: 125). The hospital is an elaborate social system, interlaced with smaller social systems and a wide variety of other occupational subcultures. Melvin Konner (1993: 29), a prominent physician-anthropologist, describes hospitals as "our modern cathedrals, embodying all the awe and mystery of modern science, all its force, real and imagined, in an imposing edifice that houses transcendent expertise and ineffable technology." Another anthropologist describes the hospital in less glowing terms by referring to it as an institution that views patients as lucrative sources of revenue as well as one that at various times functions as jail, school, factory, or resort hotel (Grossinger 1990: 28). At any rate, the hospital has become the locus of technological biomedicine. It resembles a bureaucratic assemblage of workshops that deliver a labor-intensive form of medical care. According to Georgopoulos and Mann (1979: 298), the authoritarian structure of the hospital "manifests itself in relatively sharp patterns of superordination-subordination, in expectations of strict discipline and obedience, and in distinct status differences among organizational members."

U.S. hospitals fall into one of three categories: (1) private community hospitals, (2) government hospitals, and (3) proprietary hospitals. Despite their purported nonprofit status, the first two types support capital accumulation by acting as "ideal conduits for the profits of drug companies, equipment manufacturers, construction and real estate firms, and financial institutions" (Himmelstein and Woolhandler 1984: 18). Furthermore, private community hospitals frequently share directors with profit-making health industries (Waitzkin and Waterman 1974: 109). These hospitals also provide an arena where physicians may charge high fees to their patients or third-party payers while retaining free access to sophisticated medical equipment that has been paid for at public expense through federal or state dollars.

Unfortunately, social scientific studies of hospitals have not given much attention to their governing boards of trustees. Although boards generally do not involve themselves in the day-to-day operations of hospitals, their members, however, do possess control over hospital governing policy.

In the United States, hospital boards tend to recruit members from local private elites.

Analyzing the boards of trustees of these [voluntary community] hospitals, one sees less predominance of the representatives of financial and corporate capital, and more of the upper-middle class, and primarily of the professionals—especially physicians—and representatives of the business class. Even here, the other strata and classes, the working class and lower-middle class, which constitute the majority of the U.S. population, are not represented. Not one trade union leader (even a token one), for instance, sits on any board in the hospitals in the region of Baltimore. (Navarro 1976: 154)

An example of such domination is illustrated by a project that a critical medical anthropologist worked on in 1994. The project was designed to improve the ethnic, gender, and class diversity of the boards and staff of an association of hospitals in a New England city. The effort had the official endorsement of hospital directors, and meetings took place in the hospital association's plush offices with secretarial and staff support provided by the association. Over a several-month period, a project that would have moderately changed the hitherto white male dominance of hospital boards of directors and managers while significantly improving hospital sensitivity to the ethnic heritages of patients was developed. The general need for the plan was presented at a daylong workshop with hospital trustees, managers, and leading staff. Publicly these hospital elites, most of whom were white males, gave full support for the effort to improve diversity. Based on this work, a grant proposal was written and submitted to a local community foundation to support implementation of the diversity plan. To the surprise of the project's planners, the community foundation reserved money for the grant but did not award it because they found that in their private conversations hospital elites expressed far less than full support for the proposed project.

The corporate class does not exert as much influence over the policies of hospital boards as it does over those of private health foundations, private medical schools, and even state medical schools. Its interests are represented by middle-level managers and other social actors who agree with the premises of a capitalist economy. The board of trustees has overall responsibility over the hospital and in turn delegates the day-to-day management of the organization to the hospital administration. The medical staff controls matters concerning patient care and exercises substantial influence throughout the hospital organization. This dual authority lends itself readily not only to conflict between the hospital administration and its physicians, but also to a confusion of roles among other health personnel, particularly nurses. With the growing technological and organizational complexity of hospitals, however, an increasing degree of authority is being delegated to administrators, who are more and more likely to be businessmen rather than physicians.

Indeed, a declining percentage of physicians in the United States are self-employed, and an increasing percentage of them are employees of public agencies, hospitals, medical schools, and health maintenance organizations. Some social scientists refer to this trend as the "deprofessionalization" or "proletarization" of biomedicine. By these terms they do not mean to imply that biomedical physicians resemble the typical worker. In fact, they continue to "maintain significant power by capitalizing and keeping control of patient recruitment while ceding other market-mediation functions to third parties" (Derber 1983: 591), such as insurance companies. Nevertheless, much of the work of hospital physicians, particularly in the United States, has increasingly become subject to cost controls, audits, and managerial and even patient evaluations (Schiff 2000).

Nevertheless, class struggle has become an overt aspect of the hospital. Although the trend toward unionization in U.S. hospitals first occurred among its underpaid unskilled and semiskilled workers, it also spread to technicians, nurses, and even physicians. Indeed, various surveys indicate that physicians and medical students suffer from high levels of emotional distress due to their working conditions in hospitals (Morrow 2003: 67). Factors serving to mitigate demands by unionized hospital workers, however, include the shift of the cost of higher wages to consumers and the willingness of administrators to arbitrate with unions in return for disciplined workers. Furthermore, professionalization continues to be seen by many health workers as a more viable approach for socioeconomic advancement, thus preventing them from forming an alliance with low-status health workers.

Although surgery continues to remain the focal activity of the hospitals, many U.S. community general hospitals now provide rehabilitation services, home care, and even primary care. In contrast to rural hospitals, urban hospitals have become big businesses that reflect the "segmentation of society into diverse ethnic, religious, occupational, and class groups" (Stevens 1986: 88). Indeed, an increasing percentage of urban hospitals are owned by large health care corporations oriented toward managed care—a form of health care that emphasizes cost-containment procedures that contribute to greater profit making.

Most underdeveloped countries have reproduced the pattern of hospital-based, highly technological, and curative biomedicine. National elites, which constitute the immediate beneficiaries of biomedicine, have worked in conjunction with international financial institutions and health organizations to consolidate the establishment of biomedicine in the Third World. According to Doyal with Pennell (1979: 270), "Hospital development can . . . distort the whole balance of third world health expenditure and it is not uncommon to find up to half of the recurrent budget consumed by one or two big city hospitals." Ultimately, it could be argued that biomedicine indirectly kills people in rural areas and in urban slums by diverting a large percentage of health care resources from primary care and public health projects.

Despite its centrality as an organization of medical care, the hospital as such has not been the subject of much sociological or anthropological research. Social scientists conducting research in hospitals have tended to focus primarily on more microscopic settings, such as the physician-patient relationship. Much of this research discusses the process by which patients are stripped of their identity, preferences, and decision making. Fortunately, as recounted in the following "A Closer Look," various sociologists have conducted ethnographic fieldwork in hospitals in the People's Republic of China. Gail E. Henderson, a sociologist, and Myron S. Cohen, a medical specialist on infectious disease, conducted fieldwork on the Second Attached Hospital of Hubei Provincial Medical College in the People's Republic of China (Henderson and Cohen 1984). The period from November 1979 to March 1980, when they conducted their fieldwork, is treated as the "ethnographic present," a phrase that anthropologists use to refer to the time frame of a social setting as if it exists at the present moment rather than at the time of actual investigation. Joseph W. Schneider (2001) conducted fieldwork from December 1986 to April 1987 in a hospital in a North China city.

"A Closer Look"

THE CHINESE HEALTH CARE SYSTEM AND A CHINESE HOSPITAL: A WORK UNIT IN A SOCIALIST-ORIENTED SOCIETY

Before the 1949 revolution that brought the Communist Party in China, there were few biomedical or Western-trained physicians in that country, and they generally were concentrated in large cities where they demanded high fees for their services. Except for a few missionary physicians in the countryside, the vast majority of the Chinese people obtained health care from folk practitioners who drew from traditional Chinese medicine as well as various religious healing systems. In 1949, the average life expectancy in China was only thirty-five years, comparable to that in India. The Communist government was committed to creating an elaborate health care system that emphasized both preventive and curative biomedical procedures and a revival of traditional Chinese medicine, particularly the use of medicinal herbs and acupuncture. Although Chinese physicians are trained primarily in either biomedicine or Chinese medicine, they all learn something about both systems. The Patriotic Health Movement mobilized millions of Chinese to eradicate flies, remove trash, and improve sanitation. During the first two decades following the revolution, particularly with the Great Leap Forward commencing in 1958, health institutions in China were transferred from private or foreign ownership to the Ministry of Health or to local health departments (Anson and Sun 2005). Mao introduced the barefoot doctor experiment in the countryside, under which peasants were elected by working brigade comrades to undergo three months of medical training so that they could "serve the people." During the Cultural Revolution (1966–1976), the few remaining biomedical physicians ceased practice altogether or joined public facilities. Furthermore, because biomedicine was viewed as an elitist institution, advanced biomedical education was greatly curtailed, biomedical research was halted, and many hospitals were closed. While health care in the cities suffered, basic health care in the countryside, where the majority of population lived, flourished, with almost all villages having a clinic served by two to four barefoot doctors who served populations of one to three thousand. Unfortunately, the Cultural Revolution resulted in a severe social and economic upheaval. Nevertheless, at the end of the 1970s, China had an elaborate health care network that included a Government Insurance Scheme, which covered government employees, retirees, disabled veterans, and university lecturers, staff, and students; a Labor Insurance Scheme which covered state enterprise employees, retirees, and their dependents; urban collective medical care schemes; and rural collective medical care schemes.

In this "Closer Look," we examine the Second Attached Hospital complex, which includes staff dormitories, and various auxiliary buildings situated on the outskirts of Wuhan, the fifth largest city in China. The medical college is adjacent to the hospital grounds. About two-thirds of the employees at the hospital belong to its attached *danwei*, or work unit. The *danwei* functions as a sort of "urban village" that not only provides housing and other services but serves as the center of its members' social, political, and economic life. The *danwei* is the "vehicle through which state and party health policies are implemented, and through which staff may communicate with higher-level authorities" (Henderson and Cohen 1984: 7).

About a third of the approximately 830 hospital workers live outside the complex. Furthermore, some residents of the *danwei* work outside it. The hospital complex includes day-care centers, schools, and businesses. An estimated 70 to 80 percent of the hospital and medical staff are married to each other. The standard apartment consists of a dining area, two bedrooms, and a small kitchen and bathroom. Access to desirable housing appears to be determined primarily by seniority in the work unit, luck, and a policy that attempts to restore those persecuted during the Cultural

Revolution to the equivalent of their previous quarters. In contrast to residential patterns in capitalist societies, physicians often live next door to cooks or maintenance workers.

Personnel in the hospital and associated medical school are divided into three broad occupational categories: cadres, technicians, and workers. Cadres are state administrative and professional personnel and include physicians, nurses, scientists, teachers, and accountants. The category of technicians includes the small number of lab technicians. The category of workers includes cooks, electricians, health aides, plumbers, carpenters, mechanics, laundry workers, construction workers, and unskilled manual laborers. Before and particularly during the Cultural Revolution of the 1960s health professionals routinely were sent to work on public health projects in the countryside for extended periods of time. By the late 1970s, only about 10 percent of the health professionals were given such assignments at any given point in time. The hospital is responsible for dispatching health workers for a fifteen-county area. As opposed to the past, when visiting physicians and nurses spent much time in rural communes or brigades, they now concentrate on the county hospitals that provide medical teaching for health workers in the communes and brigades.

The hospital has 580 beds and 830 staff, including some 300 physicians, 300 nurses, and 230 administrators, technicians, and workers. It consists of departments of infectious disease; surgery; internal medicine; pediatrics; obstetrics and gynecology; neurology and urology; radiology; combined Western and traditional medicine; dentistry; and ear, nose, and throat care. The hospital building is

laid out like a giant, three-story X, with a library providing a small fourth-story cap. The legs of the X are the hospital wards; at their intersection are a double staircase, auxiliary offices for radiology and laboratory tests, and a small pharmaceutical factory. Administrative offices are in a separate building. (Henderson and Cohen 1984: 47–48)

A special ward provides medical treatment for high-level cadres. A cancer unit is situated behind the hospital. In contrast to the United States, where hospital stays have been becoming shorter, the average length of stay for inpatients at the Second Attached Hospital is nineteen days. Although the hospital emphasizes biomedical treatment procedures, patients may request admission to the combined Western and traditional Chinese medicine ward. Other than two biomedically oriented physicians, the physicians on this ward are primarily practitioners of traditional medicine.

The hospital operates under the authority of the medical college, which in turn is under the authority of the provincial health and education bureaucracies. The hospital director is a Communist Party member and a physician. Vice directors head the Departments of Medical Treatment and Medical Education, and a third vice director heads the departments of administration and general affairs. The administration of the medical college parallels that of the hospital. "Ultimately, the Chinese Communist party and its basic-level organizations at the hospital and medical college direct the implementation of all political and economic policies and address local concerns ranging from personnel appointments to teaching and research" (Henderson and Cohen 1984: 69).

Although work units are hierarchical units whose staff are assigned and whose leaders are appointed, some provisions have been made for feedback from *danwei* workers, as described in the following:

The one most commonly cited is "consultation with the masses" whenever major plans or policies are being considered. These consultations may take place in small work groups such as the infectious disease ward staff. For example, at one morning report the new economic campaign was explained to the staff and their opinions solicited. Strong feelings about the proposed staff-to-bed ratio were freely offered, and the staff planned to request another physician and nurse for the ward. To our knowledge, the ratio was not changed. . . . For decisions on the ward itself, staff members are generally given a chance to participate in discussions about an upcoming change. In addition to group discussions, special days for criticism are regularly scheduled. (Henderson and Cohen 1984: 74)

Although the input sought by supervisory personnel from their subordinates hardly fulfills the socialist ideal of "proletarian democracy," it is hardly any less rigid than patterns of authority in U.S. work settings, including in hospitals. Nevertheless, as Henderson and Cohen (1984: 75) aptly observe, "such mechanisms may also conceal manipulation, acting to co-opt people into loyalty to the organization by giving them a sense of participation." Conversely, lower-echelon leaders do not generally frown upon complaints from their subordinates because they in turn can pass responsibility along to their superiors. The doctor-patient relationship follows the same basic hierarchical arrangement found among hospital personnel.

At the ward level, the doctor-nurse relationship is more egalitarian than in Western countries. In fact, with additional training, nurses may become physicians. Furthermore, health aides can become nurses, and technicians can become medical researchers. Virtually all physicians work under the direct supervision of hospital administrators. Their status in the larger society is considerably lower than it is in capitalist societies but has been increasing, because of the modernization policies of the state. Hospital and medical college administrators are generally Communist Party members and physicians, but some are not health professionals. Despite organizational constraints, physicians have a considerable amount of autonomy over their work, a pattern that undoubtedly is related to their knowledge base.

In his fieldwork on another Chinese hospital, Schneider (2001) focused on how family members and friends, referred to as *peibans*, contribute to the care of patients. In contrast to North American and European hospitals, members of the therapeutic management group cleaned patients' rooms, brought food from home, and fetched medicines and other supplies from outside the hospital, placed oxygen tanks in patients' rooms, and even delivered physicians' orders for lab tests to the appropriate places. Moreover, "if a patient was to be taken to another hospital for a special test, the work of contacting that hospital, making an appointment, and arranging transportation by means of some work unit's car all might be taken over by a family member" (Schneider 2001: 358). If the patient does not have enough family members to assist him or her, his or her work unit might send fellow workers to the hospital for this purpose. Such caretaking activities conform to both traditional Chinese familial duties as well as an emphasis on "revolutionary humanitarianism" (J. Schneider 2001: 361). In contrast to studies focusing primarily on biomedical hospitals in China, Judith Farquhar (1994) conducted ethnographic research at the Guangzhou (Canton) College of Traditional Chinese Medicine periodically during the 1980s.

Whereas the Soviet Union and the Eastern European countries, which had before the collapse of Communist regimes had highly centralized ministries of health, the Chinese health care system is a relatively decentralized one in which financing and delivery are left to local political units on the county and village levels. China spends only 3 percent of its GDP on health care, in contrast to the United States (which spends more than 16 percent) and Australia (which spends 9.6 percent), China boasts health statistics that are better than most developing societies. Between 1960 and 1998, infant mortality declined from 150 deaths per 1,000 live births in the first year of life and life expectancy increased from forty-seven to seventy-one years. With the exception of HIV/AIDS, which has been rapidly increasing in incidence over the past decade in large part due to a migratory labor force, and the Avian flu, infectious diseases have declined in incidence in China and have been replaced by chronic and lifestyle disease, with lung cancer being a big killer due to smoking. Tobacco constitutes the most important source of revenue for the Chinese government.

The Communist Party under the new leadership of Deng began to implement a program of modernization and economic reforms beginning in 1979 under the guise of a "socialist market economy," which some scholars have characterized as "state capitalism." Although these changes have propelled China into a period of tremendous economic development, a renewed emphasis on advanced biomedical education and research, and a continuation of the integration of biomedicine and traditional Chinese medicine, they have also contributed to growing socioeconomic disparities, including in terms of access to health care. The central government has drastically cut back on financial support for health care to localities, and increasingly expects provincial and local governments to generate their own revenues for health services.

There is essentially now a three-tiered system with parallel structures in the urban and rural parts of the country. The rural areas' first tier is the Village Doctors (former Barefoot Doctors) and health workers offering primary care but with a major emphasis on preventive and sanitation work; the second tier, township hospitals serving ten to thirty villages; and the third tier, county hospitals with senior doctors who deliver care for the most seriously ill. The urban counterpart begins with neighborhood and factory doctors, moves to the district hospitals, and then the municipal hospitals offering advanced services. Some of the latter are regional and national specialty centers (Rosenthal 1992: 294).

China has a number of separate insurance programs (Rosenthal 1992: 294–295). Slightly more than 2 percent of the population receives free medical care as a result of government employment or special status, such as college students and certain disabled veterans. Nearly 10 percent of the population is covered under labor insurance through national taxpaying enterprises. Whereas 48 percent of the rural population once received health care as members of medical cooperative plans, only 4.8 percent are now covered under such plans. The remainder is either enrolled in private insurance schemes or pays out of pocket.

Under Communist rule, the number of hospitals in China increased from 224 to 111,344, and the number of "county and larger hospitals" increased from 19 to 1,485 between 1952 and 1985 (Rosenthal 1992: 306). Economic reforms that began in the 1980s have contributed to the significant socioeconomic and concomitantly health differences between urban and rural areas. The ratio of expenditure in health care per capita between 1981 and the early 1990s increased from 3:1 to 5:1 (Hsiao 1995: 1053). In part due to an increased emphasis on market forces, the Chinese hospital exhibits multiple forms of ownership.

Hospital beds are not owned solely by the government; many are owned by large state enterprises. Among the 1.9 million beds in county or regional hospitals, close to 68% are owned by central and local governments, while the rest are mostly owned by various state enterprises. The Health Ministry and Provincial Health Bureaus have no regulatory jurisdiction over enterprise-owned hospitals (Hsiao 1995: 1051).

The government has encouraged groups of physicians and other health providers to assume full responsibility for running hospitals as private enterprises. Private hospitals, especially as joint ventures with foreigners, have appeared in China and charge much higher fees, sometimes ten to twenty times higher than those charged in public hospitals (Hsiao 1995: 1048). Many pharmacies now function as private businesses. Although peasants in the coastal areas often can afford a fairly high level of fee-for-service health, those in the interior generally cannot, as a result of programs of decollectivization and privatization. As Kleinman (1995: 23) observes, health care in China under the program of economic reform emphasizes "high-technology practice in urban centers and medicine as a business."

Although in theory biomedicine and traditional medicine are on an equal footing in China, in reality the former has a considerably higher status and is funded more heavily than the latter. China has about three hundred thousand practitioners, and about 13 percent of the hospitals in 1986 reportedly focused on Traditional Chinese Medicine (TCM; Zheng and Hillier 1995: 1061). At Second Attached Hospital, traditional medicine functioned largely as an adjunct to biomedicine, but it is important to note that China does have hospitals that emphasize traditional medical treatment. Biomedical physicians with some traditional training, however, are in charge. Traditional medicine is more extensively employed in remote rural areas than in urban areas or in rural county hospitals close to urban areas. According to Rosenthal (1992: 302), "Western-style is . . . the major mode of medical practice in Mainland China and dominates health care in the urban areas of the country."

Nevertheless, the People's Republic of China government continues to adhere to a policy of combining biomedicine and traditional Chinese medicine. Zheng and Hillier (1995: 1061) report that the number of TCM practitioners and in-patient beds in TCM hospitals continues to rise in China.

As is the case in China, a country that in the process of embarking on a modernization program has emulated capitalist practices and downplayed social ideals, medical pluralism in complex societies is characterized by a pattern in which biomedicine exerts dominance over alternative medical systems, whether they are professionalized or not. According to Leslie (1976: 512–513), biomedicine, regardless of the society, attempts to control the production of health specialists, define their knowledge base, regulate the biomedical division of labor, eliminate or narrowly restrict the practice of alternative healers, and deny laypeople and alternative healers access to medical technology. Despite biomedical imperialism, traditional medical systems continue to function and even thrive in the Third World. Indeed, many traditional practitioners have adopted various biomedical techniques, such as drug injections, as well as a pecuniary orientation. In his discussion of medical pluralism in Kenya, Thomas (1975: 271) observes "traditional and illegal practitioners are doing very well financially. Healing for profit is much more lucrative than growing crops and raising livestock."

MEDICAL TOURISM

In recent years, a growing number of medical anthropologists have be-gun to examine medical tourism, both in biomedical and CAM settings. Reportedly nearly half a million medical tourists travel to India each year and Singapore is attracting more than 250,000 medical tourists, almost half of them from Middle Eastern countries, each year (Womack 2010:306). Other countries engaging in medical tourism include Argentina, Cost Rica, Cuba, Jamaica, South Africa, Malaysia, Thailand, Jordan, Hungary, Latvia, Estonia, and Malta. However, even the United States can serve as the destination for patients from other countries, as Marcia C. Inhorn and her colleagues found to be the case for a couple from Italy who traveled to a major East Coast Ivy League university biomedical center in seeking assisted reproductive technologies (ARTs) treatment (Inhorn et al. 2012).

Carrera and Bridges (2006: 449) make a distinction between *health tourism* and *medical tourism* with the former referring to "the organized travel outside one's local environment for the maintenance, enhancement or restoration of an individual's well-being in mind and body" and the latter referring to "organized travel outside one's natural health care jurisdiction for the enhancement or restoration of the individual's health through medical intervention." Dahlstrom queries the generic term *medical tourism* and thus prefers the term *medical travel*:

[D]iscussions on the topic [medical tourism] have centered on it as a method for patients to receive affordable elective surgery while combining it with a vacation abroad. This undermines the importance of medical care for patients and implies tourism is the primary motivator. In actuality, the practice is largely driven by medically necessary care. For people forced to travel because they have limited access to medical services in the United States. (Dahlstrom 2012: 163)

His own ethnographic research focused on "winter Texans," most of whom are retirees, who spent part of the year residing along the US/ Mexico border in part to escape cold winters in more northerly climes and in part for recreation. In the case of his interviewees, many of whom require multiple medications and regular monitoring of medical condi-tions, residing in Ocean Valley, many of them purchased medications in the nearby Mexican town of Nuevo Progresso to get around the "Medicare 'doughnut hole,' a gap in prescription coverage that begins when the cost of a patient's prescriptions exceeds US $2700 and continues until the cost reaches US $6154" (Dahlstrom 2012: 166).

In reality, health tourism, medical tourism, and medical travel are not new phenomena. For example, patients from the Mediterranean region traveled to the shrine of Asklepios, the healing god, at Epidaurus in an-cient Greece; Romans traveled to the healing waters of Bath in Britain; and affluent Europeans visited spas in Central Europe and even on the Nile (Womack 201: 307). In 2011, Harish Naraindas and Christiana Bastos (2011) edited a special issue of *Medical Anthropology* that examines *healing holidays* at spas in several cultural settings, including Czechoslovakia/the Czech Republic, Germany, Portugal, India, and the Middle East. In seeking to generalize about what the case studies in their issue exemplify, they state:

It is evident that what makes patients itinerant in both the old and new kind of medical tourism is either a perceived shortage or constraint at 'home', or the sense of having reached a particular kind of therapeutic impasse, with the two often so intertwined that it is difficult to tell them apart. The constraint may stem from things as diverse as religious injunctions, legal hurdles, social approbation, or seasonal affliction; and the shortage can range from a lack of privacy, insurance, technology, competence, or enough therapeutic resources that can address issues and conditions that patients have. (Naraindas and Bastos 2011: 5)

Medical tourism per se is often viewed as a solution to the high cost of biomedical treatment in the United States or to delays in countries, such as Canada, the United Kingdom, and Australia, with public health plans but where there are long waits for patients seeking to undergo certain procedures, such as hip and knee replacements. The medical tourism industry entails an elaborate system of private health insurance companies, international supply chains, telecommunications, booking, transportation, and accommodation services, and government regulations. From a world systems perspective, medical tourism constitutes yet one more example of the unequal relationships between the core and semiperiphery and perhaps even periphery, although medical tourist destinations are much more likely to be found in semiperipheral countries than in peripheral ones. Turner summarizes the nature of this unequal exchange relationship as follows:

Privatization of health services in countries such as India and Thailand does not simply put access to affordable health care beyond the reach of local patients. It also undermines publicly funded health care facilities. With higher salaries in private hospitals catering to medical tourists, public health care facilities in Thailand and elsewhere have difficulty retaining health care providers. "Brain drain" occurs from publicly funded hospitals to private medical centers. As doctors and nurses leave public institutions, the differences between public hospitals and private institutions are magnified. . . . Promotion of medical tourism in such countries as India and Thailand is likely to undermine national efforts to improve health equity. (Turner 2010: 463)

Kristen Smith, a PhD student at the University of Melbourne, conducted ten months of ethnographic research of medical tourism at three biomedical hospitals in Mumbai. She argues that while the medical tourist industry bills itself as a strategy for overcoming failing public health systems, in reality the "minute you step inside the opulent surrounds of an international patient suite in a corporate or other tertiary private hospital in India, and compare it to the crumbling, overcrowded, open wards of public hospitals that in some cases stand merely blocks away, it is evident that there is something seriously amiss within the limited dominant discourses emerging from the sector" (K. Smith 2012: 3).

BIOTECHNOLOGY

Along with other medical social scientists, medical anthropologists have given increasing attention to the biotechnology (Lock and Nguyen 2010). Anthropologists have conducted studies of new reproductive technologies, organ transplants, and the mapping of the human genome. Unfortunately, the main beneficiaries of these technological innovations tend to be people in the core countries rather than people in semiperipheral and particularly peripheral countries. Poor people in the latter all too often provide the body organs that provide the affluent in both developed and developing societies a lease on life. In some extreme cases, people are killed to obtain body parts in high demand (Scheper-Hughes 2000). Due to biotechnology, many people, particularly in core countries, are what Donna Haraway (1991) refers to as modern-day cyborgs who blur the boundaries between human bodies and machines, as is seen in the case of people who carry organ transplants from animals or other humans and those with artificial body parts, such as prosthetic limbs. Julie Park and Ruth Fitzgerald (2011) seek to expand the anthropological study of biotechnology to processes by which biotechnology becomes incorporated into patient care in various contexts, including the community, the hospital, the family, and even that nation-state. Bearing these contexts in mind indicates that biomedical health care involves not only physicians, nurses, and an array of therapists, but health technicians who may operate an "X-ray machine with speed and silent compassion" or conduct blood work and DNA analysis (Park and Fitzgerald 2011: 438).

PART V

Toward an Equitable and Healthy Global System

CHAPTER 13

Health Praxis and the Struggle for a Healthy, Socially Just, and Environmentally Sustainable World System

In what we see as the first phase of its development, critical medical anthropology (CMA) struggled primarily with issues of self-definition within academic medical anthropology. Now that CMA has come of age, its proponents have begun to grapple more seriously with strategies for creating healthier environments and more equitable health care delivery systems. CMA is ultimately concerned with *praxis*, or the merger of theory and social action. Critical anthropology as the larger framework of CMA poses the questions of "anthropology for what?" and "anthropology for whom?" It wishes to move beyond an anthropology that all too often has viewed the subjects of its research as museum pieces or populations to be administered by bureaucratic organizations, such as governmental agencies and, more recently, transnational corporations. Critical anthropology strives to be part of a larger global process of liberation from the forces of economic exploitation and political oppression. At the same time, CMA seeks to grapple with the complexities of globalization, including both assessing the role of classes and corporations in driving this process, the role of governments in influencing its directions, its impacts on the health of global populations, and popular movements of resistance and response.

Like other critical medical social scientists, many critical medical anthropologists work as health activists for women's health collectives, free clinics, ethnic community health centers, environmental groups, AIDS patient advocacy efforts, antismoking pro-health groups, national health care reform groups, and nongovernmental organizations (NGOs) in the Third World. These socially active critical medical anthropologists view access to a healthy environment and comprehensive and holistic health care as a human right, not a privilege or commodity accessible to only a privileged few.

THE VISION OF DEMOCRATIC ECOSOCIALISM AS THE BASIS FOR CREATING A HEALTHY WORLD

Given the authoritarian nature of the historic Communist regimes in the Soviet Union, its satellites in Eastern Europe, China, North Korea, and other postrevolutionary societies, most North Americans, as well as many people in other societies, immediately conjure up negative images of the word socialism or find its association with the concept of democracy to be contradictory. Various commentators have interpreted the collapse of Communist regimes in most of these countries as evidence that capitalism constitutes the end of history and that socialism was a bankrupt social experiment that led to totalitarianism, forced collectivization, gulags, ruthless political purges, and inefficient centralized economies. Unfortunately, what these commentators often forget is that efforts to create socialist-oriented societies occurred by and large in economically underdeveloped countries. Russia, for instance, was an agrarian nation ruled by an absolutist czarist monarchy upon the eve of the Bolshevik Revolution in 1917. Indeed, the czarist regime did not abolish serfdom until the 1860s, as part of an effort to stabilize imperial rule in the wake of having lost the Crimean War to Britain. The efforts of Lenin, Trotsky, and other Bolsheviks to develop the beginnings of the process that they hoped would result in socialism occurred under extremely adverse conditions that included constant external threat.

In addition to economic underdevelopment and the presence of a tiny trained working class, the new Soviet republic faced a civil war and the military intervention of fifteen foreign powers, including the United States, during the period 1918–1920. Furthermore, Russia at best had only rudimentary experience with parliamentary democracy of that sort that existed in Western Europe and North America. Although the Bolsheviks, particularly under the dictatorial leadership of Stalin, managed to transform the Soviet Union into an industrial powerhouse by the 1930s, a variety of external factors, such as World War II and the arms race associated with the Cold War, and internal forces, such as a centralized command economy and a political system of one-party rule, prevented the development of socialist democracy in the Soviet Union. According to Schwartz (1991: 68), "in an isolated and relatively backward country, lacking democratic traditions, and where a militant but extremely small working class had been decimated by civil war, the bureaucracy was able to impose Stalinism as a noncapitalist crash modernization programme." With some modifications, the model of bureaucratic centralism was adopted by various other postrevolutionary societies after World War II, starting with China in 1949. The contradictory nature of Leninist regimes imploded first in Eastern Europe in 1989 and in the Soviet Union in 1991. Helping to propel the collapse of the Soviet Union was the Chernobyl nuclear plant disaster of 1986. As Mikhail Gorbachev (1996) recorded in his memoirs, "The nuclear meltdown at Chernobyl 20 years ago this month, even more than my launch of perestroika, was perhaps the real cause of the collapse of the Soviet Union five years later. Indeed, the Chernobyl catastrophe was an historic turning point: there was the era before the disaster, and there is the very different era that has followed." In the case of China, its Communist leaders embraced capitalist structures as a means of rapid development to the point that some experts argue that it now constitutes a state capitalist society in which, "though there is a high degree of public ownership, workers and peasants are exploited for the benefit of officials and managers" (Weil 1994: 17). With the loss of Soviet support, Cuba finds itself with a fragile economy that various U.S. businesspeople, including many of Cuban extraction, would like to take over. North Korea has developed into what appears to be an isolated dynastic system that in some ways resembles former archaic states. Unfortunately, as Erik Wright (2010: 106) observes, "[t]hese attempts at ruptural transformation . . . have never been able to sustain an extended process of democratic experimentalist institution-building" for a variety of complex reasons. These include internal factors such as a lack of even parliamentary democratic structures and external factors such as hostility from the powerful developed capitalist societies, particularly the United States.

Reconceptualizing Socialism

The collapse of Communist regimes has created a crisis for people on the left throughout the world. Many progressives had hoped that somehow these societies, which were characterized in a variety of ways (e.g., state socialism, transitions between capitalism and socialism, state capitalism, and new class societies), would undergo changes that would transform them into democratic and ecologically sensitive socialist societies. Various progressives have advocated shedding the concept of socialism and replacing it with other terms, including *radical democracy, economic democracy, global democracy,* and even *Earth democracy.* Stanley Aronowitz, as a major proponent of radical democracy, observes that

In contrast to conventional liberal, parliamentary democracy, radical democracy insists on *direct popular participation* in crucial decisions affecting economic life, political and social institutions, as well as everyday life. While this perspective does not exclude a limited role for representative institutions such as legislatures, it refuses the proposition according to which these institutions are conflated with the definition of democracy. In the workplace, radical democrats insist on extending the purview of participation both with respect to decisions ranging from what is to be made, to how the collective product may be distributed, as well as to how it should be produced. (Aronowitz 1994: 27)

Efforts to replace the term *socialism* with new ones are understandable given the fate of postrevolutionary or socialist-oriented societies. It is our contention that progressive people need to come to terms with both the achievements and the flaws of these societies and to reconceptualize the concept of socialism. Despite all the baggage associated with the term *socialism*, it is important to revisit the ideals of socialism and to honestly assess the social experiments that have been labeled socialist, both at national and local levels. As Amin so aptly asserts,

[T]he expression of the demands of counterculture is fraught with difficulty—because socialist culture is not there in front of our eyes. It is part of a future to be invented, a project of civilization, open to the creativity of the imagination. (Amin 2009: 2)

In other words, socialism remains very much a vision, one with which various individuals and groups seek to frame in new guises. Ultimately, of course, the issue is not the label but the social reality to be created and the principles of social relationship and environmental relationship that comprise the new reality.

According to Miliband (1994: 51), three core propositions define socialism: (1) democracy, (2) egalitarianism, and (3) socialization or public ownership of a predominant part of the economy. Although some areas of a socialist society would require centralized planning and coordination, democratic socialism recognizes the need for widespread decentralized economic, political, and social structures that would permit the greatest amount of popular participation in decision making possible. As Miliband (1994: 74) observes,

Socialist democracy would encourage the revolution of as much responsibility as possible to citizen associations at the grass roots, with effective participation in the running of educational institutions, *health facilities* [emphasis ours], housing associations and other bodies which have a direct bearing on the lives of people concerned.

In a similar vein, Boggs (1995: x) maintains that future strategies for change will need to be "more anti-bureaucratic, pluralistic, ecological, and feminist than anything experienced within the vast history of Marxian socialism." Socialist democracy would not be synonymous with total state ownership and centralized planning but could entail collective, cooperative, and individual property.

Since around the end of the twentieth century, progressives have become more sensitive to the environmental travesties that have not only occurred in both developed and developing capitalist society but also in postrevolutionary societies. As a result of this, a growing number of leftists have sought to develop an *ecosocialism*. Joel Kovel (2008: 8) provides a compelling perspective on ecosocialism in which he advocates an ecocentric perspective that entails a "decentering from our narrow species interest toward a more universal perspective that encompasses the ecosphere." Furthermore, as John Bellamy Foster so aptly argues,

[I]t is important to recognize that there is now an *ecology* as well as political economy of revolutionary change. The emergence in our times of sustainable human development, in various revolution interstices within the global periphery, could mark the beginning of a universal revolt against both world alienation and human estrangement. Such a revolt, if consistent, could have only one objective: the creation of a society of associated producers rationally regulating their metabolic relation to nature, and doing so not only in accordance with their own needs but also those of future generations and life as a whole. Today, the transition to socialism and the transition to an ecological society are one. (J. B. Foster 2009: 276)

Democratic ecosocialism, as formulated by various progressive thinkers, rejects a statist, growth-centered, or productivist ethic and recognizes that we live on an ecologically fragile planet with limited resources that must be sustained and renewed for future generations. Common ownership, which would blend elements of centralism and decentralism, has the potential to place constraints on resource depletion. McLaughlin (1990: 80–81) maintains "Socialism provides the conscious political control of those processes of interacting with nature which are left to the unconscious market processes under capitalism." The construction of democratic ecosocialism needs to be based upon a commitment to a long-term sustainable balance between sociocultural systems and the natural environment. From a medical anthropology standpoint, combining social justice and ecosocialism provides the basis for healthier human populations.

Our vision of democratic ecosocialism resembles what world system theorists Terry Boswell and Christopher Chase-Dunn (2000) term *global democracy*, a concept that entails the following components: (1) an increasing movement toward public ownership of productive forces at local, regional, national, and international levels; (2) the development of an economy oriented toward meeting social needs, such as basic food, clothing, shelter, and health care, and environmental sustainability rather than profit-making; (4) the eradication of health and social disparities and the redistribution of human resources between developed and developing countries and within societies in general; (5) the curtailment of population growth that in large part would follow from the previously mentioned conditions; (6) the conservation of finite resources and the development of renewable energy resources, such as wind, solar, and geothermal energy; (7) the redesign of settlement and transportation systems to reduce energy demands and greenhouse gas emissions; and (8) the reduction of wastes through recycling and transcending the reigning culture of consumption.

Democratic ecosocialism constitutes a vision the achievement of which will require a long-drawn-out process of struggle that will meet with resistance from the corporate class and its political allies globally. However, the maldistribution of resources on a global scale that capitalism produces is bound to keep alive ideals of equality, democracy, and socialism in oppressed classes.

Under the present world economic system, the United States, as Bodley (2008a) argues, constitutes the leading "culture of consumption."

In 2004 the United States, with less than 5 percent of the world's population, consumed 100 quadrillion BTUs [British thermal units], which represented 22 percent of the world's total consumption. In 1970 Americans accounted for 35 percent of the world's energy consumption. Worldwide economic development meant that the rest of the world was catching up with America in energy consumption; nevertheless, in 1996 total American consumption was still more than all the energy consumed by China, Japan and India combined (Bodley 2008a: 107).

However, in terms of total consumption, China, with more than four times the U.S. population, now consumes a somewhat greater amount of energy than the United States.

Although at present or in the near future the notion that democratic ecosocialism may be implemented in any society, developed or developing, or a number of societies may seem unlikely, history tells us that social changes can occur quickly once economic, political, and social structural conditions have reached a tipping point. Current patterns of ecological degradation and the mounting pressure of social inequality may well contain the fuel of social change, as continuation on the current pathway will, over time, only lead to deeper and deeper crisis. For the immediate future, a "new socialist movement" needs to "focus on concrete questions of people's welfare, democracy, and survival" (Silber 1994: 266). Needless to say, health and eradication of disease are essential components of survival. As Magdoff and Foster argue,

Everywhere radical, essentially anti-capitalist, strategies are emerging based on other ethics and forms of organization, rather than profit: ecovillages; the new urban environment promoted in Curitiba in Brazil and elsewhere; experiments in permaculture, and community-supported agriculture, farming and industrial cooperatives in Venezuela, etc. (Magdoff and Foster 2010: 25)

More recently, Fred Magdoff succinctly delineated the principles guiding the formation of an *ecological civilization*:

It must (1) provide a decent human existence for everyone: food, clean water, sanitation, health care, housing clothing, education, and cultural and recreational possibilities; (2) eliminate the domination or control of humans by others; (3) develop workers and community control of factories, farms, and other workplaces; (4) promote easy recall of elected personnel; and (5) re-create the unity between human and natural systems in all aspects of life, including agriculture, industry, transportation, and living conditions. (Magdoff 2011: 20)

The Concept of Socialist Health

Several decades ago, the authors of this book sought to introduce into medical anthropology a distinction between socialist and capitalist health (Singer and Baer 1989). A meaningful discussion of socialist health is ultimately grounded in our ability to define socialism itself. As Segall (1983: 222) argues, "The concept of socialism is of no use to people seeking solutions within capitalism, but it is essential for those interested to see that system transcended." Although disease is bound to occur under any mode of production, in that people will continue to be subject to certain hazards and infectious diseases in the natural environment and the physiological degeneration that inevitably accompanies aging, in socialist society, it may be possible to resolve the basic tension between providing for human material needs and social psychological needs and for preserving the health of the people. Ultimately, any attempt to create a socialist health system and socialism per se must not, as Erik Wright (1983: 124) asserts, focus "simply on the provision of various services by the state and various regulations of capital (as is the case under welfare capitalism), but also on the democratization of the forms of delivery of such services." In this process, CMA has an important role to play in providing careful analysis of health care systems in the social context and in contributing to the direct application of this information in improving the quality of health care, accessibility of services, and popular empowerment within the health care domain.

TOWARD HEALTH PRAXIS AND A CRITICAL BIOETHICS IN MEDICAL ANTHROPOLOGY

From its beginnings as a subdiscipline of anthropology, medical anthropology has exhibited a strong applied orientation. Indeed, Weaver (1968: 1) defined medical anthropology as "that branch of applied anthropology which deals with various aspects of health and disease." As Lindenbaum and Lock (1993: x) accurately observe, "Often confronted with human

affliction, suffering, and distress, fieldwork in medical anthropology challenges the traditional dichotomies of theory and practice, thought and action, objectivity and subjectivity."

Whereas various critical anthropologists, such as Wolf (1969) and
Stavenhagen (1971), urged the profession during the 1960s and 1970s to direct attention to establishing a theoretical framework for political engagement in the global system, anthropologists interested in health-related
issues tended to seek avenues by which their research might be acceptable
to mainstream international health agencies and biomedicine. Unfortunately, most applied anthropology historically has been and continues to
be sponsored by colonial and neocolonial (e.g., the World Bank, the International Monetary Fund, the U.S. Agency of International Development)
agencies and consequently fosters the maintenance of existing patterns of
differential power. Some time ago, Batalla (1966) asserted that much of the
research done in Latin America on problems of public health neglected the
social-structural causes of disease and malnutrition by focusing on issues
such as ethnomedical beliefs, nutritional practices, and communication
barriers between biomedical health providers and the target populations.
Elsewhere, in commenting on research on public health in Africa, Onoge
(1975: 221) made a similar criticism of the reductionist tendency of both
medical anthropologists and medical sociologists to restrict their analyses to social interaction in small groups. Other applied anthropologists,
however (e.g., Rylko-Bauer, Singer, and van Willigin 2006), have sought to
counter the reductionism of much applied anthropology.

Thus, some anthropologists have provided their research skills to com-
munity-based health organizations. After working for a few years at the El
Barrio Mental Health Center in Chicago (S. Schensul 1980), Steve and Jean
Schensul went on to become two of the founders of the Hispanic Health
Council in Hartford. While Merrill Singer served as its deputy director
and its director of research, the council evolved into a leading U.S. site of
CMA-inspired health praxis (Singer 2003).

Despite their commitment to health praxis, critical medical anthropologists need to develop this notion more fully. As Partridge (1987: 215)
observes, praxis "signifies the theories and activities that affect human
ethical and political behavior in social life." Various critical medical anthropologists in the past and particularly in recent years have noted the
need for CMA to address matters of application. Scheper-Hughes (1990:
196) calls on medical anthropologists to work "at the margins, questioning
premises, and subjecting epistemologies that represent powerful, political
interests to oppositional thinking." Subsequently, she has called on anthropologists to adopt the "idea of an active, politically committed, morally
engaged anthropology" (Scheper-Hughes 1995: 415). Contrary to Gaines's
(1991: 232) wrongheaded assertion that critical medical anthropologists

believe that "local initiatives can count for naught in the alleviation of human suffering," as has been noted, a significant number of them have been and are involved in a wide array of forms of health activism, including ones at the local level.

In ensuring health as a human right, critical medical anthropologists are strong advocates of participatory democracy in the workplace, the body politic, and health care institutions. Regardless of whether their primary work occurs in academia, in a clinical setting, a community organization, or elsewhere, they need to function as proponents of "patient power." Ultimately, as Bolough (1981: 202) states, "the problem of alienated patient cannot be overcome until medical knowledge becomes social property in practice." Under a global system organized on the basis of meeting human needs rather than on profit making, patients would in essence control the medical means of production and work in cooperation with physicians and other health experts toward the eradication of disease at both the personal and the community levels.

Conventional medical anthropologists often assume that critical praxis begins and ends with the advocacy of global transformation, because anything less would seem to amount to little more than system-maintaining reformism. Although the provision of medical care as a welfare function can serve to dampen social protest, it is nonetheless true that by placing pressure on the system real gains can be achieved, such as a cleaner environment, a safer and less alienating workplace, and improved levels of access to socially and culturally more sensitive health care. Following this line of reasoning, a distinction must be drawn between two fundamentally different categories of social and health reform. Gorz (1973) accomplished this task in his differentiation between "reformist and nonreformist reform." He used the term *reformist reform*, or what Merrill Singer (1995a) calls *system-correcting praxis*, to designate the conscious implementation of minor material improvements that avoid any alteration of the basic structure in the existing social system. Between the poles of reformist reform and complete structural transformation, Gorz identified a category of applied work that he labeled nonreformist reform.

Here he referred to efforts aimed at making permanent changes in the social alignment of power. Whereas system-correcting praxis tends to obscure the causes of suffering and sources of exploitation, system-challenging praxis is concerned with unmasking the origins of social inequity. Moreover, this latter form of praxis strives to heighten rather than dissipate social action.

System-challenging praxis that comprises the day-to-day work of critical practice constitutes a means for furthering drastic social transformation and is not an end point in change-seeking behavior. CMA praxis must emerge from recognition of a significant limitation in contemporary globalist approaches to social change. In world system, dependency, and related globalist theories, there is a tendency to assign all causality to the world capitalist system and, in the process, to ignore the impact of local-level actors. Critical medical anthropologists, in seeking to develop meaningful health praxis, attempt to identify opportunities for nonreformist reform ultimately as part and parcel of a long-drawn-out process of furthering global transformation.

As we have seen, medical anthropology has come to incorporate a wide of concerns such as the role of disease in human biological evolution, paleopathology, indigenous medical systems, the political economy of health, biomedicine, medical pluralism, national health care systems, reproduction, and specific health problems. In addressing these topics, medical anthropologists have attempted to forge links not only between physical and cultural anthropology but also with medical sociologists, medical psychologists, epidemiologists, physicians, nurses, public health people, and health policy makers. Despite these efforts at cross-fertilization, medical anthropology has only begun to enter a dialogue with bioethicists—an endeavor that has tended to be dominated by theologians, philosophers, and lawyers. Perhaps the most explicit examples of this recent development are Richard Lieban's (1990) "Medical Anthropology and the Comparative Study of Medical Ethics" and Patricia A. Marshall and Barbara Koening's (1996) review essay titled "Bioethics in Anthropology: Perspectives on Culture, Medicine and Morality." In contrast to other medical anthropology textbooks, Donald Joralemon (1999: 101–117) includes a chapter titled "Anthropology and Medical Ethics" in his introductory textbook.

From a social scientific perspective, the term *bioethics* is problematic in that it implies a concern with the ethical concerns associated with one particular medical system—namely, biomedicine (Fox 1990: 201). Jonsen (2000: 116) contends that "[t]he word bioethics had been invented in the late 1960s to designate a vision of the world in which scientific advances were linked to human and environmental values in an effort to create a global community." In keeping with anthropological interest in medical pluralism, Joralemon (1999: 103) employs the term *medical ethics* as a "cross-cultural concept that refers to the rules of conduct and underlying values that guide healing activities in each society" (Joralemon 1999: 103). Conversely, historically the term has tended to be associated with the particularistic concerns of the biomedical profession in regulating its own internal affairs and in dictating the nature of its interaction with patients and practitioners of other medical systems, such as homeopathy, osteopathy, and chiropractic. Despite various difficulties with the term *bioethics,* it is an identifier that has become well entrenched.

In this section, in conjunction with our commitment to health praxis, we wish to contribute to the development of a critical anthropological perspective on bioethics. This perspective seeks to transcend a strong tendency in bioethics to focus upon individualistic or familial concerns in a manner that conforms to Western—and perhaps more specifically, American—culture. Although individual as well as familial rights in the medical arena have their place, both bioethicists and medical anthropologists need to consider the rights of patients and their families as members of social groups, be they nation-states, social classes, racial and ethnic minorities, women, gays and lesbians, disabled people, people with AIDS, and so on. A critical bioethics incorporates the concept of *social bioethics* as delineated by Gallagher and coworkers:

Social ethics links clinical or philosophical bioethics with ethnographically oriented social science. Moreover, social ethics [as does critical medical anthropology] connects microsocial perspectives with macrosocial knowledge. From its linkage of situational with societal factors, social bioethics gains a "political" leverage that clinical bioethics lacks. (Gallagher et al. 1998: 169)

Most bioethicists who view health care as a human right tend to do so from a liberal and/or theological perspective that ultimately accepts the parameters of a capitalist political economy (McConnell 1982: 197–217; Churchill 1987; Devine 1996: 230–42; Terney 1999). To date, few U.S. bioethicists situate the struggle for universal health care within the larger endeavor of constructing an authentically democratic socialist world system or even the parameters of the U.S. political economy—one in which health care often is embedded in profit-making endeavors.

Susan Sherwin (1997: 393), a feminist bioethicist, seeks to develop a critical bioethical perspective. She argues that conventional bioethics is closely wedded to the power structures of the larger society:

For instance, work in bioethics is largely defined in terms of what may be characterized as the narrower field of medical ethics; attention is focused on the moral dilemmas that confront physicians, and the doctor's point of view is generally adopted. Problems specific to nurses are encountered far more rarely, and those that might be experienced by occupational or respiratory therapists, pharmacists, social workers, technicians, orderlies, or nursing assistants are seldom dealt with at all. (Sherwin 1992: 2–3)

The tendency on the part of bioethicists to eschew a more forceful critique of the embeddedness of biomedicine in a capitalist political economy is rather ironic given that an appreciable number of ethicists, including some in the United States, have relied on neo-Marxian analysis (Fisk 1980;

Geras 1990; Sayers 1998; Wilde 1998). Milton Fisk (2000) is one philosopher who does adopt a critical bioethical perspective. He argues that political morality entails an "element of political advocacy" (Fisk 2000: 1) and calls for a "radical politics of reform" that would require the eradication of "winner-take-all elections," given that the two mainstream parties represent primarily corporate interests, and the creation of a single-payer health care system in the United States. Last but not least, Marcio Fabri dos Anjos, a Brazilian liberation theologian, also calls for what we term a critical bioethics by arguing the following:

The poor constitute a class of persons who enter into medical encounters encumbered by health problems caused by a mesh of social relationships, including extreme poverty, hunger, lack of opportunity, and poor health care. From this perspective, medical ethics must be concerned with the causes of hunger and the diseases which have become synonymous with particular social classes. (dos Anjos 1996: 632)

Various progressive scholars have argued, however, that ultimately an incompatibility exists between capitalism and human rights due to patterns of inequality that it exhibits both internationally and within specific nation-states. Victor Sidel (1978: 348), a progressive physician, in his essay on an international perspective on the right to health care alludes to the "injustice, immorality, and ethical bankruptcy" of a world in which "the people of one country [have] relatively abundant medical care (not to speak of abundance of food, clothing, shelter, and other necessities of life) while the people of many countries have little medical care and indeed little of anything but hunger, illness and despair." Elsewhere, he delineates the following socialist principles that should underlie a national health care system:

1. health care should be oriented toward improving quality of life rather than profit making;
2. health care should not engage in the exploitation of its providers;
3. health care should "enlighten and empower people" (Sidel 1994: 559); and
4. health care "should be provided in ways that eliminate financial barriers at the time of need, permit the recipients to evaluate their care, [and] to select among alternative services" (Sidel 1994: 558).

Unfortunately, capitalism both internationally and within nation-states is characterized by patterns of social inequality. The United States exhibits the most pronounced maldistribution of wealth of all the advanced capitalist countries. A Federal Reserve research survey reported "in 1992 the richest 1/2 percent of U.S. families owned 22.8 percent of the total net wealth while the top 10 percent owned 67.2 percent" (M. Harris and Johnson 2000: 206). Furthermore, the gap between the rich and working-class

Americans widened appreciably over the course of the last three decades of the twentieth century. This gap has been growing rapidly ever since. Whereas in the United States, the gap between the average CEO pay and worker pay was 45:1 in 1982, by 2003 it had grown to 301:1 (Anderson and Cavanaugh 2005). R. Wilkinson and K. Pickett (2009) reported that in 2007 CEOs of the "largest US companies received well over 500 times the pay of their average employees." CEO compensation comes in various forms. Lee Raymond, the former head of ExxonMobil, for example, received a $398 million retirement package, pushing his earnings over a 13-year period to $686 million, or about $145,000 per day (Rumble 2006). The Global Financial Crisis or Global Recession pushed millions of Americans out of the middle class, increased poverty, and resulted in many Americans losing their dwelling unit, many of them having been forced to live in their cars, in tents, and even in water drainage canals, as in Las Vegas, the icon of American decadence.

Factors that have contributed to the enormous disparity between those at the top and those at the bottom in the United States over the course of the time since the 1980s in particular, have been the following: (1) strong corporate influence over the election of political candidates through massive campaign contributions; (2) a historically weak labor movement compared with other advanced capitalist countries; (3) the absence of relatively strong labor, social democratic, and socialist parties (e.g., such as the New Democratic Party in Canada and the Greens and the Party of Democratic Socialism in Germany); (4) a "winner-take-all" electoral system (as opposed to a system of proportional representation), which makes it extremely difficult for third-party candidates to win, particularly in national elections; (5) the existence of a large "underclass" or massive numbers of poor working-class people, particularly among African Americans, Hispanic Americans, and Native Americans; (6) the presence of a racist ideology that makes it difficult for working-class people to mobilize against the corporate class and its political allies; (7) pervasive corporate influence on hegemonic institutions, particularly the mass media and formal education; and (8) the role of the culture of consumption, organized religion, and spectator sports in deflecting attention from the pervasive corporate control of the corporate economy. At any rate, within the context of U.S. society, we argue that the pursuit of a universal health care system constitutes both a significant venue of health praxis and expression of a critical bioethics.

Indeed, Howard Waitzkin, a critical medical sociologist and biomedical physician, observes that the present U.S. corporate-driven health care system raises significant ethical concerns:

For instance, there is concern that corporate strategies lead to reduced services for the poor. While some corporations have established endowments for indigent care, the ability of such funds to assure long-term access is doubtful, especially when cutbacks occur in public-sector support. Other ethical concerns have focused on physicians' conflicting loyalties to patients versus corporations, the implications of physicians' referrals of patients for services to corporations in which the physicians hold financial interests, and the unwillingness of for-profit hospitals to provide unprofitable but needed services. (Waitzkin 2001: 19)

Ethical Issues in Medical Anthropology

In the course of their work, in (1) *basic research* (i.e., research intended to expand general knowledge about behavior and society); (2) *applied research* (i.e., research implemented as part of a social intervention, such as a needs assessment or program evaluation), as well as (3) *practice* (i.e., the use of research knowledge in advocacy, policy formation, and program development), medical anthropologists regularly confront significant ethical dilemmas or uncertainties for appropriate moral decision making and conduct. Work in medical anthropology often puts anthropologists in a position to do both considerable harm and considerable good, and it is necessary, therefore, that there be structures, training, and guidelines in place to minimize any harm and to insure maximum benefit for the lives of people touched by work in our discipline. Consequently, medical anthropologists are not only interested in the development and nature of bioethics and ethical practices in medicine as research topics but also in the development and application of ethical principles for anthropologists in all areas in which they do work (e.g., Singer et al. 2008). We consider the role of ethics and ethical challenges in each of the three arenas of anthropological activity: basic research, applied research, and practice.

Ethics in Basic Anthropological Research

The field of research ethics that has developed over the last five decades strongly emphasizes the importance of minimizing harm to research subjects. This orientation emerged initially as a reaction to gross and intentional violations of subject agency (i.e., the right to have a say in one's fate) and subject well-being by Nazi researchers prior to and during the Second World War. The establishment of generally shared standards for acceptable research with human subjects dates to the post-war Nuremberg War Crimes Trials and the Nuremberg Code. The Helsinki Declaration of 1964 (revised in 1975); the U.S. Department of Health, Education, and Welfare 1974 Guidelines; The Belmont Report on Ethical Principles and Guidelines for the Protection of Human Subjects of Research; public and researcher revulsion over the infamous Tuskegee syphilis study (White 2000); and a range of other incidents, seminal meetings, and documents have all contributed to the consolidation of contemporary thinking about research ethics with human subjects. All of these, in turn, have had an influence on thinking about the ethics of research in medical anthropology.

Traditionally, basic research in anthropology has involved the use of participant-observation ethnographic techniques within a given community, such as a village, a neighborhood, or a particular social group (e.g., patients in a hospital). Importantly, the very nature of ethnography as it defines how anthropologists should behave while conducting research raises several special ethical challenges for the discipline that may not be directly addressed by the various guidelines and discussions of ethics noted above. From the standpoint of ethics in research, ethnography as a research method is distinctive for the following reasons:

1. Its location of performance: usually ethnography is carried out in the social and geographic domain of the research subjects, on their home turf so to speak, giving the anthropologist access to aspects of the life of study participants that is not found in many other types of research (e.g., people's homes).

2. Its context of realization: data collection in ethnography is interwoven with everyday and sometimes private and quite intimate or highly emotionally charged activities of research subjects (e.g., illegal activities or secret behaviors).

3. Its investigative goals: commonly anthropologists seek to grasp the insiders' understanding and world view, to understand their behavior in social context, including what they feel, experience, and believe.

4. Its methods of data collection: to the degree possible, ethnography involves direct participation in the day-to-day activities of research subjects, as well as quite informal interviewing, and direct observation of behavior in context, activities that put anthropologists in a position to hear, see, and learn about aspects of study participants' lives that are much more extensive than other research methods.

5. Its level of personal commitment: ethnographers often do not go to work, per se; while in the field they live on the job, their work involves a full immersion into the lives of their research subjects and, as a result, during the period of research the personal lives of ethnographers are not, by design, separated from those of research participants.

6. Finally, its style of presentation: as a written document, the ethnography, typically, is a holistic narrative description of behaviors, events, and social meanings, as well as underlying patterns and associations.

One consequence of this unique approach to understanding human lifeways is that anthropologists often spend long periods of time with research subjects and commonly develop intimate knowledge of and close personal relationships with at least some of them. Not uncommonly, anthropologists have key informants among their research subjects whom they define as personal friends and with whom they maintain a relationship long after the period of research has ended. Conversely, anthropologists can develop enemies or have conflicts with people in the group under study. At the same time, from the research subject's perspective, the ethnographer as a person may be of far greater significance than the ethnographer as a researcher (a role that the subject may not well understand). Finally, a completed ethnographic account stands as a public description and assessment of aspects of the group in question. Although anthropologists often attempt to hide the name or the location of the group through the use of pseudonyms, sometimes this is not possible, and some members of the group under study may be offended by how their group is portrayed to the world. As this description makes clear, basic research in anthropology is comparatively intrusive, long-lasting, and personal. In many lines of inquiry, researcher responsibility to research subjects falls primarily within the specific context of the risks or burdens generated by the research project, but in ethnography the boundaries between research activities and other arenas of research subjects' lives may be blurry. The ethnographer contract with subjects (to protect their confidentiality and minimize harm), may, as a result, be broader than it is in biomedical, epidemiological, or other research.

These features of ethnography create critical challenges to ethical conduct in medical anthropological research. For example, because of the access anthropologists often gain to the "backstage" aspects of study participants' private lives, they are in a position to learn confidential information. In her study of female surgeons, for example, Joan Cassell (1998) learned about many private aspects of her study participants' lives, thoughts, and emotions, including deep resentments toward superiors and suggestions of improper behavior. To ensure adherence to ethical standards, in 1971 the American Anthropological Association adopted a set of Principles of Professional Responsibility (revised in 1990). These principles indicate researchers have an ethical responsibility to the following:

- the people whose lives and cultures anthropologists study (exercised by avoiding deception, ensuring voluntary consent, protecting confidentiality, avoiding exploitation, and avoiding doing harm)
- the general public (demonstrated by communicating honestly and considering consequences of communication, and by using knowledge gained through research for the public good)
- the discipline (maintained by protecting the discipline's reputation, avoiding plagiarism, justly treating colleagues, and showing them proper professional respect)
- students and trainees (shown by treating them fairly, offering appropriate assistance and guidance, giving recognition for their contributions to work, and avoiding taking advantage of them in any way)
- employers, clients, and sponsors (expressed by being honest)
- governments (evidenced by being candid with government representatives and by setting ethical limits on acceptable work assignments)

Although these are useful standards, research settings, study populations, and research goals vary considerably, and quite generalized guidelines of ethical practice, like those found in the Principles of Professional Responsibility, may be inadequate for specific research projects (e.g., Singer 1992). Moreover as Patricia Marshall (1992: 215) points out, medical anthropology researchers can be "accountable to individuals and organizations representing diverse interests, including the financial sponsor of the study, the institution or community in which the study is conducted, and the research subjects. In considering the risks and benefits at the individual and the societal level, the anthropologist must explore potential conflicts of interest and determine the most effective way to balance competing claims for allegiance."

The issue of competing claims of researcher allegiance is another arena in which social inequality is of considerable importance. In his study of "urban nomads" (homeless street-corner men) in Seattle, for example, Spradley (1970) found that his study participants were subject to inhumane treatment by the police, prison guards, and court officials. Because Spradley observed and interviewed members of all three of the later groups, they too were his research subjects. Clearly urban homeless men have considerably less power and voice in society than do the other social groups in Spradley's study. Consequently, Spradley had to confront the issue of researcher allegiance in choosing what to do with his research findings, including what to write and how to act in response to them. His choice to fully report and initiate social action to correct the abuses his research uncovered has been acclaimed as a model example of ethical behavior in anthropological research (Singer 2000).

Applied Research

All of the issues of concern in basic research are also confronted in applied research, but applied research faces some additional dilemmas. In applied research, there is a conscious commitment to making social change. The researchers involved, in other words, are not simply learning about, describing, and analyzing the world as they find it; they are attempting to use research to respond to a pressing human problem; in effect, they are attempting to use research to help fix something in human society that is deemed to be broken. A vitally important question in all applied research, therefore, is this: Who decides there is a problem in need of correcting? This is a question that goes to the heart of the critical issues of social inequality of power and decision making. For example, during the late 1970s and early 1980s, because of continued poverty, a number of developing countries began to default on their development loans from the World Bank and International Monetary Fund. A number of economic analysts who hold to what has been termed a neoliberalist philosophy came to the conclusion that the main economic problem facing poor countries is that their national governments are too deeply involved in shaping their economies (e.g., by keeping prices low on basic commodities and health care) and were inhibiting the growth of privatization, free-market activity, and a general rise in production levels that would benefit everyone. Therefore, neoliberal economists and their supporters in the Reagan administration in the United States, the Thatcher administration in Great Britain, and the Kohl administration in Germany called for a total restructuring of the economies of developing nations, involving a reduction in the role of governments in the production, sale, and purchase of goods, letting prices of goods be determined by the marketplace, and lifting protective barriers to international trade and investment. What has been the impact of these policies (developed by rich countries) on health in poor countries? Applied medical anthropology researchers at Partners in Health in Boston (Schoepf, Schoepf, and Millen 2000) have drawn the following conclusions about the impact of structural adjustment policies (SAP) on AIDS in developing countries:

Specific SAP measures, such as currency devaluation, not only shrink resources that could improve AIDS prevention and the treatment and care of persons with AIDS; they also precipitate social upheavals that accelerate the rate of HIV transmission. Poverty and SAPs have undermined the viability of rural economies, promoted mass labor migration and urban unemployment, worsened the condition of poor women, and left health systems to founder.

In short, from a critical medical anthropology perspective, applied research and planned social change must always be assessed from the standpoint of understanding who is the group proposing social change and who is the target group to be impacted by the change that is being proposed. This is a crucial question for ethical practice in applied medical anthropology research.

Another important ethical question, especially with reference to the kinds of socially subordinated populations studied by anthropologists, concerns the appropriate extent of the intervention responsibilities of researchers. In other words, when studying disadvantaged, highly at-risk and otherwise vulnerable populations, how broadly should the lines be drawn specifying the obligations of researchers to insure the welfare of the study population, especially with regard to *health and other risks that do not originate with and are not the direct result of participation in research?* Although the contemporary discourse on research ethics has tended to focus attention on the risks to human subjects that are directly created or enhanced by research procedures and activities, with highly vulnerable populations, some anthropologists have asked whether research responsibility should be expanded beyond current standards to include additional protective behaviors in light of the intimate knowledge ethnographic researchers gain about study participants.

Singer, Stopka, and coworkers (2000), for example, raised this question during a study of AIDS risk among injection drug users. During the course of the study, one of the participants, a twenty-six-year-old man of mixed Puerto Rican and Italian heritage, was shot to death by the police in an incident that the police labeled a police-assisted suicide (i.e., the man provoked the police to shoot him, by pointing a knife at them, because he wanted to die). A reexamination of various interviews conducted with the man before his death forced the research team to ask themselves whether, in light of the problematic and suggestive nature of some of his answers, they could have averted his death. They wondered, for example, whether the study should have had a mechanism in place for quickly spotting depressive symptoms among study participants or for querying them about suicidal ideation (and responding accordingly). Should the project have attempted to help educate the police or other institutions that come into contact with drug users about cultural expression of distress in the Puerto Rican community? Should all research projects that work with marginalized, low-income populations of highly at-risk drug users be required to establish a credible system of aggressive, advocated referral into drug treatment and culturally sensitive psychiatric and other medical services for all participants (even for those who do not request such assistance)? These questions, which to some degree go beyond the usual ethical standards that guide research at present, point to potential direction for the development of new standards for research on vulnerable human subjects.

Practice and Application

Almost by definition, the practical application of anthropological knowledge to engineer social change must be guided by high ethical standards. Application demands both a strong commitment to humane decision making and a keen respect for the rights of agency of the target population. Within applied anthropology, the kind of enhanced concern with professional responsibility noted above is evidenced, especially in discussions of advocacy efforts conducted by researchers. For example, Partridge (1985: 157) maintains that the appropriate level of responsibility of anthropological practitioners "requires a commitment beyond narrow professionalism to take action once analysis indicates a course of action." This "commitment to socially responsible science" is rooted in an ethic of social practice that Partridge (1985: 157) believes "contrasts vividly with the ethic of noninvolvement" characteristic of the work of many basic researchers (e.g., D'Andrade 1995). At present, work done by anthropologists can be situated along a continuum of advocatorial stances.

At the left end of this continuum . . . lies the use of the ethnographic encounter in the service of anthropologically defined goals (e.g., broadening human understanding, expanding cultural knowledge). . . . At the other end of the continuum is the use of the ethnographic encounter in the service of the Other, including defending the right to self-determination or promoting access to needed resources. (M. Singer 1990: 549)

From the perspective of critical medical anthropology, there is no contradiction between science and action, focused research and social responsibility, and morality and adherence to objective standards for knowledge generation. In other words, critical medical anthropologists argue that ultimately the discipline of anthropology must be assessed in terms of its contributions to the enhancement of human welfare broadly defined. As a result, critical medical anthropologists are finding fault with approaches that treat active response to social suffering as beyond the purview of anthropological responsibility. Although application is a particularly challenging endeavor, lack of application and social inaction when there is research-supported awareness of human risk and suffering and available courses of social response would be deemed unethical professional behavior by critical medical anthropologists.

COMPARATIVE NATIONAL HEALTH CARE SYSTEMS AS A POSSIBLE CONTRIBUTION TO CMA PRAXIS

In his teaching of Health and Development, which Hans Baer introduced into the curriculum of the Development Studies Program at the University of Melbourne, he devotes a portion of the course to the a comparison of national health care systems in both developed and developing countries. Although such an overview is not new to programs in public health, international health, global health, health policy, and even medical sociology, only a few medical anthropologists have ventured into this domain (Elling 1980). Exceptions are Linda M. Whiteford and Lois Cacivita Nixon (2000: 440), who review comparative health system research and ask "if health systems are converging on a limited number of Western-influenced models of care, or are there new and still emerging 'mosaics' of models stimulated by the conflicting forces of globalization and cultural diversity?"

Although several typologies of national health care systems exist, particularly for developed countries (see Wall 1996), we delineate a framework for both developed and developing countries which delineates four types of national health care system, at least in terms of access to biomedi-cal services: (1) largely free enterprise systems, (2) social insurance sys-tems, (3) public assistance systems, and (4) health care service systems. In the free enterprise system, health care is provided primarily by the private sectors whereby employers subscribe to health plans into which both they and their employees share expenses or patients purchase health insurance for themselves and their families. In theory, the government covers medi-cal expenses for patients who are seriously disadvantaged due to poverty, disability, or age. The United States constitutes the most explicit example of the free enterprise system, a system under which the government only theoretically covers the medical expenses of the indigent poor under a program called Medicaid and individuals over age sixty-five under a pro-gram called Medicare.

The social insurance system is a mixed system consisting of both gov-ernment contributions and employer contributions and under which bio-medical physicians are usually salaried employees of hospitals or other health organizations. Most European countries and Japan follow a variant of such a system. The public assistance system is characteristic of many developing countries where the government provides only basic pub-lic health care in hospitals and clinics where health workers, including biomedical physicians, are salaried to the masses. More affluent people usually pay for private medical care. The national health service is one in which the government assumes more or less full responsibility for health care and provide health care through tax revenues. In such a sys-tem, many biomedical physicians are public servant. Examples of such a system existed in the past in postrevolutionary societies such as the Soviet Union and the German Democratic Republic and such a system still exists in countries such as Cuba. The United Kingdom has a national health ser-vice but one in which, while most hospital specialists are public servants, general practitioners are in private practice but are responsible for a list of patients that they care for with government subsidies.

Conditions that are favorable to ensuring strong state intervention in health care provision include the presence of a strong labor move-ment and/or socialist, social democratic, or labor party; the presence of a strong centralized government as opposed to a federal system; good access to biotechnology and medical resources; national values that em-phasize collective solutions rather than individual solutions to social issues; and support or opposition of the biomedical profession to gov-ernment support for health services. Historically, however, the biomedi-cal profession has generally opposed socialized or nationalized health plans and only come to terms with them if governments make various concessions, such as allowing physicians to remain in private practice or earn high salaries.

From the CMA perspective, the health care model that would be in the best interests of most people in the United States is a single-payer health care system—one in which the government will serve as the primary funding source for health care.

The Thicket of Proposals for Health Care Reform

Proposals for national health care reform have come and gone over the course of twentieth-century U.S. history. As Ginzberg observes,

National health insurance (NHI) has been on and off this country's political agenda since 1912, when Teddy Roosevelt, running for the presidency on the Progressive ticket, first advocated its enactment. Support for NHI has reemerged periodically—in the mid-1930s, the late 1940s, and the mid-1970s—yet it has never come close to winning popular or congressional support. In the 1990s, the defects of the health care system in the United States—costliness, inefficiency, and inequitable provision to the population—have prompted health specialists and the public to turn their attention once again to NHI. (Ginzberg 1994: 51–52)

The problem of access to health insurance is no longer a concern of only the poor and the elderly, who have since the 1960s theoretically been covered under Medicaid and Medicare, respectively, but increasingly one faced by middle-class people as well. Thus, the proportion of nonelderly workers covered by employer-sponsored health insurance fell from 68 percent in 2000 to 61 percent in 2009 (Robert Wood Johnson Foundation and State Health Access Assistance Center 2011).

Aside from the issue of national health insurance in general, various single-payer proposals, all of which were opposed by the American Medical Association (AMA), have come and gone since the 1930s. The Wagner-Dingwell bill, introduced in 1943, called for the creation of a universal health care plan that would operate as part of Social Security but was defeated. President Harry Truman proposed the creation of a national health care system that would function independently of Social Security, but the AMA thwarted his proposal on the grounds that it would constitute a form of "socialized medicine" (Fisk 2000: 69). Following the defeat of the Kennedy-Griffiths Health Security Act, "Senator Edward Kennedy and his AFL-CIO [American Federation of Labor-Congress of Industrial Organizations] retreated from the single-payer concept and supported the central role of private insurance companies in paying for health services" (Bodenheimer 1993: 14). Ron Dellums, an African American congressperson from Oakland and a member of Democratic Socialists of America, prepared in 1972 the most progressive health care reform plan ever introduced before Congress. His bill called for the passage of a Health Service Act that would create a network of community-based prepaid health plans coordinated at the regional level and serviced by salaried health care providers (Rodberg 1994). Community health boards would administer local health facilities. Proponents of the Dellums bill included the American Public Health Association, the Gray Panthers, and the United Electrical Workers.

The Managed Competition Model

During his bid for the presidency in 1992, Bill Clinton inadvertently backed into the national health care reform debate under pressure from the Kerry presidential campaign. Bob Kerry, a Democratic senator from Nebraska and a proponent of a single-payer plan, made health care reform the major issue in his campaign. Although Clinton had never before shown much interest in health care reform, he became convinced that he could not ignore it. In his desire not to offend big business, Clinton turned to the managed competition model for health care reform. Alain Enthoven, a business school professor and former vice president of Litton Industries, initially developed the concept of managed competition. He presented it at a conference in Jackson Hole, Wyoming, attended by executives from the largest managed care corporations, health insurance companies, and pharmaceutical companies.

The Clinton plan called for the creation of regional Health Alliances, which would contract with insurance plans (mainly in the form of health maintenance organizations or HMOs) on behalf of small employers, the self-employed, and the unemployed. Larger employers were to provide insurance for their employees, contract directly with certified plans for coverage, or choose to pay into the Health Alliances. The Health Alliances would impose cost controls upon the insurance companies or HMOs, which would in turn discipline physicians and hospitals by denying contracts to those who would refuse to comply with insurance company cost-cutting directives. Out-of-pocket costs for covered services would be capped at $1,500 per individual and $3,000 per family. One of the positive features of the Clinton plan was a requirement that 50 percent of all residency slots be allocated to family medicine, general medicine, and general pediatrics. The plan also provided an option for states to pursue a single-payer system.

Under the Clinton plan, it was generally recognized that the big health insurance companies would dominate national health care with an elaborate system of HMOs. Navarro (1994: 207) argues that "[m]anaged competition will mean corporate assembly-line capitalism for the masses and their health care givers and continuing free choice and fee-for-service medicine for the elites." As has been the case for existing managed care operations, heavy reliance on advertising, marketing, and utilization reviewers would have made managed competition a costly way of providing national health insurance. Chief executive officers (CEOs) would have continued to be compensated extremely handsomely for transforming their companies into profitable enterprises. For example, James Lynn, CEO of Aetna, earned $23 million in 1990. Most analysts maintain that the large insurance companies would be the winners under managed competition, whereas the smaller health insurance companies would go out of business. Indeed, Aetna, Prudential, Cigna, Met Life, and Travelers' formed the Coalition for Managed Competition.

MANAGED CARE FOLLOWING THE DEMISE OF THE CLINTON PLAN

The corporate class and its political allies in the executive and legislative branches of the federal government have pushed serious discussion of some type of national health care plan on the back burner since the demise of the Clinton plan. During the 2000 presidential campaign, George W. Bush completely dismissed the idea of national health insurance, and Al Gore promised, if elected, the creation of a national health plan covering all children by 2004. In contrast, Ralph Nader, the Green Party candidate who received about 3 percent of the popular vote, spoke out in favor of a national health plan. Since the early 1990s, reforms in biomedical health care delivery have consisted of an array of piecemeal managed care arrangements that have left both health care personnel, including physicians, and patients frustrated. Critical medical sociologist Rose Weitz describes managed care as follows:

Managed care refers to any system that controls costs through closely monitoring and controlling the decisions of health care providers. Most commonly, managed care organizations (MCOs) monitor and control costs through utilization, in which doctors must obtain approval from the insurer before they can hospitalize a patient, perform surgery, order an expensive diagnostic test, or refer to a specialist outside the insurance plan. Although the terms HMO [health maintenance organization] and managed care increasingly are used interchangeably, HMOs represent only one form of managed care, and most fee-for-service insurers now also use managed care. (Weitz 2001: 230–231)

Other MCOs included preferred physician provider organizations and proprietary health corporations that operate hospitals, clinics, nursing homes, and hospices. Whereas managed care encompassed 29 percent of the health care market in 1988, by the late 1990s it had come to encompass 61 percent of it (Court and Smith 1999: 104). Managed care has become part and parcel of the profit-driven medical-industrial complex. Some two hundred corporate takeovers of nonprofit hospitals occurred between 1990 and 1996 (Court and Smith 1999: 86). Steve Wiggins (the chairperson and CEO of Oxford Health Plans), Wilson Taylor (the chairperson and CEO of Cigna Corporation), and William McGuire (the CEO of United Healthcare) earned salaries of more than $30.7 million, $12.4 million, and $8.6 million, respectively, in 1997 (Court and Smith 1999: 105). Whereas some upper-echelon HMO functionaries may be biomedical physicians, most hold MBAs or PhDs. Nurses have increasingly come to assume position as lower-echelon HMO functionaries. Purchasers of MCOs now include private sector employers, public sector employers, and public sector programs, such as Medicare and Medicaid. Despite the assertion on the part of health insurance companies and health corporations that they would provide a cheaper form of health care than a single payer system would, Fisk observes that:

The debt-laden acquisitions of the late 1990s—like the $8.8 billion Aetna buyout of U.S. Healthcare—called for cost cutting in the delivery of services but, ironically, raised health care costs for employers by adding on the expense of servicing billion-dollar debts. By 1997, less than half of the health insurers made money. Insurance rates then started going up at twice the rate of the years 1993–1996. (Fisk 2000: 278)

The medical-industrial complex has contributed to a health care system in which the United States exhibits the highest level of health expenditure as percentage of GDP of any country in the world. For example, in 2005, whereas 15.3 percent of the GDP went to health care in the United States, in Switzerland this figure was 11.6 percent, in France 11.1 percent, in Germany 10.7 percent, Canada 9.8 percent, Sweden, 9.1 percent, United Kingdom 8.3 percent, and Japan 8.0 (T. R. Reid 2009: 9). Needless to say, life expectancy was higher and infant mortality rates were lower in all of these countries compared with the United States.

In response to such developments, various consumer groups and physician organizations, including unions, have arisen in opposition to managed care (Fuentes 1997; Waitzkin 2000). Unfortunately, numerous U.S. citizens lack any form of health care coverage. Lassey, Lassey, and Jinks (1997: 27) provide figures indicating that about 15 percent of the U.S. population (40–45 million people) are uninsured and that an estimated 50 million are underinsured in that they lack sufficient insurance to "cover serious illnesses or must pay very high deductibles. T. R. Reid reports (2009: 2) that various studies indicate "that more than twenty thousand Americans die in the prime of life each year from medical problems that could be treated, because they can't afford to see a doctor."

Health Reform under President Obama

In contrast to George W. Bush during his presidency, Barrack Obama campaigned in 2008 with the promise that he would close various gaps in the U.S. health care system, particularly for the poor and the elderly. Earlier in his political career, he had even supported a single-payer health care system. Unfortunately, the private insurance industry may have shifted Obama's thinking in that "in his 2008 presidential campaign, he received approximately three times more contributions" from them than John McCain, the Republican presidential candidate (Waitzkin 2011: 182). Under his administration, employers with fifty or more employees must pay $2,000 annually per employee; health insurance companies cannot deny coverage, including for reasons based on health status, and cannot charge higher premiums for individuals with poorer health; and young people can remain on their parents' health policy until age twenty-six rather than age eighteen as in the past. The Obama administration pledged a projected decline of uninsured individuals from some 46 million people to 23 million people by 2019. Around the time that Obama assumed the U.S. presidency in January 2009, the U.S. health care system constituted the most inequitable and deficient such system in any developed country and even worse than that of a fair number of developing societies. Marmor and Oberlander report:

[T]he U.S. is the only rich democracy where a substantial portion of its residents lacks health insurance coverage. Fifty-one million Americans (nearly 17% of the population) go without health insurance at any given time. Another twenty-five million American adults are "underinsured," covered by insurance policies that inadequately protect them against the high costs of medical care. This last category of "underinsured" Americans are graphically depicted in Michael Moore's film *Sicko*. In a moving portion of the film Moore takes a boatload of patients to Guantanamo Bay where he hoped that they would receive free medical treatment as do the prisoners in the military detainee camp but is turned back. Instead, the patients are given treatment in Cuba per se and sent home with needed medicines. (Marmor and Oberlander 2011: 125)

In contrast to the Clinton administration, the Obama administration did not propose a detailed health plan and deferred to the Congress on the details of health reform. To give credit its due, some liberal Democrats proposed that the federal government serve as a vendor of health insurance and thus as a competitor to private health insurance plans, but the proposal met resistance in the Senate (G. Shaw 2010: 167). The Patient Protection and Affordable Care Act eventually managed to pass the Senate in December 2009 and the Senate in 2010 constituted a reformist reform par excellence that "creates new state health insurance exchanges, regulated marketplaces where the uninsured and small business can purchase coverage, with tax credits available on a sliding-scale to subsidize coverage (Marmor and Oberlander 2011: 127). A positive feature of the new legislation is that it prohibits private insurance companies from charging sicker persons higher premiums. Although the Patient Protection and Affordable Care Act is an improvement over what had existed previously, major provisions expanding insurance will not take effect until 2014. Even before Obama's 2008 election, Maine, Vermont, and Massachusetts enacted universal health reforms, and California and Oregon are currently considering such reforms (Smith-Nonini and Bell 2011: 510).

The Single-Payer Model

Despite the fact that the plan for a managed-competition health care system failed early on in Clinton's first presidential term, growing dissatisfaction with managed care and the failure of the existing system or what some term nonsystem to provide adequate health care to a significant portion of the American people make it apparent that health care reform will be a major societal concern now that we have begun the twenty-first century. Whereas most corporate interests and physician groups oppose the concept of a single-payer health care system, various physician groups, grassroots groups, and legislators favor it—a fact generally downplayed by the mainstream media. The single-payer concept reemerged in January 1989 with the publication of a proposal of the Physicians for a National Health Program (PHNP) in the *New England Journal of Medicine* (Himmelstein and Woolhandler 1989). PHNP, an organization with some five thousand members in thirty-four chapters in twenty-five states, advocates the creation of a single-payer Canadian-style health care system in the United States. PHNP is not a left organization per se, but much of its leadership is openly leftist and includes progressive physicians such as David Himmelstein, Steffie Woolhandler, and Vincente Navarro. Although the Canadian health care system has shortcomings of its own, it clearly is more equitable than the U.S. health care system.

The United Nations Human Development Report "ranked Canada first in the world with respect to health status, overall quality of life, and socioeconomic status" (Lassey, Lassey, and Jinks 1997: 72). Canada's three major political parties, namely the Progressive Conservatives, the Liberals, and the New Democratic Party, support a single-payer, which was approved in 1968, with strong labor support, and fully implemented in 1971 (Coburn 1999). In large part, this is because Canada exhibits a stronger "collectivist culture" than does the United States (Lemco 1994: 6). In contrast to the United States, the Canadian health care system is, according to Birenbaum (1995: 176), "accepted widely today by Canadian conservatives who oppose state intervention as well as liberals who see the state as the mediator between conflicting classes." The Canadian system is premised on the notion that health care is a right rather than a privilege.

The Canadian system, called Medicare, consists of ten provincial health plans that must abide by certain national standards and that are funded jointly by federal and provincial governments through corporate taxes, personal taxes, property taxes, and taxes on gasoline, tobacco, and liquor. The federal government exerts more control over the health care plans of the Northwest Territories and the Yukon Territory than those of the provinces. All Canadian physicians participate in the provincial or territorial health plans. The federal government prepays each province about 40 percent of medical costs, provided the provincial health insurance programs are universal, comprehensive, portable (each province recognizes the others' coverage), and publicly administered. Each province devises its own payment system for providers but is required to provide comprehensive medical services in order to obtain federal funding. The provincial governments set hospital budgets, limit the number of specialists, allocate the purchase of medical technology, and restrict costly medical procedures, such as open-heart surgery, to hospitals in large urban areas. The Canadian system charges nominal fees for medication and has administrative costs that are much lower than in the U.S. system (11% versus 25 percent; Himmelstein and Woolhandler 1994). Indeed, the 1964 Royal Commission on Health Services, the body that designed Canada's Medicare, maintained that private administration of insurance was uneconomical. Whereas about 20 percent of U.S. physicians are primary care providers, about 50 percent of their Canadian counterparts are primary care physicians. Patients choose their own physicians, most of whom are not government employees. Furthermore, most hospitals are not owned or operated by the government. Whereas U.S. citizens often feel chained to their jobs because of health care benefits, a Canadian "worker who leaves to take a job in another city or province, or with a different employer, is always completely covered" (Birenbaum 1995: 178). It is important to note that the Canadian health care system has developed serious problems over the past decade or so. Waiting periods for certain procedures can be incredibly long in Canada. Reid reports:

The waiting periods vary from province to province, and they vary according to the treatment you're waiting for. Orthopedic surgery is notorious for long waiting lines across Canada; other backed-up procedures include MRI scans, cataract surgery, coronary bypass, and radiation treatments for cancer. (T. R. Reid 2009: 128)

Furthermore, about two-thirds of working Canadians carry private health insurance to cover certain medical treatments and services not covered by Medicare, such as dental care, certain prescriptions, and childbirth classes (T. R. Reid 2009: 135). However, all provinces prohibit patients or private health plans to pay for any medical service that is covered by Medicare.

National and local coalitions of health care persuaded some thousand legislators before the Republican sweep of Congress in 1994 to cosponsor single-payer legislation. Representatives Jim McDermott (D-Washington) and John Conyers (D-Michigan) proposed a single-payer plan, called the American Health Security Act. Paul Wellstone (D-Minnesota) proposed a single-payer plan in the Senate. A Congressional Budget Office report in 1993 concluded that a single-payer system would trim up to $100 billion a year in administrative costs.

Groups supporting a single-payer system include Public Citizen, Neighbor-to-Neighbor, the Oil, Chemical and Atomic Workers, the AFL-CIO, and many other labor unions, as well as the National Medical Association (an organization of African American physicians), the Women's Medical Association, the Rainbow Coalition, and the "72 religious organizations that make up the Interreligious Health Care Access Campaign" (Navarro 1994: 211). As part of an effort to retain physician control over working conditions, which would inevitably be considerably eroded under managed competition, the College of Surgeons endorsed the Wellstone-McDermott bill. A single-payer initiative called the Health Security Act of California, which became Proposition 186, sponsored by Neighbor-to-Neighbor, garnered 1,060,000 signatures in California, ensuring a referendum on the November 8, 1994, ballot. The Health Security Act also included coverage for licensed chiropractors, acupuncturists, nurse-midwives, and mental health professionals. Heavy lobbying on the part of the health insurance industry as well as the politics of reaction that resulted in the passage of Proposition 187, which excluded undocumented workers from social and health services, contributed to the defeat of this initiative (Andrews 1995: 103–119). Furthermore, there was no unanimity nationwide among grassroots health reform groups on the issue of a single-payer system. Nevertheless, a Louis Harris poll showed that 66 percent of those surveyed preferred the Canadian health care system to the U.S. system. Other polls have also shown strong popular support for a single-payer system.

Navarro (1995) offers the following explanation as to why the large corporations oppose a single-payer plan even though they would very likely pay considerably less in fringe benefits for their employees if such a plan were implemented:

[The majority of large employers and their trade associations] most value control over their own labor force, and the employment-based health benefits coverage gives them enormous power over their employees. The United States is the only country where the welfare state is, for the most part, privatized. Consequently, when workers lose their jobs, health care benefits for themselves and their families are also lost. In no other country does this occur. . . . The United States, the only major capitalist country without government-guaranteed universal health care coverage, is also the only nation without a social-democratic or labor party that serves as the political instrument of the working class and other popular classes. (Navarro 1995: 450)

Health Care Reform Plans as System-Correcting and System-Challenging Praxis

At this point, it seems appropriate to view the two principal models for national health care reform just presented with a distinction between *system-correcting* and *system-challenging* praxis. From the CMA perspective, the managed-competition health care model constitutes by and large a reformist reform, whereas the single-payer model has a much greater potential to function as a nonreformist reform.

The Clinton plan would have contributed toward the process of concentration in the medical-industrial complex. A Prudential executive described managed competitions as the "best-case scenario for reform— preferable even to the status quo" (quoted in *In These Times*, October 18, 1993: 2). The pharmaceutical industry prefers managed competition over a single-payer system because the purchaser of drugs has much greater power to negotiate for lower prices under the latter.

A single-payer system, including one based on the Canadian health care system, appears to come much closer to system-challenging praxis. The Canadian system operates as a "publicly-funded, privately-provided, universal, comprehensive, affordable, single-payer, provincially administered national program" (Bernard 1990: 35). Canadians see the physician of their choice, 50 percent of whom are primary care providers, as opposed to the United States, where primary care providers are in scarce supply. Canada spends about 9 percent of its GNP on health care, as opposed to the United States, which spends 14 percent.

Despite its superiority to the U.S. system, the Canadian health care system itself contains contradictions, including a hierarchy in the health labor force as well as in the physician-patient relationship, little community control over health services or worker self-management within health care settings, and relatively little emphasis on prevention. Although all Canadians have access to health care, class-based inequalities persist in terms of its utilization (Schwartz 1991: 540). The Canadian system relies less on medical technology than some other advanced capitalist countries. In 2006, Canada had 378 computed tomography (CT) scan machines or 11.4 CT scan machines per million persons in the population in contrast to 32.2 per million persons in the U.S. population in 2005 and 20.6 per million people in OECD countries overall also in 2005 (Duncan, Morris, and McCarey 2010:71). Substantial waiting lists for selected surgical and diagnostic procedures occur. Conversely, it is important to note that many

American HMOs require substantial waiting periods for medical appointments. The overall rates of hospital use per capita in Canada exceed those in the United States, and patients are generally cared for in a timely manner.

Unfortunately, the Canadian health care system faces external pressures in large part because, like the American system, it is embedded in a capitalist political economy and world system (P. Armstrong and Armstrong 1996). According to Chernomas and Sepehri,

As a result of economic stagnation and conservative economic policy (e.g., deindexing the per capita grant) the federal contribution, as a percentage of the total public spending on health care, has been declining over time, while per capita health expenditures have been growing. The result is increasing pressure on the provinces and private sector to meet the financial needs of the health care system. The provinces in turn have reduced the number of services covered, and the private sector has begun to take on a larger role. (Chernomas and Sepehri 1998: 3)

In that it is reliant on profit-making operations, such as medical equipment and pharmaceutical companies, the Canadian health care system is not a utopian model. Nevertheless, a Canadian-style single-payer system holds the potential for transformation into a national health service under which the government would provide health services. As Marmor so aptly observes,

Contrary to the message of the AMA and the HIAA [Health Insurance Association of America], the Canadian system not only works reasonably well—it pays for universal access to ordinary medical care, maintains a generally high quality, is administratively efficient, and restrains the growth of health care costs far more effectively than any of the myriad cost containment schemes tried in the United States—but is as adaptable to American circumstances as one could imagine a foreign model to be. (Marmor 1994: 184)

Opposition to a single-payer health care system in the United States does not for the most part stem from the public but rather from a narrow but powerful group consisting of the insurance companies, some providers (particularly proprietary hospitals and highly paid medical specialists), and some small businesses that would be forced to pay a share of health costs for the first time. When Hillary Clinton asked David Himmelstein, a progressive physician-activist who advocates a single-payer system, how to defeat the insurance industry, he replied, "With presidential leadership and polls showing that 70 percent of Americans favor [the features of] a single-payer system" (quoted in Marmor 1994: 160). The First Lady reportedly retorted, "Tell me something interesting, David" (quoted in Marmor 1994: 160).

Although the *MacNeil/Lehrer Report* on the Public Broadcasting System included single-payer supporters on its health reform panels, the major commercial news programs consistently avoided reports on a Canadian-style single-payer health care plan (Canham-Clyde 1994). On the few occasions that they mentioned the single-payer plan, the major TV networks, the *New York Times*, and the *Washington Post* ridiculed it (Navarro 1995). Despite conservative attempts to implement significant cutbacks in Medicaid and Medicare, the demise of the Clinton plan may have inadvertently created a new opening for serious consideration of a single-payer system among health activists.

Obviously, Americans should not adopt the Canadian or any other single-payer system "lock, stock, and barrel" in creating a national health care system of their own. Various aspects of the Swedish single-payer health care system, such as county and municipal ownership and operation of hospitals, may prove to be amenable to local preferences. The creation of an American single-payer system will have to be coupled with the creation of an authentically holistic and pluralistic medical system—one that integrates biomedicine with a wide array of alternative subsystems, something that the Canadian system has not achieved (Crellin, Anderson, and Connor 1997). Although few public advisors tend to view a single-payer health care system as not falling into the scope of political pragmatism, one exception remains: Physicians for a National Health Program who attended Obama's Health Care Summit in 2009 and agreed to cancel a planned white coat demonstration in front of the White House for the privilege of attending. Despite the fact that Obama opted to support a health reform package that included the private insurance industry as an on-going major player in health care delivery, McCanne (2009: 702) asserts that a single-payer national health plan "would establish a single universal risk pool, funded equitably through progressive taxes, and it would remove financial barriers to care so that absolutely everyone could receive the care that they need, when they need it." Ultimately, however, health care systems must go beyond simply emphasizing curative medicine by creating what Smith-Nonini and Bell (2011: 508) term a *health care commons* that would "help to remedy the historically fragmented relationship between public health and medicine, and the long recognized need to integrate health planning and delivery."

Ultimately, the creation of a single-payer health care system will have to be part and parcel of other nonreformist reforms in U.S. society. In pursuing the creation of a single-payer health care system, Milton Fisk (2000: 187–206) calls for a "radical politics of reform" that would include a system of proportional representation that would make it easier for a labor or socialist-oriented party to win seats in various levels of government as well as an alliance of various working-class groups (including labor unions). At even a more profound level, however, even if the United States manages to implement a national health care program, Waitzkin (2001: 175) asserts that health policies must address social differentials in health statistics that "remain closely linked to social class, racism, gender inequalities, work hierarchies and exposures, and environmental problems." Ultimately, CMA, as well as the critical medical sociology that Waitzkin espouses, are committed to the eradication of these inequities not only in this country but internationally.

"A Closer Look"

CUBAN HEALTH CARE AT HOME AND ABROAD

A year after the Cuban revolution of 1959, Che Guevara stated in an article titled "On revolutionary medicine" that "the work that today is entrusted to the Ministry of Health and similar organizations is to provide public health services for the greatest possible number of persons, institute a program of preventive medicine, and orient the public to the performance of hygienic practices." After the revolution, the Cuban health care system was in shambles, in large part because half of the biomedical physicians left the country, many of them to the United States. Despite this, the physician/population in Cuba increased from 9.2 per 10,000 in 1958 to 58.2 per 10,000 in 1999. Whereas the United Kingdom had 1 biomedical physician for every 600 people in 2001, Cuba had 1 biomedical physician per 175 people. The Family Doctor Program provides a physician-nurse team who live in a designated community and serve about 140 families or 700 individuals (Kath 2010: 24). The family physician as the gatekeeper to the rest of the health care system and generally is situated within walking distance from patients' homes. Kath reports:

In most cases, when a patient from a family doctor's community is referred to hospital or another health institution, the doctor is required to travel to the hospital (except where provincial and national hospitals are out of the local area) to speak in person with specialists and coordinate appropriate inpatient services. Family doctors also closely follow the case thereafter ensuring that records are kept and treatment is continued. Even in emergency cases when patients bypass the family doctor's office and go directly to a hospital emergency department, the staff there are usually expected to contact the patient's family doctor to arrange follow-ups. (Kath 2010: 26)

Despite the fact that the family doctor generally functions as the point of entry into the health care system, more than 25 percent of first-contact consultations occur in the emergency rooms of hospitals and polyclinics (De Vos 2005: 201).

Sociologist Christina Perez (2008) has written a fascinating ethnography based on extensive participant-observation and qualitative interviews of community health care in Cuba. She observes in the concluding chapter of her book that "[a] moderately poor developing country like Cuba, one that is cut off from the largest funders of health care in the world (the United States, World Bank, and IMF), can create healthy bodies because the government decided that nothing is more important than the lives of the population" (Perez 2008: 270).

In contrast to many developing countries, including China, which may spend 2 to 3 percent of their GDP, Cuba spent about 16 percent of its GDP, similar to that of the United States, in 2006. The infant mortality rate of 6.33 per 1,000 in 2006 was the lowest in the Americas, along with Canada. In 2006, the live expectancy at birth was 77.23 years comparable to that of the United States, thus promoting then Secretary General of the UN Kofi Annan to comment that "Cuba demonstrates how much nations can do with the resources they have if they focus on the right priorities—health education, education, and literacy."

Cuba has achieved control of infectious diseases, including dengue fever, and eliminated "polio, neonatal tetanus, diphtheria, measles, pertussis, rubella, and mumps" (Cooper, Kennelly, and Ordunez-Garcia quoted in Mann 2010: 218). At 0.1 percent, Cuba has the lowest HIV prevalence rates in the Americas and one of the lowest in the world. The Centre for Genetic Engineering and Technology in Cuba has developed vaccines against HIV/AIDS and dengue fever, medicines to dissolve blood clots, and exported medicine and clinical supplies to forty-seven countries, including China, India, and ones in Latin America and Eastern Europe (Fitz 2012).

Whereas many developing countries export biomedical physicians and other health workers to developed countries, a phenomenon that constitutes yet another example of the unequal exchange pattern of the capitalist world system, Cuba has been exporting health workers. There are now some 52,000 Cuban biomedical workers in ninety-two countries that care for more than 70 million people. The Bolivarian Revolution in Latin America in large part spearheaded by Hugo Chavez who was elected president of Venezuela in 1998 has drawn both medical assistance and inspiration from Cuba in terms of health care reform. More than twenty thousand Cuban health workers are assisting the effort to revamp the Venezuelan health care system (de Maio 2010: 108–112). Quite in contrast, the United States in 2006 "attempted to directly sabotage Cuba's humanitarian medical missions by creating the Cuban Medical Professional Parole Program" to "lure Cuban doctors, nurses and technicians away from their foreign assignments by offering them special immigration status and speedy entry into the United States" (Brouwer 2011: 17–18). Consider that

Partners in Health has relied on Cuban health workers in Haiti. According to physician-anthropologist Paul Farmer, Partners in Health turned to Cuban health workers because it had difficulty in finding Haitian physicians "who were interested in leaving their middle-class city lifestyles to live in the primitive countryside" (Brouwer 2011: 33).

Cuban health workers provided relief in the aftermaths of the earthquakes in Pakistan and Haiti and were ready to go to New Orleans to treat the victims of Hurricane Katrina in 2005 but were refused entry by the Bush administration. At its Latin American School of Medicine which opened in 1997, with the first class graduating in 2005, Cuba trains medical workers from some forty countries, even the United States (Fitz 2012).

However, it is important to note that numerous problems exist with the Cuban health care systems, including low pay for physicians, many hospitals and clinics in disrepair, poor provision of biotechnology, frequent absence or shortage of essential medicines, and reliance on medical tourism (including for eye surgery and in the treatment of multiple sclerosis, Parkinson's disease, and various orthopedic conditions), which generates some $40 million annually. On the positive side, however, in 1990 Cuba began to integrate biomedicine and complementary and alternative medicine, including modalities such as flower essences, neural and hydromineral therapies, homeopathy, acupuncture, natural dietary supplements, yoga, and electromagnetic devices. Children are studying the multiple use of medicinal plants in primary school and are encouraged to grow them.

In their thorough overview of primary health care in Cuba, Linda M. Whiteford and Laurence G. Branch delineate ten lessons that other countries had learned from the Cuban model, although they caution that the model needs to be modified in its application to other societies:

1. "the importance of reducing disparities in health outcomes, access, opportunities, education, and access to resources" (Whiteford and Branch 2008: 111)

2. Making health care available for all, whether they reside in an urban or a rural area

3. The close proximity of health posts, polyclinics, and family physicians to people's residences

4. Widespread health promotion in the form of billboards and posters exhorting people to "save water, wash their hands, cover their food, and avoid excesses" (Whiteford and Branch 2008: 113)

5. The incorporation of community-based organizations and groups into health promotion and care

6. A sustained commitment to primary health care as part and parcel of public health

7. Primacy to preventive health care

8. Organizing a health care system for a relatively small population, such as Cuba's population of eleven million, may have implications for organizing the health care of a highly populated country, like the United States

9. The recognition of the differences between preventive health care and curative health care

10. The recognition that "curative medicine is extremely costly" (Whiteford and Branch 2008: 116)

Achieving a just, democratic, environmentally sustainable, and climate-safe world will not be easy, at either the individual or group levels, especially given the fate of earlier efforts to create more equitable and just systems (e.g., the Soviet Union and the People's Republic of China). The creation of an alternative world system will require a multifaceted effort drawing expertise and political will from many quarters, including not only mainstream political and economic institutions but also progressive social movements. Already many voices from many quarters are bucking the existing global political economic, including the anticorporate globalization or global justice, environmental, labor, indigenous and ethnic rights, peace, feminist, gay/lesbian rights, climate justice movements, and health movements. In many ways, the concerns of these various movements are not "single issues" but are intricately intertwined.

Recent years have seen the rise of the Arab Spring movement in the Middle East that began on December 18, 2010, and the Occupy Wall Street movement that began almost a year later and has spread to numerous developed societies, as well as developing societies. In terms of health issues per se, one finds organizing for health protection by sex workers in India, struggles for healthier foods, struggles against food rationing, and struggles around organ selling. As Phil Brown and colleagues (2010: 384) observe, *health social movements* "often involve citizen-science alliances in which activists collaborate with scientists and health professionals in pursuing treatment, prevention, research and expanded funding." AIDS activists, breast cancer activists, asthma activists, as well as other types of health activists have joined forces with epidemiologists, public health specialists, and medical social scientists, including medical anthropologists, on numerous occasions. Furthermore, ultimately, various other social movements, such as the social justice, environmental, climate, and indigenous rights movements, touch on health issues. In that climate change is having a profound impact on health, the climate movement plays a crucial role in drawing popular attention to the seriousness of anthropogenic climate change. Much of the climate movement in core countries, including the United States and Australia, has tended to stress climate change mitigation strategies that have come under the rubric of *ecological modernization*—that is, an emphasis on renewable sources of energy, energy efficiency, electric cars, and public transportation (Baer 2011). In contrast, the climate movement emanating from developing countries, such as India, South Africa, Bolivia, and the small Pacific Island states, has given much more attention to issues of social parity and to the fact that the core countries have historically contributed and continue to contribute much more on a per capita basis to greenhouse gas emissions than have or do the semiperipheral countries—even China, which has become the leading emitter in the world, and particularly peripheral countries. The Kimaforum that met outside of the UN Copenhagen climate change conference in December 2009 and the World People's Summit on Climate Change and the Rights of Mother Earth in Cochabamba, Bolivia, in March 2010, posited global capitalism as an economic system of production and consumption that seeks profits without limits and separates humans from nature. The latter assemblage, in particular, called for the development of an alternative world committed to social justice and environmental sustainability.

In 2000, the People's Health Movement was started by representatives from ninety-two countries at a meeting in Bangladesh. In July 2005, 1,492 people gathered at the Second People's Health Assembly in Cuenca, Ecuador, which in the Cuenca Declaration delimited the following aims and principles that have broad relevance for the building of a healthy world population (Association for Health and Environmental Development 2005):

- Solidarity with struggles in Ecuador
- Establish the right to health in an era of hegemonic globalization
- Promote health in an intercultural context
- Advance the right to health for all in the context of gender and personal diversity
- Protect the right to health in the context of environmental degradation
- Ensure workers' health and safety by defending and extending existing rights
- Defend the right to health in the face of war, militarization and violence
- Struggle for comprehensive primary health care and sustainable, quality, local and national health systems

The struggle for a healthy population around the world is intricately interwoven with many other struggles, including those for social equity and justice, environmental sustainability, a safe climate, access to clean water, public health, and the right to quality health care.

Bibliography

Abu-Lughod, Janet. 1994, ed. *From Urban Village to East Village: The Battle for New York's Lower East Side.* Cambridge, MA: Blackwell.

Ackerknecht, Erwin. 1971. *Medicine and Ethnology: Selected Essays.* Baltimore: Johns Hopkins University Press.

Action Hunger. 2007. "Interactions of: Malnutrition, Water Sanitation and Hygiene, Infections. Available at: http://www.actionagainsthunger.org.uk/fileadmin/contribution/0_accueil/pdf/Interactions%20of%20malnutrition,%20water%20sanitation%20and%20hygiene,%20infections%20-%20Version%202005%20-%20revised%202007.pdf. Accessed July 15, 2012.

Adams, Vicanne. 1998. "Suffering the Winds of Lhasa: Politicized Bodies, Human Rights, Cultural Difference, and Humanism in Tibet." *Medical Anthropology Quarterly* 12: 74–102.

Adler, Patricia. 1993. *Wheeling and Dealing: An Ethnography of an Upper-Level Drug Dealing and Smuggling Community.* New York: Columbia University Press.

Agar, Michael. 1973. *Ripping and Running: A Formal Ethnography of Urban Heroin Addiction.* New York: Seminar Press.

Agar, Michael. 1977. "Ethnography on the Street and in the Joint." In *Street Ethnography: Selected Studies of Crime and Drug Use in Natural Settings,* ed. R. S. Weppner, 143–156. Beverly Hills, CA: Sage.

Agar, Michael. 1996. *The Professional Stranger: An Informal Introduction to Ethnography,* 2nd ed. New York: Academic Press, 1996.

Alland, Alexander. 1970. *Adaptation in Cultural Evolution: An Approach to Medical Anthropology.* New York: Columbia University Press.

Allison, Ian, N. L. Bindoff, R. A. Bindschadler, P. M. Cox, N. de Noblet, M. H. England, et al. 2009. *The Copenhagen Diagnosis: Updating the World on the Latest Climate Science.* Sydney: Climate Change Research Centre, University of New South Wales.

Alster, Joseph S. 2005. "Ayurvedic Acupuncture—Transnational Nationalism: Ambivalence about the Origin and Authenticity of Medical Knowledge." In *Asian Medicine and Globalization,* ed. Joesph S. Alster, 21–44. Philadelphia: University of Pennsylvania Press.

Altman, Dennis. 2001. *Global Sex.* Chicago: University of Chicago Press.

Alvord, Katie. 2000. *Divorce Your Car: Ending the Love Affair with the Automobile.* Gabriola Island, Canada: New Society Publishers.

American Psychological Association. 2012. *Resilience in a Time of War: Warning Symptoms Checklist.* Washington, DC: American Psychological Association.

American Public Health Association. 2011. *Climate Change: Mastering the Public Health Role.* Washington, DC: American Public Health Association.

Ames, Genevieve M., Carol B. Cunradi, Roland S. Moore, and Pamela Stern. 2007. "Military Culture and Drinking Behavior among U.S. Navy Careerists." *Journal of Studies on Alcohol and Drugs* 68: 336–344.

Ames, Genevieve. 1985. "Middle-Class: Alcohol and the Family." In *The American Experience with Alcohol,* ed. Linda Bennett and Genevieve Ames, 435–458. New York: Plenum.

Amin, Samir. "Capitalism and the Ecological Footprint." *Monthly Review* 61. Available at: http://monthlyreview.org/2009/11/01/capitalism-and-the-ecological-footprint. Accessed February 15, 2013.

Amnesty International. 2010. *Deadly Delivery: The Maternal Health Crisis in the USA.* Available at: http://www.amnestyusa.org/sites/default/files/pdfs/deadlydelivery.pdf.

Anderson, A., Z. Qingsi, X. Hua, and B. Jianfeng. 2003. "China's Floating Population and the Potential for HIV Transmission: A Social-Behavioural Perspective." *AIDS Care* 15: 177–185.

Anderson, Nels. 1923. *The Hobo.* Chicago: University of Chicago Press.

Anderson, Sarah, and John Cavanaugh, with Thea Lee. 2005. *Field Guide to the Global Economy.* New York: Free Press.

Andrews, Charles. 1995. *Profit Fever: The Drive to Corporatize Health Care and How to Stop It.* Monroe, ME: Common Courage Press.

Anson, Ofra, and Shifang Sun. 2005. *Health Care in Rural China: Lessons from Hebei Province.* Aldershot, UK: Ashgate.

Appadurai, Arjun, ed. 2001. *Globalization.* Durham, NC: Duke University Press.

Archin, N., A. Liberty, A. Kashuba, S. Choudhary, J. Kuruc, J. Crooks, D. Parker. 2012. "Administration of Vorinostat Disrupts HIV-1 Latency in Patients on Antiretroviral Therapy." *Nature* 487: 482–485.

Aretxaga, Begona. 1997. *Shattering Silence: Women, Nationalism, and Political Subjectivity in Northern Ireland.* Princeton, NJ: Princeton University Press.

Arias, Enrique. 2006. *Drugs and Democracy in Rio de Janeiro.* Chapel Hill: University of North Carolina Press.

Arliss, Robert. 1997. *Against Death: The Practice of Living with AIDS.* Amsterdam: Gordon and Breach.

Armed Conflict Events Data. 2003. "Argentina's 'Dirty War' 1976–1983." Available at: http://www.onwar.com/aced/nation/all/argentina/fargentina1976.htm. Accessed January 14, 2009.

Armelagos, George J., and John R. Dewey. 1978. "Evolutionary Response to Human Infectious Diseases." In *Health and the Human Condition: Perspectives on Medical Anthropology,* eds. Michael H. Logan and Edward H. Hunt, Jr., 101–106. North Scituate, MA: Duxbury Press.

Armelagos, George J., and Kristen N. Harper. 2010. "Emerging Infectious Diseases, Urbanization, and Globalization in the Time of Global Warming." In *The New Blackwell Companion to Medical Sociology,* ed. William C. Cockerham, 291–311. Malden, MA: Wiley-Blackwell.

Armstrong, Pat, and Hugh Armstrong. 1996. *Wasting Away: The Undermining of Canadian Health Care.* New York: Oxford University Press.

Armstrong, Wilson. 2006. "Did the 'Brazilian' Kill the Pubic Louse?" *Sexually Transmitted Infections* 82: 265–266.

Arnold, David. 1993. "Medicine and Colonialism." In *Companion Encyclopedia of the History of Medicine,* Vol. 1, eds. W. F. Bynun and Roy Porter, 1393–1416. London: Routledge.

Aronowitz, Stanley. 1994. "The Situation of the Left in the United States." *Socialist Review* 23(3): 5–79.

Association for Health and Environmental Health. 2005. The Cuenca Declaration—People's Health Movement and People's Health Assembly 2, Cuenca, Ecuador.

Atkinson, Jane Monnig. 1992. "Shamanisms Today." *Annual Review of Anthropology* 21: 307–330.

Australian Academy of Sciences. 2010, August. "The Science of Climate Change: Questions and Answers." Canberra: Australian Academy of Sciences.

Australian Bureau of Meteorology. 2013. "Hottest Month on Record, Final Figures Highlight Climate Extremes." Significant Weather Media Release, February 1. Available at: http://www.bom.gov.au/climate. Accessed February 6, 2013.

Babb, Florence. 2011. *The Tourism Encounter: Fashioning Latin American Nations and Histories.* Stanford, CA: Stanford University Press.

Baer, Hans A. 1982. "On the Political Economy of Health." *Medical Anthropology Newsletter* 14: 1–2, 13–17.

Baer, Hans A. 1989. "The American Dominative Medical System as a Reflection of Social Relations in the Larger Society." *Social Science and Medicine* 28: 1103–1112.

Baer, Hans A., ed. 1996. "Critical Biocultural Approaches in Medical Anthropology: A Dialogue." Special issue of *Medical Anthropology Quarterly,* n.s. 10(4).

Baer, Hans A. 2001a. "Review of *Dying for Growth: Global Inequality and the Health of the Poor.*" *Medical Anthropology Quarterly* 15: 126–127.

Baer, Hans A. 2001b. *Biomedicine and Alternative Healing Systems in America: Issues of Class, Race, Ethnicity, and Gender.* Madison: University of Wisconsin Press.

Baer, Hans A. 2004. *Toward an Integrative Medicine: Alternative Therapies Encounter Biomedicine.* Walnut Creek, CA: AltaMira Press.

Baer, Hans A. 2009a. "A Field Report on the Critical Anthropology of Global Warming: A View from a Transplanted American Downunder." *Dialectical Anthropology* 33: 79–85.

Baer, Hans A. 2009b. *Complementary Medicine in Australia and New Zealand: Popularisation, Legitimation, and Dilemmas*. Maleny, Australia: Verdant House.

Baer, Hans. A. 2010. "The Impact of the War Machine on Global Warming and Health: A Political-Ecological Perspective. In *The War Machine and Global Health*, eds. Merrill Singer and G. Derrick Hodge, 157–178. Lanham, MA: AltaMira Press.

Baer, Hans A. 2011. "The International Climate Justice Movement: A Comparison with the Australian Climate Movement." *Australian Journal of Anthropology* 22: 256–260.

Baer, Hans A., and Merrill Singer. 2009. *Global Warming and the Political Ecology of Health: Emerging Crises and Systemic Solutions*. Walnut Creek, CA: Left Coast Press.

Baer, Hans A., Merrill Singer, and John Johnsen, eds. 1986. "Towards a Critical Medical Anthropology." Special issue of *Social Science and Medicine* 23(2).

Baer, Hans, Merrill Singer, and Ida Susser. 2004. *Medical Anthropology and the World System*. Westport, CT: Begin & Garvey.

Bailey, Robert, Stephen Moses, Corette B. Parker, Kawango Agot, Ian MacLean, John Krieger, et al. 2007. "Male Circumcision for HIV Prevention in Young Men in Kisumu, Kenya: A Randomised Controlled Trial." *The Lancet* 369: 643–656.

Balikci, A. 1963. "Shamanistic Behavior among the Netsilik Eskimos." *Southwestern Journal of Anthropology* 19: 380–396.

Balzer, Majorie Mandelstam. 1987. "Behind Shamanism: Changing Voices of Siberian Khanty Cosmology and Politics." *Social Science and Medicine* 12: 1085–1093.

Balzer, Majorie Mandelstam. 1991. "Doctors or Deceivers? The Siberian Khanty Shaman and Soviet Medicine." In *The Anthropology of Medicine: From Culture to Method*, 2nd ed., eds. Lola Romanucci-Ross, Daniel E. Moerman, and Laurence R. Tancredi, 56–80. New York: Bergin & Garvey.

Balzer, Majorie Mandelstam. 1993. "Two Urban Shamans: Unmasking Leadership in Fin-de-Soviet Siberia." In *Perilous States: Conversations on Culture, Politics, and Nation*, ed. George E. Marcus, 131–164. Chicago: University of Chicago Press.

Banerji, Debabar. 1984. "The Political Economy of Western Medicine in Third World Countries." In *Issues in the Political Economy of Health Care*, ed. John B. McKinlay, 257–282. New York: Tavistock.

Barbier, Edward B. 2010. *A Global Green Deal: Rethinking the Economic Recovery*. Cambridge, UK: Cambridge University Press.

Barker, David, and Clive Osmond. 1986. "Infant Mortality, Childhood Nutrition and Ischaemic Heart Disease in England and Wales." *The Lancet* 43: 1077–1081.

Barnes, E. 2005. *Disease and Human Evolution*. Albuquerque: University of New Mexico Press.

Barnet, Richard, and John Cavanagh. 1994. *Global Dreams: Imperial Corporations and the New World Order*. New York: Simon and Schuster.

Barrett, Ron. 2010. "Avian Influenza and the Third Epidemiological Transition." In *Plagues and Epidemics: Infected Spaces Past and Present*, eds. D. Ann Herring and Alan Swedlund, 81–94. Oxford: Berg.

Bartlett, John. 2007. "Tuberculosis and HIV Infections: Partners in Human Tragedy." *The Journal of Infectious Disease* 196(Suppl. 1): S124–S125.

Bastien, Joseph W. 1992. *Drum and Stethoscope: Integrating Ethnomedicine and Biomedicine in Bolivia*. Salt Lake City: University of Utah Press.

Batalla, G. 1966. "Conservative Thought in Applied Anthropology: A Critique." *Human Organization* 25: 89–92.

Bateson, Mary Catherine, and Richard Goldsby. 1988. *Thinking AIDS*. Reading, MA: Addison-Wesley.

Baxter, E., and Kim Hopper. 1981. *Public Places, Private Spaces*. New York: Community Service Society.

Behar, Ruth. 1996. "Introduction: Out of Exile." In *Women Writing Culture*, eds. Ruth Behar and Deborah Gordon, 1–33. Berkeley: University of California Press.

Bello, Walden. 2009. *The Food Wars*. London: Verso.

Belluck, Pam. 2012, October 15. "Hospitals Ditch Baby Formula to Promote Breast-feeding." *New York Times*, Science Section, 1.

Bennett, John. 1974. *The Ecological Transition: Cultural Anthropology and Human Adaptation*. New York: Pergamon Press.

Bennett, Linda. 2007. "Preparing Applied Anthropologists for the 21st Century." Consortium of Practicing and Applied Anthropology. Available at: http://www.copaa.info/resources_for_programs/preparing_applied_anthropologists.htm.

Bennett, Linda, and Cook, Paul. 1996. "Alcohol and Drug Studies." In *Handbook of Medical Anthropology: Contemporary Theory and Practice*, revised ed., eds. C. Sargent and T. Johnson, 235–251. Westport, CT: Greenwood Press.

Benson, Peter. 2012. *Tobacco Capitalism: Growers, Migrant Workers, and the Changing Face of a Global Industry*. Princeton, NJ: Princeton University Press.

Bentley, P. 2005. "Herbalists United to Defeat Government Aid." *Diversity* 2: 40–47.

Berger, John J. 2000. *Beating the Heat: Why and How We Must Combat Global Warming*. Berkeley, CA: Berkeley Hills Books.

Berkes, Fikret, and Dyanna Jolly. 2001. "Adapting to Climate Change: Social-Ecological Resilience in a Canadian Western Arctic Community. *Conservation Ecology* 5(2): 18. Available at: http://www.consecol.org/vol5/iss2/art18. Accessed May 22, 2011.

Berliner, Howard. 1982. "Medical Modes of Production." In *The Problem of Medical Knowledge: Examining the Social Construction of Medicine*, eds. Andrew Treacher and Peter Wright, 162–173. Edinburgh: Edinburgh University Press.

Bernard, Elaine. 1990. "The Politics of Canada's Health Care System: Lessons for the US." *Radical America* 24: 34–43.

Berndt, C. H. 1964. "The Role of Native Doctors in Aboriginal Australia." In *Magic, Faith and Healing*, ed. Ari Kiev, 264–282. New York: Free Press.

Bernstein, Jay H. 1997. *Spirits Captured in Stone: Shamanism & Traditional Medicine Among the Taman of Borneo*. Boulder, CO: Lynne Rienner.

Biehl, Joao. 2005. *Vita*. Berkeley: University of California Press.

Birenbaum, Arnold. 1995. *Putting Health Care on the National Agenda*, revised ed. Westport, CT: Praeger.

Black, Peter. 1984. "The Anthropology of Tobacco Use: Tobian Data and Theoretical Issues." *Journal of Anthropological Research* 40: 475–503.

Black, William R. 2007. "Sustainable Solutions for Freight Transfer." In *Globalized Freight Transport*, eds. T. R. Leinbach and C. Capineri, 189–216. Aldershot, UK: Edward Elgar.

Blain, Jenny, and Robert J. Wallis. 2000. "The Ergi Seidman: Contestations of Gender, Shamanism and Sexuality in Northern Religion Past and Present." *Journal of Contemporary Religion* 15: 395–411.

Bluthenthal, Ricky, and Watters, John. 1995. "Multimethod Research from Targeted Sampling to HIV Risk Environments." In *Qualitative Methods in Drug Abuse and HIV Research*, eds. E. Lambert, R. S. Ashery, and R. H. Needle (NIDA Research Monograph #157; NIH Pub. No. 95-4025), 212–230. Washington, DC: U.S. Govt. Printing Office.

Bodenheimer, Tom. 1993. "Health Care Reform in the 1990s and Beyond." *Socialist Review* 23: 13–29.

Bodley, John H. 1975. *Victims of Progress*. Menlo Park, CA: Benjamin/Cummings.

Bodley, John H. 1985. *Anthropology and Contemporary Human Problems*, 2nd ed. Palo Alto, CA: Mayfield.

Bodley, John H. 1994. *Cultural Anthropology: Tribes, States, and the Global System*. Mountain View, CA: Mayfield.

Bodley, John H. 1996. *Anthropology and Contemporary Human Problems*, 3rd ed. Mountain View, CA: Mayfield.

Bodley, John H. 2008a. *Anthropology and Contemporary Human Problems*, 5th ed. Walnut Creek, CA: AltaMira Press.

Bodley, John. 2008b. *Victims of Progress*. Lanham, MD: AltaMira Press.

Boehm, C. 1999. *Hierarchy in the Forest: The Evolution of Egalitarian Behavior*. Cambridge, MA: Harvard University Press.

Boggs, Carl. 1995. *The Socialist Tradition: From Crisis to Decline*. New York: Routledge.

Bolough, Roslyn W. 1981. "Grounding the Alienation of Self and Body: A Critical, Phenomenological Analysis of the Patient in Western Medicine." *Sociology of Health and Illness* 3: 188–206.

Bolton, Ralph. 1992. "Mapping Terra Incognita: Sex Research for AIDS Prevention—An Urgent Agenda for the 1990s." In *The Time of AIDS*, eds. Gilbert Herdt and Shirley Lindenbaum, 124–158. Newbury Park, CA: Sage.

Bolton, Ralph, and Gail Orozco. 1994. *The AIDS Bibliography: Studies in Anthropology and Related Fields*. Arlington, VA: American Anthropological Association.

Bongaarts John, Priscilla Reining, Peter Way, and Francis Conant. 1989. "The Relationship Between Male Circumcision and HIV Infection in African Populations." *AIDS* 3: 373–377.

Bonta, Bruce. 1996. "Conflict Resolution among Peaceful Societies: The Culture of Peacefulness." *Journal of Peace Research* 33: 403–420.

Bordo, Susan. 1999. "Feminism, Foucault and the Politics of the Body." In *Feminist Theory and the Body: A Reader*, eds. Janet Price and Margrit Shildrick, 246–257. London: Routledge.

Boswell, Terry, and Christopher Chase-Dunn. 2000. *The Spiral of Capitalism and Socialism*. Boulder, CO: Lynne Rienner.

Bourdieu, Pierre. 1984. *Distinction: A Social Critique of the Judgment of Taste* (Richard Nice, trans). Cambridge, MA: Harvard University Press.

Bourgois, Philippe. 2003. *In Search of Research: Selling Crack in El Barrio,* 2nd ed. Cambridge, UK: Cambridge University Press.

Bourgois, Philippe, and Jeff Schonberg. 2009. *Righteous Dopefiends.* Berkeley: University of California Press.

Bowie, Fiona. 2000. *The Anthropology of Religion: An Introduction.* Oxford, UK: Blackwell.

Boyd, Cynthia, Jonathan Darer, Chad Boult, Linda Fried, Lisa Boult, and Albert Wu. 2007. "Clinical Practice Guidelines and Quality of Care for Older Patients with Multiple Comorbid Diseases: Implications for Pay for Performance." *Journal of the American Medical Association* 294: 716–724.

Bradley, D. 1993. "Environment and Health Problems of Developing Countries." In *Environmental Change and Human Health,* 234–246 (Ciba Foundation Symposium 175). Chichester, UK: CIBA Foundation.

Brandt, T. 1989. "AIDS in Historical Perspective: Four Lessons from the History of Sexually Transmitted Disease." *American Journal of Public Health* 78: 367–371.

Brodwin, Paul. 1996. *Medicine and Modality in Haiti: The Contest for Healing Power.* Cambridge, UK: Cambridge University Press.

Brouwer, Steve. 2011. *Revolutionary Doctors: How Venezuela and Cuba Are Changing the World's Conception of Health Care.* New York: Monthly Review Press.

Brown, E. Richard. 1979. *Rockefeller Medicine Men: Medicine and Capitalism in America.* Berkeley: University of California Press.

Brown, Marilyn A., and Benjamin K. Sovacool. 2011. *Climate Change and Global Energy Security.* Cambridge, MA: MIT Press.

Brown, Peter J. 1987. "Microparasites and Macroparasites." *Cultural Anthropology* 2: 155–171.

Brown, Peter J., and Marcia C. Inhorn. 1990. "Disease, Ecology, and Human Behavior." In *Medical Anthropology: Contemporary Theory and Method,* eds. Thomas M. Johnson and Carolyn Sargent, 187–214. New York: Praeger.

Brown, Phil, Crystal Adams, Rachel Morello-Frosch, Laura Senier, and Ruth Simpson. 2010. "Health Social Movement: History, Current Work, and Future Directions." In *Handbook of Medical Sociology,* 6th ed., eds. Chloe E. Bird, Peter Conrad, Allen M. Fremont, and Stefan Timmermans, 380–394. Nashville, TN: Vanderbilt University Press.

Browner, Carole. 2001. "The Politics of Reproduction in a Mexican Village." In *Gender in Cross Cultural Perspective,* eds. Caroline Brettell and Carolyn Sargent, 460–470. Upper Saddle River, NJ: Prentice-Hall.

Buchanan, David, Merrill Singer, Susan Shaw, Wei Teng, Tom Stopka, Kaveh Khoshnood, and Robert Heimer. 2004. "Syringe Access, HIV Risk, and AIDS in Massachusetts and Connecticut: The Health Implications of Public Policy." In *Unhealthy Health Policy: A Critical Anthropological Examination,* eds. Arachu Castro and Merrill Singer, 275–285. Walnut Creek, CA: AltaMira Press.

Budrys, Grace. 2003. *Unequal Health: How Inequality Contributes to Health and Illness.* Lanham, MD: Rowman & Littlefield.

Bulled, Nicola, and Singer, Merrill. 2011. "Syringe-Mediated Syndemics." *AIDS and Behavior* 15: 1539–1545.

Burman, Stephen. 2007. *The State of the American Empire: How the USA Shapes the World*. London: Earthscan.

Butler, Barbara. 2006. *Holy Intoxication to Drunken Dissipation: Alcohol among Quichua Speakers in Otavalo, Ecuador*. Albuquerque: University of New Mexico Press.

Byg, Anja, Jan Salick, and Wayne Law. 2010. "Medicinal Plant Knowledge among Lay People in Five Eastern Tibet Villages." *Human Ecology* 38: 177–191.

Cabrol, Jean-Clement. 2011. "War, Drought, Malnutrition, Measles—A Report from Somalia." *New England Journal of Medicine* 365: 1856–1858.

Camilleri, Joseph A., and Jim Falk. 2010. *Worlds in Transition: Evolving Governance across a Stressed Planet*. Cheltenham, UK: Edward Elgar.

Campbell, Catherine. 2003. *Letting Them Die: How HIV/AIDS Prevention Programmes Often Fail*. Oxford/Cape Town: The International African Institute.

Canham-Clyde, John. 1994. "When 'Both Sides' Are Not Enough: The Restricted Debate over Health Care Reform." *International Journal of Health Services* 24: 415–419.

Cantor, N. 2002. *In the Wake of the Plague: The Black Death and the World It Made*. New York: Harper Perennial.

Capra, Fritjof. 1984. *The Tao of Physics*. Toronto: Bantam Books.

Carlson, Robert, Merrill, Singer, Richard Stephens, and Claire Sterk. 2009. "Reflections on 40 Years of Ethnographic Drug Abuse Research: Implications for the Future." *Journal of Drug Issues* 39: 57–70.

Carrera, Percivil, and John F. P. Bridges. 2006. "Globalization and Healthcare: Understanding Health and Medical Tourism." *Expert Review in Pharmacoeconomic Outcomes Research* 64: 447–454.

Cassell, Joan. 1998. *The Woman in the Surgeon's Body*. Cambridge, MA: Harvard University Press.

Cassidy, Claire. 1991. "The Good Body: When Big Is Better." *Medical Anthropology* 13: 181–214.

Castells, Manuel. 1975. "Immigrant Workers and Class Struggles in Advanced Capitalism: The Western European Experience." *Politics and Society* 5: 33–66.

Castells, Manuel. 2002. *The Castells Reader on Cities and Social Theory*, ed. I. Susser. Malden, MA: Blackwell.

Castro, Arachu, and Farmer, Paul. 2005. "Understanding and Addressing AIDS-Related Stigma: From Anthropological Theory to Clinical Practice in Haiti." *American Journal of Public Health* 951: 53–59.

Castro, Arachu, and Merrill Singer, eds. 2004. *Unhealthy Health Policy: A Critical Anthropological Examination*. Walnut Creek, CA: Altamira Press.

Caudill, William. 1953. "Applied Anthropology in Medicine." In *Anthropology Today*, ed. Alfred L. Kroeber, 771–806. Chicago: University of Chicago Press.

Cavan, Sherri. 1966. *Liquor License: An Ethnography of Bar Behavior*. Chicago: Aldine.

Cawte, J. 1974. *Medicine in the Law: Studies in Psychiatric Anthropology of Australian Tribal Societies*. Honolulu: University of Hawaii Press.

Centers for Disease Control and Prevention. 2000. "HIV-Related Knowledge and Stigma." *Morbidity and Mortality Weekly Report* 49: 1062.

Centers for Disease Control and Prevention. 2008. ATSDR Studies on Chemical Releases in the Great Lakes Region. Agency for Toxic Substances and Disease Registry. Available at: http://www.atsdr.cdc.gov/grtlakes/pdfs/2008/final/TOC_GreatLakesAOCFinal.pdf. Accessed February 15, 2013.

Chadee, D., S. Rawlins, and T. Tiwari. 2003. "Concomitant Malaria and Filariasis Infections in Georgetown, Guyana." *Tropical Medicine and International Health* 8: 140–143.

Chadwick, Douglas. 2003. Pacific suite. *National Geographic* 203(2): 104–127.

Chae, Suhong. 2003. "Contemporary Ho Chi Minh City in Numerous Contradictions: Reform Policy, Foreign Capital and the Working Class." In *Wounded Cities: Destruction and Reconstruction in a Globalized World*, eds. Jane Schneider and Ida Susser, 227–251. New York: Berg.

Chafe, Zoe. 2008. "Air Travel Reaches New Heights." In *Vital Signs 2007–2008: The Trends That Are Shaping Our Future*, ed. Linda Starke, 70–71. New York: W. W. Norton.

Changchui, He. 2012. "Why Another Hunger Summit?" Food and Agricultural Organization of the United Nations. Available at: http://www.fao.org/asiapacific/rap/home/about-assistant-director-gen/speeches/detail/en/?speech_id=4. Accessed July 19, 2012.

Chapin, Georganne, and Robert Wasserstrom. 1981. "Agricultural Production and Malaria Resurgence in Central America and India." *Nature* 293: 181–185.

Chernomas, Robert, and Ardeshir Sepehri. 1998. "Introduction." In *How to Choose: A Comparison of the U.S. and Canadian Health Care Systems*, eds. Robert Chernomas and Ardeshir Sepehri, 1–5. Amityville, NY: Baywood.

Chivers, Danny. 2009. "Climate Choices." In *People First Economics*, eds. David Ransom and Vanessa Baird, 193–209. Oxford, UK: World Changing.

Choi, A., R. Rodriquez, P. Bacchetti, D. Berenthal, P. Volberding, and A. O'Hare. 2007. "Racial Differences in End-Stage Renal Disease in HIV Infection Versus Diabetes." *Journal of the American Society of Nephrology* 18: 2968–2974.

Chopp, R. 1986. *The Praxis of Suffering*. Maryknoll, NY: Orbis.

Chrisman, Noel J., and Arthur Kleinman. 1983. "Popular Health Care, Social Networks, and Cultural Meanings: The Orientation of Medical Anthropology." In *Handbook of Health, Health Care, and the Health Professions*, ed. David Mechanic, 569–590. New York: Free Press.

Churchill, Larry R. 1987. *Rationing Health Care in America: Perceptions and Principles in Justice*. South Bend, IN: University of Norte Dame Press.

Clair, Scott, Merrill Singer, Francisco Bastos, Monica Malta, Claudia Santelices, and Naline Ebertoni. 2009. "The Role of Drug Users in the Brazilian HIV/AIDS Epidemic: Patterns, Perceptions and Prevention." In *Globalization of HIV/AIDS: An Interdisciplinary Reader*, eds. Cynthia Pope, Renée White, and Robert Malow, 50–58. New York: Routledge.

Clair, Scott, Merrill Singer, Elsa Huertas, and Margaret Weeks. 2003. "Unintended Consequences of Using an Oral HIV Test on HIV Knowledge." *AIDS Care* 15: 575–580.

Clark, Brett, and Richard York. 2005. "Carbon Metabolism: Global Capitalism, Climate Change, and Biospheric Rift." *Theory and Society* 34: 391–428.

Cleaver, Harry. 1977. "Malaria and the Political Economy of Health." *International Journal of Health Services* 7: 557–579.

Clements, Forrest. 1932. "Primitive Concepts of Disease." *University of California Publications in American Archaeology and Ethnology* 32: 185–252.

Closser, Svea. 2010. "Chasing Polio." *Anthropology Now* 2(4): 32–39

Coalition for the Homeless. 2010 http://www.coalitionforthehomeless.org/page/-/HUD%20CoC%20report%20–%20NYC%202010.pdf.

Cobb, Kurt. 2006. "Will Global Warming Create Any Winners?" *Resource Insight*. Available at: http://resource insights.blogspot.com/2006/02/will-global-warming-create-any-winners.html. Accessed July 9, 2012.

Coburn, David. 1999. "Phases of Capitalism, Welfare States, Medical Dominance, and Health in Ontario." *International Journal of Health Services* 29: 833–851.

Cohen, Mark Nathan. 1984. "An Introduction to the Symposium." In *Paleopathology at the Origins of Agriculture*, eds. Mark Nathan Cohen and George Armelagos, 1–7. New York: Academic Press.

Cohen, Mark Nathan. 1989. *Health and the Rise of Civilization*. New Haven, CT: Yale University Press.

Cohen, Robin, and Paul Kennedy. 2000. *Global Sociology*. New York: New York University Press.

Collier, Jane, and Sylvia Yanagisako, eds. 1987. *Gender and Kinship: Essays toward a Unified Analysis*. Stanford: Stanford University Press.

Comaroff, Jean. 1982. "Medicine, Symbol and Ideology." In *The Problem of Medical Knowledge: Examining the Social Construction of Medicine*, eds. Peter Wright and Andrew Treacher, 49–68. Edinburgh: University of Edinburgh Press.

Comaroff, Jean. 1993. "The Diseased Heart of Africa: Medicine, Colonialism, and the Black Body." In *Knowledge, Power & Practice: The Anthropology of Medicine and Everyday Life* (Comparative Studies of Health Systems and Medical Care), ed. Shirley Lindenbaum and Margaret Lock, 305–329. Berkeley: University of California Press.

Commoner, Barry. 1990. *Making Peace with the Planet*. New York: Pantheon Books.

Conover, S., A. Berkman, A. Gheith, R. Jahiel, D. Stanley, P. Geller, E. Valencia, and E. Susser. 1997. "Methods for Successful Follow-Up of Elusive Urban Population: An Ethnographic Approach with Homeless Men." *Bulletin of the New York Academy of Medicine* 74: 90–108.

Conrad, Peter. 1997. "Parallel Play in Medical Anthropology and Medical Sociology." *American Sociologist* 28: 90–100.

Convisier, Richard and Rutledge, John. 1989. "Can Public Policies Limit the Spread of HIV among IV Drug Users?" *Journal of Drug Issues* 19:113–128.

Coreil, Jeannine. 1990. "The Evolution of Anthropology in International Health." In *Anthropology and Primary Health Care*, eds. Jeannine Coreil and J. Dennis Mull, 3–27. Boulder, CO: Westview Press.

Counihan, C. 1990. *Food Rules, Gender Morality in the United States*. Presented at the Annual Meeting of the American Anthropological Association, New Orleans, LA.

Court, Jamie, and Francis Smith. 1999. *Making a Killing: HMOs and the Threat to Your Health*. Monroe, ME: Common Courage Press.

Courtwright, David. 1991. *Forces of Habit: Drugs and the Making of the Modern World*. Cambridge, MA: Harvard University Press.

Cowie, Jonathan. 1998. *Climate Change and Human Change: Disaster or Opportunity?* London: Parthenon.

Crellin, J. K., R. R. Anderson, and J. T. H. Connor, eds. 1997. *Alternative Health Care in Canada: Nineteenth- and Twentieth-Century Perspectives.* Toronto: Canadian Scholars' Press.

Crimp, Douglas. 1988. "How to Have Promiscuity in an Epidemic." In *AIDS: Cultural Analysis, Cultural Activism,* ed. Douglas Crimp, 237–271. Cambridge, MA: MIT Press.

Csorda, Thomas J., ed. 1994. *Embodiment and Experience: The Existential Ground of Culture and Self.* Cambridge, UK: Cambridge University Press

Currie, C., S. Gabhainn, E. Godeaum, C. Roberts, R. Smith, and D. Currie. 2008. *Inequalities in Young People's Health: HBSC International Report from the 2005/2006 Survey.* Copenhagen: WHO Regional Office for Europe.

Cushman, John. 1998. "Industrial Group Plans to Battle Climate Treat." *The New York Times.* Available at: http://www.nytimes.com/1998/04/26/us/industrial-group-plans-to-battle-climate-treaty.html?pagewanted=all&src=pm. Accessed July 19, 2012.

Dahlstrom, Matthew D. 2012. "Winter Texans and the Re-creation of the American Medical Experience in Mexico." *Medical Anthropology* 31: 162–177.

D'Andrade, Roy. 1995. "Moral Models in Anthropology." *Current Anthropology* 36: 399–408.

Das, Veena, 1995. "National Honor and Practical Kinship: Unwanted Women and Children." In *Conceiving the New World Order: The Global Politics of Reproduction,* eds. R. Rapp and F. Ginsburg, 212–234. Berkeley: University of California Press.

Das, Veena. 2008. "Violence, Gender, and Subjectivity." *Annual Review of Anthropology* 37: 283–299.

Dauvergne, Peter. 2005. "Dying of Consumption: Accidents or Sacrifice of Global Mortality?" *Global Environmental Politics* 5: 35–47.

Dauvergne, Peter, and Jane Lister. 2011. *Timber.* London: Polity.

Davies, Catriona. 2010. "Inuit Lives and Diets Change as Ice Shifts." CNN, December 30. Available at: http://edition.cnn.com/2010/WORLD/americas/12/30/inuit.impact.climate.change/index.html?hpt=C2. Accessed May 20, 2011.

Davis, Dana-Ain. 2006. *Battered Black Women and Welfare Reform: Between a Rock and a Hard Place.* Albany: State University of New York Press.

Davis, Mike. 2007. *Planet of the Slums.* New York: Verso.

Davis-Floyd, Robbie. 2001. "Gender and Ritual: Giving Birth the American Way." In *Gender in Cross-Cultural Perspective,* eds. Caroline Brettel and Carolyn Sargent, 447–460. Upper Saddle River, NJ: Prentice-Hall.

Dawson, Susan. 1992. "Navajo Uranium Mining Workers and the Effects of Occupational Illness: A Case Study." *Human Organization* 51: 389–397.

De Maio, Fernando. 2010. *Health and Social Theory.* New York: Palgrave Macmillan.

De Vos, Pol. 2005. "'No One Left Abandoned': Cuba's National Health System since the 1959 Revolution." *International Journal of Health Services* 35: 189–207.

Dehavenon, Anna Lou, ed. 1996. *There's No Place Like Home: Anthropological Perspectives on Housing and Homelessness in the United States*. Westport, CT: Bergin & Garvey.

Deleuze, Gilles. 2007. *Two Regimes of Madness, Revised Edition: Texts and Interviews 1975–1995*. Cambridge, MA: MIT Press

Dell'Amore, Christine. 2009, August 16. "Cocaine on Money: Drug Found on 90% of U.S. Bills." *National Geographic News*. Available at: http://news.nationalgeographic.com/news/2009/08/090816-cocaine-money.html. Accessed February 5, 2013.

Dentan, Robert Knox. 1968. *The Semai: A Nonviolent People of Malaya*. New York: Holt, Rinehart and Winston.

Dentan, Robert Knox. 2008. *Overwhelming Terror: Love, Fear, Peace, and Violence among Semai of Malaysia*. Lanham, MA: Rowman and Littlefield.

Department of Health and Human Services. Undated. "The Great Pandemic." Available at: http://www.flu.gov/pandemic/history/1918/index.html. Accessed July 15, 2012.

Derber, Charles. 1983. "Sponsorship and the Control of Physicians." *Theory and Society* 12: 561–601.

Devereux, George. 1956. "Normal and Abnormal: The Key Problem in Psychiatric Anthropology." In *Some Uses of Anthropology: Theoretical and Applied*, eds. Joseph B. Casagrande and Thomas Gladwin, 3–48. Washington, DC: Anthropological Society of Washington.

Devereux, George. 1957. "Dream Learning and Individual Ritual Differences in Mohave Shamanism." *American Anthropologist* 59: 10–36.

Devine, Richard J. 1996. *Good Care, Painful Choices: Medical Ethics for Ordinary People*. Malwah, NJ: Paulist Press.

Devisch, Renaat. 1986. "Belgium." *Medical Anthropology Quarterly*, o.s., 17(4): 87–89.

DeWall, C. Nathan, and Craig A. Anderson. 2011. "The General Aggression Model." In *Human Aggression and Violence: Causes, Manifestations, and Consequences*, eds. P. Shaver and M. Mikulincer, 15–33. Washington, DC: American Psychological Association.

DeWitte, S., and Wood, J. 2008. "Selectivity of Black Death Mortality with Respect to Preexisting Health." *Proceedings of the National Academy of Sciences of the United States of America* 105: 1436–1441.

Di Giacomo, Susan. 1999. "Can There Be a 'Cultural Epidemiology?'" *Medical Anthropology Quarterly* 13: 436–457.

Di Leonardo, Micaela. 1998. *Exotics at Home*. Chicago: University of Chicago Press.

Diamond, Jared. 2005. *Collapse: How Societies Choose to Fail or Succeed*. London: Penguin.

Diamond, Stanley. 1974. *In Search of the Primitive: A Critique of Civilization*. New Brunswick, NJ: Transaction.

Dicken, Peter. 2003. *Global Shift: Reshaping the Global Economic Map in the 21st Century*, 4th ed. New York: Guildford Press.

Dockery, Douglas, Arden Pope, Xiping Xu, John Spengler, James Ware, Martha Fay, Benjamin Ferris, and Frank Speizer. 1993. "An Association between Air Pollution and Mortality in Six U.S. Cities." *New England Journal of Medicine* 329: 1753–1759.

dos Anjos, Marcio Fabri. 1996. "Medical Ethics in the Developing World: A Liberation Theology Perspective." *Journal of Medicine and Philosophy* 21: 629–637.

Dow, James. 1986. "Universal Aspects of Symbolic Healing: A Theoretical Analysis." *American Anthropologist* 88: 56–69.

Doyal, Lesley (with Imogen Pennell). 1979. *The Political Economy of Health*. Boston: South End Press.

Drake, Frances. 2000. *Global Warming: The Science of Climate Change*. London: Arnold.

Draper, Patricia. 1975. "!Kung Women: Contrasts in Sexual Egalitarianism in the Foraging and Sedentary Contexts." In *Toward an Anthropology of Women*, ed. Rayna Rapp Reiter, 77–109. New York: Monthly Review Press.

Driver, Harold. 1969. *Indians of North America*. Chicago: University of Chicago Press.

Dudley, Robert. 2002. "Fermenting Fruit and the Historical Ecology of Ethanol Ingestion: Is Alcoholism in Modern Humans an Evolutionary Hangover?" *Addiction* 97: 381–388.

Dunbar, Sally. 2007. "Malnutrition and Anaemia among Somali Refugee Children in Long Term Camps." *Disasters* 8: 174–177.

Duncan, R. Paul, Michael E. Morris, and Linda A. McCarey. 2010. "Canada." In *Comparative Health Systems: Global Perspectives*, eds. James A. Johnson and Carleen, 59–82. Boston: Jones and Bartlett.

Dunn, Frederick. 1976. "Traditional Asian Medicine and Cosmopolitan Medicine as Adaptive Systems." In *Asian Medical Systems: A Comparative Study*, ed. Charles Leslie, 133–158. Berkeley: University of California Press.

Dunn, Frederick. 1977. "Health and Disease in Hunter-Gatherers: Epidemiological Factors." In *Culture, Disease, and Healing: Studies in Medical Anthropology*, ed. David, Landy, 99–107. New York: Macmillan.

Eastwood, Heather. 1997. "General Medical Practice: Alternative Medicine, and the Globalization of Health." PhD thesis, University of Queensland.

Eaton, S. Boyd, Marjorie Shostak, and Melvin Konner. 1988. *The Paleolithic Prescription: A Program of Diet and Exercise and a Design for Living*. New York: Harper and Row.

Eckert, Penelope. 1983. "Beyond the Statistics of Adolescent Smoking." *American Journal of Public Health* 73: 439–441.

Edelman, Marc. 2012. "One Third of Humanity: Peasant Rights in the United Nations." OpenDemocracy. Available at: http://www.opendemocracy.net/marc-edelman/one-third-of-humanity-peasant-rights-in-united-nations. Accessed January 27, 2013.

Edelman, Marc, and Angelique Haugerud, eds. 2005. *The Anthropology of Development and Globalization: From Classical Political Economy to Contemporary Neoliberalism*. London: Blackwell

Egwunyeng, A., J. Ajayi, O. Nmorsi, and D. Duhlinska-Popova. 2001. "Plasmodium/Intestinal Helminth Co-infections among Pregnant Nigerian Women." *Memó rias do Instituto Oswaldo Cruz* 96: 1055–1059.

Eichler, Alexander. 2012. "Mexican Drug Cartel Laundered Money through BofA, FBI Alleges." The Huffington Post. Available at: http://www.huffingtonpost.com/2012/07/09/los-zetas-laundered-money-bank-america_n_1658943.html. Accessed August 6, 2012.

Eliade, Mircea. 1964. *Shamanism: Archaic Techniques of Ecstasy*. New York: Pantheon Books.

Elling, Ray H. 1980. *Cross National Study of Health Systems*. New Brunswick, NJ: Transaction.

Elling, Ray H. 1981a. "The Capitalist World-System and International Health." *International Journal of Health Services* 11: 25–51.

Elling, Ray H. 1981b. "Political Economy, Cultural Hegemony, and Mixes of Traditional and Modern Medicine." *Social Science and Medicine* 15A: 89–99.

Engels, Friedrich. 1969 (originally published 1845). *The Condition of the Working Class in England*. London: Grenada.

Environmental Defense Fund. 2007. *Cars by the Numbers: Statistics on Automobiles and Their Global Warming Contribution*. Available at: www/edf/org. Accessed May 9, 2008.

Environmental Protection Agency. 2000. "Liquid Assets 2000: Americans Pay for Dirty Waste." Available at: http://water.epa.gov/lawsregs/lawsguidance/cwa/economics/liquidassets/dirtywater.cfm. Accessed July 20, 2012.

Environmental Protection Agency. 2012. *Water Resources and Adaptation: Climate Impacts on Water Resources*. Available online at: http://www.epa.gov/climatechange/impacts-adaptation/water.html#impacts. Accessed July 19, 2012.

Epstein, Paul R. 2002. "Climate Change and Infectious Disease: Stormy Weather Ahead. *Epidemiology* 13: 373–375.

Epstein, Paul R. 2005. "Climate Change and Public Health." *New England Journal of Medicine* 353: 1433–1436.

Epstein, Paul R., and Christine Rogers. 2004. *Inside the Greenhouse: The Impacts of CO_2 and Climate Change on Public Health in the Inner City*. Boston: The Center for Health and the Global Environment.

Ericksen, Michael, Judith Makay, and Hana Ross. 2012. *The Tobacco Atlas*, 4th ed. New York City: World Lung Foundation and American Cancer Foundation.

Erickson, Pamela. 2008. *Ethnomedicine*. Long Grove, IL: Waveland Press.

Erwin, Deborah Oates. 1987. "The Military Medicalization of Cancer Treatment." In *Encounters with Biomedicine: Case Studies in Medical Anthropology*, ed. Hans A. Baer, 201–227. New York: Gordon and Breach.

Escobar, Arturo. 1998. "Whose Knowledge, Whose Nature? Biodiversity, Conservation, and the Political Ecology of Social Movements." *Journal of Political Ecology* 5: 53–82.

Escobar, J., E. Randolph, G. Puente, F. Spiwak, J. Asamen, M. Hill, and R. Hough. 1983. "Post-traumatic Stress Disorder in Hispanic Vietnam Veterans: Clinical Phenomenology and Sociocultural Characteristics." *Journal of Nervous & Mental Disease* 171: 585–596.

Estroff, Sue. 1993. "Identity, Disability and Schizophrenia: The Problem of Chronicity." In *Knowledge, Power and Practice: The Anthropology of Medicine in Everyday Life*, eds. Shirley Lindenbaum and Margaret Lock, 247–286. Berkeley: University of California Press.

Etienne, Mona. 2001. "The Case for Social Modernity: Adoption of Children by Urban Baule Women," *Gender in Cross-cultural Perspective*, eds. Caroline Brettel and Carolyn Sargent, 32–38. Upper Saddle River, NJ: Prentice-Hall.

Evans-Pritchard, E. E. 1937. *Witchcraft, Oracles and Magic among the Azande*. Oxford, UK: Oxford University Press.

Evans-Pritchard, E. E. 1940. *The Nuer: A Description of the Modes of Livelihood and Political Institutions of Nilotic Peoples*. Oxford, UK: Clarendon Press.

Everett, Margaret. 2009. "Diabetes among Oaxaca's Transnational Indigenous Population: An Emerging Syndemic." Presented at the 2009 Congress of the Latin American Studies Association, Rio de Janeiro, Brazil June 11–14, 2009. Available at: http://lasa.international.pitt.edu/members/congress-papers/lasa2009/files/EverettMargaret.pdf.

Fabrega, Horacio. 1997. *Evolution of Sickness and Healing*. Berkeley: University of California Press.

Fagan, Brian. 2008. *The Great Warming: Climate Change and the Rise and Fall of Civilizations*. Cambridge, UK: Cambridge University Press.

Fainstein, Susan. 2001. *Property Development in New York and London, 1980–2000*, 2nd ed., revised. Lawrence: University of Kansas.

Farley, John W. 2008. "The Scientific Case for Modern Anthropogenic Global Warming." *Monthly Review* (July–August): 68–90.

Farmer, Paul. 1992. *AIDS and Accusation: Haiti and the Geography of Blame*. Berkeley: University of California Press.

Farmer, Paul. 1997. "AIDS and Anthropologists: Ten Years Later." *Medical Anthropology Quarterly* 11: 516–525.

Farmer, Paul. 1999. *Infections and Inequalities: The Modern Plagues*. Berkeley: University of California Press.

Farmer, Paul. 2003. *Pathologies of Power: Health, Human Rights, and the New War on the Poor*. Berkeley: University of California Press.

Farmer, Paul. 2009a. "'Landmine Boy' and the Tomorrow of Violence." In *Global Health in Times of Violence*, eds. Barbara Rylko-Bauer, Linda Whiteford, and Paul Farmer, 41–62. Santa Fe, NM: School of Advanced Research.

Farmer, Paul. 2009b. On Suffering and Structural Violence: A View from Below. *Race/Ethnicity. Multidisciplinary Global Perspectives* 3(1): 11–28.

Farmer, Paul. 2011. *Haiti after the Earthquake*. Jackson, TN: PublicAffairs.

Farmer, Paul, Margaret Connors, and Janie Simmons, eds. 1996. *Women, Poverty, and AIDS: Sex, Drugs and Structural Violence*. Monroe, ME: Common Courage Press.

Farmer, Paul, and John Gershman. 2012. "Jim Kim's Humility Would Serve World Bank Well." *Washington Post*, April 11. Available at http://articles.washingtonpost.com/2012-04-11/opinions/35451736_1_inclusive-growth-jim-yong-kim-world-development-report.

Farquhar, Judith. 1994. *Knowing Practic: The Clinical Encounter of Chinese Medicine*. Boulder, CO: Westview Press.

Fauci, Anthony. 2012. *Ending the HIV/AIDS Pandemic: From Scientific Advances to Public Health Implementation*. Presented at the XIX International AIDS Confections, Washington, DC.

Fee, Elizabeth, and Donald Fox. 1992. "Introduction: The Contemporary Historiography of AIDS." In *AIDS: The Making of a Chronic Disease*, eds. Elizabeth Fee and Donald Fox, 1–19. Berkeley: University of California Press.

Feinstein, A. 1970. "Pre-therapeutic Classification of Co-morbidity in Chronic Disease." *Journal Chronic Disease* 23: 455–468.

Feldman, Douglas. 1986. "Anthropology, AIDS, and Africa." *Medical Antrhopology Quarterly* 17: 38–40.

Feldman, S. 2008. "Why Overfishing = Global Warming." *Solve Climate*. Available at: http://solveclimate.com/blog/20080115/why-overfishing-global-warming. Accessed March 28, 2010.

Femia, Joseph. 1975. "Hegemony and Consciousness in the Thought of Antonio Gramsci." *Political Studies* 23: 29–48.

Ferzacca, Steve. 2001. *Healing the Modern in a Central Javanese City*. Durham, NC: Academic Press.

Feshbach, Murray, and Alfred Friendly, Jr. 1992. *Ecocide in the USSR: Health and Nature under Siege*. New York: Basic Books.

Fine, Michelle, and Jessica Ruglis. 2009. "Circuits and Consequences of Dispossession: The Realignment of the Public Sphere for U.S. Youth." *Transforming Anthropology* 17: 20–33.

Fineberg, H. 1988. "The Social Dimensions of AIDS." *Scientific American*, October, 128–134.

Finley, Erin. 2012. *Fields of Combat: Understanding PTSD among Veterans of Iraq and Afghanistan*. New York: ILFR Press.

Firth, Rose Mary. 1978. "Social Anthropology and Medicine—A Personal Perspective." *Social Science and Medicine* 12B: 237–245.

Fisk, Milton. 1980. Ethics and Society: A Marxist Interpretation of Value. New York: New York University.

Fisk, Milton. 2000. *Toward a Healthy Society: The Morality and Politics of American Health Care Reform*. Lanham, MD: University Press of America.

Fitz, Don. 2007. "What's Possible in the Military Sector? Greater than 100% Reduction in Greenhouse Gases." ZNet, April 30. Available at: http://www.zcommunications.org/whats-possible-in-the-military-sector-by-don-fitz.

Fitz, Don. 2012. "Cuba: The New Global Medicine." *Monthly Review*, September, pp. 37–46.

Fitzgerald, Ruth, and Julie Park. 2003. "Introduction: Issues in the Practice of Medical Anthropology in the Antipodes." In *Medical Anthropology: Tales from Antipodes*. Julie Park and Ruth Fitzgerald, eds. Special issue of *Sites: A Journal of Social Anthropology & Cultural Studies*, n.s. 1(1): 1–29.

Flannery, Tim. 2005. *The Weather Makers*. New York: Atlantic Monthly Press.

Flavin, Christopher, and Robert Engelmann. 2009. "The Perfect Storm." In *State of the World 2009: Confronting Climate Change*, ed. Linda Starke, 5–29. London: Earthscan.

Fleming, Douglas, and Judith Wasserheit. 1999. "From epidemiological synergy to public health policy and practice: the contribution of other sexually transmitted diseases to sexual transmission of HIV infection." *Sexually Transmitted Diseases* 75: 3–17.

Flink, James J. 1973. *The Car Culture*. Cambridge, MA: MIT Press.

Forest, James J. F., and Matthew V. Sousa. 2006. *Oil and Terrorism in the New Gulf: Framing U.S. Energy and Security Policies for the Gulf of Guinea*. Lanham, MD: Lexington Books.

Forman, Jason L., Aileen Y. Watchko, and Maria Segui-Gomez. 2011. "Death and Injury from Automobile Collisions: An Overlooked Epidemic." *Medical Anthropology* 30: 241–246.

Fortun, Kim. 2001. *Advocacy after Bhopal: Environmentalism, Disaster, and the New Global Orders*. Chicago: University of Chicago Press.

Foster, George M. 1982. "Applied Anthropology and International Health: Retrospect and Prospect." *Human Organization* 41: 189–197.

Foster, George M., and Barbara Gallatin Anderson. 1978. *Medical Anthropology*. New York: John Wiley.

Foster, John Bellamy. 2009. *The Ecological Revolution: Making Peace with the Planet*. New York: Monthly Review Press.

Foster, John Bellamy. 2010, November. "Capitalism and the Curse of Energy Efficiency: The Return of the Jevons Paradox." *Monthly Review* (November): 1–12.

Foucault, Michel. 1975. *The Birth of the Clinic: An Archaeology of Medical Perception*. New York: Vintage.

Foucault M. 1979. *Discipline and Punish: The Birth of a Prison*. New York: Vintage.

Foucault M. 1980. "Body/power." In *Power-Knowledge: Selected Interviews and Other Writings 1972–1977*, ed. C. Gordon, 55–62. New York: Pantheon.

Foucault, Michel. 1998. *The History of Sexuality*, Vol. 1. London: Penguin.

Fox, Renee. 1990. "The Evolution of American Bioethics: A Sociological Perspective." In *Social Science Perspectives on Medical Ethics*, ed. George Weisz, 201–217. Dordrecht, the Netherlands: Kluwer Academic.

Frank, Emily. 2009. "The Relation of HIV Testing and Treatment to Identity Formation in Zambia." *African Journal of AIDS Research* 8: 515–524.

Frankenberg, Ronald. 1974. "Functionalism and After? Theory and Developments in Social Science Applied to the Health Field." *International Journal of Health Services* 43: 411–427.

Frankenberg, Ronald. 1980. "Medical Anthropology and Development: A Theoretical Perspective." *Social Science and Medicine* 14B: 197–207.

Frankenberg, Ronald. 1981. "Allopathic Medicine, Profession, and Capitalist Ideology in India." *Social Science and Medicine* 15A: 115–125.

Franklin, Sarah. 2003. "Re-thinking Nature—Culture: Anthropology and the New Genetics." *Anthropological Theory* 3: 65–85.

Franklin, Sarah, and Ragone, Helena, eds. 1998. *Reproducing Reproduction*. Philadelphia: University of Pennsylvania Press.

Freedman, Andrew. 2012. "Record Summer Temperatures, by the Numbers." Available at: http://www.climatecentral.org/blogs/a-breakdown-of-record-summer-temperatures. Accessed July 24, 2012.

Freedman, Lynn. 2000. "Human Rights and Women's Health." In *Women and Health*, eds. Marlene Goldman and Maureen Hatch, 428–438. New York: Academic Press.

Freedman, Lynn, and Deborah Maine. 1993. "Women's Mortality: A Legacy of Neglect." In *The Health of Women: A Global Perspective*, eds. Marge Koblinsky, Judith Timyan, and Jill Gay, 147–171. Boulder, CO: Westview Press.

Freidson, Elliot. 1970. *Profession of Medicine*. New York: Dodd, Mead and Co.

Freudenberg, Nicolas, Marianne Fahs, Sandro Galea, and Andrew Greenberg. 2006. "The Impact of New York City's 1975 Fiscal Crisis on the Tuberculosis, HIV, and Homicide Syndemic." *American Journal of Public Health* 96: 424–434.

Freund, Peter S., and George Martin. 1993. *The Ecology of the Automobile*. Montreal: Black Rose Books.

Freund, Peter S., and Meredith B. McGuire. 1991. *Health, Illness, and the Social Body: A Critical Sociology.* Englewood Cliffs, NJ: Prentice-Hall.

Friedlander, Eva, ed. 1996. *Look at the World through Women's Eyes: Plenary Speeches, Beijing '95.* New York: NGO Forum on Women.

Friedman, Samuel, Don Des Jarlais, and Jo L. Sothern. 1986. "AIDS Health Education for Intravenous Drug Users." *Health Education Quarterly* 13: 383–393.

Frumkin, Howard. 2008. "Director's Preface." *ATSDR Studies on Chemical Releases in the Great Lakes Region.* Atlanta, GA: Agency for Toxic Substances and Disease Registry.

Fry, Douglas. 2006. *The Human Potential for Peace: An Anthropological Challenge to Assumptions about War and Violence.* New York: Oxford University Press.

Fuentes, Annette. 1997. "White Coats with Blue Collars." In *These Times* (3 March): 17–19.

Gailey, Christine Ward. 1987. "Evolutionary Perspectives on Gender Hierarchy, Analyzing Gender." In *Analyzing Gender,* ed. F. B. Hess, 32–67. Beverly Hills: Sage.

Gailey, Christine Ward. 1998. "Feminist Methods." In *Handbook of Anthropological Methods,* ed. Russell Bernard, 203–234. Washington, DC: American Anthropological Association.

Gailey, Christine Ward. 2010. *Blue Ribbon Babies and Labors of Love: Race, Class, and Gender in U.S. Adoption Practice.* Austin: University of Texas Press

Gaines, Atwood. 1987. "Shamanism and the Shaman: Plea for the Person-Centered Approach." *Anthropology and Humanism Quarterly* 12(3–4): 62–68.

Gaines, Atwood. 1991. "Cultural Constructivism: Sickness Histories and the Understanding of Ethnomedicines beyond Critical Medical Anthropologies." In *Anthropologies of Medicine: A Colloquium of Western and European Perspectives,* eds. Beatrix Pfiederer and Gilles Bibeau, 221–258. Wiesbaden, Germany: Verlag Vieweg.

Gallagher, Eugene B. 1998. "Enrich Bioethics: Add One Part Social to One Part Clinical." In *Bioethics and Society: Constructing the Public Enterprise,* eds. Raymond DeVries and Jaradan Subedi, 166–191. Upper Saddle River, NJ: Prentice Hall.

Gamburd, Michelle. 2008. *Breaking the Ashes: The Culture of Illicit Liquor in Sri Lanka.* Ithaca, NY: Cornell University Press.

Gammeltoft, Tine. 1999. *Women's Bodies, Women's Worries: Health and Family Planning in a Vietnamese Rural Community.* Surrey, UK: Curzon Press.

Garb, Paula. 2008. "Russia's Radiation Victims of Cold War Weapons Production Surviving in a Culture of Secrecy and Denial." In *Half-Lives & Half-Truths: Confronting the Radioactive Legacies of the Cold War,* ed. Barbara Rose Johnson, 249–276. Santa Fe, NM: School for Advanced Research.

Garcia, Angela. 2008. "The Elegiac Addict: History, Chronicity, and the Melancholic Subject." *Cultural Anthropology* 23: 718–746.

Garcia, Angela. 2010. *The Pastoral Clinic: Addiction and Dispossession along the Rio Grande.* Berkeley: University of California Press.

Gardner, Gary. 2008. "Aluminum Production Continues Upwards." In *Vital Signs 2007–2008: The Trends That Are Shaping Our Future,* ed. Linda Starke, 58–59, New York: W. W. Norton.

Garrett, Laurie. 1994. *The Coming Plague: Newly Emerging Diseases in a World Out of Balance*. New York: Penguin Books USA.

Gaussett, Quentin. 2001. "AIDS and Cultural Practices in Africa: The Case of the Tonga (Zambia)." *Social Science and Medicine* 52: 509–518.

Gautier, Catherine. 2008. *Oil, Water, and Climate: An Introduction*. Cambridge, UK: Cambridge University Press.

Gbowee, Leymah. 2011. *Mighty Be Our Powers*. New York: Beast Books.

Geest, Sjaak van der. 2012. "Alien Origins: Xenophilia and the Rise of Medical Anthropology in the Netherlands." *Anthropology & Medicine* 19: 9–16.

Geneva Declaration Secretariat. 2008. *Global Burden of Armed Violence*. Geneva, Switzerland: Geneva Declaration Secretariat.

Georgopoulos, Basil S., and Floyd C. Mann. 1979. "The Hospital as an Organization." In *Patients, Physicians, and Illness*, ed. E. Gartley, 296–305. New York: Free Press.

Geras, Norman. 1990. *Discourses of Extremity: Radical Ethics and Post-Marxist Extravagances*. London: Verso.

Getahun, Haileyesus, Mario Raviglione, Jay Varma, Kevin Cain, Taraz Samandari, Tanja Popovic, and Thomas Frieden. 2012. "CDC Grand Rounds: The TB/HIV Syndemic." *Morbidity and Mortality Weekly Report* 61: 484–489.

Gezon, Lisa. 2012. *Drug Effects: Khat in Biocultural and Socioeconomic Perspective*. Walnut Creek, CA: Left Coast Press

Ghalioungui, Paul. 1963. *Magic and Medical Science in Ancient Egypt*. New York: Barnes and Noble.

Gilmore, Ruth. 2007. *Golden Gulag: Prisons, Surplus, Crisis and Opposition in Globalizing California*. Berkeley: University of California Press.

Ginsburg, Faye, and Rayna Rapp. 1995. "Introduction." *Conceiving the New World Order*, ed. Faye Ginsburg and Rayna Rapp, 1–17. Berkeley: University of California Press.

Ginzberg, Eli. 1994. *Medical Gridlock and Health Reform*. Boulder, CO: Westview Press.

Girard, Françoise. 2004. "Global Implications of U.S. Domestic and International Policies on Sexuality," ed. R. Parker, ed. (Working Paper #1). New York: International Working Group on Sexuality and Social Policy.

Glantz, Michael H. 2003. *Climate Affairs: A Primer*. Washington, DC: Island Press.

Glass-Coffin, Bonnie. 1995. "Anthropology, Shamanism, and the 'New Age'." *Chronicle of Higher Education*, June 15, 1748.

Glasser, Irene. 2012. *Anthropology of Addiction and Recovery*. Long Grove, IL: Waveland Press.

Global Carbon Project. 2010. "Carbon Budget Highlights." Available at: www.globalcarbonproject.org/carbonbudget/10/hl-full.htm.

Godelier, Maurice. 1986. *The Mental and the Material: Thought Economy and Society*. London: Verso.

Goffman, Irving. 1963. *Stigma*. Englewood Cliffs, NJ: Prentice-Hall.

Goldman, Marlene, and Maureen Hatch, eds. 2000. *Women and Health*. New York: Academic Press.

Gonzalez, Alfredo. 2008, January 8. "Review of Lyon-Callo, V.: *Inequality, Poverty and Neoliberal Governance*." *Medical Anthropology Quarterly* 19(3). Article first published online.

González-Guarda, Rosa. 2009. "The Syndemic Orientation: Implications for Eliminating Hispanic Health Disparities." *Hispanic Health Care International* 7:
114–115.

González-Guarda, R., B. McCabe, A. Florom-Smith, R. Cianelli, and N. Peragallo.
2011. "Substance Abuse, Violence, HIV, and Depression: An Underlying
Syndemic Factor Among Latinas." *Nursing Research* 60: 182–189.

Good, Byron. 1994. *Medicine, Rationality, and Experience.* Cambridge, UK: Cambridge University Press.

Good, Bryon J., Michael M. J. Fischer, Sarah S. Willen, and Mary-Jo DelVecchio
Good, eds. 2010. "Introduction." In *A Reader in Medical Anthropology: Theoretical Trajectories, Emergent Realities,* 9–14. Malden, MA: Wiley-Black.

Good, Mary-Jo Delvecchio, and Byron Good. 2000. "'Parallel Sisters': Medical Anthropology and Medical Sociology." In *Handbook of Medical Sociology,* 5th
ed., eds. Chloe E. Bird, Peter Conrad, and Allen M. Fremont, 377–388. New
York: Prentice-Hall.

Goode, Judith, and Jeff Maskovsky, eds. 2001. *The New Poverty Studies: The Ethnography of Power, Politics, and the Impoverished People in the United States.* New
York: New York University Press.

Goodman, Alan, and Thomas L. Leatherman, eds. 1998. *Building a New Biocultural
Synthesis: Political-Economic Perspectives on Human Biology.* Ann Arbor: University of Michigan Press.

Goody, Jack. 1976. *Production and Reproduction: A Comparative Study of the Domestic
Domain.* Cambridge, UK: Cambridge University Press.

Goody, Jack. 1983. *The Development of Family and Marriage in Europe.* Cambridge,
UK: Cambridge University Press.

Gorbachev, Mikahail. 1996. *Memoirs.* New York: Doubleday.

Gordon, Robert. 1992. *The Bushman Myth.* Boulder, CO: Westview.

Gore, Al. 2009. *Our Choice: A Plan to Solve the Climate Crisis.* London: Bloomsbury.

Gore, Al. 2006. *An Inconvenient Truth: The Planetary Emergency of Global Warming
and What We Can Do about It.* London: Rodale.

Gorman, M., P. Morgan, and E. Lambert. 1995. "Qualitative Research Consider-
ations and Other Issues in the Study of Methamphetamine Use among
Men Who Have Sex with Other Men." In *Qualitative Methods in Drug Abuse
and HIV Research,* eds. E. Lambert, R. S. Ashery, and R. H. Needle, 156–181
(NIDA Research Monograph #157; NIH Pub. No. 95-4025). Washington,
DC: U.S. Govt. Printing Office.

Gorz, Andre. 1973. *Socialism and Revolution.* Garden City, NY: Anchor.

Gorz, Andre. 1980. *Ecology as Politics.* Boston: South End Press.

Gough, Kathleen. 1971. "Nuer Kinship: A Re-Examination." In *The Translation of
Culture: Essays to E. E. Evans-Pritchard,* ed. T. O. Beidelman, 79–121. London:
Tavistock.

Gounis, K. 1992. "Temporality and the Domestication of Homelessness." In *The
Politics of Time,* ed. H. Rutz, (Monograph Series No. 4). Washington, DC:
American Ethnological Society.

Gourevitch, Danielle. 1998. "The Paths of Knowledge: Medicine in the Roman
World." In *Western Medical Thought from Antiquity to the Middle Ages,* ed.
Mirko Grmk, 104–138. Cambridge, MA: Harvard University Press.

Gow, Peter. 1994. "River People: Shamanism and History in Western Amazonia." In *Shamanism, History, and the State*, eds. Nicholas Thomas and Caroline Humphrey, 90–113. Ann Arbor: University of Michigan Press.

Gowan, Teresa. 2010. *Hobos, Hustlers, and Backsliders: Homeless in San Francisco*. Minneapolis: University of Minnesota Press.

Graham, A., T. Lamb, A. Read, and J. Allen. 2005. "Malaria-Filaria Coinfection in Mice Makes Malarial Disease More Severe Unless Filarial Infection Achieves Patency." *Journal of Infectious Diseases* 191: 410–421.

Gran, Peter. 1979. "Medical Pluralism in Arab and Egyptian History: An Overview of Class Structures and Philosophies of the Main Phases." *Social Science and Medicine* 13B: 339–348.

Green, Traci, Ricky Bluthenthal, Merrill Singer, Leo Beletsky, Lauretta Grau, Patricia Marshall, and Robert Heimer. 2010. "Prevalence and Predictors of Transitions to and Away from Syringe Exchange Use over Time in 3 US Cities with Varied Syringe Dispensing Policies." *Drug and Alcohol Dependence* 111: 74–81.

Greenberg, Paul. 2010, October. "Time for a Sea Change." *National Geographic*. Available at: http://ngm.nationalgeographic.com/2010/10/seafood-crisis/greenberg-text. Accessed February 8, 2013.

Griffith, David. 2009. "The Moral Economy of Tobacco." *American Anthropologist* 111(4): 432–442.

Grossinger, Richard. 1990. *Planet Medicine: From Stone Age Shamanism to Post-Industrial Healing*. Berkeley, CA: North Atlantic Books.

Gruenbaum, Ellen. 1983. "Struggling with the Mosquito: Malaria Policy and Agricultural Development in Sudan." *Medical Anthropology* 7: 53–62.

Gupta, Akhil. 1998. *Postcolonial Developments: Agriculture in the Making of Modern India*. Durham, NC: Duke University Press.

Guyer, Jane. 1991. "Female Farming in Anthropology and African History." In *Gender in the Crossroads of Knowledge: Feminist Anthropology in the Postmodern Era*, ed. Micaela di Leonardo, 257–278. Berkeley: University of California Press.

Habermas, Juergen. 1991. "What Does Socialism Mean Today? The Revolutions of Recuperation and the Need for New Thinking." In *After the Fall: The Failure of Communism and the Future of Socialism*, ed. Robin Blackburn, 25–46. London: Verso.

Hahn, Robert A. 1983. "Biomedical Practice and Anthropological Theory: Frameworks and Directions." *Annual Review of Anthropology* 12: 305–333.

Hahn, Robert. 1995. *Sickness and Healing: An Anthropological Perspective*. Ann Arbor: University of Michigan Press.

Hahn, Robert A., and Marcia Inhorn, eds. 2009. *Anthropology and Public Health: Bridging Differences in Culture and Society*, 2nd ed. Oxford, UK: Oxford University Press.

Hahn, Robert A., and Marcia Inhorn, eds. 2010. *Anthropology and Public Health: Bridging Differences in Culture and* Society, 2nd ed. Oxford: Oxford University Press.

Haire, Doris. 1978. "The Cultural Warping of Childbirth." In *The Cultural Crisis of Modern Medicine*, ed. John Ehrenreich, 185–200. New York: Monthly Review Press.

Han, G. S. 2000. "Traditional Herbal Medicine in the Korean Community in Australia: A Strategy to Cope with the Health Demands of Immigrant Life." *Health* 4: 426–454.

Handelbaum, Don. 1977. "The Development of a Washo Shaman." In *Culture, Disease, and Healing: Studies in Medical Anthropology*, ed. David Landy, 427–438. New York: Macmillan.

Hanson, Bill, George Beschner, James Walters, and Elliot Bovelle. 1985. *Life with Heroin: Voices from the Inner City*. New York: Lexington Books.

Haraway, Donna. 1991. *Simians, Cyborgs, and Women*. New York: Routledge.

Harding, Scott, and Libal, Kathryn. 2008. "War and the Public Health Disaster in Iraq." In *The War Machine and Global Health: A Critical Medical Anthropology Examination of the Human Costs of Armed Conflict and the International Violence Industry*, eds. Merrill Singer and G. Derrick Hodge, 59–88. Lantham, MA: Altamira Press.

Hare, W. L. 2009. "A Safe Landing for the Climate." In *State of the World: Confronting Climate*, ed. Linda Starke, 13–29. London: Earthscan.

Harmless, A. 1990. "Developmental Impact of Combat Exposure: Comparison of Adolescent and Adult Vietnam Veterans." *Smith College Studies in Social Work* 60: 185–195.

Harner, Michael. 1968. *The Jivaro*. Berkeley: University of California Press.

Harner, Michael 1980. *The Way of the Shaman: A Guide to Power and Healing*. New York: Bantam Books.

Harrington, Michael. 1962. *The Other America*. New York: Simon and Schuster.

Harris, Anna. 2009. "Overseas Doctors in Australian Hospitals: An Ethnographic Study of How Degrees of Difference Are Negotiated in Medical Practice." PhD thesis, Centre of Health and Society, University of Melbourne.

Harris, Marvin, and Orna Johnson. 2000. *Cultural Anthropology*. Boston: Addison-Wesley.

Harris, Marvin, and Eric Ross. 1987. *Death, Sex, and Fertility: Population Regulation in Preindustrial and Developing Societies*. New York: Columbia University Press.

Harris, Paul G. 2010. *World Ethics and Climate Change: From International to Global Justice*. Edinburgh: Edinburgh University Press.

Hart, Jason, and Bex Tyrer. 2006. "Research with Children Living in Situations of Armed Conflict: Concepts, Ethics & Methods." Refugee Studies Center, Working Paper No. 30. Oxford, UK: Department of International Development, University of Oxford Press.

Haug, M. 1975. "The Deprofessionalization of Everyone?" *Sociological Focus* 8: 197–213.

Harvey, D. 2003. *Paris: Capital of Modernity*. New York: Routledge.

Harvey, D. 2005. *A Brief History of Neoliberalism*. New York: Oxford University Press.

Hayden, Dolores. 2002. *Redesigning the American Dream*. New York: W. W. Norton.

Heath, Dwight. 1987. "Cultural Studies on Drinking: Definitional Problems." In *Cultural Studies on Drinking and Drinking Problems*, eds. P. Paakkanen and P. Sulkunen, 5–40. Helsinki: Social Research Institute of Alcohol Studies.

Heath, Dwight. 1990. "Cultural Factors in the Choice of Drugs." In *Recent Developments in Alcoholism* 8: 245–254.

Heath, Dwight. 1991. "Continuity and change in Drinking Patterns of the Bolivian Camba." In *Society, Culture and Drinking Patterns Reexamined* (Alcohol, Culture and Social Control Monograph Series), eds. D. Pittman and H. White, 78–86. New Brunswick, NJ: Rutgers Center for Alcohol Studies.

Heath, Dwight. 2000. *Drinking Occasions: Comparative Perspectives on Alcohol and Culture*. Philadelphia: Taylor and Francis.

Heath, Dwight. 2004. "Camba (Bolivia) Drinking Patterns: Changes in Alcohol Use, Anthropology, and Research Perspectives." In *Drug Use and Cultural Contexts: Beyond the West*, eds. R. Coomber and N. South, 119–136. London: Free Association Books.

Heggenhougen, Kris. 1986. "Scandinavia." *Medical Anthropology Quarterly*, o.s., 17(4): 94–95.

Heinberg, Richard. 2006. *The Oil Depletion Protocol: A Plan to Avert Oil, Wars, Terrorism and Economic Collapse*. Gabriola Island, BC: New Society Publishers.

Heise, Lori. 1993. "Violence against Women: The Missing Agenda." In *The Health of Women: A Global Perspective*, eds. Marge Koblinsky, Judith Timyan, and Jill Gray, 171–197. Boulder, CO: Westview Press.

Helman, Cecil. 1994. *Culture, Health, and Illness: An Introduction for Health Professionals*, 3rd ed. Oxford, UK: Butterworth-Heinemann.

Henderson, Gail E., and Myron S. Cohen. 1984. *The Chinese Hospital: A Socialist Work Unit*. New Haven, CT: Yale University Press.

Hendryx, Michael. 2009. "Mortality from Heart, Respiratory and Kidney Disease in Coal Mining Areas of Appalachia." *International Archives of Occupational and Environmental Health* 82: 243–249.

Hendryx, Michael, Katheryn O'Donnell, and Kimberly Horn. 2008 Lung cancer mortality is elevated in coal-mining areas of Appalachia. *Lung Cancer* 62: 1–7.

Henrici, Jane. 2010. *Women in New Orleans: Race, Poverty, and Hurricane Katrina*. Institute for Women's Policy Research Fact Sheet D490. Available at: http://www.iwpr.org/publications/pubs/women-in-new-orleans-race-poverty-and-hurricane-katrina. Accessed January 27, 2013.

Henrici. J. 2010, October. "A Gendered Response to Disaster in the Aftermath of Haiti's Earthquake." *Anthropology News* 5.

Herdt, Gilbert. 1987. *The Sambia: Ritual and Gender in New Guinea*. New York: Holt, Rinehart, and Winston.

Herdt, Gilbert. 2001. "Stigma and the Ethnographic Study of HIV: Problems and Prospects." *AIDS and Behavior* 5: 141–149.

Herrnstein, Richard J., and Charles Murray. 1994. *The Bell Curve: Intelligence and Class Structure in American Life*. New York: Free Press.

Herring, D. Ann. 2008. "Viral Panic, Vulnerability and the Next Pandemic." In *Health, Risk and Adversity*, eds. Catherine Panter-Brick and Agustín Fuentes, 78–100. Oxford, UK: Berghahn Books.

Herring, D. Ann, and Lisa Sattenspiel. 2007. "Social Contexts, Syndemics, and Infectious Disease in Northern Aboriginal Populations." *American Journal of Human Biology* 19: 190–202.

Hertsgaard, Mark. 2011. *Hot: Living through the Next Fifty Years on Earth*. Boston: Houghton Mifflin Harcourt.

Hewlitt, Barry, and Bonnie Hewlitt. 2008. *Ebola, Culture, and Politics: The Anthropology of an Emerging Disease*. Belmont, CA: Thompson Higher Education.

Hickel, Jason. 2012. The World Bank and the Development Delusion. Aljazeera. Available online at: http://www.aljazeera.com/indepth/opinion/2012/09/201292673233720461.html. Accessed December 12, 2012.

Hill, Carole E., ed. 1991. *Training Manual in Medical Anthropology*. Washington, DC: American Anthropological Association.

Himmelgreen, David, Nancy Romero-Daza, David Turkon, Sharon Watson, Ipolto Okello-Uma, and Daniel Sellen. 2009. "Addressing the HIV/AIDS-Food Insecurity Syndemic in Sub-Saharan Africa." *African Journal of AIDS Research* 8: 401–412.

Himmelstein, David U., and Steffie Woolhandler. 1984. "Medicine as Industry: The Health-Care Sector in the United States." *Monthly Review* 35(11): 13–25.

Himmelstein, David U., and Steffie Woolhandler. 1989. "A National Health Program for the United States: A Physician's Proposal." *New England Journal of Medicine* 320: 102–108.

Himmelstein, David U., and Steffie Woolhandler. 1994. *The National Health Program Book: A Source Guide for Advocates*. Monroe, ME: Common Courage Press.

Hindustan Times. 2012. "Bengal Heat Wave Toll Crosses 100." Available at: http://www.hindustantimes.com/India-news/Kolkata/Bengal-heat-wave-toll-crosses-100/Article1-867072.aspx. Accessed February 6, 2013.

Hippler, Arthur. 1976. "Shamans, Curers, and Personality: Suggestions toward a Theoretical Model." In *Culture-Bound Syndromes, Ethnopsychiatry, and Alternate Therapies*, ed. William Lebra, 103–113. Honolulu: University of Hawaii Press.

Hirsch, Jennifer, Holly Wardlow, Daniel Jordan Smith, Harriet M. Phinney, Shanti Parikh, and Constance J. Nathanson. 2010. *The Secret: Love, Marriage and HIV*. Nashville, TN: Vanderbilt University Press.

Ho, John. 1996. "The Influence of Coinfections on HIV Transmission and Disease Progression." *The AIDS Reader* 6: 114–116.

Hoffer, Lee. 2006. *Junkie Business: The Evolution and Operation of a Heroin Dealing Network*. Belmont, CA: Thomson/Wadsworth.

Hogan, David, and Jonathan Burstein. 2002. *Disaster Medicine*. London: Wolters Kluwer.

Hogue, Carol J. Rowland. 2000. "Gender, Race, and Class: From Epidemiologic Association to Etiologic Hypotheses." In *Women and Health,* eds. Marlene Goldman and Carolyn Sargent, 15–25. New York: Academic Press.

Honigmann, John, and Irma Honigmann. 1965. "How Baffin Island Eskimo Have Learned to Use Alcohol." *Social Forces* 44: 73–83.

Hoppal, Mihaly, and Keith D. Howard, eds. 1993. *Shamans and Cultures*. Los Angeles: International Society for Trans-Oceanic Research.

Hopper, Kim. August 1992. "Counting the Homeless: S-Night in New York." *Evaluation Review* 16: 376–388.

Hopper, Kim. 2003. *Reckoning with Homelessness*. Ithaca, NY: Cornell University Press.

Hopper, K., E. Susser, and S. Conover. 1987. "Economics of Makeshift: Deindustrialization and Homelessness in New York City." *Urban Anthropology* 14: 183–236.

Hopper, Kim, and L. Cox. 1982. "Litigation in Advocacy for the Homeless: The Case of New York City." *Development: Seeds of Change* 2: 57–62.

Horowitz, Leah. 2012. "Power, Profit, Protest: Grassroots Resistance to Industry in the Global North." *Capitalism Nature Socialism* 23: 20–34.

Howell, Nancy. 2000. *Demography of the Dobe !Kung*. Hawthorne, UK: Aldine-DeGruyter.

Hsiao, William C. 1995. "The Chinese Health Care System: Lessons for Other Nations." *Social Science and Medicine* 41: 1047–1055.

Hughes, Charles C. 1978. "Ethnomedicine." In *Health and the Human Condition: Perspectives on Medical Anthropology*, eds. Michael H. Logan and Edward E. Hunt, Jr., 150–158. North Scituate, MA: Duxbury Press.

Hughes, Donald H. 1975. *The Ecology of Ancient Civilizations*. Albuquerque: University of New Mexico Press.

Human Security Research Group. 2009. *Human Security Research Report: The Shrinking Costs of War*. Vancouver, Canada: School for International Studies, Simon Fraser University.

Hunt, Edward E., Jr. 1978. "Evolutionary Comparisons of the Demography, Life Cycles, and Health Care of Chimpanzee and Human Populations." In *Health and the Human Condition: Perspectives on Medical Anthropology*, eds. Michael H. Logan and Edward E. Hunt, Jr., 52–57. North Scituate, MA: Duxbury Press.

Hunt, Geoffrey, and Judith Barker. 2001. "Socio-Cultural Anthropology and Alcohol and Drug Research: Towards a Unified Theory." *Social Science & Medicine* 53: 165–188.

Hunt, Geoffrey, Kristin Evans, and Faith Kares. 2007. "Drug Use and Meanings of Risk and Pleasure." *Journal of Youth Studies* 10: 73–96.

Hunter, Susan S. 1985. "Historical Perspectives on the Development of Health Systems Modeling in Medical Anthropology." *Social Science and Medicine* 21: 1297–1307.

Hutchinson, Sharon, and Jok Madut Jok. 2002. "Gendered Violence and the Militarisation of Ethnicity: A Case Study from South Sudan." In *Postcolonial Subjectivities in Africa*, ed. Richard Werbner, 84–109. New York: Zed Books.

Ingman, Stanley R., and Anthony E. Thomas, eds. 1975. *Topias and Utopias in Health: Policy Studies*. The Hague: Mouton.

Ingstad, B. 1990. "The Cultural Construction of AIDS and Its Consequences for Prevention in Botswana." *Medical Anthropology Quarterly* 4: 28–40.

Inhorn, Marcia. 2006. "Defining Women's Health: A Dozen Messages from More than 150 Ethnographies." *Medical Anthropology Quarterly* 20: 345–378.

Inhorn, Marcia C., and Peter J. Brown. 1990. "The Anthropology of Infectious Disease." *Annual Review of Anthropology* 19: 89–117.

Inhorn, Marcia C., Pankaj Shrivastav, and Pasquale Patrizio. 2012. "Assisted Reproductive Technologies and Fertility 'Tourism': Examples from Global Dubai and the Ivy League." *Medical Anthropology* 31: 249–265.

Inhorn, Marcia, and Emily A. Wentzell, eds. 2012. *Medical Anthropology at the Intersections*. Durham, NC: Duke University Press.

Institute for Population and Social Research. 2005. *Youth at Odds: Thai Youth's Precarious Futures in a Globalizing World*. Princeton, NJ: Princeton University.

Intergovernmental Panel on Climate Change. 2007. *A Report of Working Group I of the Intergovernmental Panel on Climate Change: Summary for Policymakers*. Available at: http://www.ipcc.ch/pdf/assessment report.

Jacka, Judy. 1998. *Natural Therapies: A Bridge between Ancient Wisdom and New Edges Science*. Melbourne: Lothian.

Jacobsen, Kathryn H. 2008. *Introduction to Global Health*. Sudbury, MA: Jones and Bartlett.

Jacobson, Mark, and Hoever, John Ten. 2012. "Worldwide Health Effects of the Fukushima Daiichi Nuclear Accident." *Energy and Environmental Science* 5: 8743–8757.

Jacoby, Russell. 1975. *Social Amnesia: A Critique of Contemporary Psychology from Adler to Laing*. Boston: Beacon Press.

Jakobson, Merete Demant. 1999. *Shamanism: Traditional and Contemporary Approaches to the Mastery of Spirits and Healing*. New York: Berghahn.

Janes, Craig R., and Kitty K. Corbett. 2011. "Global Health." In *A Companion to Medical Anthropology*, eds. Merrill Singer and Pamela I. Erickson, 135–157. Malden, MA: Wiley-Blackwell.

Janzen, John M. 1978. *The Quest for Therapy in Lower Zaire*. Berkeley: University of California Press.

Jelin, Elizabeth. 2004. "The Family in Argentina: Modernity, Economic Crisis and Politics." In *Handbook of World Families*, eds. Bert Adams and Jan Trost, 391–413. Thousand Oaks, CA: Sage.

Jewkes, Rachel. 2002. "Intimate Partner Violence: Causes and Prevention." *The Lancet* 359: 1423–1429.

Johansen, Bruce E. 2006. *Global Warming in the 21st Century, Volume 2: Melting Ice and Warming Seas*. Westport, CT: Praeger.

Johnson, Bruce, Paul Goldstein, Edward Preble, J. Schmeidler, Doug Lipton, Barry Spunt, and T. Miller. 1985. *Taking Care of Business: The Economics of Crime by Heroin Abusers*. New York: Lexington Books.

Johnson, Thomas M. 1987. "Practicing Medical Anthropology: Clinical Strategies for the Work in the Hospital." In *Applied Anthropology in America*, 2nd ed., eds. Edith M. Eddy and William L. Partridge, 316–339. New York: Columbia University Press.

Johnson, Barbara Rose, Susan Dawson, and Gary Madsen. 2007. "Uranium Mining and Milling: Navajo Experiences in the American Southwest." In *Half-Lives & Half-Truths: Confronting the Radioactive Legacies of the Cold War*, ed. Barbara Rose Johnson, 97–116. Santa Fe, NM: School for Advanced Research.

Jones, Chaunetta. 2011. "'If I Take My Pills I'll Go Hungry': The Choice between Economic Security and HIV/AIDS Treatment in Grahamstown, South Africa." *Annals of Anthropological Practice* 35: 67–80.

Jonsen, Albert R. 2000. *A Short History of Medical Ethics*. New York: Oxford University Press.

Joralemon, Donald. 1990. "The Selling of the Shaman and the Problem of Informant Legitimacy." *Journal of Anthropological Research* 46: 105–118.

Joralemon, Donald. 2010. *Exploring Medical Anthropology*, 2nd ed. Boston: Prentice Hall.

Judt, Tony. 2010. *Ill Fares the Land*. New York: Penguin Books.

Justice, Judith. 1986. *Policies, Plans, and People: Culture and Health Development in Nepal.* Berkeley: University of California Press.

Kabeer, Naila. 1985. "Do Women Gain from High Fertility?" In *Women, Work, and Ideology in the Third World,* ed. Haleh Afshar, 66–83. London: Tavistock.

Kalofonos, Ippolytos Andreas. 2010. "'All I Eat Is ARVs': The Paradox of AIDS Treatment Interventions in Central Mozambique." *Medical Anthropology Quarterly* 24: 363–380.

Kalweit, Holger. 1992. *Shamans, Healers, and Medicine Men.* Boston: Shambhala.

Kamat, Vinay. 2009. "The Anthropology of Childhood Malaria in Tanzania." In *Anthropology and Public Health: Bridging Differences in Culture and Society,* eds. Robert Hahn and Marcia Inhorn, 35-63. Oxford: Oxford University Press.

Kamin, Leon. 1995. "Behind the Curve." *Scientific American* 272(2): 99–103.

Kant, L. 2003. "Diabetes Mellitus-Tuberculosis: The Brewing Double Trouble." *Indian Journal of Tuberculosis* 50: 83–84.

Kaplan, G., E. Pamuck, J. Lynch, R. Cohen, and J. Balfour. 1996. "Inequality in Income and Mortality in the United States: Analysis of Mortality and Potential Pathways." *British Medical Journal* 312: 999–1003.

Karbuz, Sohbet. 2011. A Look at US Military Energy Consumption. OilPrice.com. Available at: http://oilprice.com/Energy/Energy-General/A-Look-At-US -Military-Energy-Consumption.html. Accessed July 13, 2012.

Kath, Elizabeth. 2010. *Social Relations and the Cuban Health Miracle.* New Brunswick, NJ: Transaction.

Katz, Richard. 1982. *Boiling Energy: Community Healing among the Kalahari !Kung.* Cambridge, MA: Harvard University Press.

Kaufert, Leyland, and J. M. Kaufert. 1978. "Alternative Courses of Development: Medical Anthropology in Britain and North America." *Social Science and Medicine* 12B: 255–261.

Kaufert, Patricia, and John O'Neil. 1993. "Analysis of a Dialogue on Risks in Childbirth: Clinicians, Epidemiologists and Inuit Women." In *Knowledge, Power and Practice: The Anthropology of Medicine and Everyday Life,* ed. Shirley Lindenbaum and Margaret Lock, 32–55. Berkeley: University of California Press.

Kawachi, Ichiro. 1997. "Social Capital, Income Inequality, and Mortality." *American Journal of Public Health* 87: 1491–1498.

Kawachi, Ichiro, Bruce P. Kennedy, Richard G. Wilkinson. 1999. *The Society and Population Health Reader.* New York: The New Press.

Kjetland, Eyrun, Patricia Ndhlovu, Exeneviab Gomo, Takafira Mduluza, Nicholas Midzi, Lovemore Gwanzura, et al. 2006. "Association between Genital Schistosomiasis and HIV in Rural Zimbabwean Women." *AIDS* 20: 593–600.

Keesing, Roger. 1983. *Elota's Story: The Life and Times of a Solomon Islands Big Man.* New York: Holt, Rinehart, and Winston.

Kehoe, Alice Beck. 2000. *Shamans and Religion: An Anthropological Exploration in Critical Thinking.* Prospect Heights, IL: Waveland Press.

Kelman, Sander. 1975. "The Social Nature of the Definition Problem in Health." *International Journal of Health Services* 5: 625–642.

Khan, Omar, and Gregory Pappas, eds. 2011. *Megacities and Global Health.* Washington, DC: American Public Health Association.

Kidder, Tracy. 2003. *Mountains beyond Mountains.* New York: Random House.

Kiev, Ari, ed. 1966. *Magic, Faith and Healing: Studies in Primitive Psychiatry Today*. New York: Free Press of Glencoe.

Kim, Jim Yong, Joyce V. Millen, Alec Irwin, and John Gershman, eds. 2000. *Dying for Growth: Global Inequality and the Health of the Poor*. Monroe, ME: Common Courage Press.

King, D., L. King, D. Foy, and D. Gudanowski. 1996. "Prewar Factors in Combat-Related Posttraumatic Stress Disorder: Structural Equation Modeling with a National Sample of Female and Male Vietnam Veterans." *Journal of Consulting and Clinical Psychology* 64: 520–531.

Kingfisher, Catherine. 2007. "Discursive Constructions of Homelessness in a Small City in the Canadian Prairies: Notes on Destructuration, Individualization, and the Production of (Raced and Gendered) Unmarked Categories." *American Ethnologist* 34: 91–107.

Kingsolver, Ann. 2011. *Tobacco Town Futures: Global Encounters in Rural Kentucky*. Long Grove, IL: Waveland Press.

Klare, Michael T. 2007, December 7. "Iraq and Climate Change." *Foreign Policy in Focus*.

Klare, Michael T. 2008. *Rising Powers, Shrinking Planet: The New Geopolitics of Energy*. New York: Metropolitan Books.

Klein, Dorie. 1983. "Ill and against the Law: The Social and Medical Control of Heroin Users." *Journal of Drug Issues* 13: 31–55.

Klein, Hugh. 2011. "Using a Syndemics Theory Approach to Study HIV Risk Taking in a Population of Men Who Use the Internet to Find Partners for Unprotected Sex." *American Journal of Men's Health* 5: 466–476.

Klein, Naomi. 2007. *The Shock Doctrine*. New York: Henry Holt and Co.

Klein, Norman. 1979. "Introduction." In *Culture, Curers and Contagion*, ed. Norman Klein, 1–4. Novato, CA: Chandler and Sharp.

Kleinman, Arthur. 1977. "Lessons from a Clinical Approach to Medical Anthropological Research." *Medical Anthropology Newsletter* 8: 5–8.

Kleinman, Arthur. 1978. "Problems and Prospects in Comparative Cross-Cultural Medical and Psychiatric Studies." In *Culture and Healing in Asian Societies: Anthropological, Psychiatric and Public Health Studies*, eds. Arthur Kleinman, Peter Kunstadter, E. Russell Alexander, and James L. Gale, 329–374. Cambridge, MA: Schenkman.

Kleinman, Arthur. 1995. *Writing at the Margin: Discourse Between Anthropology and Medicine*. Berkeley: University of California Press.

Kleinman, Arthur. 2009. Foreword. In *Anthropology and Public Health: Bridging Differences in Culture and Society*, 2nd ed., eds. R. Hahn and M. Inhorn, v–viii. Oxford, UK: Oxford University Press.

Kleinman, Arthur, Veena Das, and Margaret Lock, eds. 1997. *Social Suffering*. Berkeley. University of California Press.

Kligman, Gail. 1995. "Political Demography: The Banning of Abortion in Ceausescu's Romania." In *Conceiving the New World Order: The Global Politics of Reproduction*, eds. R. Rapp and F. Ginsberg, 234–255. Berkeley: University of California Press.

Koester, Stephen. 1994. "Copping, Running, and Paraphernalia Laws: Contextual Variables and Needle Risk Behavior among Injection Drug Users in Denver." *Human Organization* 53: 287–295.

Kolbert, Elizabeth. 2006. *Field Notes from a Catastrophe: Man, Nature, and Climate Change*. New York: Holtzbrinck.

Konadu, Kwask. 2007. *Indigenous Medicine and Knowledge in African Society*. New York: Routledge.

Konner, Melvin. 1993. *Medicine at the Crossroads: The Crisis in Health Care*. New York: Pantheon Books.

Kornfield, R., and S. Babalola. 2008. "Gendered Responses to Living with AIDS: Case Studies in Rwanda." In *AIDS, Culture, and Africa*, ed. Douglas A. Feldman, 35–56. Gainesville: University Press of Florida.

Kovel, Joel. 2008. "Ecosocialism, Global Justice, and Climate Change." *Capitalism, Nature, Socialism* 19: 4–14.

Krause, Elliot. 1977. *Power and Illness: The Political Sociology of Health and Medical Care*. New York: Elsevier.

Krause, Elliot. 1996. *Death of the Guilds: Professions, States, and the Advance of Capitalism, 1930 to the Present*. New Haven, CT: Yale University Press.

Kreniske, John. 1997. "AIDS in the Dominican Republic: Anthropological Reflections on the Social Nature of Disease." In *AIDS in Africa and the Caribbean*, eds. George C. Bond, John Kreniske, Ida Susser, and Joan Vincent, 33–51. Boulder, CO: Westview Press.

Krieger, Nancy. 2001. "Theories for Social Epidemiology in the Twenty-First Century: An Ecosocial Perspective." *International Journal of Epidemiology* 30: 668–677.

Krieger, Nancy. 2005. *Health Disparities and the Body*. Boston: Harvard School of Public Health.

Kroeber, Alfred. 1941. "Salt, Dogs, Tobacco." *Anthropological Records* 6: 1–20.

Kurtz, Steven. 2008. "Unexpected Additional Evidence for Syndemic Theory." *Journal of Psychoactive Drugs* 40: 513–521.

Kutalek, Ruth, Verena C. Muenzenmeir, and Armin Prinz. 2012. What about *Ethnomedicin*? Reflections on the Early Days of Medical Anthropologies in German-Speaking Countries." *Anthropology & Medicine* 19: 39–47.

Kwong, Peter, Coproducer. 2010. *China's Un-natural Disaster: Tears of Sichuan Province*. HBO Documentary Films.

LaBarre, Weston. 1972. "Hallucinogens and the Shamanic Origins of Religion." In *Flesh of the Gods: The Ritual Use of Hallucinogens*, ed. Peter T. Furst, 261–278. New York: Praeger.

Lafeuillade, Alain. 2011. "Potential Strategies for an HIV Infection Cure." *HIV Clinical Trials* 12: 121–130.

Lamphere, Louise. 1987. *From Working Daughters to Working Mothers: Immigrant Women in a New England Industrial Community*. Ithaca, NY: Cornell University Press.

Lamphere, Louise, and Michelle Zimbalist Rosaldo, eds. 1974. *Women, Culture and Society*. Stanford, CA: Stanford University Press.

Lamphere, Louise, Helena Ragone, and Patricia Zavella, eds. 1997. *Situated Lives: Gender and Culture in Everyday Life*. New York: Routledge.

Lan, David. 1985. *Guns and Rain: Guerrillas and Spirit Mediums in Zimbabwe*. Berkeley: University of California Press.

Landesman, S. 1993. "Commentary: Tuberculosis in New York City—The Consequences and Lessons of Failure." *American Journal of Public Health* 83: 766–768.

Landy, David. 1977. "Introduction." In *Culture, Disease, and Healing: Studies in Medical Anthropology*, ed. David Landy, 1–9. New York: Macmillan.

Landy, David. 1983. "Medical Anthropology: A Critical Appraisal." In *Advances in Medical Social Science*, Vol. 1, ed. Julio L. Ruffini, 185–314. New York: Gordon and Breach.

Langdon, E. 1992. "Introduction: Shamanism and Anthropology." In *Portals of Power: Shamanism in South America*, eds. E. Langdon, Jean Matteson, and Gerhard Baer, 1–21. Albuquerque: University of New Mexico Press.

Langwick, Stacey S. 2011. *Bodies, Politics, and African Healing: The Matter of Maladies in Tanzania*. Bloomington: Indiana University Press.

Lassey, Marie L., William R. Lassey, and Martin J. Jinks, eds. 1997. *Health Care Systems Around the World: Characteristics, Issues, Reforms*. Upper Saddle River, NJ: Prentice Hall.

Latour, Bruno, and Steve Woolgar. 1986. *Laboratory Life: The Construction of Scientific Facts*. Princeton, NJ: Princeton University Press.

Laughlin, William S. 1963. "Primitive Theory of Medicine: Empirical Knowledge." In *Man's Image in Medicine and Anthropology*, ed. Iago Galdston, 116–140. New York: International Universities Press.

Lawinski, Terese. 2010. *Living on the Edge in Suburbia: From Welfare to Workfares*. Nashville, TN: Vanderbilt University Press.

Lazarus, Ellen. 1988. "Theoretical Considerations for the Study of the Doctor–Patient Relationship: Implications of a Perinatal Study." *Medical Anthropology Quarterly*, n.s., 2: 34–59.

Leacock, Eleanor Burke. 1972. "Introduction." In *The Origins of the Family, Private Property and the State*, ed. Eleanor Burke Leacock, 7–69. New York: International Publishers.

Leacock, Eleanor, and Mona Etienne, 1980. *Women and Colonization*. New York: Bergin & Garvey.

Leacock, Eleanor Burke, and Richard B. Lee, eds. 1982. *Politics and History in Band Societies*. Cambridge, UK: Cambridge University Press.

Lee, Richard B. 1979. *The !Kung San: Men, Women and Work in a Foraging Society*. Cambridge, UK: Cambridge University Press.

Lee, Richard, and Susser, Ida. 2008. "Confronting Conventional Wisdom: The Ju/'hoansi." In *AIDS, Culture, and Africa*, ed. D. Feldman, 18–34. Gainesville: University Press of Florida.

Lee, Richard B., and Irven DeVore. 1976. *Kalahari Hunter-Gatherers*. Cambridge, MA: Harvard University Press.

Lee, Richard. 2012. *The Dobe Ju/'hoansi*. Belmont, CA: Wadsworth.

Leeds, Anthony. 1971. "The Concept of the 'Culture of Poverty': Conceptual, Logical, and Empirical Problems, with Perspectives from Brazil and Peru." In *The Culture of Poverty: A Critique*, ed. Eleanor Burke Leacock, 226–284. New York: Simon and Schuster.

Leeson, Joyce. 1974. "Social Science and Health Policy in Preindustrial Society." *International Journal of Health Services* 4: 429–440.

Leff, Laurel. 2005. *Buried by the Times: The Holocaust and America's Most Important Newspaper*. New York: Cambridge University Press.

Leibowitch, J. 1985. *Strange Virus of Unknown Origin*. New York: Ballantine Books.

Lemco, Jonathan. 1994. "Introduction." In *National Health Care: Lessons from the United States and Canada*, ed. Jonathan Lemco, 1–41. Ann Arbor: University of Michigan Press.

Lerner, B. 1993. "New York City's Tuberculosis Control Efforts: The Historical Limitations of the 'War on Consumption.'" *American Journal of Public Health* 83: 758–766.

Leshner, Alan. 2003. Addiction Is a Brain Disease and It Matters. *Focus* 1: 190–193.

Leslie, Charles. 1974. "The Modernization of Asian Medical Systems." In *Rethinking Modernization*, ed. John Poggie, Jr., and Robert N. Lynch, 69–107. Westport, CT: Greenwood Press.

Leslie, Charles. 1976. "Introduction." In *Asian Medical Systems: A Creative Study*, ed. Charles Leslie, 1–12. Berkeley: University of California Press.

Leslie, Charles. 1977. "Medical Pluralism and Legitimation in the Indian and Chinese Medical Systems." In *Culture, Disease, and Healing: Studies in Medical Anthropology*, ed. David Landy, 511–517. New York: Macmillan.

Leslie, Charles. 1992. "Interpretations of Illness: Syncretism in Modern Ayurveda." In *Paths to Asian Medical Knowledge*, eds. Charles Leslie and Allan Young, 177–208. Berkeley: University of California Press.

Levin, Betty Wolden. 1990. "International Perspectives in Decision Making in Neonatal Intensive Care." *Social Science and Medicine* 30: 901–912.

Lewis, Gilbert. 2007. "Medical System and Questions in Fieldwork.' In *Knowing and Not Knowing*, ed. Ron Littlewood, 28–38. Walnut Creek, CA: Left Coast Press.

Lewis, I. M. 1989. *Ecstatic Religion: A Study of Shamanism and Possession*. 2nd ed. London: Routledge.

Li, Bigqin. 2007. "Floating Population or Urban Citizens? Status, Social Provision and Circumstances of Rural–Urban Migrants in China." *Social Policy and Administration* 40: 174–195.

Li, Minqi. 2008. "Climate Change, Limits to Growth and the Imperative for Socialism." *Monthly Review*, July–August: 51–67.

Lieban, Richard W. 1990. "Medical Anthropology and the Comparative Study of Medical Ethics." In *Social Science Perspectives in Medical Ethics*, ed. George Weisz, 221–239. Dordrecht, the Netherlands: Kluwer Academic.

Lindemann, Mary. 2010. *Medicine and Society in Early Modern Europe*. Cambridge, UK: Cambridge University Press.

Lindenbaum, Shirley. 1998. "Images of Catastrophe: The Making of an Epidemic." In *Political Economy of AIDS*, ed. Merrill Singer, 33–58. Amityville, NY: Baywood.

Lindenbaum, Shirley. 1987. "The Mystification of Female Labors." In *Gender and Kinship: Essays toward a Unified Analysis*, ed. Jane Fishburne Collier and Sylvia Junko Yanagisako, 221–243. Stanford, CA: Stanford University Press.

Lindenbaum, Shirley, and Margaret Lock. 1993. "Preface." In *Knowledge, Power and Practice: The Anthropology of Medicine and Everyday Life*, ed. Shirley Lindenbaum and Margaret Lock, ix–xv. Berkeley: University of California Press.

Lindenbaum, Shirley. 1998. "Images of Catastrophe: The Making of an Epidemic." In *Political Economy of AIDS*, ed. Merrill Singer, 33–58. Amityville, NY: Baywood.

Lindstroem, Christine, and Martin Lindstroem. 2006. "'Social Capital,' GNP Per Capita, Relative Income, and Health: An Ecological Study of 23 Countries. *International Journal of Health Services* 36: 679–696.

Lipuma, J. 2005. "Update on the Burkholderia cepacia complex." *Current Opinion in Pulmonary Medicine* 11: 528–533.

Little, Amanda. 2009. *Power Trip: From Oil Wells to Solar Cells—Our Ride to the Renewable Future*. London: Harper Press.

Littleton, Judith, and Julie Park. 2009. "Tuberculosis and Syndemics: Implications for Pacific Health in New Zealand." *Social Science and Medicine* 69: 1674–1680.

Liu, Shao-hua. 2011. *Passage to Manhood: Youth Migration, Heroin and AIDS in Southwest China*. Stanford, CA: Stanford University Press.

Liu, Yingling. 2008. "Steel Production Soars." In *Vital Signs 2007–2008: The Trends That Are Shaping Our Future*, ed. Londa Starke, 56–57. New York: W. W. Norton.

Livingstone, Frank B. 1958. "Anthropological Implications of Sickle Cell Gene Distribution in West Africa." *American Anthropologist* 60: 533–562.

Lock, Margaret. 1980. *East Asian Medicine in Urban Japan*. Berkeley: University of California Press.

Lock, Margaret. 1993. "Cultivating the Body: Anthropology and Epistemologies of Bodily Practice and Knowledge." *Annual Reviews of Anthropology* 22: 133–155.

Lock, Margaret, and Vinh-Kim Nguyen. 2010. *An Anthropology of Biomedicine*. Malden, MA: Wiley-Blackwell.

Lock, Margaret, and Nancy Scheper-Hughes. 1990. "A Critical-Interpretive Approach in Medical Anthropology: Rituals and Routines of Discipline and Dissent." In *Medical Anthropology: Contemporary Theory and Method*, eds. Thomas M. Johnson and Carolyn F. Sargent, 47–72. Westport, CT: Praeger.

Lomnitz, Claudio. 2003. "The Depreciation of Life During Mexico City's Transition into 'the Crisis.'" In *Wounded Cities: Destruction and Reconstruction in a Globalized World*, eds, Jane Schneider and Ida Susser, 47–71. New York: Berg.

Loudon, J. B. 1976. "Preface." In *Social Anthropology and Medicine*, ed. J. B. Loudon. London: Academic Press, pp. v–viii.

Lovell, Ann. 2011. "Debating Life after Disaster: Charity Hospital Babies and Bioscientific Futures in Post-Katrina New Orleans." *Medical Anthropology Quarterly* 25: 254–277.

Lubkemann, Stephen. 2008. *Culture in Chaos: An Anthropology of the Social Condition of War*. Chicago: University of Chicago Press.

Lueng, Big. 2008. *Traditional Chinese Medicine: The Human Dimension*. Maleny, Australia: Verdant House.

Luke, Tim. 2008. "Climatologies as Social Critiques: The Social Construction/Creation of Global Warming, Global Dimming, and Global Cooling." In *Political Theory and Global Climate Change*, ed. Steve Vanderheiden, 121–152. Cambridge, MA: MIT Press.

Lurie, Peter, Percy C. Hintzen, and Robert A. Lowe. 2004. "Socioeconomic Obstacles to HIV Prevention and Treatment in Developing Countries: The Roles of the International Monetary Fund and the World Bank." In *HIV and AIDs in Africa: Beyond Epidemiology*, eds. Ezekiel Kalipeni, Susan Craddock, Joseph R. Oppong, and Jayati Ghosh, 204–212. Malden, MA: Blackwell.

Lynas, Mark. 2004. *High Tide: The Truth about Our Climate Crisis*. New York: Picador.

Lyon-Callo, Vincent. 2004. *Inequality, Poverty, and Neoliberal Governance: Activist Ethnography in the Homeless Sheltering Industry* (Teaching Culture: UTP Ethnographies for the Classroom). Toronto: University of Toronto Press.

MacAndrew, Craig, and Robert Edgerton. 1969. *Drunken Comportment: A Social Explanation*. Chicago: Aldine.

Machel, Graça. 1996. *Promotion and Protection of the Rights of Children: Impact of Armed Conflict on Children*. United Nations/UNICEF. Available at: http://www.unicef.org/graca/a51-306_en.pdf. Accessed January 15, 2009.

Mack, John. 2011. "Healing Word: Becoming a Spirit-Host in Madagascar." *Medical Anthropology* 18: 231–243.

Macpherson, Cluny, and La'avasa Macpherson. 1990. *Samoan Medical Belief & Practice*. Auckland: Auckland University Press.

Magdoff, Fred. 2011. "Ecological Civilization." *Monthly Review* 62(10): 1–25.

Magdoff, Fred, and John Bellamy Foster. 2010. "What Every Environmentalist Needs to Now about Capitalism." *Monthly Review* 61: 1–30.

Magnant, Cheryl. 2011. "Women in War and Peace. Ethnoscopes: Tracks of an Anthropologist Blog." Available at: http://ethnoscopes.blogspot.com/2011/12/women-war-peace-movie.html. Accessed June 2, 2012.

Magner, Lois N. 1992. *A History of Medicine*. New York: Marcel Dekker.

Mahmood, Shakeel ahmen Ibne. 2011. "Air Pollution Kills 15,000 Bangladeshis Each Year: The Role of Public Administration and Government's Integrity." *Journal of Public Administration and Policy Research* 3: 129–140.

Maia, Suzana. 2012. *Transnational Desires: Brazilian Erotic Dancers in New York*. Nashville, TN: Vanderbilt University Press.

Mamdani, Mahmood. 1972. *The Myth of Population Control*. New York: Monthly Review Press.

Manderson, Lenore, and M. Matthews. 1985. "Care and Conflict: Vietnamese Medical Beliefs and the Australian Health Care System." In *Immigration and Ethnicity in the 1980s*, eds. I Barclay, S. Encel, and G. McCall. Melbourne: Longman-Cheshire.

Mann, Jonathan, Daniel Tarantola, and Thomas Netter. 1992. *AIDS in the World*. Cambridge, MA: Harvard University Press.

Mann, Scott. 2010. *Bioethics in Perspective: Corporate Power, Public Health and Political Economy*. Melbourne: Cambridge University Press.

Marcus, Anthony. 2006. *Where Have All the Homeless Gone: The Making and Unmaking of a Crisis*. New York: Berghahn Press.

Marketing News. 2002, October 28. "Global Youth United: Homogeneous Group Prime Target for U.S. Marketers," 49.

Marks, G., and W. Beatty. 1976. *Epidemics*. New York: Charles Scribner's Sons.

Marmor, Theodore R. 1994. *Understanding Health Care Reform*. New Haven, CT: Yale University Press.

Marmor, Theodor, and Jonathan Oberlander. 2011. "The Patchwork: Health Reform, American Style." *Social Science and Medicine* 72: 125–128.

Marmot, Michael, and Richard G. Wilkinson. 2000. *The Social Determinants of Health.* Oxford: Oxford University Press.

Marshall, Mac. 1979. *Weekend Warriors: Alcohol in a Micronesian Culture.* Mountain View, CA: Mayfield.

Marshall, Mac. 1990. *Silent Voices Speak: Women and Prohibition in Truk.* Belmont, CA: Wadsworth Modern Anthropology Library.

Marshall, Mac. 2005. "Carolina in the Carolines: A Survey of Patterns and Meanings of Smoking on a Micronesian Island." *Medical Anthropology Quarterly* 19: 365–382.

Marshall, Mac. 2013. *Drinking Smoke: The Tobacco Syndemic in Oceania.* Honolulu: University of Hawai'i Press.

Marshall, Mac, Genevieve Ames, and Linda Bennett. 2001. "Anthropological Perspectives on Alcohol and Drugs at the Turn of the New Millennium." *Social Science & Medicine* 53: 153–164.

Marshall, Patricia. 1991. "Research Ethics in Applied Medical Anthropology." In *Training Manual in Applied Medical Anthropology,* ed. Carole Hill, 213–235. Washington, DC: American Anthropological Association.

Marshall, Patricia A. and Barbara A. Koenig. 1996. "Bioethics in Anthropology: Perspectives on Culture, Medicine and Morality." *Medical Anthropology: Contemporary Theory and Method,* revised ed., ed. Carolyn F. Sargent and Thomas M. Johnson, 349–373. Westport, CT: Praeger.

Martin, Emily. 1987. *The Woman in the Body: A Cultural Analysis of Reproduction.* Boston: Beacon Press.

Martin, Emily 1990. "Toward an Anthropology of Immunology: The Body as Nation State." *Medical Anthropology Quarterly,* n.s., 4: 410–426.

Martin, Emily. 1996. *Flexible Bodies.* Boston: Beacon Press.

Mascie-Taylor, C. G. N. 1993. "The Biology of Disease." In *The Anthropology of Disease,* ed. C. G. N. Mascie-Taylor, 1–72. Oxford, UK: Oxford University Press.

Maskovsky, Jeff. 2013. "Diversifying AIDS Activism: Lessons Learned from ACT UP/Philadelphia." In *Global HIV/AIDS politics, policy, and activism: Persistent challenges and emerging issues: Vol. 3. Activism and community mobilization,* ed. R. A. Smith. Santa Barbara, CA: Praeger.

Maslin, Mark. 2009. "Hot or Cold Future?" In *The Complete Ice Age: How Climate Change Shaped the World,* ed. Brian Fagan, 206–231. London: Thames & Hudson.

Matveychuk, Wasyl. 1986. "The Social Construction of Drug Definitions and Drug Experiences." In *Culture and Politics of Drugs,* ed. Peter Park and Wasyl Matveychuk, 7–12. Dubuque, IA: Kendall/Hunt.

Mayer, Jane. 2010. "Covert Operations: The Billionaire Brothers Who Are Waging a War against Obama." *The New Yorker,* August 30.

McCanne, Don R. 2009. "The Organization for Economic Cooperation and Development and Health Care Reform in the United States." *International Journal of Health Services* 39: 699–704.

McCombie, Susan. 1990. "AIDS in Cultural, Historic, and Epidemiologic Context." In *Culture and AIDS,* ed. D. Feldman, 9–28. New York: Praeger.

McConnell, Terrence C. 1982. *Moral Issues in Health Care: An Introduction to Medical Ethics.* Monterey, CA: Wadsworth.

McCoy, Alfred. Undated. "Opium History, Basic Terms." Available at: http://opioids.com/opium/index.html. Accessed August 2, 2012.

McElroy, Ann. 1996. "Should Medical Ecology Be Political?" *Medical Anthropology Quarterly*, n.s., 10: 519–22.

McElroy, Ann, and Patricia K. Townsend. 1979. *Medical Anthropology in Ecological Perspective.* Boulder, CO: Westview Press.

McElroy, Ann, and Patricia K. Townsend. 1989. *Medical Anthropology in Ecological Perspective*, 2nd ed. Boulder, CO: Westview Press.

McElroy, Ann, and Patricia K. Townsend. 1996. *Medical Anthropology in Ecological Perspective*, 3rd ed. Boulder, CO: Westview Press.

McElroy, Ann, and Patricia K. Townsend. 2009. *Medical Anthropology in Ecological Perspective*, 5th ed. Boulder, CO: Westview Press.

McFarland, Lynne. 1995. "Epidemiology of Infectious and Iatrogenic Nosocomial Diarrhea in a Cohort of General Medicine Patients." *American Journal of Infection Control* 23: 295–305.

McGovern, Theresa. 2007. Building Coalitions to Support Women's Health and Rights in the United States: South Carolina and Florida. *Reproductive Health Matters* 15(29): 119–129.

McGrath, J. W., C. B. Rwabukwali, D. A. Schumann, J. Pearson-Marks, S. Nakayiwa, B. Namande, L. Nakyobe, and R. Mukasa. 1993. "Anthropology and AIDS: The Cultural Context of Sexual Risk Behaviour among Urban Baganda Women in Kampala, Uganda." *Social Science & Medicine* 36: 429–439.

McGraw, Sarah, Kevin Smith, Jean Schensul, and J. Emilio Carillo. 1991. Sociocultural factors associated with smoking behavior by Puerto Rican adolescents in Boston. *Social Science & Medicine* 33: 1355–1364.

McKinlay, John B. 1976. "The Changing Political and Economic Content of the Patient-Physician Encounter." In *The Doctor–Patient Relationship in the Changing Health Scene* (DHEW Pub. No. [NIH] 78-183), ed. Eugene B. Gallagher, 155–188. Washington, DC: U.S. Government Printing Office.

McKinlay, John B., and Joan Arches. 1985. "Towards the Proletarianization of Physicans." *International Journal of Health Services* 15: 161–195.

McLaughlin, Andrew. 1990. "Ecology, Capitalism, and Socialism." *Socialism and Democracy* 10: 69–102.

McMichael, Anthony J. 1993. *Planetary Overload: Global Environmental Change and the Health of the Human Species.* Cambridge, UK: Cambridge University Press.

McMichael, A. J., and C. D. Butler. 2011. "Promoting Global Population Health While Constraining the Environmental Footprint." *Annual Review of Public Health* 32: 179–197.

McNeill, William. 1976. *Plagues and Peoples.* New York: Anchor Books.

Meadows, Donella, Dennis I., Jorgen Randers, and William H. Behrens, III. 1972. *The Limits to Growth.* New York: Universe Books.

Meadows, Donella, Dennis I., Jorgen Randers, and William H. Behrens, III. 2004. *The Limits to Growth: The 30-Year Update.* New York: Chelsea Green.

Mechanic, David. 1976. *The Growth of Bureaucratic Medicine.* New York: John Wiley and Sons.

Medicine, Beatrice. 2007. *Drinking and Sobriety among the Lakota Sioux*. Lanham, MA: AltaMira Press.

Mehrabadi, A. 2005. "Patients and Innovations in Biotechnology: From a Satellite Looking down at Our Use of Patients in the Great Planetary Scheme of Things." *Science Creative Quarterly* 1: 22–33.

Meier, Matt, and Rivera, Feliciano. 1972. *The Chicanos*. New York: Hill and Wang.

Melville, Kate. 2003. "Globally, 90% of Large Fish Are Gone." Available at: http://www.scienceagogo.com/news/20030414203530data_trunc_sys.shtml. Accessed July 19, 2012.

Mendenhall, Emily. 2011. *The VIDDA Syndemic: Distress and Diabetes in Social and Cultural Context*. PhD dissertation, Department of Anthropology, Northwestern University.

Mendenhall, Emily. 2012. *Syndemic Suffering: Social Distress, Depression, and Diabetes among Mexican American Women*. Walnut Creek, CA: Left Coast Press.

Mendelsohn, N. 2008. "A Different Face of Eating Disorders: Diabulimia." Available at: http://www.savvyhealth.com/disp.asp?doc_id=25. Accessed March 8, 2008.

Merchant, Carolyn. 1992. *Radical Ecology: The Search for a Livable World*. New York: Routledge.

Mering, Otto von. 1970. "Medicine and Psychiatry." In *Anthropology and the Behavioral and Health Sciences*, eds. Otto von Mering and Leonard Kasdan, 272–307. Pittsburgh, PA: University of Pittsburgh Press.

Merry, Sally, and Setha Low. 2010. "Engaged Anthropology: Diversity and Dilemmas." *Current Anthropology* 51(Suppl. 2): S203–S226.

Metraux, Alfred. 1972. *Voodoo in Haiti*. New York: Schocken Books.

Mettler, Fred. 2004. "Chernobyl's Living Legacy." *International Atomic Energy Agency Bulletin* 47/2. Available at: http://www.iaea.org/Publications/Magazines/Bulletin/Bull472/htmls/chernobyls_legacy2.html. Accessed July 18, 2012.

Metz, Bert. 2010. *Controlling Climate Change*. Cambridge, UK: Cambridge University Press.

Meyers, Carol. 2003. "International Commodity Markets, Local Land Markets and Class Conflict in a Provincial Mexican City." In *Wounded Cities: Destruction and Reconstruction in a Globalized World*, eds. Jane Schneider and Ida Susser, 71–91. New York: Berg.

Michaelson, Karen L., ed. 1988. *Childbirth in America: Anthropological Perspectives*. South Hadley, MA: Bergin & Garvey.

Micozzi, Marc S., ed. 2007. *Fundamentals of Complementary and Alternative Medicine*, 3rd ed. New York: Churchill Livingstone.

Miles, Anne. 1998. "Science, Nature, and Tradition: The Mass-Marketing of Natural Medicine in Urban Ecuador." *Medical Anthropology Quarterly* 12: 206–225.

Miliband, Ralph. 1994. *Socialism for a Skeptical Age*. London: Courage Press.

Milkman, Ruth. 1987. *Gender at Work*. Urbana: University of Illinois Press.

Miller, Barbara D. 2000. "Female Infanticide and Child Neglect in Rural North India." In *Gender in Cross-Cultural Perspective*, eds. Caroline Brettel and Carolyn Sargent, 492–507. Upper Saddle River, NJ: Prentice-Hall.

Miller, C., E. Wood, P. Spittal, K. Li, J. Frankish, P. Braitstein, J. Montaner, and M. Schechter. 2004. "The Future Face of Coinfection: Prevalence and Incidence of HIV and Hepatitis C Virus Coinfection among Young Injection Drug Users." *Journal of Acquired Immune Deficiency Syndrome* 36: 743–749.

Mills, C. Wright. 1959. *The Sociological Imagination*. New York: Grove Press.

Millstein, Bobby. 2001. *Introduction to the Syndemics Prevention Network*. Atlanta, GA: Centers for Disease Control and Prevention.

Miner, Horace. 1979. "Body Ritual among the Nacirema." In *Culture, Curers and Contagion*, ed. Norman Klein, 9–14. Novato, CA: Chandler and Sharp.

Mintz, Sidney. 1985. *Sweetness and Power*. New York: Penguin Books.

Moerman, Daniel E. 1979. "Anthropology of Symbolic Healing." *Current Anthropology* 20: 59–80.

Mohan, S., A. S. Pradeepkumar, C. U. Thresia, K. R. Thankappan, W. S. Poston, C. K. Haddock, et al. 2006. "Tobacco Use among Medical Professionals in Kerala, India: The Need for Enhanced Tobacco Cessation and Control Efforts." *Addictive Behaviors* 31: 2313–2318.

Molina, R., L. Gradoni, and J. Alvar. 2003. "HIV and the Transmission of Leishmania." *Annals of Tropical Medicine and Parasitology* 97(Suppl. 1): S29–S45.

Montaigne, Fen. 2007, April. "Still Waters, the Global Fish Crises." *National Geographic*. Available at: http://ngm.nationalgeographic.com/2007/04/global-fisheries-crisis/montaigne-text. Accessed February 8, 2013.

Montgomery, Scott L. 2010. *The Powers That Be: Global Energy for the Twenty-First Century and Beyond*. Chicago: University of Chicago Press.

Morens, David M., and Anthony S. Fauci. 2007. "The 1918 Influenza Pandemic: Insights for the 21st Century." *Journal of Infectious Diseases*, 195: 1018–1028.

Morgan, Lynn M. 1987. "Dependency Theory in the Political Economy of Health: An Anthropological Critique." *Medical Anthropology Quarterly*, n.s., 1: 131–155.

Morgen, Sandra, and Jeff Maskovsky. 2003. "The Anthropology of Welfare Reform." *Annual Review of Anthropology* 32: 315–338.

Morgen, Sandra. 1987. "'It's the Whole Power of the City Against Us!': The Development of Political Consciousness in a Women's Health Care Coalition." In *Women and the Politics of Empowerment*, eds. Ann Bookman and Sandra Morgen, 97–105. Philadelphia: Temple University Press.

Morgen, Sandra. 2002. *Into Our Own Hands: The Women's Health Movement in the United States, 1969–1990*. New Brunswick, NJ: Rutgers University Press.

Morley, Peter. 1978. "Culture and the Cognitive World of Traditional Medical Beliefs: Some Preliminary Considerations." In *Culture and Curing: Anthropological Perspectives on Traditional Medical Beliefs and Practices*, eds. Peter Morley and Roy Wallis, 1–18. Pittsburgh: University of Pittsburgh Press.

Morris, Brian. 2011. "Medical Herbalism in Malawi." *Medical Anthropology* 18: 245–255.

Morrow, Carol Tupperman. 2003. "Sick Doctors: The Social Construction of Professional Deviance." In *Health and Health Care as Social Problems*, eds. Peter Conrad and Valerie Letter, 297–316. Toronto, Canada: Rowann and Lexington.

Morse, Stephen. 1992. "AIDS and Beyond: Defining the Rules for Viral Traffic." In *AIDS: The Making of a Chronic Disorder*, eds. Elizabeth Fee and Daniel Fox, 23–48. Berkeley: University of California Press.

Morse, David. 2005. *War of the Future: Oil Drives the Genocide in Darfur*. Common Dreams. Available at: http://www.commondreams.org/views05/0819-26.htm. Accessed July 12, 2012.

Morsy, Soheir. 1979. "The Missing Link in Medical Anthropology: The Political Economy of Health." *Reviews in Anthropology* 6: 349–363.

Morsy, Soheir. 1990. "Political Economy in Medical Anthropology." In *Medical Anthropology: Contemporary Theory and Method*, eds. Thomas M. Johnson and Carolyn F. Sargent, 26–46. New York: Praeger.

Moss, A. 2000. "Epidemiology and the Politics of Needle Exchange." *American Journal of Public Health* 90: 1385–1387.

Muir, John. 1911. *My First Summer in the Sierra*. Boston: Houghton Mifflin.

Mullings, Leith. 2003. "After Drugs and the 'War on Drugs': Reclaiming the Power to Make History in Harlem, New York." In *Wounded Cities: Destruction and Reconstruction in a Globalized World*, eds. Jane Schneider and Ida Susser, 173–203. New York: Berg.

Mullings, Leith, and Alika Wali. 2001. *Stress and Resilience: The Social Context of Reproduction in Central Harlem*. New York: Kluwer Academic Press.

Murdock, George Peter. 1980. *Theories of Illness: A World Survey*. Pittsburgh, PA: University of Pittsburgh Press.

Murphy, Jane. 1964. "Psychotherapeutic Aspects of Shamanism on St. Lawrence Island, Alaska." In *Magic, Faith, and Healing*, ed. Ari Kiev, 53–83. New York: Free Press.

Murphy, Pat. 2008. *Plan C: Community Survival Strategies for Peak Oil and Climate Change*. Gabriola Island, Canada: New Society.

Mustanski, Brian, Robert Garofalo, Amy Herrick, and Geri Donenberg. 2007. "Psychosocial Health Problems Increase Risk for HIV among Urban Young Men Who Have Sex with Men: Preliminary Evidence of a Syndemic in Need of Attention." *Annals of Behavioral Medicine* 34: 37–45.

Myers, R., J. Baum, T. Shepherd, S. Powers, and C. Peterson. 2007. "Cascading Effects of the Loss of Apex Predatory Sharks from a Coastal Ocean. *Science* 315: 1846–1850.

Myers, Ransom, and Worm, Boris. 2003. "Rapid Worldwide Depletion of Predatory Fish Communities." *Nature* 423: 280–283.

Naraindas, Harish, and Christiana Bastos. 2011. "Healing Holidays? Itinerant Patients, Therapeutic Locales, and the Quest for Health." *Medical Anthropology* 18: 1–6.

National Council of Research on Women. 2004. *Missing: Information about Women's Lives* (pp. 1–24). New York: National Council for Research on Women.

National Geographic. September 2004. "Global Warming: Bulletin from a Warmer World." Washington, DC: National Geographic Society.

National Science Foundation. 1998. "Nature's Complex." Available at: http://www.nsf.gov/news/frontiers_archive/5-98/5nature.jsp. Accessed July 14, 2012.

NOAA National Climatic Data Center. 2012. State of the Climate: National Overview for Annual 2012. http:ncdc.noaa.gov/sotc/national/2012/2012/13.

Navarro, Vincente. 1976. *Medicine under Capitalism*. New York: Prodist.

Navarro, Vincente. 1986. *Crisis, Health and Medicine: A Social Critique*. New York: Tavistock.

Navarro, Vincente. 1994. *The Politics of Health Policy: The US Reforms, 1980–1994.* Oxford: Blackwell.

Navarro, Vincente. 1995. "Enact Health Care Reform." *Journal of Health Politics, Policy and Law* 20: 455–462.

Navarro, Vincente. 2011. "Why We Don't Spend Enough on Public Health: An Alternative View." *International Journal of Health Services* 41: 117–120.

Needle, Richard, Susan Coyle, Helen Cesari, Robert Trotter, Michael Clatts, Stephen Koester, and Laurie Price. 1998. "HIV Risk Behaviors Associated with the Injection Process: Multiperson Use of Drug Injection Equipment and Paraphernalia in Injection Drug User Networks." *Substance Use and Misuse* 33: 2403–2423.

Nellemann, Christian, Stefan Hain, and Jackie Alder, eds. 2008. *In Dead Water—Merging of Climate Change with Pollution, Over-Harvest, and Infestations in the World's Fishing Grounds.* Arendal, Norway: United Nations Environment Programme.

New York Times. 2012. "More Children in Homeless Shelters." September 26, 2012: A26.

Ngokwey, N. 1987. "Varieties of Palm Wine among the Lele of Kasai." In *Constructive Drinking: Perspectives on Drink from Anthropology,* ed. Mary Douglas, 113–120. New York: Routledge.

Nichter, Mark. 2003. "Smoking: What Does Culture Have to Do With It?" *Addiction* 98(Suppl. 1): 139–145.

Nichter, Mark. 2006. "Introducing Tobacco Cessation in Developing Countries: An Overview of Project Quit Tobacco International." *Tobacco Control* 15(Suppl. 1): i12–i17.

Nichter, Mark. 2008. *Global Health: Why Cultural Perceptions, Social Representations, and Biopolitics Matter.* Tucson: University of Arizona Press.

Nichter, Mark, and Elizabeth Cartwright. 1991. "Saving the Children for the Tobacco Industry." *Medical Anthropology* 5: 236–256.

Nichter, Mark, and Mimi Nichter. 1991. Hype and weight. *Medical Anthropology* 13: 249–271.

Nichter, Mark, Mimi Nichter, and David Van Sickle. 2004. "Popular Perceptions of Tobacco Products and Patterns of Use among Male College Students in India." *Social Science and Medicine* 59: 415–431.

Nichter, Mark, Mimi Nichter, Pamela J. Thompson, Saul Shiffman, and Anna-Barbara Moscicki. 2002. Using qualitative research to inform survey development on nicotine dependence among adolescents. *Drug and Alcohol Dependence* 68: S41–S56.

NIH News. 2012. "NIH-Funded Study Finds High HIV Infection Rates among Gay and Bisexual Black Men in the U.S." Available at: http://www.niaid.nih.gov/news/newsreleases/2012/Pages/HPTN061.aspx. Access July 27, 2012.

Nordstrom, Carolyn. 1996. "Rape: Politics and Theory in War and Peace." *Australian Feminist Studies* 11: 147–162.

Nordstrom, Carolyn. 1997. *A Different Kind of War Story.* Philadelphia: University of Pennsylvania Press.

Nordstrom, Carolyn. 1998. "Terror Warfare and the Medicine of Peace." *Medical Anthropology Quarterly* 12(1): 103–121.

Noymer, A., and M. Garenne. 2000. "The 1918 Influenza Epidemic's Effects on Sex Differentials in Mortality in the United States." *Population Development Review* 26: 565–581.

Nunn, John Francis. 1996. *Ancient Egyptian Medicine*. Norman: University of Oklahoma Press.

Nuttall, Mark. 2009. "Living in a World of Movement: Human Resilience to Environmental Instability in Greenland." In *Anthropology and Climate Change: From Encounters to Actions*, eds. Susan Crate and Mark Nuttall, 292–310. Walnut Creek, CA: Left Coast Press.

Nyamnjoh, Francis. 2002. "'A Child Is One Person's Only in the Womb': Domestication, Agency and Subjectivity in the Cameroonian Grassfields." In *Postcolonial Subjectivities in Africa*, ed. Richard Werbner, 111–139. New York: Zed Books.

O'Connor, James. 1989. "The Political Economy of Ecology of Socialism and Capitalism." *Capitalism, Nature, Socialism* 3: 93–127.

Officer, Charles, and Jake Page. 2009. *When the Planet Rages: Natural Disasters, Global Warming, and the Future of the Earth*. Oxford, UK: Oxford University Press.

Ohnuki-Tierney, Emiko. 1980. "Shamans and Imu among Two Ainu Groups: Toward a Cross-Cultural Model of Interpretation." *Ethos* 8: 204–228.

Ohnuki-Tierney, Emiko. 1984. *Illness and Culture in Contemporary Japan*. Cambridge, UK: Cambridge University Press.

Oliver, Douglas. 1961. *The Pacific Islands*. Garden City, NY: Anchor Books.

Olivier, M., R. Bararo, F. Medrano, and J. Moreno. 2003. "The Pathogenesis of Leishmania/HIV Co-infection: Cellular and Immunological Mechanisms." *Parasitology* 97(Suppl. 1): S79–S98.

Olshansky, S. Jay, Toni Antonucci, Lisa Berkman, Robert H. Binstock, Axel Boersch-Supan, John T. Cacioppo, et al. 2012. "Differences in Life Expectancy Due to Race and Educational Differences Are Widening, and Many May Not Catch Up." *Health Affairs (Millwood)* 31: 1803–1813.

Omidian, Patricia, and Kevin Miller. 2006. "Addressing the Psychosocial Needs of Women in Afghanistan." *Critical Half* 4: 17–21.

Ong, Aihwa. 1987. *Spirits of Resistance and Capitalist Discipline*. Albany: State University of New York Press.

Onoge, Omafume F. 1975. "Capitalism and Public Health: A Neglected Theme in the Medical Anthropology of Africa." In *Topias and Utopias*, eds. Stanley R. Ingman and Anthony E. Thomas, 219–232. The Hague: Mouton.

Oreskes, Naomi. 2004. "The Scientific Consensus on Climate Change." *Science* 306: 1686.

Oreskes, Naomi, and Erik Conway. 2010. *Merchants of Doubt: How a Handful of Scientists Obscured the Truth on Issues from Tobacco Smoke to Global Warming*. New York: Bloomsbury Press.

Oths, Kathryn. 1999. "Debilidad: A Biocultural Assessment of an Embodied Andean Illness." *Medical Anthropology Quarterly* 13: 286–315.

Ouellet, Lawrence, Wayne Weibel, and Antonio Jimenez. 1995. "Team Research Methods for Studying Intranasal Heroin Use and Its HIV Risks." In *Qualitative Methods in Drug Abuse and HIV Research*, eds. E. Lambert, R. S. Ashery, and R. H. Needle (NIDA Research Monograph #157; NIH Pub. No. 95-4025). Washington, DC: U.S. Govt. Printing Office.

Page, J. Bryan. 1999. "Historical Overview of Other Abusable Drugs." In *Prevention and Societal Impact of Drug and Alcohol Abuse,* eds. R. Ammerman, P. Ott, and R. Tarter, 47–63. Mahwah, NJ: Erlbaum.

Page, J. Bryan. 2011. "Anthropology and the Study of Illicit Drug Use." In *A Companion to Medical Anthropology,* eds. Merrill Singer and Pamela E. Erickson, 357–377. Malden, MA: Wiley-Blackwell.

Page, J. Bryan, and Sian Evans. 2003. "Cigars, Cigarillos, and Youth: Emergent Patterns of Subcultural Complexes." *Journal of Ethnicity in Substance Abuse* 2: 63–76.

Page, J. Bryan, Prince C. Smith, and Normie Kane. 1990. "Shooting Galleries, Their Proprietors, and Implications for Prevention of AIDS." *Drugs and Society* 5: 69–85.

Page, J. Bryan, and Merrill Singer. 2010. *Comprehending Drug Use: Ethnographic Research at the Social Margins.* New Brunswick, NJ: Rutgers University Press.

Panayotakis, Costas. 2006. "Working More, Selling More, Consuming More: Capitalism's 'Third Contradiction'." In *Coming to Terms with Nature,* eds. Leo Panitch and Colin Leys, 254–272. London: Merlin Press.

Pandolfi, Mariella, and Deborah Gordon. 1986. "Italy." *Medical Anthropology Quarterly,* o.s., 17(4): 90.

Panter-Brick, Catherine. 2010. "Conflict, Violence, and Health: Setting a New Interdisciplinary Agenda." *Social Science and Medicine* 70: 1–6.

Pappas, Gregory. 2010. "Pakistan's Hygiene Hijinks." *Anthropology Now* 2: 140–147.

Pappas, Gregory, Susan Queen, Wilbur Hadden, and Gail Fisher. 1993. "The Increasing Disparity of Mortality between Socio-Economic Groups in the United States, 1960–86." *New England Journal of Medicine* 329: 103–109.

Parenti, Michael. 1980. *Democracy for the Few.* New York: St. Martin's Press.

Park, Julie, and Ruth Fitzgerald. 2011. "Biotechnologies of Care." In *A Companion to Medical Anthropology,* eds. Merrill Singer and Pamela I. Erickson, 425–441. Malden, MA: Wiley-Blackwell.

Parker, Richard, and Peter Aggleton. 2003. "HIV and AIDS-Related Stigma and Discrimination: A Conceptual Framework and Implications for Action." *Social Science & Medicine,* 57: 13–24.

Parkinson, Stuart. 2007. "Guns and Global Warming: War, Peace and the Environment." Web version of presentation given at the Network for Peace AGM, London, February, Scientists for Global Responsibility. Available at: http://www.sgr.org.uk/resources/guns-and-global-warming-war-peace-and-environment.

Parsons, Howard L., ed. 1977. *Marx and Engels on Ecology.* Westport, CT: Greenwood.

Partridge, William. 1985. "Toward a Theory of Practice." *American Behavioral Scientist* 29: 139–163.

Partridge, William L. 1987. "Toward a Theory of Practice." In *Applied Anthropology in America,* eds. Elizabeth M. Eddy and William L. Partridge, 211–233. New York: Columbia University Press.

Patterson, Matthew. 2007. *Automobile Politics: Ecology and Cultural Political Economy.* Cambridge, UK: Cambridge University Press.

Paul, Benjamin. 1969. "Anthropological Perspectives on Medicine and Public Health." In *Cross-Cultural Approach to Health Behavior,* ed. R. Lynch, 26–42. Madison, NJ: Fairleigh Dickinson University Press.

Paul, James A. 1978. "Medicine and Imperialism." In *The Cultural Crisis of Modern Medicine*, ed. John Ehrenreich, 271–286. New York: Monthly Review Press.

Pawlowski, A., M. Jansson, M. Sköld, M. Rottenberg, and G. Källenius. 2012. "Tuberculosis and HIV Co-Infection." *PLoS Pathog* 8: e1002464. Available at: http://www.plospathogens.org/article/info%3Adoi%2F10.1371%2Fjournal.ppat.1002464. Accessed February 15, 2013.

Payer, Lynn. 1988. *Medicine and Culture: Varieties of Treatment in the United States, England, West Germany and France.* New York: Henry Holt.

Pearce, Fred. 2006. *The Last Generation: How Nature Will Take Her Revenge for Climate Change.* London: Transworld.

Peattie, Lisa. 1984. "Normalizing the Unthinkable." *Bulletin of the Atomic Scientists* 40: 32–56.

Peck, Jamie A., and Adam Tickell. 2002. "Neoliberalizing Space: The Free Economy and the Penal State." In *Spaces of Neoliberalism: Urban Restructuring in North America and Western Europe* (Antipode Book Series), eds. Neil Brenner and Nik Theodore, 380–404. Oxford: Blackwell.

Pederson, Duncan. 2006. "Reframing Political Violence and Mental Health Outcomes: Outlining a Research and Action Agenda for Latin America and the Caribbean Region." *Ciência & Saúde Coletiva* 11: 293–302.

People's Health Movement 2005. *Global Health Watch 2005–2006.* London: Zed Books.

Pepin, Jacques. 2012. *The Origins of AIDS.* Cambridge, UK: Cambridge University Press.

Perera, Liz. 2011, Fall. "Climate Change May Be Hazardous to Your Health." *Catalyst.* Union of Concerned Scientists. Available at: http://www.ucsusa.org/publications/catalyst/fall11-climate-change-health.html. Accessed January 27, 2013.

Perez, Christina. 2008. *Caring for Them from Birth to Death: The Practice of Community-Based Cuban Medicine.* Lanham, MD: Lexington Books.

Permanent Secretariat of Nobel Peace Laureates Summits. 2009. *Charter for a World Without Violence.* Available at: http://www.nobelforpeace-summits.org/wp-content/uploads/2009/07/charter-EN1.pdf. Accessed December 30, 2009.

Petchesky, Rosalind P. 2000. "Sexual Rights: Inventing a Concept, Mapping an International Practice." In *Framing the Sexual Subject: The Politics of Gender, Sexuality, and Power*, eds. Richard Parker, Regina Maria Barbosa, and Peter Aggleton, 81–104. Berkeley: University of California Press.

Petchesky, Rosalind Pollack. 2003. *Global Prescriptions: Gendering Health and Human Rights.* London: Zed Books.

Petryna, Adriana. 2002. *Life Exposed: Biological Citizens after Chernobyl.* Princeton, NJ: Princeton University Press.

Pfeiderer, Beatrix, and Wolfgang Bichman. 1986. Germany. *Medical Anthropology Quarterly* 17: 89–90.

Pfeiffer, James, and Mark Nichter. 2008. "What Can Critical Medical Anthropology Contribute to Global Health? A Health Systems Perspective." *Medical Anthropology Quarterly* 22: 410–415.

Pilote, Louise, Robert M. Califf, Shelly Sapp, Dave P. Miller, Daniel B. Mark, W. Douglas Weaver et al. 1999. "Regional Variation across the United States in the Management of Acute Myocardial Infarction." *New England Journal of Medicine* 333: 565–572.

Pine, Adrien. 2008. *Working Hard, Drinking Hard*. Berkeley: University of California Press.

Piot, Peter. 2001. "A Gendered Epidemic: Women and the Risks and Burdens of HIV." *Journal of the American Medical Women's Association* 56: 90–91.

Pittock, A. Barrie. 2008. "Ten Reasons Why Climate Change May Be More Severe than Projected." In *Sudden and Disruptive Climate Change: Exploring the Real Risks and How We Can Avoid Them*, eds. By Michael C. McCracken, Frances Moore, and John C. Topping, Jr., 11–27. London: Earthscan.

Piven, Frances, and Richard Cloward. 1971. *Regulating the Poor*. New York: Vintage.

Pollack, Donald. 1992. "Culina Shamanism: Gender, Power, and Knowledge." In *Portals of Power: Shamanism in South America*, eds. E. Langdon, Jean Matteson, and Gerhard Baer, 25–40. Albuquerque: University of New Mexico Press.

Poole, Robert, and Wenzel Gessler. 2005. *Medical Anthropology: Understanding Public Health*. Maidenhead, UK: Open University Press.

Preble, Edward, and John J. Casey. 1969. "Taking Care of Business: The Heroin User's Life on the Streets." *International Journal of the Addictions* 15: 329–337.

Preston, Richard. 1994. *The Hot Zone*. New York: Random House Publishers.

Prussing, Erica. 2011. *White Man's Water: The Politics of Sobriety in a Native American Community*. Tucson: University of Arizona Press.

Queeley, Andrea. 2011. "She jes' gits hold of us dataway": The Greens and Blues of Neighborhood Recovery in Post-Katrina New Orleans." *Transforming Anthropology* 19: 21–32.

Quinlan, Marsha B. 2011. "Ethnomedicine." In *A Companion to Medical Anthropology*, eds. Merrill Singer and Pamela I. Erickson, 381–403. San Francisco: Wiley-Blackwell.

Quintero, Gilbert, and Sally M. Davis. 2002. "Why Do Teens Smoke? American Indian and Hispanic Adolescent's Perspectives on Functionalist Values and Addiction." *Medical Anthropology Quarterly* 16: 439–457.

Quintero, Gilbert, and Mark Nichter. 2011. "Generation RX: Anthropological Research on Pharmaceutical Enhancement, Lifestyle Regulation, Self-Medication, and Recreational Drug Use." In *A Companion to Medical Anthropology*, eds. Merrill Singer and Pamela I. Erickson, 339–355. Malden, MA: Wiley-Blackwell.

Raffel, Marshall W., and Norma K. Raffel. 1994. *The U.S. Health System: Origins and Functions*, 4th ed. Albany, NY: Delmar.

Raikhel, Eugene. 2009. "Institutional Encounters: Identification and Anonymity in Russian Addiction Treatment (and Ethnography)." In *Being There: The Fieldwork Encounter and the Making of Truth*, eds. John Borneman and Abdella Hammoudi, 201–236. Berkeley: University of California Press.

Rakel, David, and Andrew Weil. 2003. "Philosphy of Integrative Medicine." In *Integrative Medicine*, ed. David Rakel, 3–9. Philadelphia: Saunders.

Ramin, Brodie. 2007. "Anthropology Speaks to Medicine: The Case of HIV/AIDS in Africa." *McGill Journal of Medicine* 10: 127–132.

Raphael, Dennis. 2006. "Social Determinants of Health: Present Status, Unanswered Questions, and Future Directions." *International Journal of Health Services* 36: 651–677.

Rapp, Rayna. 2000. *Testing Women, Testing the Fetus: The Social Impact of Amniocentesis in America*. New York: Routledge.

Reichard, Gladys. 1950. *Navaho Religion: A Study of Symbolism*. New York: Stratford Press.

Reid, Janice. 1983. *Sorcerers and Healing Spirits: Continuity and Change in an Aboriginal Community*. Canberra, Australian Capital Territory: Australian National University Press.

Reid, T. R. 2009. *The Healing of America: A Global Quest for Better, Cheaper, and Fairer Health Care*. New York: Penguin Press.

Reiter, Rayna Rapp, ed. 1975. *Toward an Anthropology of Women*. New York: Monthly Review Press.

Reitmanova, S., and D. Gustafson. 2012. "Coloring the White Plague: A Syndemic Approach to Immigrant Tuberculosis in Canada." *Ethnicity and Health* 17: 403–418.

Renner, Michael. 1997. "Environmental and Health Effects of Weapons Production, Testing, and Maintenance." In *War and Public Health,* eds. Barry S. Levy and Victor W. Sidel, 117–136. New York: Oxford University Press.

Resistance. 1999. *Environment, Capitalism & Socialism*. Sydney: Resistance Books.

Reynolds, Vernon, and Ralph Tanner. 1995. *The Social Ecology of Religion*. New York: Oxford University Press.

Rheinberger, Hans-Jörg. 1997. *Toward a History of Epistemic Things: Synthesizing Proteins in the Test Tube*. Stanford, CA: Stanford University Press.

Rhodes, Lorna. 2004. *Total Confinement*. Berkeley: University of California Press.

Rhodes, Nancy, David R. Roskos-Ewoldsen, Aime Edison, and Mary Beth Bradford. 2008. "Attitude and norm accessibility affect processing of anti-smoking messages." *Health Psychology* 29(Suppl. 3): S224–S232.

Ribera, Joan Muela, and Susanna Hausmann-Muela. 2011. "The Straw That Breaks the Camel's Back: Redirecting Health-Seeking Behavior Studies on Malaria Vulnerability." *Medical Anthropology Quarterly* 25: 103–121.

Richman, Douglas, David Margolis, Martin Delany, Warner Greene, Daria Hazuda, and Roger Pomerantz. 2009. "The Challenge of Finding a Cure for HIV Infection." *Science* 323: 1304–1307.

Richter, Burton. 2010. *Beyond Smoke and Mirrors: Climate Change and Energy in the 21st Century*. Cambridge, UK: Cambridge University Press.

Ripinsky-Naxon, Michael. 1993. *The Nature of Shamanism: Substance and Function of a Religious Meta*. Albany: State University of New York Press.

Rittenbaugh, Cheryl. 1991. "Body Size and Shape: A Dialogue of Culture and Biology." *Medical Anthropology* 13: 173–180.

Rivers, W. H. R. 1924. *Medicine, Magic, and Religion*. London: Kegan, Paul, Trench, Trubner.

Robb, J. 1986. "Smoking as an Anticipatory Rite of Passage: Some Sociological Hypotheses on Health-Related Behaviour." *Social Science and Medicine* 23: 621–627.

Robbins, Richard. 2002. *Global Problems and the Culture of Capitalism*. Boston: Allyn and Bacon.

Robert Wood Johnson Foundation and State Health Access Data Assistance Center. 2011. "State-Level Trends in Employer-Sponsored Health Insurance." Available at: http://www.rwjf.org/files/research/72528shadac201106.pdf.

Roberts, J. Timmons, and Bradley C. Parks. 2007. *A Climate of Injustice: Global Inequality, North-South Politics, and Climate Policy.* Cambridge, MA: MIT Press.

Roberts, J. Timmons, Peter E. Grimes, and Jodie L. Manale. 2003. "Social Roots of Global Environmental Change: A World-Systems Analysis of Carbon Dioxide Emissions." *Journal of World-Systems Research* 9: 227–315.

Robotham, Don. 2009. "Liberal Social Democracy, Neo-Liberalism and Neo-Conservatism: Some Genealogies." In *Rethinking America,* eds. Jeff Maskovsky and Ida Susser. Boulder, CO: Paradigm.

Rock, Melanie, Bonnie Buntain, Jennifer Hatfield, and Benedikt Hallgrimsson. 2009. "Animal-Human Connections, 'One Health,' and the Syndemic Approach to Prevention." *Social Science & Medicine* 68: 991–995.

Rodberg, Leonard S. 1994. "Anatomy of a National Health Program: Reconsidering the Dellums Bill after 10 Years." In *Beyond Crisis: Confronting Health Care in the United States,* ed. Nancy F. McKenzie, 610–615. New York: Meridian.

Rogers, Spencer L. 1982. *The Shaman: His Symbols and His Healing Power.* Springfield, IL: Charles C Thomas.

Rogers, Stephanie. 2011. *Top 10 American Global Warming Deniers.* Ecosalon. Available at: http://ecosalon.com/top-10-american-global-warming-deniers-292. Accessed July 20, 2012.

Romanucci-Ross, Lola. 1977. "The Hierarchy of Resort in Curative Practices: The Admiralty Islands, Melanesia." In *Culture, Disease, and Healing: Studies in Medical Anthropology,* ed. David Landy, 481–487. New York: Macmillan.

Room, Robin. 1984. "Alcohol and Ethnography: A Case of Problem Deflation?" *Current Anthropology* 25: 169–178.

Rosa, Eugene A., and Thomas Dietz. 2010. "Global Transformations: Passage to a New Ecological Era." In *Human Footprints on the Gobal Environment: Threats to Sustainability,* eds. Eugene A. Rosa, Andreas Dielmannn, Thomas Dietz, and Carlo Jaeger, 1–45. Cambridge, MA: MIT Press.

Roseman, Marina. 1991. *Healing Sounds from the Malaysian Rainforest: Temiar Music and Medicine.* Berkeley: University of California Press.

Rosenthal, Marilynn M. 1992. "Modernization and Health Care in the People's Republic of China: The Period of Transition." In *Health Care Systems and Their Patients: An International Perspective,* eds. Marilynn M. Rosenthal and Marcel Frenkel, 293–315. Boulder, CO: Westview Press.

Rothstein, Frances. 1982. *Three Different Worlds: Women, Men and Children in an Industrializing Community.* Westport, CT: Greenwood Press.

Rothstein, Frances. 2007. *Globalization in Rural Mexico: Three Decades of Change.* Austin: University of Texas Press.

Roy, Anupom. 2012. "Tobacco Consumption and the Poor: An Ethnographic Analysis of Hand-Rolled Cigarette (*Bidi*) Use in Bangladesh." *Ethnography* 13: 162–188.

Rubin, Gayle. 1975. "The Traffic in Women: Notes on a 'Political Economy' of Sex." In *Toward an Anthropology of Women,* ed. Rayna Rapp Reiter, 157–210. New York: Monthly Review Press.

Ruddiman, William F. 2005. *Plows, Plagues and Petroleum: How Humans Took Control of Climate*. Princeton, NJ: Princeton University Press.

Rudowitz, Robin, Diane Rowland, and Adele Shartzer. 2006. "Health Care in New Orleans before and after Katrina." *Health Affairs* 25: 393–406.

Rumble, Eric. 2006. "Explaining National Climate Change Policies." *Global Environmental Change* 5: 235–249.

Ruppert, Michael C. 2009. *Confronting Collapse: The Crisis of Energy and Money in a Post Peak Oil Change—A 25-Point Program for Action*. White River Junction, VT: Chelsea Green.

Ruyle, Eugene. 1977. "A Socialist Alternative for the Future." In *Cultures of the Future*, eds. Magorah Maruyma and Arthur M. Harkins, 613–628. The Hague: Mouton.

Rwabukwali, Charles. 2008. "Gender, Poverty, and AIDS Risk: Case Studies from Rural Uganda." In *AIDS, Culture, and Africa*, ed. Douglas A. Feldman, 239–254. Gainesville: University Press of Florida.

Rylko-Bauer, Barbara, and Merrill Singer. 2011. "Political Violence, War and Medical Anthropology." In *A Companion to Medical Anthropology*, eds. Merrill Singer and Pam Erickson, 219–249. San Francisco: Wiley.

Rylko-Bauer, Barbara, Merrill Singer, and John van Willigen. 2006. "Reclaiming Applied Anthropology: Its Past, Present, and Future." *American Anthropologist* 108: 178–190.

Sachs, Jeffrey D. 2008. *Common Wealth: Economics for a Crowded Planet*. New York: Allen Lane.

Sahlins, Marshall. 1972. *Stone Age Economics*. Chicago: Aldine.

Saillant, Francine and Serge Genest, eds. 2007. *Medical Anthropology: Regional Perspectives and Shared Concerns*. Malden, MA: Blackwell.

Saks, Michael. 1994. "The Alternatives to Medicine." In *Challenging Medicine*, eds. Jonathan Gabe, David Kelleher, and Gareth Williams, 84–102. London: Routledge.

Salkend, Ellen J. 2005. "Holistic Physicians' Clinical Discourse on Risk: An Ethnographic Study." *Medical Anthropology* 24: 325–347.

Sample, Ian. 2007. "Scientists Offered Cash to Dispute Climate Study." Available at: http://www.guardian.co.uk/environment/2007/feb/02/frontpagenews .climatechange. Accessed July 19, 2012.

Sanders, Barry. 2009. *The Green Zone: The Environmental Costs of Militarism*. Oakland, CA: AK Press.

Santa Barbara, Joanna. 2008. "The Impact of War on Children." In *War and Public Health*, eds. Barry Levy and Victor Sidel, 179–192. Washington, DC: American Public Health Association.

Santelli, John, Mary Ott, Maureen Lyon, Jennifer Rogers, Daniel Summers, and Rebecca Schliefer. 2006. "Abstinence and Abstinence-Only Education: A Review of US Policies and Programs." *Journal of Adolescent Health* 38: 72–87.

Sargent, Carolyn, and Thomas M. Johnson, eds. 1996. *Medical Anthropology and Contemporary Theory and Method*, rev. ed. Westport, CT: Praeger.

Sattenspiel, Lisa, and D. Ann Herring. 2010. "Emerging Themes in Anthropology and Epidemiology: Geographic Spread, Evolving Pathogens and

Syndemics." In *A Companion to Biological Anthropology,* eds. Clark Spencer Larsen, 167–178. Malden, MA: Wiley.

Sayers, Sean. 1998. *Marxism and Human Nature.* London: Routledge.

Scaruffi, Piero. 2009. "Wars and Genocides of the 20th Century." Available at: http://www.scaruffi.com/politics/massacre.html. Accessed January 18, 2012.

Schacker, T. 2001. "The Role of HSV in the Transmission and Progression of HIV." *Herpes* 8: 46–49.

Schanzer, Bella, Boanerges Dominguez, Patrick E. Shrout, and Carol L. M. Caton. 2007. "Homelessness, Health Status, and Health Care Use." *American Journal of Public Health* 97: 464–469.

Scheffler, Harold. 1991. "Sexism and Naturalism in the Study of Kinship." In *Gender at the Crossroads of Knowledge: Feminist Anthropology in the Postmodern Era,* ed. Micaela di Leonardo, 361–383. Berkeley, CA: University of California Press.

Schensul, Jean, Judith Levy, and William Disch. 2003. "Individual, Contextual, and Social Network Factors Affecting Exposure to HIV/AIDS Risk Among Older Residents Living in Low-Income Senior Housing Complexes." *Journal of Acquired Immune Deficiency Syndromes* 33(Suppl. 2): S138–S152.

Schensul, Jean, Margaret Weeks, and Merrill Singer. 1999. "Building Research Partnerships." In *Research Roles and Research Partnerships, Book 6, The Ethnographer's Toolkit,* eds. Margaret LeCompte, Jean Schensul, Margaret Weeks, and Merrill Singer, 85–164. Walnut Creek, CA: Altamira Press.

Schensul, Stephen L. 1980. "Anthropological Fieldwork and Sociopolitical Change." *Social Problems* 27: 309–319.

Schensul, Stephen L. 2011, March. "The Medical Anthropologist as Interventionist: Culturally-Based Approaches to Public Health Problems." *Anthropology News,* 41.

Scheper-Hughes, Nancy, and Margaret Lock, 1987. "The Mindful Body: A Prolegomenon to Future Work in Medical Anthropology." *Medical Anthropology Quarterly,* n.s., 1: 6–41.

Scheper-Hughes, Nancy. 1990. "Three Propositions for a Critically Applied Medical Anthropology." *Social Science and Medicine* 30: 189–197.

Scheper-Hughes, Nancy. 1992. *Death without Weeping: The Violence of Everyday Life.* Berkeley: University of California Press.

Scheper-Hughes, Nancy 1995. "The Primacy of the Ethical: Propositions for a Militant Anthropology." *Current Anthropology* 36: 409–420.

Scheper-Hughes, Nancy. 2000. "The Global Traffic in Organs." *Current Anthropology* 41: 191–224.

Scheper-Hughes, Nancy, and Margaret Lock. 1986. "Speaking 'Truth' to Illness: Metaphors, Reification, and a Pedagogy for Patients." *Medical Anthropology Quarterly,* o.s., 17(5): 137–140.

Schiff, Gordon. 2000. "Fatal Distraction: Finance Versus Vigilance in U.S. Hospitals." *International Journal of Health Services* 30: 739–743.

Schneider, David. 1968. *American Kinship: A Cultural Account.* Chicago: University of Chicago.

Schneider, David, and R. T. Smith. 1982. *Class Differences and Sex Roles in American Kinship and Family Structure.* Chicago: University of Chicago Press.

Schneider, Jane. 1971. "Of Vigilance and Virgins: Honor, Shame and Access to Resources in Mediterranean Societies." *Ethnology* 9: 1–24.

Schneider, Jane, and Ida Susser, eds. 2003. *Wounded Cities: Destruction and Reconstruction in a Globalized World*. New York: Berg.

Schneider, Jane, and Peter Schneider. 1996. *Festival of the Poor: Fertility Decline and the Ideology of Class in Sicily, 1860–1980*. Tucson: University of Arizona Press.

Schneider, Joseph W. 2001. "Family Care Work and Duty in a 'Modern' Chinese Hospital." In *Readings in Medical Sociology*, ed. Duanne A. Matcha, 354–371. Boston: Allyn and Bacon.

Schoepf, Brooke Grudfest. 1988. "Women, AIDS, and Economic Crisis in Central Africa." *Canadian Journal of African Studies* 22: 625–644.

Schoepf, Brooke Grundfest. 2004. "AIDS in Africa: Structure, Agency, and Risk." In: *HIV and AIDS in Africa: Beyond Epidemiology*, eds. Ezekiel Kalipeni, Susan Craddock, Joseph R. Oppong, and Jayati Ghosh, 121–131. Malden, MA: Blackwell.

Schoepf, Brooke, Claude Schoepf, and Joyce Millen. 2000. "Theoretical Perspectives, Remote Remedies: SAPs and the Political Ecology of Poverty and Health in Africa." In *Dying for Growth: Global Inequality and the Health of the Poor*, eds. Jim Kim, Joyce Millen, Alec Irwin, and John Gershman, 91–126. Monroe, ME: Common Courage Press.

Schor, Juliet. 2010. *Plentitude: The New Economics of True Wealth*. New York: Penguin.

Schwartz, Justin. 1991. "A Future for Socialism in the USSR." In *Communist Regimes—The Aftermath: The Socialist Register 1991*, eds. Ralph Miliband and Leo Panitch, 67–94. London: Merlin.

Scotch, Norman. 1963. "Medical Anthropology." In *Biennial Review of Anthropology*, ed. Bernard J. Siegel. Stanford, CA: Stanford University Press, 30–68.

Seaman, Gary, and Jane S. Day. 1994. *Ancient Traditions: Shamanism in Central Asia and the Americas*. Niwot: University Press of Colorado.

Seefeld, Andrew W., and Adam Landman. 2008. "Navigating the ER." *UCLA Magazine* 19(2): 16–17.

Segall, M. 1983. "On the Concept of a Socialist Health System: A Question of Marxist Epidemiology." *International Journal of Health Services* 13: 221–225.

Seppilli, Tullio. 2012. "Itineraries and Specificities of Italian Medical Anthropology." *Anthropology & Medicine* 19: 17–25.

Sexton, Randall, Ellen Anne Buljo Stabbursvik. 2010. "Healing in the Sámi North." *Culture, Medicine and Psychiatry* 34: 571–589.

Shannon, Thomas R. 1996. *An Introduction to the World-System Perspective*, 2nd ed. Boulder, CO: Westview Press.

Sharff, Jagna. 1998. *King Kong on 4th Street: Families and the Violence of Poverty on the Lower East Side*. Boulder, CO: Westview Press.

Sharon, Douglas. 1978. *Wizard of the Four Winds: A Shaman's Story*. New York: Free Press.

Sharp, Leslie A. A. 2006. *Strange Harvest: Organ Transplants, Denatured Bodies, and the Transformed Self*. Berkeley: University of California Press.

Shaw, Christopher. 2010. "Dangerous Limits: Climate Change and Modernity." In *History at the End of the World: History, Climate Change and the Possibility of Closure*, eds. Mark Levene, Rob Johnson, and Penny Roberts, 95–111. Penrith, UK: Humanities-Ebooks.

Shaw, Greg M. 2010. *The Health Care Debate: Controversial Issues in America*. Santa Barbara, CA: Greenwood Press.

Sherwin, Susan. 1992. *No Longer Patient: Feminist Ethics and Health Care*. Philadelphia: Temple University Press.

Sherwin, Susan. 1997. "Gender, Race, and Class in the Delivery of Health Care." In *Bioethics: An Introduction to the History, Methods, and Practice*, eds. Nancy S. Jecker, Albert R. Jonsen, and Robert A. Pearlman, 392–401. Boston: Jones and Bartlett.

Sherwood, Peter. 2004. "Evolution of Natural Medicine and Biomedicine and Their Future Roles in Health Care." PhD thesis, Faculty of Human Development, Victoria University, Melbourne.

Shilts, Randy. 1987. *And the Band Played On*. New York: St. Martin's Press.

Shiva, Vandana. 2008. *Soil Not Oil: Environmental Justice in an Age of Climate Crisis*. Boston: South End Press.

Sidel, Victor. 1978. "The Right to Health Care: An International Perspective." In *Bioethics and Human Rights: A Reader for Health Professionals*, eds. Elsie L. Bandman and Betram Bandman, 341–350. Boston: Little, Brown.

Shostak, Marjorie. 1981. *Nisa: The Life and Words of a !Kung Woman*. Cambridge, MA: Harvard University Press.

Sidel, Victor. 1994. "Health Care for a Nation in Need." In *Beyond Crisis: Confronting Health Care in the United States*, ed. Nancy F. McKenzie, 559–573. New York: Meridian.

Sidel, Victor W., and Ruth Sidel. 1982. *The Health of China*. Boston: Beacon Press.

Siegel, Ronald. 2005. *Intoxication: Life in the Pursuit of Artificial Paradise*. Rochester, VT: Park Street Press.

Silber, Irwin. 1994. *Socialism: What Went Wrong? An Inquiry into the Theoretical and Historical Sources of the Socialist Crisis*. London: Pluto Press.

Silverblatt, Irene. 1991. "Interpreting Women in States: New Feminist Ethnohistories." In *Gender at the Crossroads of Knowledge: Feminist Anthropology in the Postmodern Era*, ed. Micaela di Leonardo, 140–175. Berkeley: University of California Press.

Singer, Elyse, and Schensul, Jean. 2011. "Negotiating Ecstasy Risk, Reward, and Control: A Qualitative Analysis of Ecstasy-Using Urban Young Adults." *Substance Use & Misuse* 46: 1675–1689.

Singer, Merrill. 1986. "Toward a Political-Economy of Alcoholism: The Missing Link in the Anthropology of Drinking." *Social Science and Medicine* 23: 113–130.

Singer, Merrill. 1990. "Another Perspective on Advocacy." *Current Anthropology* 31: 548–549.

Singer, Merrill. 1992. "AIDS and U.S. Ethnic Minorities: The Crisis and Alternative Anthropological Responses." *Human Organization* 51: 89–95.

Singer, Merrill. 1994. "Community Centered Praxis: Toward an Alternative Non-dominative Applied Anthropology." *Human Organization* 53: 336–344.

Singer, Merrill. 1995a. "Beyond the Ivory Tower: Critical Praxis." *Medical Anthropology Quarterly*, n.s., 9: 80–106.

Singer, Merrill. 1995b. "Providing Substance Abuse Treatment to Puerto Rican Clients Living in the Continental U.S." In *Substance Abuse Treatment in the Era of AIDS*, Vol. 2. ed. Omowale Amuyleru-Marshal, 93–114. Rockville, MD: Center for Substance Abuse Treatment.

Singer, Merrill. 1996a. A dose of drugs, a touch of violence, a case of AIDS: Conceptualizing the SAVA syndemic. *Free Inquiry in Creative Sociology* 24: 99–110.

Singer, Merrill. 1996b. "Farewell to Adaptationism: Unnatural Selection and the Politics of Biology." *Medical Anthropology Quarterly*, 10: 496–575.

Singer, Merrill. 1998a. "The Development of Critical Medical Anthropology: Implications for Biological Anthropology." In *Building a New Biocultural Synthesis: Political-Economic Perspectives in Human Biology*, eds. Alan Goodman and Thomas Leatherman, 93–123. Ann Arbor: University of Michigan Press.

Singer, Merrill. 1998b. "Articulating Personal Experience and Political Economy in the AIDS Epidemic: The Case of Carlos Torres." In *The Political Economy of AIDS*, ed. Merrill Singer, 61–73. Amityville, NY: Baywood.

Singer, Merrill. 2000. "Introduction." *You Owe Yourself a Drunk,* ed. James Spradley, xiii–xxvii. Prospect Heights, IL: Waveland Press.

Singer, Merrill. 2003. "The Hispanic Health Council: An Experiment in Applied Anthropology." *Practicing Anthropology* 25(3): 2–7.

Singer, Merrill. 2006a. *Something Dangerous: Emergent and Changing Illicit Drug Use and Community Health*. Prospect Heights, IL: Waveland Press.

Singer, Merrill. 2006b. "A Dose of Drugs, a Touch of Violence, a Case of AIDS, Part 2: Further Conceptualizing the SAVA Syndemic." *Free Inquiry in Creative Sociology* 34(1): 39–56.

Singer, Merrill. 2008. *Drugging the Poor: Legal and Illegal Drug Industries and the Structuring of Social Inequality*. Prospect Heights, IL: Waveland Press.

Singer, Merrill. 2009a. *Introduction to Syndemics: A Systems Approach to Public and Community Health*. San Francisco, CA: Jossey-Bass.

Singer, Merrill. 2009b. "Desperate Measures: A Syndemic Approach to the Anthropology of Health in a Violent City." In *Global Health in the Time of Violence*, eds. Barbara Rylko-Bauer, Linda Whiteford, and Paul Farmer. Sante Fe, NM: SAR Press.

Singer, Merrill. 2009c. "Doorways in Nature: Syndemics, Zoonotics, and Public Health: A Commentary on Rock, Buntain, Hatfield & Hallgrímsson." *Social Science and Medicine* 68: 996–999.

Singer, Merrill. 2009d. "Pathogens Gone Wild?: Medical Anthropology and the 'Swine Flu' Pandemic." *Medical Anthropology* 28: 199–206.

Singer Merrill. 2009e. "Beyond Global Warming: Interacting Ecocrises and the Critical Anthropology of Health." *Anthropology Quarterly* 82:795-820.

Singer, Merrill. 2010a. "Atmospheric and Marine Pluralea Interactions and Species Extinction Risks." *Journal of Cosmology* 8: 1832–1837.

Singer, Merrill. 2010a. "Ecosyndemics: Global Warming and the Coming Plagues of the 21st Century." In *Plagues: Models and Metaphors in the Human 'Struggle' with Disease*, eds. D. Ann Herring and Alan C. Swedlund, 21–38. London: Berg.

Singer, Merrill. 2010b. "Pathogen-Pathogen Interaction: A Syndemic Model of Complex Biosocial Processes in Disease." *Virulence* 1(1): 10–18.

Singer, Merrill. 2011a. "Double Jeopardy: Vulnerable Children and the Possible Global Lead Poisoning/Infectious Disease Syndemic." In *Routledge Handbook in Global Health*, eds. Richard Parker and Marni Sommer, 154–161. New York: Routledge.

Singer, Merrill 2011b "Toward a Critical Biosocial Model of Ecohealth in Southern Africa: The HIV/AIDS and Nutrition Insecurity Syndemic." *Annals of Anthropology Practice* 35: 8–27.

Singer, Merrill. 1999. "Studying Hidden Populations." In *Mapping Networks, Spatial Data and Hidden Populations, Book 4, The Ethnographer's Toolkit*, 2nd ed., eds. Jean Schensul, Margaret LeCompte, Robert Trotter, Ellen Cromley, and Merrill Singer, 125–191. Walnut Creek, CA: Altamira Press.

Singer, Merrill, and Hans A. Baer. 1989. "Toward an Understanding of Capitalist and Socialist Health." *Medical Anthropology* 11: 99–109.

Singer, Merrill, and Hans A. Baer. 1995. *Critical Medical Anthropology*. Amityville, NY: Baywood Press.

Singer, Merrill, and Hans A. Baer. 2012. *Introducing Medical Anthropology: A Discipline in Action*. Lanham, MD: AltaMira Press.

Singer, Merrill, Hans A. Baer, and Ellen Lazarus, eds. 1990. *Critical Medical Anthropology: Theory and Research*. Special Issue of *Social Science and Medicine* 30(2).

Singer, Merrill, and Maria Borrero. 1984. "Indigenous Treatment for Alcoholism: The Case for Puerto Rican Spiritism." *Medical Anthropology* 8: 246–272.

Singer, Merrill, and Scott Clair. 2003. "Syndemics and Public Health: Reconceptualizing Disease in Bio-Social Context." *Medical Anthropology Quarterly* 17: 423–441.

Singer, Merrill, Lani Davison, and Gina Geddes. 1988. "Culture, Critical Theory and Reproductive Illness Behavior in Haiti." *Medical Anthropology Quarterly* 2: 370–385.

Singer, Merrill, and Pamela Erickson, eds. 2011. *A Companion to Medical Anthropology*. San Francisco: Wiley-Blackwell.

Singer, Merrill, Pamela Erickson, Louise Badiane, Rosemary Diaz, Dueidy Ortiz, Traci Abraham, and Anne Marie Nicolaysen. 2006. "Syndemics, Sex and the City: Understanding Sexually Transmitted Disease in Social and Cultural Context." *Social Science and Medicine* 63: 2010–2021.

Singer, Merrill, D. Ann Herring, Judith Littleton, and Melanie Rock. 2011. "Syndemics in Global Health." In *A Companion to Medical Anthropology*, eds. Merrill Singer and Pamela I. Erickson, 219–249. Malden, MA: Wiley-Blackwell.

Singer, Merrill, and G. Derrick Hodge, eds. 2009. *The War Machine and Global Health*. Malden, MA: AltaMira/Roman Littlefield.

Singer, Merrill, Else Huertas, and Glen Scott. 2000. "Am I My Brother's Keeper?: A Case Study of the Responsibilities of Research." *Human Organization* 59: 389–400.

Singer, Merrill, and Zhongke Jia. 1993. "AIDS and Puerto Rican Injection Drug Users in the U.S." In *Handbook on Risks of AIDS: Injection Drug Users and Their Sexual Partners*, eds. Barry Brown and George Beschner, 227–255. Westport, CT: Greenwood Press.

Singer, Merrill, and Greg Mirhej. 2004. "The Understudied Supply Side: Public Policy Implications of the Illicit Drug Trade in Hartford, CT." *Harvard Health Policy Review* 5(2): 36–47.

Singer, Merrill, Patricia Marshall, and Michael Clatts. 1999. "Frontiers in AIDS and Drug Abuse Prevention Research—Toward the Integration of Anthropological and Epidemiological Approaches." In *Cultural, Observational, and Epidemiological Approaches in the Prevention of Drug Abuse and HIV/AIDS*, eds. Patricia Marshall, Merrill Singer, and Michael Clatts, 1–25. Bethesda, MD: National Institute on Drug Abuse.

Singer, Merrill, Greg Mirhej, Derrick Hodge, Hassan Salaheen, Celia Fisher, and Meena Mahadevan. 2008. "Ethical Issues in Research with Hispanic Drug Users: Participant Perspectives on Risks and Benefits." *Journal of Drug Issues* 38: 351–372.

Singer, Merrill, Greg Mirhej, J. Bryan Page, Erica Hastings, Hassan Salaheen, and Giorelly Prado. 2007. "Black 'N Mild and Carcinogenic: Cigar Smoking among Inner City Young Adults in Harford, CT." *Journal of Ethnicity and Substance Abuse* 6: 81–94.

Singer, Merrill, Nancy Romero-Daza, Margaret Weeks, and Pushpender Pelia. 1995. "Ethnography and the Evaluation of Needle Exchange in the Prevention of HIV Transmission." In *Qualitative Methods in Drug Abuse and HIV Research*, eds. E. Lambert, R. S. Ashery, and R. H. Needle, 231–257 (NIDA Research Monograph #157; NIH Pub. No. 95-4025). Washington, DC: National Institute on Drug Abuse.

Singer, Merrill, Claudia Santelices, G. Derrick Hodge, Zahíra Medina, and Marisa Solomon. 2010. "Assessing and Responding to a Community Health Risk: Second-Hand Smoking in Puerto Rican Households." *Practicing Anthropology* 32: 4–8.

Singer, Merrill, Glen Scott, Wilson Scott, Delia Easton, and Margaret Week. 2001. "War Stories: AIDS Prevention and the Street Narratives of Drug Users." *Qualitative Health Research* 11: 589–602.

Singer, Merrill, and Elyse Singer. 2008. "Eating Disorders." In *Encyclopedia of Epidemiology*, Vol. 1, ed. S. Boslaugh, 293–295. Thousand Oaks, CA: Sage.

Singer, Merrill, T. Stopka, C .Siano, K. Springer, G. Barton, K. Khoshnood, A. Gorry de Puga, and R. Heimer. 2000. "The Social Geography of AIDS and Hepatitis Risk: Qualitative Approaches in Sterile-Syringe Access among Injection Drug Users." *American Journal of Public Health* 90: 1049–1056.

Singer, Merrill, and Elizabeth Toledo. 1995. "Oppression Illness: Critical Theory and Intervention with Women at Risk for AIDS." Paper presented at the American Anthropological Association Meeting, Washington, DC.

Singer, Philip. 1977. "Introduction: From Anthropology and Medicine to 'Therapy' and Neo-Colonialism." In *Traditional Healing: New Science or New Colonialism*, ed. Philip Singer, 1–25. London: Conch Magazine Limited.

Siraisi, Nancy G. 1990. *Medieval and Early Renaissance Medicine: An Introduction.* Chicago: University of Chicago Press.

Sirkin, Susannah, James Cobey, and Eric Stover. 2008. "Landmines." In *War and Public Health*, eds. Barry Levy and Victor Sidel, 102–116. Washington, DC: American Public Health Association.

Siskin, Edgar E. 1984. *Washo Shamans and Peyotists: Religious Conflict in an American Indian Tribe.* Salt Lake City: University of Utah Press.

Skeer, M., M. Land, D. Cheng, and M. Siegel. 2004. "Smoking in Boston Bars before and after a 100% Smoke-Free Regulation: An Assessment of Early Compliance." *Journal of Public Health Management and Practice* 10: 501–507.

Smith, Barbara Ellen. 1981. "Black Lung: The Social Production of Disease." *International Journal of Health Services* 11: 343–359.

Smith, Gar. 1990–1991, Winter. "How Fuel-Efficient Is the Pentagon? Military's Oil Addiction." *Earth Island Journal.* Available at: http://www.envirosagainstwar.org/know/read.php?itemid+593m. Accessed June 12, 2008.

Smith, Gavin A. 1999. *Confronting the Present: Towards a Politically Engaged Anthropology.* Oxford, UK; New York: Berg.

Smith, Kristen. 2012. "The Problemization of Medical Tourism: A Critique of Neo-liberalism." *Developing World Bioethics* 12: 1–8.

Smith, M. G. 1968. "Secondary Marriage among Kadera and Kagoro." In *Marriage, Family, and Residence,* ed. Paul Bohannon and John Middleton, 109–130. Garden City, NJ: Natural History Press.

Smith, Neil. 1996. *The New Urban Frontier: Gentrification and the Revanchist City.* New York: Routledge.

Smith, Neil. 2010. *Uneven Development: Nature, Capital and Production of Space,* 3rd ed. London: Verso.

Smith-Nonini, Sandy, and Beverly Bell. 2011. "Operationalizing a Right to Health: Theorizing a National Health System as a 'Commons'." In *A Companion to Medical Anthropology,* eds. Merrill Singer and Patricia I. Erickson, 493–514. San Francisco: Wiley-Blackwell.

Snyder, Mariah, and Ruth Lindquist, eds. 2006. *Complementary/Alternative Therapies in Nursing,* 5th ed. New York: Springer.

Sontag, Deborah. 2012. "Years after Haiti Quake, Safe Housing Is a Dream for Many." *New York Times,* August 15, A1

Sovacool, Benjamin K. 2010. "A Transition to Plug-In Hybrid Electric Vehicles (PHEVs): Why Public Health Professionals Must Care." *Journal of Epidemiology and Community Health* 64: 185–187.

Spence, Christopher. 2005. *Global Warming: Personal Solutions for a Healthy Planet.* New York: Palgrave.

Sperling, Daniel, and Deborah Gordon. 2010. *Two Billion Cars: Driving Toward Sustainability.* New Haven, CT: Yale University Press.

Spicer, Paul. 1997. "Toward a (Dys)functional Anthropology of Drinking: Ambivalence and the American Indian Experience with Alcohol." *Medical Anthropology Quarterly* 11: 306–323.

Spicer, Paul. 2001. "Culture and the Restoration of the Self among Former American Indian Drinkers." *Social Science and Medicine* 53: 227–240.

Spiegel, Paul, and Peter Salama. 2000. "War and Mortality in Kosovo, 1998–99: An Epidemiological Testimony." *The Lancet* 355: 2204–2209.

Spiro, Melford. 1967. *Burmese Supernaturalism.* Englewood Cliffs, NJ: Prentice-Hall.

Sponsel, Leslie E. 2009. "Reflections on the Possibilities of a Nonkilling Society and Nonkilling Anthropology." In *Toward a Nonkilling Paradigm,* ed. Joám Evans Pim, 35–70. Honolulu, HI: Center for Global Nonkilling. Available at: http://www.nonkilling.org. Accessed December 29, 2009.

Spradley, James. 1970. *You Owe Yourself a Drunk: An Ethnography of Urban Nomads.* Prospect Heights, IL: Waveland Press.

Stack, Carol. 1974. *All Our Kin.* Boston: Beacon Press.

Stall, Ron, Mark Friedman, and Joseph A. Catania. 2007. "Interacting Epidemics and Gay Men's Health: A Theory of Syndemic Production among Urban Gay Men." In *Unequal Opportunity: Health Disparities Affecting Gay and Bisexual Men in the United States,* eds. Richard J. Wolitski, Ron Stall, and Ronald O. Valdiserri, 251–274. Oxford, UK: Oxford University Press.

Stall, Ron, Thomas Mills, John Williamson, Trevor Hart, Greg Greenwood, Jay Paul, et al. 2003. "Association of Co-occurring Psychosocial Health Problems and Increased Vulnerability to HIV/AIDS Among Urban Men Who Have Sex with Men." *American Journal of Public Health* 93: 939–942.

Stanley, Laura. 1999. "Transforming AIDS: The Moral Management of Stigmatized Identity." *Anthropology and Medicine* 6: 103–120.

Stavenhagen, Rodolfo. 1971. "Decolonizing Applied Social Science." *Human Organization* 30: 333–357.

Stebbins, Kenyon. 1987. "Tobacco or Health in the Third World? A Political-Economic Analysis with Special Reference to Mexico." *International Journal of Health Services* 17: 523–538.

Stebbins, Kenyon. 1990. "Transnational Tobacco Companies and Health in Underdeveloped Countries: Recommendations for Advancing a Smoking Epidemic." *Social Science and Medicine* 30: 227–235.

Stebbins, Kenyon. 2001. "Going Like Gangbusters: Transnational Tobacco Companies 'Making a Killing' in South America." *Medical Anthropology Quarterly* 15: 147–170.

Stein, Howard. 1990. *American Medicine as Culture.* Boulder, CO: Westview Press.

Stein, Leonard I. 1967. "The Doctor-Nurse Game." *Archives of General Psychiatry* 16: 699–703.

Stein, Zena, Mervyn Susser, Gerhard Saenger, Frank Marolla. 1975. *Famine and Human Development: The Dutch Hunger Winter of 1944–1945.* New York: Oxford University Press.

Sterk, Claire. 1995. "Determining Drug Use Patterns among Women: The Value of Qualitative Research Methods." In *Qualitative Methods in Drug Abuse and HIV Research,* eds. E. Lambert, R. S. Ashery, and R. H. Needle (NIDA Research Monograph #157; NIH Pub. No. 95-4025), 65–83. Washington, DC: U.S. Govt. Printing Office.

Sterk, Claire. 2000. *Tricking and Tripping: Prostitution in the Era of AIDS.* Putnam Valley, NY: Social Change Press.

Stern, Nicholas, 2007. *The Economics of Climate Change: The Stern Review.* Cambridge, UK: Cambridge University Press.

Stern, Pamela R. 2010. *Daily Life of the Inuit.* Santa Barbara, CA: Greenwood Press.

Stevens, Rosemary. 1986. "The Changing Hospital." In *Applications of Social Science to Clinical Medicine and Health Policy,* eds. Linda H. Akin and David Mechanic, 80–99. New Brunswick, NJ: Rutgers University Press.

Stillo, Jonathan. 2012. "Who Cares for the Caregivers: Romanian Women's Experiences with Tuberculosis." *Anthropology Now* 4: 10–17.

Stolcke, Verena. 2012. "Homo Clonicus." *Thamyris/Intersecting: Place, Sex and Race* 25: 25–43.

Stoler, Ann Laura. 1991. "Carnal Knowledge and Imperial Power: Gender, Race, and Mortality in Colonial Asia." In *Gender at the Crossroads of Knowledge: Feminist Anthropology in the Postmodern Era*, ed. Micaela di Leonardo, 51–102. Berkeley: University of California Press.

Strathern, Andrew, and Pamela J. Stewart. 2010. *Culture and Healing: Medical Anthropology in Global Perspective*, 2nd ed. Durham, NC: Carolina Press.

Strathern, Marilyn. 1992. *Reproducing the Future: Anthropology, Kinship, and the New Reproductive Technologies*. Manchester, UK: Manchester University Press

Streefland, Pieter. 1986. "The Netherlands." *Medical Anthropology Quarterly*, o.s., 17(4): 91.

Striffler, Steve. 2005. *Chicken: The Dangerous Transformation of America's Favorite Food*. New Haven, CT: Yale University Press

Strohmaier, Gotthard. 1998. "Reception and Tradition: Medicine in the Byzantine and Arab World." In *Western Medical Thought from Antiquity to the Middle Ages*, ed. Mirko Grmek, 139–169. Cambridge, MA: Harvard University Press.

Strunin, Lee. 2001. "Assessing Alcohol Consumption: Developments from Qualitative Research Methods." *Social Science & Medicine* 53(2): 215–226.

Sun, Helen. 2010. "Zijin Mining Officials Fined 1.16 Million Yuan for Waste Spills in Fujian." Bloomberg.com. Available at: http://www.bloomberg.com/news/2010-12-28/zijin-mining-officials-fined-1-16-million-yuan-for-waste-spills-in-fujian.html. Accessed July 20, 2012.

Surin, Kenneth. 2009. *Freedom Not Yet: Liberation and the Next World Order*. Durham, NC: Duke University Press.

Susser, E., E. Valencia, and S. Conover. 1993. "Prevalence of HIV Infection among Psychiatric Patients in a Large Men's Shelter." *American Journal of Public Health* 83: 568–570.

Susser, Ida. 1985. "Union Carbide and the Community Surrounding It: The Case of a Community in Puerto Rico." *International Journal of Health Services* 15: 561–583.

Susser, I. 1988. "Anthropology of Health and Industry," Special Issue of *Medical Anthropology Quarterly* 2(3).

Susser, Ida. 1991a. "The Separation of Mothers and Children. In *The Dual City*, eds. J. Mollenkopf and M. Castells, 207–225. Newbury Park, CA: Sage.

Susser, Ida. 1991b. "Women as Political Actors in Rural Puerto Rico: Continuity and Change." In *Anthropology and the Global Factory*, eds. F. Rothstein and M. Blim, 206–219. New York: Bergin & Garvey.

Susser, Ida. 1993. "Creating Family Forms: The Exclusion Men and Teenage Boys from Families in the New York City Shelter System, 1987–91." *Critique in Anthropology* 13: 267–283.

Susser, Ida. 1996. "The Construction of Poverty and Homelessness in U.S. Cities." *Annual Reviews in Anthropology* 25: 411–425.

Susser, Ida. 1997. "The Flexible Woman: Regendering Labor in the Informational Society." *Critique of Anthropology* 17: 389–402.

Susser, Ida. 1998. "Inequality, Violence and Gender Relations in a Global City." *New York. Identities* 5: 219–247.

Susser, Ida 1999. "Creating Family Forms: The Exclusion of Men and Teenage Boys from Families in the New York City Shelter System, 1987–91." In *Theorizing the City: The New Urban Anthropology Reader*, ed. Setha Low, 67–83. New Brunswick, NJ: Rutgers University Press.

Susser, Ida. 2001. "Sexual Negotiations in Relation to Political Mobilization: The Prevention of HIV in Comparative Context." *The Journal of AIDS and Behavior* 5: 163–172.

Susser, Ida. 2002a. "The Health Rights of Women in the Age of AIDS." *International Journal of Epidemiology* 31: 45–48.

Susser, Ida. 2002b. "Losing Ground: Advancing Capitalism and the Relocation of Working Class Communities." In *Time and Space: Global Restructurings, Politics, and Identity*, ed. David Nugent, 274–290. Stanford, CA: Stanford University Press.

Susser, Ida. 2006, March. "Global Visions and Grassroots Movements: An Anthropological Perspective." *International Journal of Urban and Regional Research* 30: 212–218.

Susser, Ida. 2007. "Women and AIDS in the Second Millennium." *Women Studies Quarterly* 35: 336–344.

Susser, Ida. 2009a. *AIDS, Sex and Culture: Global Politics and Survival in Southern Africa*. Malden, MA: Wiley-Blackwell.

Susser, Ida. 2009b. "Imperial Moralities." In *Rethinking America: The Imperial Homeland in the 21st Century*, eds. J. Maskovsky and I. Susser, 83–101. Boulder, CO: Paradigm.

Susser, Ida. 2010. "The Anthropologist as Social Critic: Working Toward a More Engaged Anthropology." *Current Anthropology* 51(Suppl. 2): 227–235.

Susser, Ida. 2011. "Organic intellectuals, crossing scales, and the emergence of social movements with respect to AIDS in South Africa" (Presidential Address). *American Ethnologist* 38: 733–742.

Susser, Ida. 2012. *Norman Street, Updated Edition. "Claiming a Right to New York City."* New York: Oxford University Press.

Susser, Ida, and Richard Lee. 2008. "Women's Autonomy Combats AIDS in the Kalahari." *Anthropology Now* 1(1): 36–43.

Susser, Ida, and M. Alfredo González. 1992. "Sex, Drugs and Videotape: The Prevention of AIDS in a New York City Shelter for Homeless Men." In *Rethinking AIDS Prevention*, ed. Ralph Bolton and Merrill Singer, 169–184. Philadelphia: Gordon and Breach Science.

Susser, Ida, and J. Schneider. 2003. "Wounded Cities: Destruction and Reconstruction in a Globalized World." In *Wounded Cities*, eds. J. Schneider and I. Susser, 1–25. Oxford, UK: Berg.

Susser, Ida, and Zena Stein. 2000. "Culture, Sexuality, and Women's Agency in the Prevention of HIV/AIDS in South Africa." *American Journal of Public Health* 90: 1042–1048.

Susser, Mervyn. 1993. "Health as a Human Right: An Epidemiologist's Perspective on Public Health." *American Journal of Public Health* 83: 418–426.

Susser, Mervyn, and Zena Stein. 2009. *Eras in Epidemiology: The Evolution of Ideas*. Oxford, UK: Oxford University Press.

Susser, Mervyn, and William Watson. 1962. *Social Medicine: Sociology in Medicine*. Oxford, UK: Oxford University Press.

Susser, Mervyn, and William Watson. 1971. *Social Medicine: Sociology in Medicine*, 2nd ed. Oxford: Oxford University Press.

Susser, Mervyn, William Watson, and Kim Hopper. 1985. *Social Medicine: Sociology in Medicine*, 3rd ed. Oxford: Oxford University Press.

Sutter, A. 1966. "The World of the Righteous Dope Fiend." *Issues in Criminology* 196: 177–222.

Sweezy, Paul. 1973. "Cars and Cities." *Monthly Review* 24(11): 1–18.

Symond, Carolyn, Lelani Arris, and Bill Heal, eds. 2004. *Arctic Climate Impact Assessment*. Cambridge, UK: Cambridge University Press.

Syndemics Prevention Network. 2005. "Syndemics Overview: What Principles Characterize a Syndemic Orientation?" Available at: http://www.cdc.gov/syndemics/overview-principles.htm. Accessed January 8, 2006.

Synott, John. 2004. *Global and International Studies: Transdisciplinary Perspectives*. Southbank, Australia: Social Science Press Australia.

Tabuchi, Hiroko. 2012. "Inquiry Declares Fukushima Crisis a Man-Made Disaster." *New York Times*, July 5, 2012, A1.

Taussig, Michael. 1987. *Shamanism, Colonialism, and the Wild Man*. Chicago: University of Chicago Press.

Taylor, Carl E. 1976. "The Place of Indigenous Medical Practitioners in the Modernization of Health Services." In *Asian Medical Systems: A Comparative Study*, ed. Charles Leslie, 285–299. Berkeley: University of California Press.

Taylor, Graeme. 2008. *Evolution's Edge: The Coming Collapse of Our World*. Gabriola Island, Canada: New Society.

Taylor, L., S. Latham, and M. Woolhouse. 2001. "Risk Factors for Human Disease Emergence." *Philosophical Transactions of the Royal Society of London* 356: 983–989.

Terney, Robert M. 1999. "Challenge to Universal Access to Health Care with Limited Resources." In *The American Medical Ethics Revolution: How the AMA's Code of Ethics Has Transformed Physicians' Relationship to Patients, Professionals, and Society*, ed. John B. Baker et al., 252–259. Baltimore: Johns Hopkins University Press.

Thomas, Anthony E. 1975. "Health Care in Ukambani Kenya: A Socialist Critique." In *Topias and Utopias*, eds. Stanley Ingman and Anthony E. Thomas, 266–281. The Hague: Mouton.

Thornton, Robert. 2009. "Sexual Networks and Social Capital: Multiple and Concurrent Sexual Partnerships as a Rational Response to Unstable Social Networks." *African Journal of AIDS Research* 8: 413–421.

Tickell, Oliver. 2008. *Kyoto2: How to Manage the Global Greenhouse*. London: Zed Books.

Topley, Marjorie. 1976. "Chinese Traditional Etiology and Methods of Cure in Hong Kong." In *Asian Medical Systems: A Comparative Study*, ed. Charles Leslie, 243–265. Berkeley: University of California Press.

Townsend, Joan B. 1999. "Shamanism." In *Anthropology of Religion: A Handbook*, ed. Stephen D. Glazier, 429–469. Westport, CT: Praeger.

Trostle, James. 1986. "Early Work in Anthropology and Epidemiology: From Social Medicine to the Germ Theory, 1840 to 1920." In *Anthropology and*

Epidemiology: Interdisciplinary Approaches to the Study of Health and Disease,
eds. Craig R. Janes, Ron Stall, and Sandra M. Gifford, 59–94. Dordrecht, the
Netherlands: Reidel.

Trostle, James A., and Johannes Sommerfeld. 1996. "Medical Anthropology and
Epidemiology." *Annual Reviews in Anthropology* 25: 253–274.

Trostle, James A. 2005. *Epidemiology and Culture.* Cambridge, UK: Cambridge University Press.

Trotter, Robert. 1985. "Greta and Azarcon: A Survey of Episodic Lead Poisoning
from a Folk Remedy." *Human Organization* 44: 64–72.

Trotter, Robert. 1995. "Drug Use, AIDS, and Ethnography: Advanced Ethnographic
Research Methods Exploring the HIV Epidemic." In *Qualitative Methods in
Drug Abuse and HIV Research,* eds. E. Lambert, R. S. Ashery, and R. H. Needle
(NIDA Research Monograph #157; NIH Pub. No. 95-4025), 38–64. Washington,
DC: U.S. Govt. Printing Office.

True, William. 1996. "Epidemiology and Medical Anthropology." In *Medical Anthropology: Contemporary Theory and Method,* 2nd ed., eds. Carol Sargent and
Thomas Johnson, 325–346. New York: Praeger.

Turner, Leigh. 2010. "'Medical Tourism' and the Global Marketplace in Health Services: U.S. Patients, International Hospitals, and the Search for Affordable
Health Care." *International Journal of Health Services* 40: 443–467.

Turshen, Meredith. 1977. "The Political Ecology of Disease." *Review of Radical Political Economics* 9: 45–60.

Turshen, Meredith. 1984. *The Political Ecology of Disease in Tanzania.* New Brunswick,
NJ: Rutgers University Press.

Turshen, Meredith. 1989. *The Politics of Public Health.* New Brunswick, NJ: Rutgers
University Press.

Tuttle, Heather. 2011, Fall. "He Can't Quit Fighting for Nuclear Safety." *Catalyst.*
Union of Concerned Scientists. Available at: http://www.ucsusa.org/
publications/catalyst/fa11-interview.html. Accessed January 27, 2013.

UNAIDS. 2010. *Global Report: UNAIDS Report on the Global AIDS Epidemic 2010.*
Geneva: WHO.

UNFPA, UNICEF, WHO, and World Bank. 2012. *Trends in Maternal Mortality
1990–2010.* Geneva: World Health Organization. Available at: http://www
.unfpa.org/public/home/publications/pid/10728.

UNICEF. 2005. "World Water Day 2005: 4,000 Children Die Each Day from a Lack
of Safe Water." Available at: http://www.unicef.org/wash/index_25637
.html. Access July 20, 2012.

United Nations Children's Fund. 1996. *The State of the World's Children.* Oxford,
UK: Oxford University Press.

United Nations Development Programme. 1999. *Human Development Report 1999.*
New York: Oxford University Press.

United Nations Population Fund. 2002. *The Impact of Armed Conflict on Women
and Girls: A Consultative Meeting on Mainstreaming Gender in Areas of Conflict and Reconstruction.* Bratislava, Slovakia: United Nations Population
Fund.

United Nations Programme on HIV/AIDS. 2000. *UNAIDS Report on the Global
HIV/AIDS Epidemic.* Geneva, Switzerland.

United Nations Research Institute for Development. 2005. Politics and the Political Economy of AIDS. Available at: http://www.unrisd.org/80256B3C 005BB128/(httpProjects)/0642D1AB78D1505BC1256E43005C9BA4? OpenDocument. Accessed July 26, 2012.

Unshuld, Paul U. 1985. *Medicine in China: A History of Ideas*. Berkeley: University of California Press.

U.S. Conference of Mayors. 1987. *Status Report on Homeless Families in America's Cities: A 29-City Survey*. Washington, DC: U.S. Conference on Mayors.

U.S. Government Annual Report on Homelessness. 2010. Available at: https://www .onecpd.info/resources/documents/2010homelessassessmentreport.pdf.

Van Spall, Harriette, Andrew Toren, Alex Kiss, and Robert Fowler. 2007. "Eligibility Criteria of Randomized Controlled Trials Published in High-Impact General Medical Journals: A Systematic Sampling Review." *Journal of the American Medical Association* 297: 1233–1240.

van Willigen, John, and Susan Eastwood. 1998. *Tobacco Culture: Farming Kentucky's Burley Belt*. Lexington: The University Press of Kentucky.

Vanderbilt, Tom. 2008. *Traffic: Why We Drive the Way We Do (and What It Says about Us)*. London: Penguin Books.

Vaughn, Megan. 1991. *Curing Their Ills: Colonial Power and African Illness*. Stanford, CA: Stanford University Press.

Velimirovic, Boris. 1990. "Is Integration of Traditional and Western Medicine Really Possible?" In *Anthropology and Primary Health Care*, eds. Jeannine Coreil and J. Dennis Mull, 51–78. Boulder, CO: Westview Press.

Vincent, Joan. 1982. *Teso in Transformation*. Berkeley: University of California.

Vine, Alex. 1995. *Still Killing: Landmines in Southern Africa*. Washington, DC: Human Rights Watch.

Virchow, Rudolf. 1879. *Gesammelte Ahandlungen aus dem Gebeit der Oeffentlichen Medizin under Seuchenlehre*. Vol. 1. Berlin: Hirschwald.

Virchow, Rudolph. 1985. "The Epidemics of 1848." In *Rudolf Virchow: Collected essays on public health and epidemiology*, ed. L. J. Rather, 113–136. Canton, MA: Science History/Watson Publishing International.

Vitebsky, Piers. 1995a. *The Shaman*. Boston: Little, Brown.

Vitebsky, Piers. 1995b. From "Cosmology to Environmentalism: Shamanism as all Knowledge in a Global Setting." In *Counterworks: Managing the Diversity of Knowledge*, ed. Richard Farah, 182–204. London: Routledge.

Vogt, Dawne, Rachel Glickman, Mark Schultz, Mark Drainoni, Mari-Lynn Elwy, and Susan Eisen. 2011. "Gender Differences in Combat-Related Rani Stressors and Their Association with Postdeployment Mental Health in a Nationally Representative Sample of U.S. OEF/OIF Veterans." *Journal of Abnormal Psychology* 120: 797–806.

Wackernagel, M., and William Rees. 1996. *Our Ecological Footprint: Reducing Human Impact on the Earth*. Gabriola Island, BC: New Society.

Waldram, James, D. Ann Herring, and T. Kue Young. 2006. *Aboriginal Health in Canada: Historical, Cultural, and Epidemiological*. Toronto: University of Toronto Press.

Wagner, Amy W., Jessica Wolfe, Andrea Rotnitsky, Susan Proctor, and Darin J. Erickson. 2000. "An Investigation of the Impact of Posttraumatic Stress Disorder on Physical Health." *Journal of Trauma Stress* 13: 41–55.

Wagner, D. 1993. *Checkerboard Square*. Boulder, CO: Westview Press.

Waitzkin, Howard. 1983. *The Second Sickness: Contradictions of Capitalist Health Care*. New York: Free Press.

Waitzkin, Howard. 2000. "Choosing Patient-Physician Relationships in the Changing Health-Policy Environment." In *Handbook of Medical Sociology*, 5th ed., eds. Chloe E. Bird, Peter Conrad, and Allen Fremont, 271–283. Upper Saddle River, NJ: Prentice-Hall.

Waitzkin, Howard. 2001. *At the Front Lines of Medicine: How the Health Care System Alienates Doctors and Mistreats Patients and What We Can Do about It*. Lanham, MD: Rowman & Littlefield.

Waitzkin, Howard 2011. *Medicine and Public Health at the End of Empire*. Boulder, CO: Paradigm.

Waitzkin, Howard, and Barbara Waterman. 1974. *The Exploitation of Illness in Capitalist Society*. Indianapolis: Bobbs-Merrill.

Wall, Ann, ed. 1996. *Health Care Systems in Liberal Democracies*. London: Routledge.

Wall, Derek. 2010. *The Rise of the Green Left: Inside the Worldwide Ecosocialist Movement*. London: Pluto Press.

Wallace, Deborah, and Roderick Wallace. 1998. *A Plague on Your Houses: How New York Was Burned Down and National Public Health Crumbled*. New York: Verso.

Wallerstein, Immanuel. 1979. *The Capitalist World-Economy: Essays*. New York: Cambridge University Press.

Wallerstein, Immanuel. 2004. *World-Systems Analysis: An Introduction*. Durham, NC: Duke University Press.

Wallis, Robert J. 2003 *The International Climate Justice Movement: A Comparison with the Australian Climate Movement. Shamans/Neo-Shamans: Ecstasy, Alternative Archaeologies and Contemporary Pagans*. London: Routledge.

Walsh, Roger N. 1997. "The Psychological Health of Shamans: A Reevaluation." *Journal of the American Academy of Religion* 45: 101–120.

Walsh, Roger N. 1990. *The Spirit of Shamanism*. New York: G. P. Putnam's Sons.

Walt, Gill. 1994. *Health Policy: An Introduction to Process and Power*. London: Zed Books.

Ward, Peter D. 2010. *The Flooded Earth: Our Future in a World without Ice Caps*. New York: Basic Books.

Wasserheit, Judith. 1992. "Epidemiological Synergy. Interrelationships between Human Immunodeficiency Virus Infection and Other Sexually Transmitted Diseases." *Sexually Transmitted Diseases* 19: 61–77.

Waterston, Alisse. 1993. *Street Addicts in the Political Economy*. Philadelphia: Temple University Press.

Watkins, J. 1997. *Briefing on Poverty*. Oxford, England: Oxfam Publications.

Watt-Cloutier, Sheila. 2005. "Petition to the Inter-American Commission on Human Rights to Oppose Climate Change Caused by the United States of America." Inuit Circumpolar Council. Available at: http://www.inuitcircumpolar.com/index.php?ID=316&Lang=En. Accessed July 19, 2012.

Weaver, Thomas. 1968. "Medical Anthropology: Trends in Research and Medical Education." In *Essays in Medical Anthropology*, ed. Thomas Weaver, 1–12. Athens: University of Georgia Press.

Weidman, Hazel H. 1986. "Origins: Reflections on the History of the SMA and Its Official Publication." *Medical Anthropology Quarterly*, o.s., 17: 115–124.

Weil, Robert. 1994. "China at the Brink: Contradictions of 'Market Socialism,' Part I." *Monthly Review* 46: 10–35.

Weiner, A. 1988 *The Trobrianders of Papua New Guinea*. New York: Holt, Rinehart and Winston.

Weitz, Rose. 2001. *The Sociology of Health, Illness, and Health Care: A Critical Approach*, 2nd ed. Belmont, CA: Wadsworth.

Werner, E. 2012. "Children and War: Risk, Resilience, and Recovery." *Developmental Psychology* 24: 553–558.

Wertz, Richard, and Dorothy Wertz. 1979. *Lying-In: A History of Childbirth in America*. New York: Schocken Books.

Westing, Arthur. 2008. "The Impact of War on the Environment." In *War and Public Health*, eds. Barry Levy and Victor Sidel, 69–84. Washington, DC: American Public Health Association.

Whelehan, Patricia. 2009. *The Anthropology of AIDS: A Global Perspective*. Gainesville: The University of Florida Press.

White, Leslie A. 2008. *Modern Capitalist Culture*, eds. Burton J. Brown, Benjamin Urish, and Robert L. Carneiro. Walnut Creek, CA: Left Coast Press.

White, Robert. 2000. "Unraveling the Tuskegee Study of Untreated Syphilis." *Archives of Internal Medicine* 160: 585–598.

Whiteford, Linda. 1996. "Political Economy, Gender and the Social Production of Health and Illness." In *Gender and Health: An International Perspective*, ed. Carolyn Sargent and Caroline Brettel, 242–256. Upper Saddle River, NJ: Prentice-Hall.

Whiteford, Linda M., and Laurence G. Branch. 2008. *Primary Health Care in Cuba: The Other Revolution*. Lanham, MD: Rowman & Littlefield.

Whiteford, Linda M., and Lois Lacivita Nixon. 2000. "Comparative Health Systems: Emerging Convergences and Globalizaton." In *Handbook of Social Studies in Health and Medicine*, eds. Gary L. Albrecht, Ray Fitzpatrick, and Susan C. Scrimshaw, 440–453. Thousand Oaks, CA: Sage.

Wigand, Jeffrey. 2007. Testimony before the House Subcommittee on Workforce Protections. Washington, DC. Available at: http://www.jeffreywigand .com/WigandTestimonyFinal2.pdf.

Wilde, Lawrence. 1998. *Ethical Marxism and Its Radical Critics*. New York: St. Martin's Press.

Wilkinson Richard. 1986. *Class and Health*. London: Tavistock.

Wilkinson Richard, and Kate Pickett. 2010. *The Spirit Level: Why Greater Equality Makes Societies Stronger*. New York: Bloomsbury Press.

Willis, Evan. 1989. *The International Climate Justice Movement: A Comparison with the Australian Climate Movement. Medical Dominance: The Division of Labour in Australian HealthCare*, 2nd ed. Sydney: Allen and Unwin.

Winkelman, Michael James. 1992. *Shamans, Priests and Witches: A Cross-Cultural Study of Magico-Religious Practitioners* (Anthropological Research Papers #44). Tempe: Arizona State University.

Winkelman, Michael James. 2000. *Shamanism: The Neural Ecology of Consciousness and Healing*. Westport, CT: Bergin & Garvey.

Witherspoon, Gary. 1977. *Language and Art in the Navajo Universe*. Ann Arbor: University of Michigan Press.

Wohl, Stanley. 1984. *Medical Industrial Complex*. New York: Harmony Books.

Wolf, Eric. 1982. *Europe and the People without History*. Berkeley: University of California Press.

Wolf, Eric. 1969. "American Anthropologists and American Society." In *Concepts and Assumptions in Contemporary Anthropology*, ed. Stephen Tyler, 3–11. Athens: University of Georgia Press.

Wolfe, N., W. Switzer, J., Carr, V., Bhullar, V., Shanmugam, U., Tamoufe, A., et al. 2004. "Naturally Acquired Simian Retrovirus Infections in Central African Hunters." *The Lancet* 363: 932–937.

Wolpe, Paul B. 2002. "Medical Culture and CAM Culture: Science and Ritual in the Academic Medical Center." In *The Role of Complementary and Alternative Medicine: Accommodating Pluralism*, ed. Daniel Callahan, 163–171. Washington, DC: Georgetown University Press.

Womack, Mari. 2010. *The Anthropology of Health and Healing*. Lanham, MD: AltaMira Press.

Wood, Corinne Shear. 1979. *Human Sickness and Health: A Biocultural View*. Palo Alto, CA: Mayfield.

Wood, Kate. 2008. "Coded Talk, Scripted Omissions: The Micropolitics of AIDS Talk in an Affected Community in South Africa." *Medical Anthropology Quarterly* 22: 213–233.

Woolhandler, Steffie, and David Himmelstein. 1989. "Ideology in Medical Science: Class in the Clinic." *Social Science and Medicine* 28: 1205–1209.

World Bank. 2006. *Bangladesh Country Environmental Analysis*. Bangladesh Development Series Paper No. 12. Dhaka, Bangladesh: World Bank.

World Health Organization. 2010. *ATLAS on Substance Use Resources for the Prevention and Treatment of Substance Use Disorders*. Geneva: WHO.

World Health Organization. 2011. "Tackling the Global Clean Air Challenge." Available at: http://www.who.int/mediacentre/news/releases/2011/air_pollution_20110926/en/index.html. Accessed July 20, 2012.

World Health Organization. 2012a. *Chronic Respiratory Diseases; Scope: Asthma*. Available at: http://www.who.int/respiratory/asthma/scope/en/index.html. Accessed July 10, 2012.

World Health Organization. 2012b. *Schistosomiasis Fact Sheet* #115. Available at: http://www.who.int/mediacentre/factsheets/fs115/en/. Accessed July 14, 2012.

World Water Assessment Programme. 2009. *WWDR: Water in a Changing World*. Available at: http://www.unesco.org/new/en/natural-sciences/environment/water/wwap/wwdr/wwdr3-2009. Accessed July 20, 2012.

Worobey, Michael, Marlea Gemmel, Dirk Teuwen, Tamara Haselkorn, Kevin Kunstman, Michael Bunce, Jean-Jacques Muyembe, Jean-Marie Kabongo, Raphaël Kalengayi, Eric Van Marck, M. Thomas P. Gilbert, and Steven M. Wolinsky. 2008. "Direct Evidence of Extensive Diversity of HIV-1 in Kinshasa by 1960." *Nature* 455: 661–664.

Wright, Beverley. 2011. "Race, Place, and the Environment in the Aftermath of Katrina." *Anthropology of Work Review* XXXII: 4–8.

Wright, Erik O. 1983. "Capitalism's Future." *Socialist Review* 13: 77–126.

Wright, Erik O. 2010. *Envisioning Real Utopias*. New York: Verso.

Xia, X., J. Luo, J. Bai, and R. Yu. 2008. "Epidemiology of Hepatitis C Virus Infection among Injection Drug Users in China: Systematic Review and Meta-Analysis." *Public Health* 122: 990–1003.

Yih, Katherine. 1990. "The Red and the Green." *Monthly Review* 42: 16–27.

Young, Allan. 1976. "Some Implications of Medical Beliefs and Practices for Medical Anthropology." *American Anthropologist* 78: 5–24.

Young, Allan. 1978. "Rethinking the Western Health Enterprise." *Medical Anthropology* 2: 1–10.

Zheng, Xiang, and Sheila Hillier. 1995. "The Reforms of the Chinese Health Care System: County Level Changes: The Jiangxi Study." *Social Science and Medicine* 41: 1057–1064.

Zierler, Sally, Nancy Krieger, Yuren Tang, William Coady, Erika Siegfried, Alfred DeMaria, and John Auerbach. 2000. "Economic Deprivation and AIDS Incidence in Massachusetts." *American Journal of Public Health* 90: 1064–1073.

Zimmering, Paul, James Toolan, Renate Safrin, and Bernard Wortis. 1951. "Heroin Addiction in Adolescent Boys." *Journal of Nervous and Mental Diseases* 114: 19–34.

Zinn, Howard. 1980. *People's History of the United States*. New York: Harper and Row.

Zola, Irving Kenneth. 1978. "Medicine as an Institution of Social Control." In *The Cultural Crisis of Modern Medicine*, ed. John Ehrenreich, 80–100. New York: Monthly Review Press.

About the Authors

HANS A. BAER, PhD, earned his PhD in anthropology at the University of Utah in 1976. He is an associate professor in the School of Social and Political Sciences at the University of Melbourne. Baer has held permanent and visiting positions at various universities in the United States, at Humboldt University in the former German Democratic Republic, and at the Australian National University. His areas of research have included Mormonism, African American religion, socio-political life in East Germany, critical medical anthropology, medical pluralism in the US, UK, and Australia, the critical anthropology of climate change; and climate politics and the climate movement in Australia. Baer has published 18 books and some 180 book chapters and journal articles. His most recent books have included *Global Warming and the Political Ecology of Health* (2009, with Merrill Singer); *Complementary Medicine in Australia and New Zealand*, and *Global Capitalism and Climate Change: The Need for an Alternative Medical System* (2012). In 1994 he was a recipient of the Rudolf Virchow Award. Baer has served on the editorial board of *Medical Anthropology*, the *Medical Anthropology Quarterly*, and *Complementary Health Review*.

MERRILL SINGER, PhD, a medical anthropologist, is a professor in the departments of anthropology and community medicine, and a senior research scientist at the Center for Health, Intervention, and Prevention at the University of Connecticut. Additionally, he is on the faculty of the Center for Interdisciplinary Research on AIDS at Yale University. Over his career, his research and writing have focused on HIV/AIDS in highly vulnerable and disadvantaged populations, illicit drug use and drinking behavior, community and structural violence, health disparities, and the political ecology of health. Dr. Singer has published over 250 articles and book chapters and has authored or edited 25 books. He is a recipient of the Rudolph Virchow Prize, the George Foster Memorial Award for Practicing Anthropology, the AIDS and Anthropology Paper Prize, the Prize for Distinguished Achievement in the Critical Study of North America, the Solon T. Kimball Award for Public and Applied Anthropology and the Career Award in Anthropology and AIDS.

IDA SUSSER, PhD (Columbia 1980), professor of anthropology at CUNY Graduate Center and Hunter College, adjunct-professor of socio-medical sciences at the HIV Center, Columbia University, has conducted ethnographic research with respect to urban displacement and social movements in the United States and the gendered politics, local, national, and global, of the AIDS epidemic in New York City, Puerto Rico, and southern Africa. Her most recent books are *Norman Street, Updated Edition. "Claiming a Right to New York City."* (Oxford, 2012), *AIDS, Sex and Culture: Global Politics and Survival in Southern Africa* (Wiley-Blackwell, 2009), and the co-edited *Rethinking America* (2009). Among her other publications are *Wounded Cities: Destruction and Reconstruction in a Globalized World* (co-edited 2003*)*, and *The Castells Reader on Cities and Social Theory.* She received an award for Distinguished Achievement in the Critical Study of North America, was president of the American Ethnological Society, founding president of the Society for the Anthropology of North America and is a founding member of Athena: Advancing Gender Equity and Human Rights in the Global Response to HIV/AIDS.

Index

Abiotic environment, 37
Aboriginal peoples, 39–40, 352–353
Abortion, 175, 185, 195
Abstinence-only programs, 192, 193
Academic programs, in medical
    anthropology, 22
Acid rain, 98
Ackerknecht, Erwin, 20
Acquired immunodeficiency
    syndrome (AIDS).
    See HIV/AIDS
Adaptation, 36–38, 197
Addiction, 227, 230–232, 265–266
    See also Drug use
Adler, Patricia, 262
Adoption, 185, 195
Affordable Care Act, 163, 164
Affordable housing, 149–150
Afghanistan War, 205–206, 219–220
Africa, 84, 123, 145, 156
    See also specific countries
    colonialism in, 360–361
    malaria in, 93, 312, 322–323
    medical pluralism in, 366
    patterns of disease in, 156–157
    schistosomiasis in, 318–320

African Americans, 37, 60, 61, 122,
    141, 183, 259, 261, 278, 283, 286,
    295, 409
African National Congress (ANC),
    161–162
Agar, Michael, 238
Aging populations, 185
Agrarian state societies, 71, 79–81,
    176, 333
Agribusiness, 94, 157
Agriculture, 69, 70, 80, 81, 93, 116–118,
    147, 157–158, 176
AIDS. See HIV/AIDS
AIDS and Anthropology Research
    Group (AARG), 287–288
Air pollution, 97–98, 122, 128,
    134, 136
Air travel, 114
Alaska, 118
Alcohol, 76, 227, 228
Alcohol use, 249–254
    anthropology of, 251–254
    cultural model of, 232–236
    study of, 232–233
Alland, Alexander, 37
Allergens, 18–19

Allopathic medicine, 361–362, 363
  See also Biomedicine
Alternative medicine, 49, 368, 369–374
Aluminum, 115
Amala, 156
Amazon rain forest, 117–118
American Anthropology Association
  (AAA), 59, 287–288
American Enterprise Institute, 46, 125
American Holistic Medical
  Association, 370
American Medical Association
  (AMA), 359, 367, 418
American Petroleum Institute, 125
Ames, Genevieve, 251
Amphetamines, 227
Antarctica, 107, 110
Anthropology, 63
  See also Medical anthropology
  of alcohol use, 251–254
  of drug use, 225–263
  of HIV/AIDS, 287–296, 300
  of illicit drugs, 256–263
  of syndemics, 325–330
  of tobacco use, 244–249
Antimalarial campaigns, 93–95
Antiretroviral treatment, 293
Apartheid, 184, 209
Appalachia, 133–134, 148
Apple, 140
Applied medical anthropology, 35, 58
Applied research ethics, 413–415
Arab Spring, 432
Arab states, 356–357
Arctic Climate Impact Assessment,
  118–119
Argentina, 207–208
Arias, Enrique, 263
Armed conflicts. See War
Aronowitz, Stanley, 399–400
Arthritis, 281
Asia, 84
Assisted reproduction, 48, 189, 392
Association of Social Anthropologists
  (ASA), 23
Asthma, 18–19, 122, 136
Asymmetrical wars, 205–206

Atlantic Ocean currents, 110
Attractiveness, 54–55
Australia, 40, 107–108, 352–353
Australian Broadcasting
  Corporation, 46
Australian College of Natural
  Medicine (ACNM), 370
Autoarcheology, 379
Automobile accidents, 98–99
Automobile industry, 95–97, 113
Automobiles, health dangers of,
  95–100
Ayahuasca shamanism, 376–377
Ayurvedic medicine, 17, 49, 358,
  363–364, 374
Azande, 6, 336

Baby formulas, 158–159
Back injuries, 99
Baer, Hans, 23, 42, 212, 369, 416
Balienism, 378
Bambuti, 333
Bangladesh, 186, 214, 246
Barbiturates, 227
Bartlett, John, 302
Basic research ethics, 410–413
Bastien, Joseph Q., 380
Beach erosion, 118
Beauvoir, Simone de, 170
Beck, Glenn, 125
Behavioral adaptations, 37–38
Belgium, 25
The Bell Curve (Herrnstein and
  Murray), 60
Bennett, John, 71
Benson, Peter, 248
Benzopyrene, 98
Bias, 60
Biehl, Joao, 159–160
Big Pharma, 48
Bioethics, 402–416
Biofuels, 122
Biomedicine, 6, 10, 12–15, 28,
  301–303, 334
  capitalism and, 46
  CMA and, 44–45
  emergence of, 360–362

hegemony of, 16–17, 20, 48–50,
     359–394
hospitals and, 381–391
medical tourism and, 392–394
neoliberalism and, 48
Biopolitics, 155, 159, 195
Biopower, 194–195
Biosocial approach, 306
Biosocial facts, 206
Biotechnology, 48, 167, 189–191,
     196–197, 394
Biotic environment, 37
Birth experience, 15–16
Black, Peter, 244, 245
Black Drive, 40
Black-lung disease, 92
Black Plague, 27, 311
Bloodletting, 311
Blood pressure, 76
Blood sugar, 76
Boas, Franz, 19, 61, 170
Bodily organs, market for, 48, 195, 394
Bodley, John H., 5, 70, 71, 87
Body
     commodification of, 55–56, 195
     connection between mind and, 7–8
     medicalization of, 56
     mindful, 8, 51–52, 57, 194
     reproduction and the, 193–197
     sociocultural construction of, 52–55
Body image, 8, 54–56
Body piercing, 55
Body processes, 3
Body shaping, 55–56
Body weight, 54–55
Bolshevik Revolution, 398
Bolton, Ralph, 296–297
Bordo, Susan, 195
Borneo, 378
Boswell, Terry, 401
Bourdieu, Pierre, 55
Bourgois, Philippe, 155, 239
Brazil, 117
Breastfeeding, 158–159, 175
Brink, Stuart, 309
Britain. See Great Britain
British Empire, 360

British Medical Anthropology
     Society, 23
Brodwin, Paul, 365
Brown, E. Richard, 14–15
Brown, Peter, 80
Brown, Phil, 31, 34
Browner, Carole, 186
Bubonic plague, 27, 311
Bush, George W., 192, 193, 420

Cacivita, Lois, 416
Calderon Palomino, Eduardo, 375–376
Callister, Margaret, 310
Camba, 232–234, 235
Cambodia, 213
Cameroon, 176
Campbell, Catherine, 160
Canada, 114
Canadian health care system, 423–428
Cancer, 78, 129, 130
Cancer treatment, 13, 14
Capital accumulation, 88
Capitalism, 5, 14, 43, 45–47, 62, 71, 408
     climate change and, 104, 110–113
     drug, 263–265
     emergence of, 359
     global inequalities and, 137–165
     green, 104
     health and the environment under,
          81–92
     impact on environment, 81–83
     reliance on fossil fuels, 113–116
     women and, 170
Capitalist class, 83
Caplan, Arthur, 127
Capra, Fritjof, 303, 304
Carbon dioxide, 104–109, 111–113,
     115–117, 213
Carnegie Foundation, 14–15
Carpenter, John, 220
Cars. See Motor vehicles
Castaneda, Carlos, 379–380
Casualties, of war, 203–204, 207–208
Caudill, William, 20
CDC. See Centers for Disease Control
     and Prevention (CDC)
Cement, 115

Centers for Disease Control and
    Prevention (CDC), 28, 275, 317
Chadwick, Douglas, 303
Chamberlain, Joseph, 360
Chase-Dunn, Christopher, 401
Chernobyl nuclear accident, 101,
    129–130, 159, 211, 399
Chicago School, 139
Childbirth, 179, 180, 186–187,
    188, 195
    See also Reproduction
Childrearing, in indigenous
    societies, 174
Children
    homeless, 151
    household roles of, 186
    impact of war on, 215, 219
    intestinal infections in, 324
    malnutrition in, 214–215
China, 85, 93
    allopathic medicine in, 361–362
    automobiles in, 95–96, 99
    communism in, 399
    consumption in, 402
    Cultural Revolution in, 386–387
    earthquake in, 143
    economy of, 85, 389–390
    floating population, 271–272
    greenhouse gas emissions, 109,
        111–112
    health care system in, 385–391
    hospitals in, 385–391
    industrialization in, 140
    medical pluralism in, 355–356
    middle class in, 116
    social services in, 140
Chinese Boxer Rebellion, 203
Chinese medicine, 17, 337, 353,
    355–356, 358, 361–362, 363, 391
Chiropractic medicine, 49
Chlorofluorocarbons, 108, 109
Cholera, 27, 123, 139
Cholesterol, 76
Chronic disease, 48, 77, 157
Church, 179
Cigarettes, 158, 242–249
Cirrhosis, 250

Cities, 80
    challenges of, 138–139
    in crisis, 142–143
    gentrification of, 142, 145, 146, 182
    growth of, 137
    homelessness in, 143–147
    informal settlements surrounding,
        145, 160–163
    migration to, 157
    poverty in, 143–151
    Third World, 156–161
    wounded, 138
Citizenship, 159
Civilians, in wars, 204, 208
Civilization, 81
Civil society, 47
Civil wars, 203–204, 205
Class. See Social class
Class relations, 46, 49
Class struggle, 50–51
Cleaver, Harry, 94
Clements, Forrest, 20, 336–337
Climate change, 19, 23, 103–136, 433
    awareness of, 103–104
    capitalism as generator of, 104,
        110–113
    causes of, 104–105
    current state of, 106–107
    denial of, 124–127
    evidence for, 103
    fossil fuels and, 113–116
    greenhouse gas emissions, 104,
        108–111, 113–118
    health and, 121–136
    human-induced, 105–110
    impacts of, 118–136, 322–324
    planned doubt about, 125
    projections, 105
    tipping points, 110
    war and, 212–213
    winners and losers, 127–129
Climate refugees, 118, 323–324
Clinical anthropology, 21
Clinical gaze, 12
Clinton, Bill, 64, 419–420
Clinton health plan, 419–420, 426
Clinton River, 132–133

Club drugs, 257
Club of Rome, 88
CMA. *See* Critical medical
    anthropology (CMA)
Coal, 114
Coalition for the Homeless, 149–150
Coal Mine Health and Safety Act, 92
Coal miners, 92
Coastal cities, 118
Coastal ecosystems, 118
Cobb, Kurt, 129
Coinfections, 325
Cold War, 21, 96, 210–211
Collateral damage, 206–220
Colonialism, 80, 81, 156, 180, 191, 195,
    203, 360–362
Commodification
    of the body, 195
    of drugs, 263–265
Commodities, 116
Communism, 398–399
Comorbidity, 302–303, 304
Complementary and alternative
    medicine (CAM), 369–374
Concrete, 115
Confucianism, 356
Consumer culture, 116
Consumption, 402
Contraception, 181–182, 192, 194
Conway, Erik, 126–127
Cooptation, 63–66
The Copenhagen Diagnosis, 108,
    109–110
Coping mechanisms, 78
Coral, 135
Core countries, 83–84, 86
Core-periphery model, of world
    system, 83–84
Corporations, 46, 83, 87
Cosmopolitan medical systems, 11
Costa Rica, 327
Coterminous body injection, 308–309
Counter-syndemic, 304
Courtwright, David, 263
Crack cocaine, 239
Crichton, Michael, 125
Criminal economy, 138

Critical anthropological realism, xii
Critical anthropology, viii, 397
Critical anthropology of global
    warming, 23
Critical biocultural anthropology, 91
Critical bioculturalism, 17
Critical bioethics, 402–416
Critical epidemiology, 31
Critical medical anthropology (CMA),
    viii, 4, 24, 25, 31, 35, 36, 42–66,
    397–398
  biomedicine and, 44–45
  cooptation and, 63–66
  cultural interpretive theory and, 41
  drug use and, 239–240
  health praxis and, 403–420
  levels of health care systems, 45–59
  medical ecology theory and, 38–39
  precursors of, 42–44
  science and, 59–61
  social origin of disease and, 61–62
Critical tipping points, 110
Crops, 79
Cuba, 85
Cuban health care, 429–433
Cultural brokers, 38
Cultural constructivist approach, 35
Cultural environment, 37
Cultural epidemiology, 25–26
Cultural interpretive theory, 40–41
Cultural model, of drug use, 232–236
Cultural relativism, xii
Culture, xii, 38, 237
  alcohol use and, 232–236
  body image and, 54–56
  consumer, 116
  of consumption, 402
  global youth, 270–271
  homogenization of, 271
Cunning folk, 357–358
Cycling, 100

Dam construction, 82
Darfur, 205
Das, Veena, 204
Davis, Mike, 158
DDT, 93–94

Debilidad, 57
Deepwater Horizon oil spill, 264
Deforestation, 89, 108, 116–118
Deindustrialization, 150, 154, 155
Deleuze, Gilles, 240
Dellums, Ron, 418–419
Democratic ecosocialism, 398–403
Demographic patterns, 181
Dengue fever, 27, 123
Deregulation, 139
Developing countries
    asthma rates in, 19
    chronic disease in, 48
    cities of, 156–161
    reproduction in, 187–189
    therapeutic alliance in, 380–381
Development projects, 82
Diabetes, 309
Diamond, Stanley, 81
Diarrhea, 324
Diet
    in foraging societies, 75–78
    in horticultural village societies, 79
    industrial workers, 158
    Paleolithic, 75–76
    U.S., 75–76
Dinka, 177
Diphtheria, 27
Discordance hypothesis, 77
Disease(s)
    See also Infectious diseases
    biosocial approach to, 306
    chronic, 48, 77, 157
    of climate change, 121–122
    comorbid, 302–303, 304
    concept of, 6–7
    cultural perspective of, 40–41
    environment and, 72
    etiological theories of, 335–340
    interactions among, 17–18
    isolation of, 301–302
    nature of, 301–303
    neglected tropical, 292–293
    political economy of, 156
    reductionist model of, 51
    social context of, 7, 17, 30–31
    social origins of, 61–62, 313–315

    spread of, 138
    sufferer experience of, 7–8
    susceptibility to, 74, 80
    syndemics of, 218–220, 303–330
    transmission of, 308
    vector-borne, 80, 123
    waterborne, 124
Disease theory system, 10
Doctor-patient relationship, 16, 21, 51
Domestic animals, 78, 82, 117
Domestic violence, 191
Dopamine, 228
Dos Anjos, Marcio Fabri, 408
Down syndrome, 189–190
Dowry, 179–180
Drinking water, 140
Driver safety regulations, 98–99
Drought, 118, 128
Drug classification, 227–228
Drug policies, 259
Drug resistance, 93, 94
Drug-resistant pathogenic species, 27
Drug trade, 255–256, 263–265
Drug use, 225–266
    abuse, addiction, and, 230–232
    alcohol, 249–254
    altered minds, 225–229
    among hidden populations, 236
    anthropology of, 226–263
    critical medical anthropology
        model of, 239–240
    cultural model of, 232–236
    emergent, 229–230
    experiential model of, 240–241
    history of, 226–227
    HIV/AIDS and, 226–227, 256–257
    illegal drugs, 254–263
    lifestyle model of, 237–239
    models of, 232–241
    recreational drugs, 228–229
    research on, 241–263
    tobacco, 242–249
Drug-user narratives, 297–300
DuBois, Cora, 20
Dunn, Frederick, 73–74
Durack, David, 275
Dying for Growth (Kim et al.), 65

Eastwood, Susan, 248
Eating patterns, 75–78, 79
Eaton, S. Boyd, 75
Ebola virus, 26–27, 28, 30
Ecological approach, 35, 36–40
Ecological civilization, 403
Ecological footprint, 89, 90–91
Ecological modernization, 432–433
Economic growth, 87
Ecosocial epidemiology, 33
Ecosocialism, 398–403
Ecosyndemics, 321–325
Ecstasy, 231, 257
Edelman, Marc, 157–158
Egypt, ancient, 354–355
Electricity, 114
Elling, Ray H., 21, 46
Emerging diseases, 26–27, 30
Emotional distress, war and, 215
Emotional pathways, of disease, 309
Emotional trauma, of war, 216–218
Empiricism, 60
Enclosure Laws, 147
Endangered species, 119
Endeavour College of Natural
    Medicine, 369–374
Energy consumption, 88–89,
    113–116, 212–213
Engagement, 163–165
Engels, Friedrich, 7, 16, 42, 62,
    81–82, 170
England, 14
Enthoven, Alain, 419
Entitlement programs, 148
Environment, 37–39
    in capitalist system, 87–88
    health and, 69–101
    human interaction with, 69
    impact of automobiles on, 97–98
    impact of industrialization on, 81–83
    in preindustrial societies, 71–75
    social, 69
Environmental degradation, 71, 84,
    87, 88, 89
    in postrevolutionary societies,
    100–101
    from war, 209–213

Environmental refugees, 118
Epidemics, 80, 123, 139, 179, 279,
    325–327
Epidemiological synergism, 303
Epidemiology, 25–32, 33
Epstein, Paul R., 121
Escherichia coli, 27
Estroff, Sue, 281
Ethical issues, 410–416
Ethiopia, 214
Ethnic cleansing, 204
Ethnomedical systems, 10
Ethnomedicine, 311–312, 334–335,
    340, 372
Etiological theories, in indigenous
    societies, 335–340
Eugenics movement, 184
Europe, 111, 357–358
European expansion, 80
European Union, 47, 114
Exclusion, 159–160
Experiential health, 4–5
Experiential model, of drug use,
    240–241
ExxonMobile, 125

Fabrega, Horacio, 339–340
Factory workers, 139, 158
Fagan, Brian, 104
Families, 182–183, 196
Family planning, 183, 184–185, 186
Family size, 181–182, 184–185
Famine, 157
Farmer, Paul, 63–66
Farming, 69, 70
Fatherhood, 182
Fat intake, 76
Fatness, 54–55
Fauci, Anthony, 268
Femininity, 170
Feminist theory, 168
Fertility, 176, 181, 185
Fertilizers, 117
Feudalism, 147
F-gas family, 109
Fiber, 78
Filarial worm infection, 323

Finley, Eric, 218
Fires, 128
Firth, Rosemary, 23
Fishing, 130–132, 135
Fisk, Milton, 408, 428
Flink, James J., 95
Floating population, 271–272
Flooding, 104, 118, 127, 128–129
Folk practices, 311–312, 352–353, 354
Food crisis, 122
Food security, impact of climate
    change on, 118–121
Food supply, 80
Foraging societies, 69–78, 88, 172–177,
    333, 348
    See also Indigenous societies
Forced sterilization, 184
Forcings, 105–106
Fortes, Meyer, 23
Fortun, Kim, 160–161
Fossil fuel industry, climate change
    denial and, 125
Fossil fuels, 88, 104, 106, 109, 113–116,
    117, 136
Foster, George, 20
Foster, John Bellamy, 105
Foucault, Michel, 12, 154, 155, 159,
    194–195, 382
France, 14
Frankenberg, Ronald, 21, 24–25
Frankfurt School, 42
Freedman, Lynn, 191
Free enterprise system, 417
Free markets, 157–158
French-Algerian War, 203
French-Vietnam War, 203
Freshwater, 118, 132–134, 140
Friedman, Milton, 139
Fukushima Dai-ichi nuclear accident,
    129–130, 143
Functional health, 4–5

G20, 47
G7, 47
G8, 47
Gailey, Christine, 171, 197
Gallo, Robert, 276

Gamburd, Michele, 254
Gammeltoft, Tine, 188
Garb, Paula, 211
Garcia, Angela, 240–241
Gastric ulcers, 27
Gay-related immune deficiency
    (GRID), 275–276
Gbowee, Leynah Roberta, 221–222
Gender, 168
    in indigenous societies, 172–178
    in state societies, 178–181
Gender inequality, 168–170, 178–181,
    184–185
Gender roles, 171, 175, 177, 184
Gene mixing, among pathogens, 309
General Motors, 96
Genest, Serge, 22–23
Genocide, 40, 203, 205
Gentrification, 142, 145, 146, 182
Germany, 14, 25, 49, 111
Germ theory of disease, 15
Ghana, 372
Glacial melting, 110, 118
Global capitalism.
    See Capitalism
Global culture, 70, 71
Global democracy, 401–402
Global dimming, 106
Global economy, 45–47
Global health, 32–34
Global inequalities, 137–165
Globalization, 46–47, 82, 87, 113, 150,
    156, 157, 183, 191, 255–256,
    270, 397
Global marine capture, 130
Global South, experimentation in,
    195–196
Global temperature, 105–108, 110,
    122, 138
Global warming.
    See Climate change
Global youth culture, 270–271
Gluckman, Max, 24
Gnau, 5–6, 336
Goldman, Emma, 170
Gonzalez, Alfredo, 154
Good, Byron J., 35, 40, 41, 59

Goody, Jack, 179
Gorbachev, Mikhail, 399
Gore, Al, 103–104, 125, 420
Gorz, Andre, 87, 405
Gough, Kathleen, 177
Gramsci, Antonio, 16
Grassroots organizing, 160
Great Britain
    greenhouse gas emissions, 111
    Industrial Revolution in, 81
    medical anthropology in, 23–24
    poorhouses in, 147–148
Great Depression, 148
Greco-Roman era, 356
Green capitalism, 104
Greenhouse effect, 106
Greenhouse gas emissions, 97–98,
    104–106, 108–111, 114–116,
    213, 433
    from agriculture and deforestation,
    116–118
    from fossil fuels, 113–116
Greenland, 107, 110, 120
Green movement, 100, 101
Green Revolution, 116–117
Griffith, David, 248–249
Group for Medical Anthropology
    (GMA), 22
Growth paradigm, 65
Gruben Glacier, 118
Gruenbaum, Ellen, 94

H1N1 influenza, 27
Habermas, Juergen, 71
Hahn, Robert, 35
Haiti, 53, 64, 142–143, 365–366
Hansen, James, 110
Hantavirus disease, 27
Harner, Michael, 378–379
Harrington, Michael, 148
Harris, Anna, 23
Harvey, David, 46
Hayden, Dolores, 182
Hayek, Friedrich, 139
Hazardous waste, 134–135
Healers, 8, 10, 334, 343–352, 354–358,
    374–381

Healing
    in indigenous societies, 340–343
    symbolic, 342–343
Health
    alcohol and, 250
    climate change and, 121–136
    concept of, 4–6
    functional vs. experiential, 4–5
    global, 32–34
    impact of war on, 207–222
    impacts on, 3
    pluralea and, 18–19, 135–136
    political ecology of, 91–92
    political economy of, 43, 44,
    57–58, 59
    politics and, 164–165
    reproduction and, 167–168
    social determinants of, 43–44
    socialist, 403
    in South Africa, 161–163
    in Third World cities, 156–161
    tobacco use and, 243
Health and the environment,
    69–101
    in agrarian state societies, 79–81
    in capitalist world system, 81–92
    in foraging societies, 69–78
    in horticultural village societies,
    78–79
    in postrevolutionary societies,
    100–101
    in preindustrial societies, 71–75
Health care, access to, 138, 151,
    163, 314
Health care commons, 428
Health care reform, 418–429
Health care systems, 8–10
    alternative, 49
    biomedicine, 359–394
    Canadian, 423–428
    comparative, 416–420
    in indigenous societies, 333–353
    levels of, 45–59
    in precapitalist states, 353–358
    as reflection of social relations,
    362–369
    types of, 10–11

Health issues
  of homeless populations, 151–156
  of women, 168
Health maintenance organizations
  (HMOs), 50, 419–420
Health policy, 47
Health praxis, 403–420
Health research, 23
Health social movements, 432–433
Health tourism, 392
Health visitor, 21
Health workers, 50–51, 384
Heat exhaustion, 122
Heath, Dwight, 232–234, 235, 253
Heat waves, 104, 122
Heckler, Margaret, 276
Hegemony, 16–17, 20, 42, 48–49,
  359–394
Height, 56
Helicobacter pylori, 27
Helman, Cecil, 32
Helminths, 74, 75, 78, 323
Hemorrhagic colitis, 27
Herbal medicine, 11, 341–342, 352, 353
Herdt, Gilbert, 282–283
Heritage Foundation, 46
Heroin, 227, 237, 257, 262
Herpes simplex virus (HSP), 308
Herring, Ann, 325–327
Herrnstein, Richard, 60, 61
Hewlett, Barry, 27, 30
Hewlett, Bonnie, 27, 30
Hidden populations, of drug
  users, 236
Hierarchy, 11–12, 16, 50, 54
Himmelgreen, David A., 327–329
Hispanic Americans, 259, 409
HIV/AIDS, 26, 38, 141, 178, 267–300,
  306, 327–329
  among homeless population,
    151–154
  anthropology of, 287–296, 300
  beginnings of pandemic, 274–277
  breastfeeding and, 159
  current status of, 267–272
  drug use and, 226–227, 256–257
  epidemic, 87

functional cure of, 269–270
funding for, 286–287
leishmanisis and, 220
lessons from, 285–287
narratives of, 297–300
origins of pandemic, 272–274
politics and, 40
prevention, 29, 269–270, 293–295
reproduction and, 188
risk for, 271
risk groups, 291
schistosomiasis and, 318–320
sexual relations and, 296–297
social aspects of, 277–280
stigma of, 280–284
as syndemogenic disease, 320–321
transmission of, 188–189, 276, 292
treatment of, 268–269, 270, 286
Hobos, 148
Holisitic health, 370–371
Holocaust, 208–209
Homelessness, 143–151, 154–156, 182
Homeless populations
  characteristics of, 150–151
  health issues of, 151–156
  mentally ill, 152–154
Homeopathy, 359–360
Honigmann, Irma, 235
Honigmann, John, 235
Hookworm, 93
Hoover, Herbert, 148
Hoovervilles, 148
Horticultural societies, 176–177,
  333, 334
Horticultural village societies, 78–79
Horticulture, 70, 77, 93
Hospital ethnography, 23
Hospitals, 49–51, 381–391
Household roles, 186
Housing, 116
Hughes, Charles, 334
Human aggression, 202–203
Human body. *See* Body
Human-environmental
  relationship, 39
Human immunodeficiency virus
  (HIV). *See* HIV/AIDS

Hurricane Isaac, 142
Hurricane Katrina, 104, 141–142
Hutu, 209–210
Hydrofluorocarbons, 109

Iatrogenic pathways, 309–310
Ice Age, 106
Illegal drugs, 227, 228
  anthropology of, 256–263
  use of, 254–256
Illicit Drug Anti-Proliferation Act, 230
Immune system, 53–54
Incarceration, 139
Income inequality, 44, 84, 137, 144,
  150, 163–165, 408–409
India, 49, 96, 107
  economy of, 139–140
  food crisis in, 122
  greenhouse gas emissions, 109
  health disparities in, 140
  medical pluralism in, 363–364
  medical tourism to, 392
  tobacco use in, 247
  Union Carbide, 160–161
Indigenous people, 39–40, 118–121
Indigenous societies, 5, 43
  ethnomedicine in, 334–335, 340
  healers in, 343–352, 374–381
  healing methods in, 340–343
  medical systems in, 333–353
  reproduction in, 172–178
  theories of disease etiology in,
    335–340
Individual level, of health care
  systems, 51–59
Indonesia, 117, 180
Industrial disasters, 160–161
Industrialization, 81–82, 106, 140, 179
Industrial Revolution, 81, 82, 88, 103,
  104, 106
Industrial societies, 71
  health care in, 10
  reproduction in, 179–181
Inequality, 84–85, 137–165, 240,
  408–409
  gender, 168–170, 178–181,
    184–185

impact on health and disease,
    313–315
  reproduction and, 168–170
  structural factors, 246
Infant formulas, 158–159
Infant mortality, 85, 161, 164, 179, 180
Infectious diseases, 74
  in agrarian state societies, 179
  appearance of new, 26–27
  in cities, 138–139
  domestic animals and, 78
  reemergent, 27, 82
  in sedentary societies, 79
  spread of, 82, 156
  susceptibility to, 81
  vector-borne, 80, 123
  war and, 214–215
  waterborne, 124
Influenza, 307–308, 326, 327
Influenza pandemic (1918-1919), 18,
  306, 310
Informal settlements, 145, 160–163
Infrastructure destruction, 213–214
Inheritance, 179
Inhofe, James, 125
Injection doctors, 48
Injuries, war-related, 216–218
Insects, 128
Institute of Public Affairs, 46
Integrative medicine, 370–371, 373
Intellectual property rights, 137
Intergovernmental Panel on Climate
  Change (IPCC), 106–107, 110
Intermediate level, of health care
  systems, 49–51
Internally displaced persons,
  213, 216
International health, 32
  See also Global health
International health field, 20–21
International Monetary Fund (IMF),
  31, 46, 47, 191
Interpretive approach, 35
Intestinal infections, 324
Intoxication, 225–226
Intravenous drug users (IDUs),
  283–284, 289, 292

Intuit, 119, 347
Inuit, 77, 119–121, 235, 336
IQ, 60
Iraq War, 115, 205–206, 208, 212
Irrigation systems, 80
Islamic medicine, 356–357

Janjaweed, 205
Japan, 11, 111, 114
    Fukushima Dai-ichi nuclear
        accident, 129–130, 143
    medical pluralism in, 365
Jivaro, 9
Jones, Clive, 304
Joralemon, 43
Junk food, 120, 158

Kamat, Vinay, 312
Kamin, Leon, 60
Kanpo, 11, 365
Kaposi's sarcoma, 275
Kark, Sydney, 24
Katz, Richard, 348–350
Kelman, Sander, 4–5
Kennedy, Edward, 418
Kenya, 214
Kim, Jim, 63, 64–66
Kimaforum, 433
Kingfisher, Catherine, 155
Kingsolver, Ann, 248
Kinship, 171, 176–179, 196, 197
Klein, Dorie, 259
Klein, Norman, 4
Kleinman, Arthur, 21, 40–41
Koch, Charles, 126
Koch, David, 125–126
Koester, Stephen, 257–258
Kollontai, Alexandra, 170
Konner, Melvin, 382
Kopper, Kim, 24
Kopple, Barbara, 92
Kosovo War, 204, 212
Kovel, Joel, 401
Krieger, Nancy, 33, 313
Kroeber, Alfred Louis, 245
!Kung, 348–350, 375
Kyoto Protocol, 114

Labor, division of, 83
Labor and childbirth, 186–187
Labor force, women in, 182, 184
Landes, Ruth, 170
Landmines, 209–210
Land reclamation, 82
Landy, David, viii, 22
Large-scale cultures, 70
Lassa, 26
Latin America, 123
Lead exposure, 311–312
Lee, Richard, 178
Leeson, Joyce, 24
Legal drugs, 227
Legionnaires' disease, 27
Leighton, Alexander, 21
Leighton, Dorothea, 21
Leishmaniasis, 219–220
Leprosy, 281
Leshner, Alan, 231
Leslie, Charles, 17, 362–363
Lesotho, 327–329
Levittown, 182–183
Lewis, Charles, 126
Lewis, Gilbert, 336
Liberia, 221–222
Lieban, Richard, 406
Life expectancy, 87, 164, 179, 180
    in capitalist world system, 85, 86
    in preindustrial societies, 72–73, 76
    in U.S., 140, 180–181
Life-span perspective, 33–34
Lifestyle model, of drug use, 237–239
Limits to Growth project, 88
Littleton, Judith, 23
Lived experience, 58
Liver cirrhosis, 250
Livestock, 117
Livingstone, Frank, 93
Local biology, 33–34
Local health behaviors, 30–31
Local knowledge, 234
Local medical systems, 10, 11
Lock, Margaret, 7–8, 33, 193–194, 365
Lomnitz, Claudio, 140
London, 138, 147
Los Angeles, 97

Lovell, Ann, 141
Luxemberg, Rosa, 88
Luxembourg, 127
Lyme disease, 26, 27, 325
Lynn, James, 420

Macomb County, Michigan, 132–133
Macro-level disease interactions, 313–315
Macro-micro connections, 57–58
Macroparasitism, 80, 285–286
Macrosocial level, of health care systems, 45–49
Madagascar, 343
Magdoff, Fred, 403
Magic, 6, 9, 357–358
Magnant Cheryl, 216
Maladaptation, 39, 40
Malaria, 37, 74, 80, 82, 92–95, 123, 312–313, 322
Malawi, 341–342
Maldives, 118
Malnutrition, 80, 81, 122, 139, 156, 214–215, 314, 324
Managed care, 419–421
Managed competition model, 419–420
Mano, 37
Manufacturing, 115–116
Marburg virus, 26
Marcos, Ferdinand, 94
Marine environments, 135–136
Marine transport, 114–115, 136
Market economy, 71
Marriage, 171, 174, 177–180
Marshall, Mac, 245, 329–330
Martin, Emily, 13, 167
Marx, Karl, 16, 42, 62, 81, 82, 170, 177
Masai, 341
Masculinity, 170
Mass media, 46
Maternal mortality, 169, 170, 179, 180
Mayer, Jane, 126
Mbeki, Thabo, 163
Mbuti pygmies, 333
McCoy, Alfred, 264
McElroy, Ann, 35, 37, 38, 39, 77
McGuire, Meredith, 21

McGuire, William, 421
McMichael, Tony, 121, 123
McNeill, William H., 80, 285
Mead, Margaret, 170
Measles, 80, 326
Meat consumption, 75–76
Meat production, 117
Mechanical medicine, 335
Medical anthropology
    See also Critical medical anthropology (CMA)
    central concepts, 3–19
    epidemiology and, 25–32
    ethical issues in, 410–416
    field of, vii–viii, 22–23, 31–32
    history of, 19–34
    theoretical perspectives on, 35–66
    war and, 222–223
Medical Anthropology Newsletter, 22
Medical ecology theory, 36–40
Medical education, 41
Medical ethics, 406
    See also Bioethics
Medical hegemony, 15–17, 20
Medical hierarchy, 50
Medical-industrial complex, 48, 367–368, 421
Medicalization, 15–17, 51, 56, 187
Medical missionaries, 360
Medical pluralism, 10–12, 48–49, 353–358, 359–394
Medical profession, dominance of, 49–50
Medical sociology, 21–22
Medical systems. See Health care systems
Medical tourism, 392–394
Medications, 302
Medicinal herbs, 137
Medicine, as cultural construct, 9–10
Medicine, Beatrice, 252
Mehrabadi,, 48
Meme, 339–340
Men, household roles of, 186
Mental illness, 150, 152–154
Mering, Otto von, 19, 21

Meso-level disease interactions,
    310–313
Mesolithic era, 72, 78
Methane, 108, 109, 110, 117
Mexican drug cartels, 256
Mexico, 47
Mexico City, 97, 140, 145, 157
Microlevel
    disease interactions, 307–310
    of health care systems, 51–52
Microparasites, 285–286
Middle class, 138, 140
Midwives, 16, 187
Militaries, 83, 212–213
Militaristic imagery, 13–14, 53–54
Military operations, 115
Milkman, Ruth, 182
Milloy, Steve, 125
Mills, C. Wright, 42
Mind-altering drugs, 254–263
    See also Drug use
Mind-body duality, 7–8, 51–52
Mindful body, 8, 51–52, 57, 194
Miner, Horace, 9
Mining, 133–134
Mintz, Sidney, 158, 264
Money laundering, 256
Mongols, 80
Montagnier, Luc, 276
Montana, 118
Moral economy, 248–249
Morgan, Lewis Henry, 170
Morley, Peter, 337–338
Morning-after pills, 190, 192
Morsy, Soheir, 42
Mosquitoes, 123
Moss, A., 29
Motherhood, 171, 182, 183, 184, 189
Mothers of the Plaza de Mayo, 208
Motor vehicles
    accidents, 98–99
    in China, 95–96, 99
    emissions from, 106
    energy consumption by, 114
    health dangers of, 95–100
    impacts of, 96, 97
    traffic congestion, 97

Mozambique, 204
Muir, John, 303–304
Multidisciplinarity, 317–318
Multinational corporations, 83, 87
Murdock, George Peter, 338–339
Murngin, 336
Murray, Charles, 60, 61
Mustanski, Brian, 316
Mutations, 27, 37

Nacirema, 9
Nader, Ralph, 99, 420
Nano, 96
Narcotics, 255
National health insurance, 418–420
Nation-states, 47
Native Americans, 14, 245,
    252–253, 375
Natural disasters, 141–143
Natural gas, 113–114
Naturalism, 336
Naturalistic systems, 10, 337
Natural medicine, 49
Natural medicine colleges, 369–374
Natural resources, 82–83
Nature, 69, 79, 80, 303–304
    See also Environment
Naturopathy, 49
Navajo-Cornell Field Health
    Project, 21
Navajo Nation, 210–211, 343, 352
Navarro, Vincente, 30, 42, 49
Nazis, 61, 184, 208–209, 410
Needle sharing, 257–258
Neglected tropical diseases, 292–293
Neoliberalism, 23, 46, 47, 48, 65, 87,
    138–140, 145, 146, 154–156, 163
Neolithic era, 78–79, 80
Neo-shamanism, 378–380
Netherlands, 25
New, Peter Kong-Ming, 21
New Agers, 378–379
New Deal, 148
New Orleans, 141–142
New World, spread of disease to, 80
New York City, 143–146, 148–152, 239
New Zealand, 118

NGOs. *See* Nongovernmental
    organizations (NGOs)
Nicaragua, 213–214
Nichter, Mark, 33–34, 56, 306
Nichter, Mimi, 56
Nicotine, 227
Ninth International Congress for
    Anthropological and Ethnological
    Sciences, 42
Nipah virus disease, 27
Nitrous oxide, 108, 109, 114, 136
Nongovernmental organizations
    (NGOs), 47, 49
Nonopportunistic infections, 320
Nordstrom, Carolyn, 204
North American Free Trade
    Agreement (NAFTA), 157
Nossal Institute for Global Health, 33
Nuclear accidents, 101, 129–130, 143,
    159, 211, 399
Nuclear family, 196, 197
Nuclear threat, 129–130
Nuer, 177
Nurses, 50, 51
Nuttall, Mark, 120
Nyamnjoh, Francis, 176

Obama, Barack, 65, 163, 193, 292,
    421–423
Objectivity, 60
Occupational diseases, 92
Occupational hazards, 140
Occupy Wall Street movement,
    155–156
Ocean
    acidification of, 135
    currents, 110
    overfishing, 130–132, 135
    pollution, 136
Oil, 113, 115
Oliver, Douglas, 39–40
Opportunistic infections, 320
Oppression illness, 262
Oreskes, Naomi, 126–127
Organ farming, 195, 394
Organized crime, 262–263
Ottoman Empire, 203

Outbreak ethnography, 27
Outsourcing, 113
Overcrowding, 139
Overfishing, 130–132, 135
Ozone, 108, 122, 136

Paleolithic diet, 75–76
Paleolithic era, 72
Pan American Health
    Organization, 47
Pandemics, 279
Paper production, 117–118
Pappas, Gregory, 160
Parasites, 74, 75, 78
Parenti, Michael, 258
Paris, 138–139
Park, Julia, 23
Parsons, Elsie Clewes, 170
Parsons, Howard L., 91
Partners in Health (PIH), 63, 64
Pastoralists, 77, 88
Pastoral societies, 176–177, 179
Pathogens, 82
Patient Protection and Affordable
    Care Act, 422–423
Patients, 8, 10
Patrilineage, 177, 179
Paul, Benjamin, 20
Paul, James, 47
Payer, Lynn, 14
Peasants, 88, 157–158
Peccei, Auerlio, 88
Pedestrian deaths, 99
Pentagon, 115
People's Health Movement, 433
Perez, Christina, 430
Perfluorocarbons, 109
Periphery, 83–84, 86, 137, 159–160
Personalistic systems, 10, 337
Personal Responsibility and Work
    Opportunity Reconciliation Act
    (PRWORA), 144, 183
Pesticides, 78, 113
Petryna, Adriana, 159
Pharmaceutical industry, 48, 94–95,
    256, 426
Pharmaceutical medicine, 335, 341

Philippines, 94
Physical environment, 37
Physician-patient relationship, 16,
    21, 51
Physicians
    ancient, 354–355
    Chinese, 385–386, 388–389
    constraints on, 50
    deprofessionalization of, 367
    in early modern Europe, 357–358
    as employees, 384
Physicians for National Health
    Program (PHNP), 423
Pittock, A. Barrie, 108
Plague, 27, 311
Plastic surgery, 55–56
Pluralea, 18–19, 135–136
Political ecological orientation, 41
Political ecology, 91–92
Political ecology of health, 91–92
Political economic medical
    anthropology, 36
Political economy, 42, 259
Political economy of disease, 156
Political economy of health, 43, 44,
    57–59
Politics, 9, 29–30, 40
    health and, 164–165
    South Africa, 161–163
Pollutants, 19
Pollution, 82, 87, 156–157
    air, 97–98, 122, 128, 134, 136
    ocean, 136
    water, 132–134
Poor, 77, 85, 138, 146
    health care for, 314
    increase in, 150
    reproduction among the, 187–189
Poorhouses, 147–148
Popular epidemiology, 31, 33, 34
Population
    density, 80
    increases, 157, 176, 179
    state regulation of, 183–186
Postrevolutionary societies,
    environmental devastation in,
    100–101

Poststructuralism, 57–58
Post-traumatic stress disorder (PTSD),
    217–218
Poverty, 137–138, 147–148
    disease and, 314
    homelessness and, 143–156
    population growth and, 184–185
    in Third World cities, 156–161
    women and, 169–170
Power differences, 42
Power relations, 44, 45, 49, 50, 51
Praxis, 397, 403–420
Precapitalists societies, 353–358
Pregnancy
    exposure to toxins during, 189–190
    folk practices, 188
    medicalization of, 187
Preindustrial societies
    health and environment in, 71–75
    health care in, 9, 10
    life expectancies in, 72–73
Primates, 74
Primitive medicine, 20
Privatization, 87, 139
Processed food, 120, 158
Production processes, 115–116
Professional class, 83
Project on the Predicament of
    Mankind, 88
Protozoa, 74, 75, 78
Psychophysiological healing, 335
Psychosomatic ailments, 11
Public assistance programs, 148
Public Broadcasting System, 46
Public health, 164, 302
    politics of, 29–30
    in South Africa, 161–162
Public transportation, 99
Puerto Ricans, 261–262, 295

Qatar, 112

Racism, 184
Radical democracy, 399–400
Radical social constructionism, 60
Raikhel, Eugene, 241
Rain forest, 117–118

Rape, 216
Raphael, Dennis, 44
Reagan, Ronald, 145
Realism, xii
Recreational drugs, 228–229
Reductionist model of disease, 51
Reformist reform, 405
Refugees, 38, 118, 213–216, 323–324
Regional medical systems, 10–11
Regional variations, in medical practice, 14
Religious right, 193
Reproduction
    among poor populations, 187–189
    anthropological perspectives on, 170–172
    biotechnology of, 189–191, 196–197
    body and, 193–197
    class and, 181–183
    decisions about, 186
    health and, 167–168
    in indigenous societies, 172–178
    inequality and, 168–170
    labor and childbirth, 186–187
    morality and, 192–193
    social context of, 183–187
    state regulation of, 183–186
    in state societies, 178–181
Reproductive health, 138
Reproductive rights, 172, 191, 192, 194
Reproductive tourism, 195
Research ethics, 410–416
Resilience, 38, 220–223
Respiratory ailments, 122, 136
Rind, David, 128
Rio de Janeiro, 145
Rivers, W. H. R., 19
Road construction, 82
Rockefeller Foundation, 14–15, 93, 362
Romania, 184, 185
Romans, 356
Romanucci-Ross, Lola, 12
Romero-Daza, Nancy, 327–329
Room, Robin, 234–235
Roosevelt, Franklin D., 148
Rotavirus, 27
Ruling class, 79, 80, 88

Rupert, Henry, 346
Russia, 109, 111, 398
Rwanda, 209–210, 216

Sahlins, Marshall, 70
Saillant, Francine, 22–23
Same-sex relationships, 196
Samoa, 351–352
San, 76–77, 172–178, 336
SARS (severe acute respiratory syndrome), 27
Sas Balen, 119
SAVA, 316–317
Scandinavia, 25
Schensul, Stephen, 164–165
Scheper-Hugher, Nancy, 7–8, 58
Schistosomiasis, 80, 82, 318–320
Schneider, David, 196
Schneider, Jane, 179, 181
Schneider, Peter, 181
Schonberg, Jeff, 155
Schreiner, Olive, 170
Science, 59–61
Science and technology studies, 48
Scientific method, 60
Scotch, Norman, 20
Seafood, 130–132
Sea level rise, 107, 118
Sedentary lifestyle, 75, 326
Seeds, 137
Self-medicating, 240
Semiperiphery, 83–84, 86
September 11, 2001, 286–287
Settlement patterns, impact of climate change on, 118–121
Sex education, 192, 193
Sex tourism, 141, 195
Sexual behavior, HIV/AIDS and, 296–297
Sexuality, 177, 192
Sexually transmitted diseases (STDs), 141, 178, 308
Sexual orientation, 172
Shamans/shamanism, 9, 335, 343–350, 365, 374–381
Shantytowns, 145
Sharon, Douglas, 379

Shaw, Christopher, 110
Shellfish, 135
Shellfish poisoning, 124
Shelters, 149–151
Sherwin, Susan, 407
Shinto, 365
Shiva, Vandana, 122
Shostak, Marjorie, 75
Sick role, 51
Sidel, Victor, 408
Siegel, Ronald, 226
Singapore, 96, 392
Singer, Merrill, 22, 29, 42, 260–262,
    321–322, 405
Singer, Phillip, 380–381
Single-payer system, 418, 423–429
Sleeping sickness, 156
Slimness, 54–55
Slums, 81
Small cultures, 70
Smallpox, 214
Smeed's Law, 98
Smith, Kristen, 393–394
Smoking, 158, 242–249, 329–330
Social capital, 44
Social class, 46, 49
    body differences and, 55–57
    reproduction and, 181–183
    self-image and, 55
    toxic exposures and, 56–57
Social context, 17, 30–31
    of disease, 7
    of reproduction, 183–187
Social control, 16, 79
Social determinants of health, 43–44
Social environment, 69
Social epidemiology, 25
Social insurance systems, 417
Socialism
    democratic ecosocialism, 398–403
    reconceptualizing, 399–403
Socialist health, 403
Socialist market economy, 85,
    389–390
Social justice, 163–165
Social Medicine
    (Susser and Watson), 24

Social movements, 47, 138, 145,
    155–156, 163–164, 432–433
Social origin of disease, 61–62,
    313–315
Social relations, embodiment of, 57
Social Security Act, 148
Social services, 138, 139, 148–149, 150
Social stratification, 79, 81, 84
Social suffering, 239
Social support networks, 314
Society for Medical Anthropology
    (SMA), vii, viii, 22
Sociocultural adaptive strategies,
    37–38
Sociocultural evolution, 71–92
Somalia, 214
Songbirds, 128
South Africa, 145
    apartheid regime in, 184, 209
    health in, 161–163
    HIV/AIDS in, 295
    political change in, 161–163
Southern School of Southern
    Therapies, 369–374
Soviet Union, 15, 100–101, 211,
    377–378, 389, 398–399
Spain, 85
Specialization, 13, 367
Spicer, Paul, 235–236, 252–253
Spirits, 337, 343, 377
Spiritual medicine, 335
Stall, Ron, 316–317
Stanley, David, 118
State societies
    gender and reproduction in,
        178–181
    medical systems in, 353–358
St. Clair River, 132–133
Stebbins, Kenyon, 245–246
Steel, 115
Stein, Leonard, 50
Sterilization, 184
Sterly, Joachim, 25
Stern, Nicholas, 104
Stewart, Pamela J., 35
Stigmatization, of HIV/AIDS, 280–284
Stillo, Jonathan, 159

Stolcke, Verena, 197
Stone age diet, 75–76
Stopes, Marie, 193
Strathern, Andrew, 35
Street drug users, 237–238, 259–260, 262–263
Stress, 99
Stroke, 122
Structural adjustment programs, 31, 87, 191
Sub-Saharan Africa, 84, 87, 327
    HIV/AIDS in, 327–329
    malaria in, 93, 312
    schistosomiasis in, 318–320
Subsistence, impact of climate change on, 118–121
Substance abuse, 138, 150
Suburbs, 99
Sudan, 94, 177, 205
Sufferer experience, 7–8, 51–52
Sulphur hexafluroide, 109
Sumer, 354
Supernatural causes, of disease, 338
Super-wealthy, 84–85
Surveillance, 194
Susser, Ida, 144, 161–162, 165, 178, 193
Susser, Mervyn, 24
Susser, Zena Stein, 24
Symbolic healing, 342–343
Syndemics, 23, 279
    anthropological origins of, 315–317
    anthropologists working on, 325–330
    concept of, 17–18, 303–307
    ecosyndemics, 321–325
    future of, 330
    HIV/AIDS and, 320–321
    macro-level disease interactions, 313–315
    meso-level disease interactions, 310–313
    micro-level disease interactions, 307–310
    model, 305, 306–307
    multidisciplinarity and, 317–318
    multiplying effects of, 313
    social origins of, 313–315

tick-borne, 324–325
    understanding, 318–320
    of war, 218–220
Syphilis, 156
System-challenging praxis, 426–429
System-correcting praxis, 426–429

Taiwan, 11
Taman shamanism, 378
Tanzania, 361
Taosim, 356, 365
Tariffs, 157
Tasmania, 39, 40
Tata, 96
Tattooing, 55
Taussig, Michael, 376
Taylor, Charles, 222
Taylor, Wilson, 421
Technological innovation, 69
Temiar, 351
Temperature increases, 105–108, 110, 122
Temporary Assistance to Needy Families, 150
Thailand, 271
Theoretical perspectives, 35–66
    critical, 36
    critical medical anthropology, 42–66
    cultural interpretive theory, 40–41
    medical ecology theory, 36–40
Therapeutic alliance, 380–381
Thermohaline circulation, 110
Think tanks, 46
Third World. See
        Developing countries
Third World cities, 156–161
TIbetan medicine, 17
Tibetan medicine, 52, 342
Tick-borne syndemics, 324–325
Tobacco use, 242–249, 329–330
Toledo, Elizabeth, 262
Tourism, 140–141
Townsend, Patricia, 35, 37, 38, 39, 77
Toxic exposure, 56–57
Toxic waste, 133, 134–135
Trade agreements, 157
Traditional medicine, 372–373

Traffic congestion, 97
Transnational states, 47
Transportation, energy consumption
    by, 114–115
Trauma, 216–218, 314
Trephination, 341
Trilateral Commission, 47
Trophic cascades, 131–132
Tropical diseases, 122
Trostle, James A., 25–26
Truman, Harry, 418
Trypanosomiasis, 82
Tuberculosis (TB), 27, 139, 151–152,
    159, 320–321, 326, 327
Tutsi, 209–210
Tuvalu, 118

Uganda, 214
Unani, 49
Unano, 363
Undocumented immigrants, 163
Unemployment, 148, 157
Unhealthy behaviors, 78
UNICEF, 34
Union Carbide, 160–161
Unionization, of health workers,
    50–51, 384
United Kingdom. See Great Britain
United States, 14, 47
    auto industry in, 96–97
    automobile culture in, 99–100
    ecological footprint, 89
    greenhouse gas emissions, 109, 111
    health care reform in, 418–429
    health care system in, 409–410, 417
    health disparities in, 140, 144–145,
      180–181
    homelessness in, 143–151
    hospitals in, 382
    inequalities in, 137, 163–165,
      408–409
    life expectancy in, 180–181
    maternal mortality in, 169–170
    military of, 115, 212–213
    morality and reproductive health
      in, 192–193
    political systems of, 409

    social inequality in, 85
    temperatures in, 107
    wars by, 205–206
    women's health movement in, 189
University of Melbourne, 33
Uranium mining, 210–211
Urbanization, 81, 87, 106, 137, 158
Urban life, 138
Urban migration, 157
Urban sprawl, 89
U.S. diet, 75–76

Vaccinations, 160, 161, 214
Vagrancy, 147
Vanport City, 182
Van Willigen, John, 248
Vector-borne diseases, 80, 123
Vibrio vulnificus, 124
Vietnam, 140
Vietnam War, 201, 217, 218
Violence
    See also War
    domestic, 191
    encountering, 201–202
    as inherent to human species,
      202–203
Virchow, Rudolf, 7, 9, 19, 62, 201
Virgin complex, 179
Volkow, Nora, 231

Wage labor, 147, 157
Wagner, David, 149
Wagner-Dingwell bill, 418
Waitzkin, Howard, 46–47, 409–410
Wall, Derek, 84
Wallerstein, Immanuel, 83
Wallis, Robert J., 379
War, 201–203
    See also Violence
    asymmetrical, 205–206
    as biosocial disease, 206–221
    causalities from, 203–204, 207–208
    children and, 215, 219
    collateral damage from, 206–220
    environmental, 209–213
    health impact sof, 207–222
    human resilience in face of, 220–223

impacts of, 204, 206–220
infectious disease and, 214–215
infrastructure destruction in,
   213–214
malnutrition and, 214–215
medical anthropology and, 222–223
syndemics of, 218–220
traumas of, 216–218
in twenty-first century, 205–206
women and, 216
War machine, 206
War motif, 53–54
War on cancer, 13, 14
War on drugs, 14
Washington consensus, 156
Washo Indians, 375
Waste removal, 80
Wastewater, 132
Water, 80, 140
Waterborne diseases, 124
Water pollution, 132–134
Water sources, 118
Waterston, Allise, 259–260
Water vapor, 108
Watson, William, 24
Wealthy, 84–85
Weber, Max, 351
Weitz, Rose, 420
Welfare reform, 144, 150, 183
Welfare state, 137, 140, 148
Wellin, Edward, 20
Wellness, 4
Western medicine, 365
   See also Biomedicine
   spread of, 360–362
West Nile virus, 123
Whiteford, Linda M., 416
WHO. See World Health Organization
   (WHO)
Whooping cough, 326–327
Wigand, Jeffrey, 249
Wiggins, Steve, 420–421

Wikler, Abraham, 231
Witchcraft, 6, 9, 336
Wolf, Eric, 264
Wollstonecraft, Mary, 170
Women
   access to reproductive health, 138
   autonomy of, 183, 191
   domestic violence and, 191
   health issues of, 168
   household roles of, 186
   inequality and, 168–170, 178–181,
      184–185
   in labor force, 182, 184
   poor, 169–170, 183
   in poverty, 142
   resilience in, 220–223
   war and, 216
Women in Peacebuilding Network
   (WIPNET), 221
Working class, 77, 83, 139, 150
Working poor, 150
Workplace, toxic exposures in, 56–57
World Bank, 31, 34, 46, 47, 65, 87, 191
World Health Organization (WHO), 4,
   20, 27, 34, 64, 93, 227, 313
World Lung Foundation (WLF), 243
World system theory, 57, 59
World Trade Organization, 47, 137
World War I, 203
World War II, 182, 203, 208–209
Wounded cities, 138
Wright, Erik, 403

Yang, 337, 356
Yellow fever, 27, 123
Yersinia pestis, 311
Yin, 337, 356
Youth drug revolution, 226

Zambia, 295
Zimbabwe, 377
Zuma, Nkosazane, 162